Toward a Science of Consciousness II
The Second Tucson Discussions and
Debates

Complex Adaptive Systems
John H. Holland, Christopher G. Langton, and Stewart W. Wilson, advisors

Toward a Science of Consciousness II
The Second Tucson Discussions and Debates

Edited by
Stuart R. Hameroff
Alfred W. Kaszniak
Alwyn C. Scott

A Bradford Book
The MIT Press
Cambridge, Massachusetts
London, England

This book was set in Palatino on the Monotype "Prism Plus" PostScript Imagesetter by Asco Trade Typesetting Ltd., Hong Kong and was printed and bound in the United States of America.

Library of Congress Cataloging-in-Publication Data

Toward a science of consciousness: the first Tucson discussions and debates /
   edited by Stuart R. Hameroff, Alfred W. Kaszniak, Alwyn C. Scott.
      p.   cm.—(Complex adaptive systems)
   "A Bradford book."
   Includes index.
   ISBN 0-262-08249-7 (alk. paper)
      1. Consciousness—Congresses.   I. Hameroff, Stuart R.
   II. Kaszniak, Alfred W., 1949–   III. Scott, Alwyn, 1931–
   IV. Series.
   QP411.T68   1996
   612.8'2—dc20   95-26556
                                                              CIP

Predicate Questions

Carol Ebbecke

"To ask the hard question is simple."
—W. H. Auden, "#12"

Ask the both/and question again, if you please.
the one exquisitely implicit in intellectual mutterings—
the keenest sensibility, however evasive, reveals itself
in flickering, shimmering; we are surprised

at the concomitant flurry, the circumvented logic:
an astronishing invention, that hair dryer.
David the Golem; cool glass beads—a night sky full
of aeronautic radiance—yet so much else rains,

won't come under the ethereal umbrella.
Endless trial tracks in the desert landscape
evade desire, *are* the grail; our disconnectedness
haunts. Such ghosts pass, collapse in still another state—

oh the nights we've spent collecting the dreams
of zombies, the flash and dare of what gathers
returning again and again, at last dissipating,
at last re-emerging in the breath of the skittish

dark javelinas posed in front of the museum,
the natural gallery to contain those
slippery thoughts we're desperate to savor,
even in their fleeting.

Contents

Acknowledgments

This book is a product of the Tucson II conference ("Toward a Science of Consciousness 1996") made possible by support and advice generously offered by all members of the Scientific Program Committee. Skilled and steady management contributed by Jim Laukes from the Conference Services of UA's Extended University was essential. For the book itself, David Chalmers and Petra Stoerig provided invaluable editorial advice and analysis in their areas of expertise. The whelming task of putting the manuscript into final form was accomplished by the tireless efforts of Carol Ebbecke with timely encouragements from Harry Stanton of MIT Press. Special artwork was created by Cindi Laukes and Dave Cantrell. Our families and academic colleagues supported our efforts.

We are also grateful to all who attended Tucson II and the growing community of interdisciplinary students of consciousness. The field is indebted to the Fetzer Institute for its support of both the conference and the fledgling Center for Consciousness Studies at The University of Arizona.

We dedicate this volume to the memory of Harry Bradford Stanton and Euan J. Squires.

Contributors

Syed Mustafa Ali
Brunel University
Uxbridge, United Kingdom

Geoffrey L. Ahern
Department of Neurology
University of Arizona
Tucson, Arizona

Michael T. Alkire
Department of Anesthesiology, Pediatrics,
and Neurology
University of California—Irvine Medical
Center
Orange, California

Beatrice Axelrod
Department of Psychiatry
University of Arizona
Tucson, Arizona

Bernard J. Baars
The Wright Institute
Berkeley, California

Talis Bachmann
Department of Psychology
University of Portsmouth
Portsmouth, United Kingdom

Andrew Bailey
Department of Philosophy
University of Calgary
Calgary, Alberta, Canada

Friedrich Beck
Institut fur Kernphysik
Technische Hochschule Darmstadt
Darmstadt, Germany

Colin G. Beer
Department of Psychology
Rutgers University
Newark, New Jersey

Dick Bierman
University of Amsterdam
Amsterdam, The Netherlands

Susan Blackmore
Department of Psychology
University of the West of England
Bristol, United Kingdom

Ned Block
Departments of Philosophy and Psychology
New York University
New York, New York

Paul Bloom
Department of Psychology
University of Arizona
Tucson, Arizona

Joseph E. Bogen
University of Southern California
Pasadena, California

David J. Chalmers
Department of Philosophy
University of California, Santa Cruz
Santa Cruz, California

Patricia Smith Churchland
Department of Philosophy
University of California, San Diego
La Jolla, California

Allen Combs
Department of Psychology
University of North Carolina at Asheville
Asheville, North Carolina

Richard J. Davidson
Departments of Psychology and Psychiatry
University of Wisconsin
Madison, Wisconsin

Daniel C. Dennett
Center for Cognitive Studies
Tufts University
Medford, Massachusetts

Carol Ebbecke
Department of English
University of Arizona
Tucson, Arizona

James H. Fallon
Department of Anatomy and Neurobiology
University of California—Irvine Medical
Center
Orange, California

Peter Farleigh
The Australian Association for Process
Thought
University of Sidney
New South Wales, Australia

Hans Flohr
Brain Research Institute
University of Bremen
Bremen, Germany

Robert K.C. Forman
Program in Religion
Hunter College
New York, New York

Nicholas P. Franks
Imperial College of Science, Technology, and
Medicine
London, United Kingdom

Jeffrey A. Gray
Department of Psychology
Institute of Psychiatry
London, United Kingdom

Susan A. Greenfield
Department of Pharmacology
University of Oxford
Oxford, United Kingdom

Richard J. Haier
Departments of Pediatrics and Neurology
University of California—Irvine Medical
Center
Orange, California

Stuart R. Hameroff
Departments of Anesthesiology and
Psychology
University of Arizona
Health Sciences Center
Tucson, Arizona

Danny Hillis
Walt Disney Imagineering
Glendale, California

J. Allan Hobson
Department of Psychiatry
Laboratory of Neurophysiology
Harvard Medical School
Boston, Massachusetts

David Hodgson
Supreme Court of New South Wales
Queens Square
New South Wales, Australia

Timothy L. Hubbard
Department of Psychology
Texas Christian University
Fort Worth, Texas

Piet Hut
School of Natural Sciences
Institute of Advanced Study
Princeton, New Jersey

Ezio M. Insinna
Schoeller Elektronik
Bureau de Liason Sud/Est
Bussy-Saint-Georges, France

Alumit Ishai
Department of Neurobiology
Weizmann Institute of Science
Rehovot, Israel

Syoichi Iwasaki
Psychology Unit
Department of Humanities and Social Sciences
Fukushima Medical Center
Fukushima, Japan

Paul K. Johnston
Department of English
State University of New York, Plattsburgh
Plattsburgh, New York

Alfred W. Kaszniak
Department of Psychology
University of Arizona
Tucson, Arizona

Aaron King
Department of Mathematics
University of Arizona
Tucson, Arizona

James E. King
Department of Psychology
University of Arizona
Tucson, Arizona

Stanley A. Klein
School of Optometry
University of California, Berkeley
Berkeley, California

Stanley Krippner
The Saybrook Institute
San Francisco, California

Stephen LaBerge
Department of Psychology
Stanford University
Stanford, California

Richard D. Lane
Departments of Psychiatry and Psychology
University of Arizona
Tucson, Arizona

Jaron Lanier
Department of Computer Science
Columbia University
New York, New York

David A. Leopold
Division of Neuroscience
Baylor College of Medicine
Texas Medical Center
Houston, Texas

Daniel S. Levine
Department of Psychology
University of Texas at Arlington
Arlington, Texas

William R. Lieb
Imperial College of Science, Technology, and
Medicine
London, United Kingdom

Michael Lockwood
Green College
Oxford University
Oxford, United Kingdom

Nikos K. Logothetis
Max Planck Institute for Biological
Cybernetics
Tubingen, Germany

Bruce Mangan
Institute of Cognitive Studies
University of California, Berkeley
Berkeley, California

Edwin May
The Laboratories for Fundamental Research
Science Applications International Co.
Palo Alto, California

James Newman
Colorado Neurological Institute
Denver, Colorado

Lis Nielsen
Psychological Laboratory
University of Copenhagen
Klampenborg, Denmark

Victor Norris
IFR Systemes Integres Laboratoire de
Microbiologie
Universite de Rouen
Mont Saint Aignan, France

Van A. Reidhead
Department of Anthropology
University of Missouri, St. Louis
St. Louis, Missouri

Eric N. Reiman
Department of Psychiatry
The University of Arizona Health Sciences
Center
Tucson, Arizona

Diana Reiss
Department of Psychology
Rutgers University
Newark, New Jersey

Gregg H. Rosenberg
Artificial Intelligence Programs
University of Georgia
Athens, Georgia

Duane M. Rumbaugh
Language Research Center
Georgia State University
Atlanta, Georgia

E. Sue Savage-Rumbaugh
Department of Biology
Georgia State University
Atlanta, Georgia

Dov Sagi
Department of Neurobiology
Weizmann Institute of Science
Rehovot, Israel

Prestor A. Saillant
Department of Neuroscience
Brown University
Providence, Rhode Island

Marilyn Schlitz
Institute of Noetic Sciences
Sausalito, California

Gary E. Schwartz
Department of Psychology
University of Arizona
Tucson, Arizona

Alwyn C. Scott
Program in Applied Mathematics
University of Arizona
Tucson, Arizona

John R. Searle
Department of Philosophy
University of California, Berkeley
Berkeley, California

Roger N. Shepard
Department of Psychology
Stanford University
Stanford, California

James A. Simmons
Department of Neuroscience
Brown University
Providence, Rhode Island

Euan J. Squires (deceased)
Department of Mathematical Sciences
University of Durham
Durham, United Kingdom

Henry P. Stapp
Lawrence Berkeley Laboratory
University of California
Berkeley, California

Petra Stoerig
Institut fur Physiologisch Psychologie
Heinrich Heine Universitat
Düsseldorf, Germany

Charles T. Tart
Institute of Transpersonal Psychology
Palo Alto, California

John G. Taylor
Department of Mathematics
King's College
London, United Kingdom

Nigel J.T. Thomas
Department of Humanities
Rio Hondo College
Whittier, California

Francisco J. Varela
LENA—Neuroscience Cognitives et Imagerie
Cerebrale
Hopital de la Salpetriere
Paris, France

Max Velmans
Department of Psychology
Goldsmiths, University of London
London, United Kingdom

Giuseppe Vitiello
Departimento de Fisica
Universita degli Studi di Salerno
Salerno, Italy

Roger Walsh
Department of Psychiatry and Human
Behavior
University of California, Irvine
Irvine, California

Lawrence Weiskrantz
Department of Experimental Psychology
University of Oxford
Oxford, United Kingdom

John B. Wolford
Department of Anthropology
University of Missouri, St. Louis
St. Louis, Missouri

Lang-Sheng Yun
Department of Computer Science
University of Arizona
Tucson, Arizona

Robert M. Zimmer
Brunel University
Uxbridge, United Kingdom

Introduction

One hundred years after publication of the classic *Principles of Psychology* by the celebrated American psychologist and philosopher William James, and at the close of a century dominated by the limited perspectives held by American psychologist John B. Watson, a robust field of consciousness studies is beginning to spring Phoenix-like from behaviorism's ashes. It is an exciting time. Philosophers and mathematical physicists, computer scientists and electrophysiologists, biochemists and psychiatrists, neurologists and ethnologists, among other professional disciplines, are communicating and jointly trying to comprehend the nature of conscious experience.

What is consciousness? Although we have as yet no clear answer to this vexing question, recent attempts to find one have motivated two inter-disciplinary conferences sponsored by the University of Arizona. This book is a selection of invited papers from the second, "Toward a Science of Consciousness 1996" (affectionately called "Tucson II"), which was held at Tucson in April 1996. In the spirit of these two conferences, the *Journal of Consciousness Studies,* and the fledgling Center for Consciousness Studies at the University of Arizona, the book—and indeed the field of consciousness studies itself—is quintessentially interdisciplinary.

Where is the common ground for such a cooperative effort? The questions currently being addressed in consciousness studies fall very roughly along an axis defined by responses to the "hard problem," which was defined by philosopher David Chalmers as a challenge to reductionist neuroscience. Can the intimate experiences of consciousness be fully explained by firing patterns of the brain's neurons? Are feelings, sensations—our inner lives—direct consequences of neural synaptic connections and network firing patterns? Is even complete understanding of all the brain's mechanisms—from the cultural to the molecular level (and perhaps to the quantum level)—sufficient to comprehend consciousness?

Reductionists like philosopher Daniel Dennett insist that consciousness arises wholly and directly from neural activities. What else could be involved? Chalmers, on the other hand, believes consciousness may be an irreducible, fundamental property of the universe—in the same category as space and time or mass and electric charge. Although these positions are good reference points for other views—opposite poles terminating some sort of axis—the field is much more intricate than a linear axis would suggest, and a host of questions arise. For example, to what extent are differences of opinion, however strongly expressed, real disagreements rather than mere verbal misunderstandings? Can opposing views be understood as the result of seeing the problem from different perspectives? How can real progress be made? Where are we now? Because the Tucson conferences and the *Journal of Consciousness Studies* have been focal points for recent interdisciplinary efforts to answer such questions, here is a brief history of these efforts.

Following an enthusiastic response to Tucson I in April 1994, heated interdisciplinary debate on consciousness filled internet discussion groups PSYCHE-D and jcs-online. The *Journal of Consciousness Studies* blossomed and the University of Arizona organizers (the editors of this volume together with Jim Laukes of the Extended University's Conference Services) looked ahead to an expanded follow-up conference two years later. Because the Tucson I participants completely filled the 350-seat Duval Auditorium at the University of Arizona Medical Center, Tucson II was moved downtown to the Tucson Convention Music Hall; a modern 2200-seat concert hall and home of the Tucson Symphony. Rooms in an adjacent Convention Center building and hotel were reserved to house parallel speaking sessions, poster sessions, book exhibits, and a space devoted to "consciousness art" and quiet conversation that was ably organized by Tucson artist Cindi Laukes.

To more fully and efficiently cover the spectrum of approaches toward consciousness, the scientific program committee for Tucson II was significantly expanded from the three volume editors in autumn 1994. Joining the committee were David Chalmers (a philosopher at the University of California, Santa Cruz), Christof Koch (a biophysicist at the California Institute of Technology), Marilyn Schlitz (the Research Director at the Institute of Noetic Sciences), Petra Stoerig (a neuropsychologist at the University of Munich and now at the University of Düsseldorf), and Keith Sutherland (Publisher of the *Journal of Consciousness Studies*).

The augmented committee defined five major categories into which papers, talks, and sessions would be organized: (1) Philosophy, (2) Cognitive science, (3) Neuroscience, (4) Mathematics and Physics, and (5) Phenomenology and Culture. Themes for thirteen interdisciplinary plenary sessions were then chosen, and forty-five distinguished plenary speakers were invited, of whom forty-two accepted. The response to a call for abstracts was encouraging (if not overwhelming), and in September 1995 the committee began evaluating more than 500 submissions, selecting 120 for concurrent talks and assigning the balance to poster sessions. Keith Sutherland at the *Journal of Consciousness Studies*, in collaboration with David Chalmers and other committee members, further classified the abstracts, more carefully elaborating the major themes. Their classification scheme, along with the number of abstracts assigned to each category, appears in an appendix to this book.

Thus the stage was set for Tucson II. On April 8, 1996, a beautiful spring day in the Sonoran Desert, well over 1000 "consciousness scientists" assembled from 27 countries in Tucson's Music Hall to begin their participation. Following brief opening remarks, a short piano recital by recording artist (and plenary speaker) Jaron Lanier set the tone for the next few days, and the first plenary session began. The following narrative account by Keith Sutherland, Jean Burns, and Anthony Freeman for the *Journal of Consciousness Studies*, is reprinted here in lightly edited form with their permission.

Monday April 8

The conference started off with a session on the "hard problem" chaired by David Chalmers. It seemed nothing short of remarkable that a clear consensus appeared among the speakers (with one exception) that consciousness cannot be explained within the paradigms of our current science.

The first speaker was Michael Lockwood, who argued in "the enigma of sentience" that the scientific view of the brain cannot account for qualia. Then Jeffrey Gray gave a résumé of his recent article in *Brain and Behavioral Sciences* on the neuropsychology of the content of consciousness. He proposed an experimental program to determine whether functional or structural brain features were responsible for the content, but concluded that neither this (nor any other program he could think of) can tell us why any brain processes should give rise to conscious experience.

The next speakers, Roger Shepard and Piet Hut, proposed to turn the hard problem upside down, suggesting that brains arise out of consciousness rather than the other way around. The mystery is not our own conscious experience (this is the only thing we know), but the physical world, and the theory dismisses the common observation that consciousness is a product of complexity. What is complex about a simple quale like a pain or the smell of a rose? They reviewed various psychological evidence from blindsight to jokes in dreaming, before moving on to review the sort of physics that would be needed to make sense of conscious experience.

The only dissenter from the mysterians on the panel was philosopher Daniel C. Dennett, who felt "like a policeman at Woodstock." In his early career he had viewed himself as a radical, and it amused him now to find himself defending orthodox reductive materialism against a solid front of mysterians. He argued his now-familiar case by metaphor and analogy with his customary charm and panache. Although it was a great performance, many of the participants remained unconvinced.

Tuesday, April 9

The morning plenary shifted to the neural correlates of consciousness, in which Rodolfo Llinás, J. Allan Hobson, Joe Bogen, and Susan Greenfield presented their own very different angles from the perspective of brain research. Llinás reviewed the evidence for binding as a result of temporal synchronization and Hobson outlined his conscious-states paradigm, related to work on sleep and dreaming as mediated by changes in the brain stem. Joe Bogen, a veteran colleague of Roger Sperry (and sounding a dead ringer for desert denizen John Wayne), put forward the thalamic intralaminar nuclei as the best candidate for an area in the brain most closely associated with conscious experience. Susan Greenfield took issue with this proposition, arguing that consciousness was more likely to be associated with global brain gestalts than any particular anatomical area. Both Bogen and Greenfield took pains to emphasize that their work showed only correlation and they could not say how any brain state might give rise to conscious experience. Greenfield argued that this is one question we should not even ask, for such knowledge might give rise to attempts to manipulate other people's consciousness.

The next plenary session, on folk psychology, was a showdown between a professor of physiology, Colin Blakemore, and an Australian Supreme Court judge, David Hodgson. Blakemore revealed a wealth of evidence showing that our folk-psychological notions of conscious control are an illusion. Unfortunately he spent so much time presenting the evidence that the discussion was a bit thin, concluding that the folk-psychological underpinnings of the law were a thinly veiled coverup for an Old Testament desire for vengeance and punishment. David Hodgson made a quietly passionate plea for scientific and philosophical elites to consider the social and ethical consequences of their theorizing. Because the Western legal and ethical systems are entirely based on notions of free will and volition, theorists are obliged to consider their evidence very carefully. He concluded that the case against folk psychology was at the moment unproved, but that we needed a new understanding of causality that would find a place for volition and intentionality within our understanding of physics and psychology. He then outlined his own candidate for such a theory.

One of the most exciting panels was on machine consciousness. The moderator, Christof Koch, instructed speakers to keep it short, leaving a delightful 45 minutes for wrangling. Dave Rumelhart, one of the pioneers in connectionism, pointed out that cognition in general and emotion in particular must be viewed in an embodied context. He presented a model of emotion based on the sympathetic-parasympathetic nervous system, but admitted that was all it was—a model—and remained skeptically agnostic about whether any such model might be conscious. Danny Hillis took a much more upbeat approach, arguing that skeptics about machine consciousness were guilty of lacking imagination. He did not explain, however, why it was any more valid to "imagine" that consciousness might result from some as-yet-unconstructed computational system rather than any other slice of the physical universe. Jaron Lanier seemed to win over the audience with a delightful roast of computationalism, but his humor hid a deeply serious agenda. Lanier has argued in the *Journal of Consciousness Studies* (2(1): 76–81) that the artificial intelligence (AI) research program has damaged our view of ourselves and our culture. Roger Penrose finished the prepared talks with a spirited defense of his own theory that human understanding is independent of algorithmic processes.

Then the fun started. Although Christof felt the chair's responsibility to stir up a good argument, he need not have worried. Dan Dennett was first to the microphone, replying to Lanier's *JCS* piece. Happy to agree with Lanier's view of his zombie philosophy, Dennett challenged us all to clarify what it is that we claimed "we" are over and above our own "zimbo" computational mental processes. He also agreed with Lanier's observation that the ascendancy of AI has been correlated with a return to religious fundamentalism, but he said that this connection was no reason for scientists and philosophers to exercise some sort of self-censorship. Susan Blackmore then launched a passionate attack on another of Lanier's claims. But the most memorable part of the session was an exchange between Penrose and Hillis during which the back and forth of the table microphone was reminiscent of a center-court tennis rally at Wimbledon.

Wednesday, April 10

The third day started with a panel on language and interspecies communication, which moderator Colin Beer introduced in a short survey of some controversies in recent ethology. In 1976, Donald Griffin had proposed that we try to communicate with animals in their own tongues, but this approach was not found to be effective and has mostly been replaced by attempts to teach animals to use human speech and communication systems.

Sue Savage-Rumbaugh began by showing how the Cartesian view of animals as devoid of consciousness has suggested an innate grammar module in human beings but not in other animals. The communication systems of all nonhuman animals were thought to be closed (hard-wired) and informative to others of the same species only in an unconscious or unintentional sense. But her own work among bonobo apes has led her to the view that apes can spontaneously acquire a human language system if properly exposed from an early age, and that conscious intentional language usage is clearly within the ape's cognitive competence. One of the most interesting experiments that she outlined was a Piagetian test showing that bonobos have a "theory of mind" that is as good as that of human 4-year-olds. Because her bonobos use symbols in novel and context-dependent ways, she suggested that we have come to myopic conclusions on the true nature of language by focusing tightly on syntax and human speech.

Diana Reiss outlined some of the work being done with dolphins. Although this species is far removed from the human, they show clear evidence of linguistic systems. Although we recognize a danger in reading too much into anecdotal evidence, her own observations and those from other laboratories on mirror use and play suggest evidence of self-awareness and self-monitoring.

Irene Pepperberg presented extraordinary experimental evidence from two decades of work with a gray parrot named Alex. The avian Einstein has shown a highly developed grasp of categories such as color, shape, identity, size, quantity, and even confounded number sets. He was able to apply these categories to novel objects with consistent accuracy of about 75 percent. Pepperberg had puzzled for some time whether such cognitive abilities could be said to indicate consciousness, but felt reassured upon hearing Colin Blakemore define human consciousness as purely cognitive. Many participants at this conference, however, were unhappy with such an operational definition.

Paul Bloom finished the session with "language and consciousness," a paper highly relevant to some recent debates on jcs-online. Starting with Darwin's question—Is our rich mental life the result of language?—he went on to address the classical theories of Whorf, Hobbes, and Quine that language is essential for concept formation. Bloom acknowledged that words can motivate categorization via labeling and can give rise to distinctions that we would not otherwise be conscious of, an example being the training of wine tasters, but he felt the conclusion that experience is in some way "created" by language is overstated. He referred to observations by William James and Oliver Sacks that abstract thought is perfectly possible without words. Susan Shaller's work among deaf isolates indicated a rich prelinguistic mental life. Upon finally learning words, they pick them up very rapidly. Bloom's interpretation of the Helen Keller case was that she learned to apply labels to prexisting experiential categories. Commenting that prelinguistic infants are perfectly capable of abstract object individuation, he concluded that language is not essential for creating concepts.

The next two sessions, on transpersonal psychology and conscious vision in the striate cortex, indicated how diverse is the consciousness debate. In the first session, Charley Tart presented a critique of science as a social phenomenon. He argued that science had been very successful in some areas, but we need to reconsider methodological issues before it can deal effectively with the full range of human experience. Roger Walsh presented a brief history of transpersonal psychology, concluding that for a movement that was only 25 years old, great progress has been made.

The contrast with the afternoon session could not have been more pronounced. Three distinguished researchers—Petra Stoerig, Robert Turner, and Dov Sagi—all addressed the function of primary visual cortex (V1) in conscious vision. In the context rich in functional MRI and other data, it was interesting to sample the continuing debate on the binding problem. According to Llinás's talk on Tuesday, binding is a bottom-up process, derived from temporal synchronization among cells in diverse cortical areas. Robert Turner argued in his talk that it is inappropriate to view area V1 as some sort of passive sensory mapping of the external world because clear evidence shows that V1 is subject to top-down modulation from higher cognitive set-determining regions (typically frontal).

An interesting addition to this panel was philosopher Ned Block, who pointed out a confusion among psychologists in using the word "consciousness." Block delineated his distinction between phenomenal experience (p-consciousness) and access (a-consciousness), the latter dealing with global control of action, decision making, reporting, and so on. He claims to find some confusion among these terms, particularly in recent work by Crick and

Koch. He suggests that their claim that V1 is not conscious (because it is not connected to frontal areas) is actually dealing with a-consciousness and is at best an empty tautology, telling us nothing about p-consciousness. Dan Dennett, who does not accept Block's distinction, was first to the microphone to challenge him, and the episode showed how essential it is to include philosophers in even the most hands-on areas in brain research.

Thursday April 11

The fourth day opened with a session on medicine and consciousness. Nicholas Franks spoke on the molecular mechanisms in general anesthesia, giving evidence for the view that general anesthetics act much more specifically than had previously been thought: at hydrophobic pockets in a select group of neural receptors.

Andrew Weil pleaded eloquently on behalf of the body's capacity for self-healing, suggesting that clinicians in training spend far too much time with very sick people. They gain a distorted picture, for by definition these are the cases in which natural healing mechanisms have failed. In consequence, the medical profession pays far too little heed to the significance of their patients' states of consciousness as a way of accessing the body's natural healing capacity.

The hall was full for the next session on quantum processes in the brain, and when chairman Euan Squires called for an audience vote on the relevance of quantum theory to consciousness, skeptics won easily. The session kicked off with Friedrich Beck describing his recent work with Sir John Eccles on quantum influences on the release of neurotransmitter vesicles. It seems that only about 15 percent of action potentials cause neurotransmitter-vesicle release from axon terminals. The occurrences are thought to be random, or probabilistic. Beck and Eccles argue that quantum indeterminacy is at play. That this claim has potential we see in recent evidence that "probabilistic" release may be a key cognitive factor. Dimitri Nanopoulos followed Beck with a discussion of fairly technical material, attempting to relate super-string theory (from the reaches of high-energy physics) to the properties of microtubules.

The next speaker, philosopher Patricia Churchland, was expected to attack the Penrose-Hameroff (Orch OR) microtubule theory, but instead went after David Chalmers's hard problem as an *argumentum ad ignorantiam.* Whenever researchers present a new piece of work on some aspect of cognition, she lamented, someone inevitably gets up to say, Okay, but what about the hard problem? Stuart Hameroff followed, first disposing of some criticisms of the microtubule theory that had come from Churchland and Dennett. He went on with a good, if hurried account of the Penrose-Hameroff theory of orchestrated objective reduction in microtubules (Orch OR) which is an attempt to address the hard problem through the physics of "funda-mental" space-time geometry.

Friday, April 12

Much current experimental work on consciousness is being done on vision, for reasons laid out clearly by Francis Crick in his recent *Astonishing Hypothesis*. Having addressed the primary visual area of the occipital lobe (V1) on Wednesday, we now turned to the extrastriate cortex's function in conscious vision. Christof Koch said that he and Crick were finding evidence for coding in individual neurons of the macaque monkey and are looking for antibodies to activate these neurons. Roger Tootell described functional MRI maps of activities related to consciousness, leading to a "dicing apart" of cortical areas, and Nikos Logothetis presented evidence suggesting that more than 90 percent of the occipital neurons are active during visual perception. Finally, Larry Weiskrantz defined two types of blindsight, with corresponding changes in the retina.

In a session on integrative perspectives, David Chalmers displayed his prototype "consciousness meter" for the first time during a debate with Paul Churchland. (Although the thing looked like an ordinary hair dryer, it can't have been that because the qualia-detection light shone brightly when the machine was directed toward ordinary mortals and only flickered when pointed at strict reductionists.) Humor aside, Chalmers's presentation went beyond a statement of his "hard problem" to clarify the implicit philosophical assumptions underlying the search for neural correlates of consciousness. Paul Churchland followed this act with a review and status report on perceptions in classical neural-network theory, suggesting that reentrant networks (those with closed causal loops) must be considered to provide a basis for conscious phenomena.

The panel on phenomenology and experiential approaches was very carefully structured, beginning with an exchange of views between John Searle and Max Velmans on scientific method. Although they disagreed on details (is a pain in the finger actually a pain in the head?), they agreed that the hard line between subjectivity and objectivity is not justified. Searle pointed out that although consciousness is ontologically subjective, it can be accessed and studied in ways that are epistemologically objective, given sufficient methodological rigor. Francisco Varela filled in some of the detail on this program with a paper on "Neurophenomenology," pointing out that the Husserl tradition provides a toolbox for studying subjective states but requires many years of rigorous training.

Phenomenology of meditation practice was discussed by religion professor Robert Forman, who argued that nature should be studied in its simplest form and then extrapolated to more complex systems. In the same way as a biologist might choose to study the paramecium or *E. coli*, consciousness should be studied starting with the "pure consciousness event," which many mystical traditions argue is the ground state for conscious awareness.

Remarkable agreement appeared on the scope and methodology appropriate for investigating consciousness. Searle commented that since the seventeenth century we have lived in a demystified world and thus, in principle, nothing is beyond scientific inquiry's reach; the important requirement is that the methods have intersubjective rigor. Because consciousness is puzzling, we should not rule out any approach to gaining understanding a priori.

Saturday April 13

The morning session was on current directions in parapsychology. Sparsely represented at Tucson I, such "psi" effects were deemed sufficiently controversial to require a representative skeptic to ensure a balanced presentation. This role was assumed by Susan Blackmore, a former parapsychologist and vocal opponent of current research on the subject. Psychologist Daryl Bem began by describing the extensive *ganzfeld* experiments, in which a subject hears white noise with Ping-Pong-ball halves taped over his eyes. After relaxing, the subject reports his mental impressions for 30 minutes, while a "sender" gazes at a film clip or something of the sort. Correlations are judged blindly and analysis shows statistically significant identification by the ganzfeld subject of the content in whatever the sender was observing. The experimental procedures and analytical methods have been debated for some years. Bem (who is also a magician who routinely fakes mind reading as an entertainment), was originally skeptical, but is now convinced that they are valid.

Susan Blackmore started out believing that parapsychology could help her understand the nature of mind, but after a time with unrewarding experiments of her own, together with suspicion about results reported by another experimenter, she went on to generalize that psi effects are unlikely to exist. She also claims that even if it does exist, psi involves nonconscious brain effects.

Roger Nelson presented results of PK (psychokinesis) experiments using random-number generators as indicators of mass-consciousness levels. Deviations from randomness occurred at the time of the O. J. Simpson verdict, for example, and also during peak television viewing (but not during the advertising periods). Dick Bierman showed that PK effects can occur even if the target is randomly chosen after the experiment has been done, and suggested that the explanation relied on quantum effects.

In a session on functions of consciousness, V. S. Ramachandran described stroke patients who experience neglect and denial of their own limbs or injury. Even a patient whose left arm is paralyzed may vehemently deny it. Ramachandran explored this effect, for example, by asking a patient to clap her hands. The patient clapped with one hand, while claiming she was doing it with both (the sound of one hand clapping!). Ramachandran also described a "cold caloric midbrain stimulation test," which involved pouring icewater into the ear of one such neglect patient. Accompanying the expected rapid eye movement, the patiently suddenly realized she was paralyzed. Because neglect occurs with stroke only in the nondominant right hemisphere (with left-side paralysis), Ramachandran suggests a link between neglect and Freudian denial and repression theory.

Dan Schacter talked about memory. He read a list of words to the audience, such as sugar, sour, taste, and honey, then asked how many remembered the word "taste" being on the list. About half the audience raised their hands. He then asked how many remembered the word "sweet" on the list. Almost as many raised their hands (but of course sweet wasn't on the list). He went on to explain this effect in the context of his theory of implicit memory.

The final plenary session was on consciousness and the physical world. Henry Stapp claimed that consciousness can be explained by quantum mechanics, because the quantum-mechanics formulation inherently refers to conscious experience. In his writings, Stapp describes conscious events as "Heisenberg quantum events." Avi Elitzur suggested that current physics is unable to adequately discuss consciousness. He pointed out that according to Einstein's theory of relativity, all events that happen to a person must be considered to exist on a world line, along which conscious experience simply moves. Furthermore, the conscious experiences of different people do not necessarily move synchronously. When you talk to someone, that person may simply be a zombie, whose conscious experience has moved on. Finding this view untenable, Elitzur concludes that we must expand our understanding of physical laws.

Alwyn Scott ended the conference by restating his view of consciousness as emerging not from a single level of description but—like life—from all the relevant levels of dynamic activity. From this perspective he suggested that we may come to see consciousness as a phenomenon that reaches seamlessly from protein biochemistry through the algorithmic jungles of neural-network theory and the psychological laboratories to the configurations of culture and the ecstatic mysteries of the human spirit. If he is correct, an interdisciplinary approach to consciousness studies is surely needed.

Beyond these plenary sessions, excitement was high at the concurrent speaking sessions and poster sessions, some of it stimulated by the extensive media coverage that the conference received. This attention included substantial reports in *The New York Times, New Scientist, The Calcutta Telegraph,* and *The Times Higher Education Supplement.* Special video clips appeared on CBC TV (Canada) and German television, and the Japan Broadcasting Corporation (NHK) prepared a two-hour documentary on Tucson II, which aired on Japanese television on May 13 and 14, 1996.

Perhaps the conference's most remarkable and creative aspect was that so many people with starkly differing intuitions, insights, and professional backgrounds came together and debated the subject of consciousness responsibly, during the concurrent and poster presentations as well as after the plenary sessions. Intense discussions rattled through the concert hallways, spilling out beneath Tucson's blue skies and palm trees and continuing both under the stars and into the bars. Keith Sutherland, for example, reported a conversation in which Robert Turner (Institute of Neurology, London), who had earlier presented his MRI research on the visual cortex, drew the attention of Bob Forman (Religion, City University of New York) to writings by the Sufi divine, Ibn Arabi. Christof Koch (who normally hangs out with macaque monkeys) spent much of his Tucson time talking to the transpersonal psychologists, and Paul Johnston (English, State University of New York) almost converted Al Scott to the subtle theory of predestination developed in the eighteenth century by American theologian Jonathan Edwards. Although one participant reported overhearing an intense discussion about the proper nature of psychological research between John Watson and William James at the back of the Cushing Street Bar after Wednesday night's reception, this sighting could not be confirmed. The light was poor and lots of elderly people live in Tucson, but it *was* that kind of week.

This book is a sequel to the Tucson I proceedings, *Toward a Science of Consciousness: The First Tucson Discussions and Debates* (Cambridge, MIT Press, 1996). Because it was not possible to publish all available manuscripts in one volume, the editors invited contributions selected from concurrent and poster presentations as well as plenary talks, to cover the spectrum of presentations as faithfully as possible. This selection resulted in a collection of sixty-four chapters arranged in fifteen sections, each preceded by a short introduction.

Although the problem of consciousness may not soon be solved, it is becoming clear that a robust interdisciplinary field of consciousness studies is beginning to take shape.

I Phenomenology and Epistemology

OVERVIEW

Although the broad aim of the Tucson conferences is to develop a science of consciousness, some suggest that the nature of science must be expanded to capture the essential qualities of mind. This is not a trivial matter. Changing the ways in which one conceptualizes and investigates reality—even pushing the envelope of current practice—requires modifications in habits of thought that go to the core of cultural perception. The chapters in Part I propose ways in which current scientific practice might be modified to encompass subjective mental phenomena.

John Searle sets the stage by discussing nine standard objections to the scientific study of consciousness. Although he finds the most challenging objection to be the difficulty of representing subjective perception (qualia) in terms of neural firing patterns, this objection has the most simple answer: We know in fact that it happens. Searle also provides responses to persons who dismiss consciousness as merely epiphenomenal without evolutionary significance, and he criticizes overreliance on the reductive and informational aspects of current scientific practice.

A radically new approach to the scientific study of consciousness is proposed by Francisco Varela, who calls his method "neurophenomenology." Taking subjective experience seriously as the central object of study, this approach aims to develop methods that are appropriate to study first-hand experience. The approach is likely to become familiar to a growing community of researchers.

Along somewhat the same lines, Max Velmans insists that consciousness cannot be understood unless it is accurately described and that reductive approaches are inherently inappropriate to this descriptive task. Why? Because mere correlations between subjective experiences and neural activities (e.g., as indicated by brain scans) is not equivalent to ontological identity.

Robert Forman describes a fully nonreductionist approach to the study of consciousness by focusing attention on various accounts of mystical experience, which exemplifies the relevant phenomena in more simple forms. The pure conscious event achieved through the practice of standard meditation may evolve into a dualistic mystical state in which one experiences unity with the world beyond the self. Such widely reported experiences suggest that awareness is more evolved than are the processes of ordinary sensation or thinking.

Finally, from recent perspectives of mathematical science, Alwyn Scott observes that the reductive approach seems inadequate to describe the essential natures of life and mind because they emerge from interactions among many levels of the dynamic hierarchies of body and brain.

1 How to Study Consciousness Scientifically

John R. Searle

The neurosciences have now advanced to the point that we can address—and, in the long run, perhaps even solve—the problem of consciousness as a scientific problem like any other. However, there are a number of philosophical obstacles to this project. This chapter addresses and tries to overcome some of those obstacles.

Because the problem of giving an adequate account of consciousness is a modern descendant of the traditional mind–body problem, I will begin with a brief discussion of the traditional problem. The mind–body problem can be divided into two problems—the first is easy to solve, the second is much more difficult. The first problem is this: What is the *general* character of the relations between consciousness and other mental phenomena on the one hand and the brain on the other. The solution to the easy problem can be given with two principles: First, consciousness and all mental phenomena are *caused by lower level neurobiological processes in the brain*; and, second, consciousness and other mental phenomena are *higher level features of the brain*. I have expounded this solution to the mind–body problem in a number of writings, so I won't say more about it here.[1]

The more difficult problem is to explain in detail how it actually works in the brain. I believe that a solution to the second problem would be the most important scientific discovery of the present era. When—and if—it is made it will be an answer to this question: "How exactly do neurobiological processes in the brain cause consciousness?" Given our present models of brain functioning it would be an answer to the question, "How exactly do the lower-level neuronal firings at synapses cause all of the enormous variety of our conscious, (subjective, sentient, aware) experiences?" Perhaps we are wrong to think that neurons and synapses are the right anatomical units to account for consciousness, but we do know that some elements of brain anatomy must be the right level of description for answering our question. We know that, because we know that brains do cause consciousness, in a way that elbows, livers, television sets, cars and commercial computers do **not**. Therefore the special features of brains, features that they do not have in common with elbows, livers, etc., must be essential to the causal explanation of consciousness.

Explaining consciousness is essential for explaining most of the features of our mental life because in one way or another they involve consciousness. How exactly do we have visual and other sorts of perceptions? What exactly is the neurobiological basis of memory? Of learning? What are the mechanisms by which nervous systems produce sensations of pain? What, neurobiologically speaking, are dreams? Why do we have dreams? Even, why does alcohol make us drunk? Why does bad news make us feel depressed? In fact I do not believe we can have an adequate understanding of *unconscious* mental states until we know more about the neurobiology of consciousness.

Our ability to get an explanation of consciousness—a precise neurobiology of consciousness—is in part impeded by a series of philosophical confusions. This is an area of science—and they are actually more common than you might suppose in which scientific progress is blocked by philosophical error.

Because it may seem presumptuous for a philosopher to advise scientists in an area outside his special competence, I begin by discussing the relation of philosophy to science and the nature of the problem we are concerned with. The words "philosophy" and "science" do not name distinct subject matters in the way that "molecular biology", "geology", and "the history of Renaissance painting" name distinct subject areas; rather, at the abstract level at which I am now considering these issues, there is no distinction of subject matter because, in principle at least, both are universal in subject matter and, of the various parts of this universal subject matter, each aims for knowledge.

When knowledge becomes systematic, we are more inclined to call it scientific knowledge, but knowledge as such contains no restrictions on subject matter. "Philosophy" is in large part the name for all the questions that we do not know how to answer in the systematic way that is characteristic of science. These questions include, but are not confined to, the large family of conceptual questions that have traditionally occupied philosophers— What is truth? Justice? Knowledge? Meaning?

For the purposes of this discussion, the only important distinction between philosophy and science is this: Science is systematic knowledge; philosophy is, in part, an attempt to get us to the point at which we can have systematic knowledge. This is why science is always right and philosophy is always wrong—as soon as we think we really know something, we stop calling it philosophy and start calling it science. Beginning in the seventeenth century, the area of systematic knowledge, that is, scientific knowledge, increased with the growth of systematic methods for acquiring knowledge. Unfortunately, most questions that bother us have not yet been amenable to the methods of scientific investigation. But we do not know how far we can go with scientific methods, and we should be reluctant to say a priori that particular questions are beyond the reach of science. I will have more to say about this issue later, because many scientists and philosophers think that the whole subject of consciousness is somehow beyond the reach of science.

A consequence of these points is that there are no "experts" in philosophy in the way that there are in the sciences. There are experts on the history of philosophy and experts in certain specialized corners of philosophy such as mathematical logic, but for most central philosophical questions there is no such thing as an established core of expert opinion. I remark on this because I frequently encounter scientists who want to know what philosophers think about a particular issue. Scientists ask these questions in a way that suggests that they think a body of expert opinion exists, which they hope to consult. But in the way that there is an answer to the question "What do neurobiologists currently think about LTP (long-term potentiation)?" there is no comparable answer to the question "What do philosophers currently think about consciousness?" Another consequence of these points is that you have to judge for yourself whether what I say in this chapter is true. I cannot appeal to a body of expert opinion to back me up. If I am right, what I say should seem obviously true, once I have said it and once you have thought about it.

The method I use in my attempt to clear the ground of various philosophical obstacles to the examination of the question, "How exactly do brain processes cause consciousness?" is to present a series of views that I think are false or confused, and then, one by one, try to correct each view by explaining why I think it is false or confused. In each case I discuss views I have found to be widespread among practicing scientists and philosophers.

THESIS 1

Consciousness is not a suitable subject for scientific investigation because the very notion is ill defined. We do not have anything like a scientifically acceptable definition of consciousness, and it is not easy to see how we could get one because consciousness is unobservable. The whole notion of consciousness is at best confused and at worst mystical.

Answer to Thesis 1

We need to distinguish analytic definitions, which attempt to tell us the essence of a concept, from common-sense definitions, which just make clear what we are talking about. An example of an analytic definition is:

Water = df. H_2O

A common-sense definition of the same word is, for example:

Water is a clear, colorless, tasteless liquid. It falls from the sky in the form of rain, and it is the liquid found in lakes, rivers, and seas.

Notice that analytic definitions typically come at the *end*, not the beginning, of a scientific investigation. At this point in our discussion we need a common-sense definition of consciousness and such a definition is not hard to give:

John R. Searle: How to Study Consciousness Scientifically

"Consciousness" refers to the states of *sentience* or *awareness* that typically begin when we wake from a dreamless sleep and they continue through the day until we fall asleep again, die, go into a coma, or otherwise become "unconscious". Dreams are also a form of consciousness, though in many respects they are quite unlike normal waking states.

Such a definition, whose job is to identify the target of scientific investigation but not to provide an analysis, is adequate, and indeed is exactly what we need to begin our study.

Because it is important to be clear about the target, I want to note several consequences of the definition. First, consciousness so defined is an inner, qualitative, subjective state typically present in humans and the higher mammals. We do not at present know how far down the phylogenetic scale this state goes; until there is an adequate scientific account of consciousness, it is not useful to worry about, for example, whether snails are conscious.

Second, consciousness so defined should not be confused with *attention* because in this sense of consciousness there are many things one is conscious of that one may not pay attention to, such as the feeling of the shirt on one's back for example.

Third, consciousness so defined should not be confused with self-consciousness. As I am using the word, consciousness refers to *any* state of sentience or awareness; but self-consciousness, in which the subject is aware of himself or herself, is a very special form of consciousness, perhaps peculiar to humans and the higher animals. Forms of consciousness such as feeling pain do not necessarily involve consciousness of a self as a self.

Fourth, one can experience one's own conscious states but cannot experience or observe conscious states of other humans or animals. But the fact that the consciousness of others is unobservable does not by itself prevent one from developing a scientific account of consciousness. For example, electrons, black holes, and the Big Bang theory are not observable by anybody, but that does not prevent their scientific investigation.

THESIS 2

Science, by definition, is objective, but on the definition of consciousness you have provided, you admit it is subjective. Thus, it follows from your definition that there cannot be a science of consciousness.

Answer to Thesis 2

I believe that this thesis reflects several centuries of confusion about the distinction between objectivity and subjectivity. It would be a fascinating exercise in intellectual history to trace the vicissitudes of the objective–subjective distinction. In Descartes's writings in the seventeenth century, "objective" meant nearly the opposite of its current meaning.[2] Sometime between the seventeenth century and the present the objective–subjective distinction rolled over in bed.

For present purposes, we need to distinguish between the epistemic sense of the objective–subjective distinction and the ontological sense of the distinction. In the epistemic sense, objective claims are objectively verifiable or objectively knowable in that they can be known to be true or false in a way that does not depend on the preferences, attitudes, or prejudices of particular human subjects. Thus, if I say, "Rembrandt was born in 1606," the truth or falsity of the statement does not depend on the particular attitudes, feelings or preferences of human subjects. It is, as they say, a matter of objectively ascertainable fact that Rembrandt was born in 1606. This statement is epistemically objective.

However, subjective claims cannot be known in this way. For example, if I say, "Rembrandt was a better painter than Rubens," the claim is epistemically subjective because, as we would say, it is a matter of subjective opinion. There is no objective test—nothing independent of the opinions, attitudes, and feelings of particular human subjects—which would be sufficient to establish that Rembrandt was a better painter than Rubens. I hope the distinction between objectivity and subjectivity in the epistemic sense is intuitively clear.

But another distinction related to the *epistemic* objective–subjective distinction should not be confused with it: the distinction between *ontological* objectivity and subjectivity. Some entities have a subjective mode of existence; some have an objective mode of existence. For example, the present feeling of pain in my lower back is ontologically subjective in the sense that it only exists as experienced by me. In this sense, all conscious states are ontologically subjective because to exist they have to be experienced by a human or animal subject. In this respect, conscious states differ from, for example, mountains, waterfalls, or hydrogen atoms. Such entities have an objective mode of existence because to exist they do not have to be experienced by a human or animal subject.

Given the distinction between the *ontological* sense of the objective–subjective distinction and the *epistemic* sense of the distinction, one can see the ambiguity of the claim made in Thesis 2. Science is indeed objective in the epistemic sense. Science seeks truths that are independent of the feelings and attitudes of particular investigators. Thus, whether an investigator likes it or does not like it, hydrogen atoms have one electron. It is not a matter of opinion. The fact that science seeks objectivity in the epistemic sense should not blind us to the fact that there are ontologically subjective entities that are as much a matter of scientific investigation as are any other biological phenomena. One can have epistemically objective knowledge of domains that are ontologically subjective. In the epistemic sense, for example, that I have pains in my lower back is an objective matter of fact—not a matter of anybody's opinion—but the existence of the pains themselves is ontologically subjective.

The answer to Thesis 2 is that the requirement that science be objective does not prevent us from developing an epistemically objective science in a domain that is ontologically subjective.

THESIS 3

There is no way that we could ever give an intelligible causal account of how anything subjective and qualitative could be caused by anything objective and quantitative, such as neurobiological phenomena. There is no way to make an intelligible connection between objective, third-person phenomena such as neuron firings and qualitative, subjective states of sentience and awareness.

Answer to Thesis 3

Of all the theses we are considering, this one seems the most challenging. In the hands of some authors, such as Thomas Nagel,[3] the thesis is presented as a serious obstacle to getting a scientific account of consciousness using anything like our existing scientific apparatus. The problem, according to Nagel, is that we have no idea how objective phenomena, such as neuron firings, could necessitate or make it unavoidable that there be states of subjective awareness. Our standard scientific explanations have a kind of necessity that seems to be absent from any imaginable account of subjectivity in terms of neuron firings. For example, what fact about neuron firings in the thalamus could necessitate that anybody who has the firings in that area of the brain must feel a pain?

Although I think this thesis is a serious problem for philosophical analyses, for the purpose of the present discussion, there is a rather swift answer to it: We know in fact that brain processes cause consciousness. The fact that we do not have a theory that explains now it is possible that brain processes could cause consciousness is a challenge for philosophers and scientists. But it is by no means a challenge to the fact that brain processes do in fact cause consciousness because we know independently of any philosophical or scientific argument that they do. The mere fact that it happens is enough to tell us that we should be investigating the form of its happening, not challenging the possibility of its happening.

I accept the unstated assumption behind Thesis 3 that, given our present scientific paradigms, it is not clear how consciousness could be caused by brain processes, but I see that assumption as analogous to these explanations: Within the explanatory apparatus of Newtonian mechanics, it is not clear how a phenomenon such as electromagneticism could exist or within the explanatory apparatus of nineteenth-century chemistry, it is not clear how there could be a nonvitalistic, chemical explanation of life. In other words, I see the problem as analogous to earlier, apparently unsolvable problems in the history of science. The challenge is to forget about how one thinks a process ought to work and, instead, figure out how it in fact works.

My own guess is that when we develop a general theory of how brain processes cause consciousness, our sense that the process is arbitrary or mysterious will disappear. For example, it is clear how the heart causes the pumping of blood. Our understanding of the heart allows us to see the necessity of the process—given the contractions of the heart, blood must flow through the arteries. What we lack so far for the brain is an analogous account of how the brain causes consciousness.

Our sense of mystery has changed since the seventeenth century. To Descartes and the Cartesians, it seemed mysterious that a physical impact on our bodies caused a sensation in our souls. But we have no trouble sensing the necessity of pain given certain sorts of impacts on our bodies. We do not think it at all mysterious that a man whose foot is caught in the punch press is suffering terrible pain. We have moved the sense of mystery inside. Now it seems mysterious that neuron firings in the thalamus should cause sensations of pain. I am suggesting that a thorough neurobiological account of exactly how and why it happens would remove the sense of mystery.

THESIS 4

Within the problem of consciousness we need to separate the qualitative, subjective features of consciousness from the measurable, objective aspects that can be studied scientifically. The subjective features, sometimes called "qualia," can be left to the side, that is, the problem of qualia should be separated from the problem of consciousness. Because consciousness can be defined in objective, third-person terms, the qualia can be ignored. In fact, the best neurobiologists are separating the general problem of consciousness from the special problem of qualia.

Answer to Thesis 4

I did not think that the thesis that consciousness could be treated separately from qualia was commonly held until I discovered it in several recent books on consciousness.[4] The basic idea is that the problem of qualia can be carved off from consciousness and treated separately or, better still, simply brushed aside. This idea seems to me to be profoundly mistaken. There are not two problems—the problem of consciousness and a subsidiary problem, the problem of qualia. *The problem of consciousness is identical with the problem of qualia because conscious states are qualitative states right down to the ground.* Take away the qualia and there is nothing there. This is why I seldom use the word "qualia," except in sneer quotes, because it suggests that there is something else to consciousness in addition to qualia, and that is not true. By definition, conscious states are inner, qualitative, subjective states of awareness or sentience.

Of course, anybody could define the terms in other ways and use the word "consciousness" for something else. But we would still have the problem of what I call "consciousness"—the problem of accounting for the existence of our ontologically subjective states of awareness. The problem of consciousness and the problem of qualia is the same problem; one cannot evade the identity by treating consciousness as a third-person, ontologically objective phenomenon and setting qualia aside because to do so is simply to change the subject.

THESIS 5

Even if consciousness did exist in the form of subjective states of awareness or sentience, it could not make a real difference to the real physical world. Consciousness would just be a surface phenomenon that did not matter causally to the behavior of the organism in the world. To use current philosophical jargon, consciousness would be epiphenomenal. It would be like surface reflections on the water of the lake or the froth on the wave coming to the beach. Science can offer an explanation for why there are surface reflections and why the waves have a froth. In our basic account of how the world works, these surface reflections and a bit of froth are themselves caused, but they are are causally insignificant in producing further effects. For example, in doing computer models of cognition, two computers might perform cognitive tasks but the second computer might be lit up with a purple glow. That is what consciousness amounts to: a scientifically irrelevant, luminous, purple glow. The proof is that for any apparent explanation in terms of consciousness a more fundamental explanation can be given in terms of neurobiology. For every explanation of the form, for example, my conscious decision to raise my arm caused my arm to go up, there is a more fundamental explanation in terms of motor neurons, acetylcholine, and the like.

Answer to Thesis 5

It might turn out that in our final scientific account of the biology of conscious organisms, the consciousness of these organisms plays only a small or negligible role in their life and survival. This is logically possible in the sense that, for example, it might turn out that DNA is irrelevant to the inheritance of biological traits. It might turn out that way, but it is most unlikely, given what we already know. Nothing in Thesis 5 is a valid argument in favor of the causal irrelevance of consciousness.

There are indeed different levels of causal explanation in any complex system. When I consciously raise my arm, there is a macrolevel of explanation in terms of conscious decisions and a microlevel of explanation in terms of synapses and neurotransmitters. But, as a perfectly general point about complex systems, the fact that the macrolevel features are themselves caused by the behavior of the microelements and realized in the system composed of the microelements does not show that the macrolevel features are epiphenomenal. Consider, for example, the solidity of the pistons in a car engine. The solidity of the piston is entirely explainable in terms of the behavior of the molecules of the metal alloy of which the piston is composed; and for any macrolevel explanation of the workings of the car engine given in terms of pistons, the crank shaft, spark plugs, and the like, there will be microlevels of explanation given in terms of molecules of metal alloys, the oxidization of hydrocarbon molecules, and so forth. But this explanation does not show that the solidity of the piston is epiphenomenal. On the contrary, such an explanation shows why you can make effective pistons of steel and not of butter or papier mache. Far from showing that the macrolevel is epiphenomenal, the microlevel of explanation explains, among other things why the macrolevels are causally efficacious. That is, in such cases, the bottom up causal explanations of macrolevel phenomena show why the macrophenomena are not epiphenomenal. An adequate science of consciousness should analogously show how my conscious decision to raise my arm causes my arm to go up by showing how the consciousness, as a biological feature of the brain, is grounded in microlevel neurobiological features.

The point I am making here is quite familiar: it is basic to our world view that higher-level or macrofeatures of the world are grounded in or implemented in microstructures. The grounding of the macrofeature in the microstructures does not by itself show that the macrophenomena are epiphenomenal. Why then is it difficult to accept this point with regard to consciousness and the brain?

I believe the difficulty is that we are still in the grip of a residual dualism. The claim that mental states must be epiphenomenal is supported by the assumption that because consciousness is nonphysical, it cannot have physical effects. The thrust of my argument rejects this dualism. Consciousness is an ordinary biological, and therefore physical, feature of the organism, as much as are digestion or photosynthesis. The fact that consciousness is a physical, biological feature does not prevent its being an ontologically subjective mental feature. The fact that consciousness is both a higher-level and a mental feature is no argument that it is epiphenomenal, any more than any other higher-level biological feature is epiphenomenal. To repeat, consciousness might turn out to be epiphenomenal, but no valid, a priori, philosophical argument that shows that it must turn out that way has yet been given.

THESIS 6

The discussion so far fails to answer the crucial question about the causal role of consciousness, that is: What is the evolutionary function of consciousness? No satisfactory answer has ever been proposed to that question, and it is not easy to see how one will be forthcoming, because it is easy to imagine beings behaving just like us, who lack these "inner, qualitative" states you have been describing.

Answer to Thesis 6

I find this point very commonly made, but it is a very strange claim to make. Suppose someone asked, "What is the evolutionary function of wings on birds?" The obvious answer is that for most species of birds wings enable them to fly and flying increases their genetic fitness. The matter is a little more complicated because not all winged birds are able to fly (e.g., penguins) and, more interestingly, according to some accounts, the earliest wings were really stubs that stuck out of the body and functioned to help the organism keep warm. But there is no question that, relative to their environments, seagulls, for example, are immensely aided by having wings with which they can fly.

Suppose somebody objected by saying that we could imagine the birds flying just as well without wings. What are we supposed to imagine—that birds are born with rocket engines? The evolutionary question only makes sense given certain background assumptions about how nature works. Given the way that nature works, the primary function of the wings of most speces of birds is to enable them to fly. And the fact that we can imagine a science-fiction world in which birds fly just as well without wings is really irrelevant to the evolutionary question.

Similarly, the way that human and animal intelligence works is through consciousness. We can easily imagine a science-fiction world in which unconscious zombies behave exactly as we do. Indeed, I actually constructed such a thought experiment to illustrate certain philosophical points about the separability of consciousness and behavior.[5] But that is irrelevant to the actual causal role of consciousness in the real world.

When one forms a thought experiment to test the evolutionary advantage of some phenotype, what are the rules of the game? In examining the evolutionary functions of wings, no one would think it allowable to argue that wings are useless because we can imagine birds flying just as well without wings. Why is it supposed to be allowable to argue that consciousness is useless because we can imagine humans and animals behaving just as they do now but without consciousness? As a science-fiction thought experiment, that is possible, but it is not an attempt to describe the actual world in which we live. In our world, the question "What is the evolutionary function of consciousness?" is like the question "What is the evolutionary function of being alive?" After all, we could imagine beings who outwardly behaved much as we do but who are made of cast iron, reproduce by smelting, and are quite dead.

I believe that the standard way in which the question is asked reveals fundamental confusions. In the case of consciousness, the question "What is the evolutionary advantage of consciousness?" is asked in a manner that reveals that we are making the Cartesian mistake. The form of the question reveals thinking of consciousness not as part of the ordinary physical world of wings and water, but as a mysterious, nonphysical phenomenon that stands outside the world of ordinary biological reality. If we think of consciousness biologically, and if we then try to take the question seriously, the question boils down to "What is the evolutionary function of being able to walk, run, sit, eat, think, see, hear, speak a language, reproduce, raise the young, organize social groups, find food, avoid danger, raise crops, and build shelters?" *For humans all these activities, as well as countless others essential for our survival, are conscious activities.* In other words, "consciousness" does not name a phenomenon isolable from all other aspects of life, but rather the mode in which humans and the higher animals conduct the major activities of their lives.

This is not to deny that there are interesting biological questions about the specific forms of our consciousness. For example, what evolutionary advantages, if any, do we derive from the fact that our color discriminations are conscious and our digestive discriminations in the digestive tract are typically not conscious? But as a general challenge to the reality and efficacy of consciousness, the skeptical claim that consciousness serves no evolutionary function is without force.

THESIS 7

Causation is a relation between discrete events ordered in time. If brain processes really cause conscious states, the conscious states would have to be separate events from the brain processes and the result would be a form of dualism—a dualism of brain and consciousness. Any attempt to postulate a causal explanation of consciousness in terms of brain processes is necessarily dualistic and therefore incoherent. The correct scientific view is to see that consciousness is nothing but patterns of neuron firings.

Answer to Thesis 7

This thesis expresses a common mistake about the nature of causation. Certainly there are many causal relations that fit this paradigm. For example, in the statement, "The shooting caused the death of the man," one describes a sequence of events—first, the man was shot; then he died. But many causal relations are not discrete events; they are permanent causal forces operating through time. Think of gravitational attraction. It is not the case that there is first gravitational attraction and then, later, chairs and tables exert pressure against the floor. Rather, gravitational attraction is a constant operating force, and at least in these cases, the cause is cotemporal with effect.

More importantly, there are many forms of causal explanation that rely on bottom-up forms of causation. Two examples are solidity and liquidity. A table is capable of resisting pressure and is not interpenetrated by solid objects. But, like other solid objects, the table actually consists entirely of clouds of molecules. How is it possible that these clouds of molecules exhibit the causal properties of solidity? The theory is that solidity is caused by the behavior of molecules. Specifically, when the molecules move in vibratory movements within lattice structures, the object is solid. Somebody might therefore say, "Then solidity consists in nothing but the behavior of the molecules," and, in a sense, the person would be right.

However, solidity and liquidity are causal properties in addition to the summation of the molecule movements. Some philosophers find it useful to use the notion of an "emergent property". I do not find this a very clear notion because its explanation seems confused in the literature. But if we are careful, we can give a clear sense to the idea that consciousness, like solidity and liquidity, is an emergent property of the behavior of the microelements of a system that is composed of those microelements. An emergent property, so defined, is a property that is explained by the behavior of the microelements but cannot be deduced simply from the composition and the movements of the microelements. I use the notion of a "causally emergent property"[6]; in that sense, liquidity, solidity, and consciousness are all causally emergent properties caused by the microelements of the system of which they are themselves features.

The point I am eager to insist on is simply this: The fact that there is a causal relation between brain processes and conscious states does not imply a dualism of brain and consciousness any more than does the fact that the causal relation between molecule movements and solidity implies a dualism of molecules and solidity. I believe the correct way to view the problem is to see that consciousness is a higher-level feature of the system, the behavior of whose lower-level elements causes it to have that feature. This claim leads to the next problem—reductionism.

THESIS 8

Science is by its very nature reductionistic. A scientific account of consciousness must show that consciousness is an illusion in the same sense in which heat is an illusion. There is nothing to the heat of a gas except the mean kinetic energy of the molecule movements. Similarly, a scientific account of consciousness will show that there is nothing to consciousness except the behavior of the neurons. This is the death blow to the idea that there will be a causal relation between the behavior of the microelements, in this case neurons, and the conscious states of the system.

Answer to Thesis 8

The concept of reduction is one of the most confused notions in science and philosophy. In the literature of the philosophy of science, I found at least a half dozen different concepts of reductionism. It seems to me that the notion has probably outlived its usefulness. What we want from science are general laws and causal explanations. Typically, when we have a causal explanation, we redefine the phenomenon in terms of the cause and thereby reduce the phenomenon to its cause. For example, instead of defining measles in terms of its symptoms, we redefine it in terms of the virus that causes the symptoms. Thus, measles is reduced to the presence of a certain kind of virus. There is no factual difference between saying, "The virus causes the symptoms that constitute the disease," and saying, "The presence of the virus is the presence of the disease, and the disease causes the symptoms." The facts are the same in both cases. The reduction is just a matter of different terminology. What we want to know is: What are the facts?

In the case of reduction and causal explanations of the sort I just gave, it seems that there are two sorts of reductions—those that eliminate the phenomenon being reduced by showing that there is really nothing there in addition to the features of the reducing phenomena and those that do not eliminate the phenomenon but simply give a causal explanation for it. This distinction is not very precise, but examples may make it intuitively clear. In the case of heat, we need to distinguish between movement of the molecules with a certain kinetic energy and subjective sensations of heat. There is nothing there except the molecules moving with a certain kinetic energy. This motion causes the sensations that we call sensations of heat. The reductionist account of heat carves off the subjective sensations and defines heat as the kinetic energy of the molecule movements. We have an eliminative reduction of heat because there is no objective phenomenon there except the kinetic energy of the molecule movements. Analogous remarks can be made about color. There is nothing there but the differential scattering of light. The scattering causes the experiences that we call color experiences. But there is no color phenomenon beyond that of light reflectances and their subjective effects on us.

In such cases, we can have eliminative reductions of heat and color. We can say they are nothing but physical causes and that these produce the subjective experiences. Such reductions are eliminative reductions in that they get rid of the phenomenon that is being reduced. But in this respect they differ from the reductions of solidity to the vibratory movement of molecules in lattice structures. Solidity is a causal property of the system and cannot be eliminated by the reduction of solidity to the vibratory movements of molecules in lattice-type structures.

Why can we not do an eliminative reduction of consciousness in the way that we did for heat and color? The pattern of the facts is parallel—for heat and color we have physical causes and subjective experiences; for consciousness we have physical causes in the form of brain processes and the subjective experience of consciousness. Thus, it seems we should reduce consciousness to brain processes. Of course, in this trivial sense, we could. We could also redefine the word "consciousness" to mean the neurobiological causes of our subjective experiences. But if we did these things, we would have the subjective experiences left over.

The point of having the concept of consciousness is to have a word to name the subjective experiences. The other reductions were based on carving off the subjective experience of heat and color and redefining the notion in terms of the causes of the experiences. Because the phenomenon that we are discussing *is* the subjective experience itself, one cannot carve off the subjective experience and redefine the notion in terms of its causes without losing the point of the concept. The asymmetry between heat and color on the one hand and consciousness on the other has not to do with the facts in the world, but rather with our definitional practices. We need a word to refer to ontologically subjective phenomena of awareness or sentience. If we redefined the word in terms of the causes of our experiences, we would lose that feature of the concept of consciousness.

One cannot make the appearance–reality distinction for conscious states themselves as one can for heat and color because for conscious states the existence of the appearance is the reality in question. If it seems to me I am conscious, then I am conscious. That is not an epistemic point. It does not imply that we have certain knowledge of the nature of our conscious states.

John R. Searle: How to Study Consciousness Scientifically

On the contrary, we are frequently mistaken about our own conscious states, for example, in the case of phantom limb pains. The statement is a point about the ontology of conscious states.

When we study consciousness scientifically, I believe we should forget our obsession with reductionism and seek causal explanations. The obsession with reductionism is a hangover from an earlier phase in the development of scientific knowledge. What we want is a causal explanation of how brain processes cause our conscious experience.

THESIS 9

Any genuinely scientific account of consciousness must be an information process-ing account. That is, we must see consciousness as consisting of a series of informa-tion processes; And the standard apparatus for accounting for information process-ing in terms of symbol manipulation by a computing device must form the basis of any scientific account of consciousness.

Answer to Thesis 9

Actually, in a number of earlier publications, I have answered this objec-tion in detail.[7] For present purposes, the essential thing to remember is that consciousness is an intrinsic feature of certain human and animal nervous systems. The problem with the concept of "information processing", is that information processing is typically in the mind of an observer. For example, we treat a computer as a bearer and processor of information, but, intrin-sically, the computer is simply an electronic circuit. We design, build, and use such circuits because we can interpret their inputs, outputs, and inter-mediate processes as information-bearing. However, the information in the computer is in the eye of the beholder; it is not intrinsic to the computational system.

The same explanation applies a fortiori to the concept of symbol manipu-lation. The electrical-state transitions of a computer are symbol manipula-tions only relative to the attachment of a symbolic interpretation by some designer, programmer, or user. The reason we cannot analyze consciousness in terms of information processing and symbol manipulation is that con-sciousness is intrinsic to the biology of nervous systems—information pro-cessing and symbol manipulation are relative to the observer. For this reason, any system can be interpreted as an information-processing system—the stomach processes information about digestion, the falling body processes information about time, distance, and gravity, and so on.

The exceptions to the claim that information processing is relative to the observer are cases in which some conscious agent is thinking. For example, if I as a conscious agent think, consciously or unconsciously, "$2 + 2 = 4$," information processing and symbol manipulation are intrinsic to my mental processes because they are the processes of a conscious agent. But in that respect my mental processes differ from that of my pocket calculator adding

2 + 2 and getting 4. Thus, the addition in the calculator is not intrinsic to the circuit, but the addition in me is intrinsic to my mental life.

To make the distinction between the cases that are intrinsically information bearing and symbol manipulating from those that are observer relative we need the notion of consciousness. Therefore, we cannot explain the notion of consciousness in terms of information processing and symbol manipulation.

CONCLUSION

We need to take consciousness seriously as a biological phenomenon. Conscious states are caused by neuronal processes, they are realized in neuronal systems, and they are intrinsically inner, subjective states of awareness or sentience. We want to know how these states are caused by and how they are realized in the brain. Perhaps they can be caused by a type of chemistry different from that of brains altogether, but until we know how brains produce the chemistry, we are not likely to be able to reproduce it artificially in other chemical systems.

The mistakes to avoid are those of changing the subject—thinking that consciousness is a matter of information processing or behavior, for example—or not taking consciousness seriously on its own terms. Perhaps above all, we need to forget about the history of science and get on with producing what may turn out to be a new phase in that history.

NOTES

1. See, for example, Searle, J. R. 1984. *Minds, Brains and Science.* Cambridge: Harvard University Press and Searle, J. R. 1992. *The Rediscovery of the Mind.* Cambridge: MIT Press.

2. For example, Rene, Descartes's *Meditations on First Philosophy*, especially Third Meditation. "But in order for a given idea to contain such and such objective reality, it must surely derive it from some cause which contains at least as much formal reality as there is objective reality in the idea." In J. Cottingham, R. Stoothoff, and D. Murdoch, trans., Meditations on first philosophy. *The Philosophical Writings of Descartes*, vol. II. Cambridge: Cambridge University Press, 1984.

3. See, for example, Nagel's 1974 article, What is it like to be a bat? *Philosophical Review* 83:435–450.

4. For example, Crick, F. 1994. *The Astonishing Hypothesis: The Scientific Search for the Soul.* New York: Simon & Schuster; Edelman, G. 1989. *The Remembered Present: A Biological Theory of Consciousness.* New York: Basic Books.

5. Chapter 3 of Searle (1992).

6. Chapter 5 of Searle (1992). pp. 111ff.

7. See Searle, J. R., 1980. "Minds, Brains and Programs", *Behavioral & Brain Sciences*, 3:417–458; Chapter 3 of Searle 1992, and Searle, J. R. 1984.

2

A Science of Consciousness as If Experience Mattered

Francisco J. Varela

WHY WE NEED A RADICALLY NEW APPROACH

A science of consciousness requires a significant reframing of the way that is usually posed within cognitive science and in the Anglo-American philosophy of mind. We need to turn to a systematic exploration of the only link between mind and consciousness that seems both obvious and natural: *the structure of human experience itself* (Varela 1996).[1] Practically speaking, this means taking the tradition of phenomenology as a science of experience seriously and linking it skillfully with modern science. My purpose in this chapter is to sketch for the scientific study of consciousness a research direction that is radical in the way in which methodological principles are linked to scientific studies to seek a productive marriage between modern cognitive science and a disciplined approach to human experience. I call this approach *neurophenomenology*.[2] No piecemeal empirical correlates or purely theoretical principles help at this stage. Yet, a skillful bridge-building between science and experience stands in stark contrast to what most people at the Tucson Conference presented.

Three axes seem to capture the essential orientations in the current boom of discussion on consciousness. These orientations are analogous to those in politics—the center, the right, and the left. The right, best represented by P. S. Churchland and F. Crick, is close to the spontaneous philosophy of a significant percentage of my colleagues in neuroscience, and is appropriately labeled as neuroreductionism or eliminitivism. As is well known, this view seeks to solve the "hard problem" by eliminating the pole of experience in favor of some form of neurobiological account that generates consciousness.

At the center position are a variety of proposals that can be labeled functionalistic. They are identified as the most popular ecology of ideas active today, and include a number of well-developed proposals such as Jackendorff's (1987) "projective mechanism," Baars's (1992) "global workspace," Dennett's (1991) "multiple drafts," Calvin's (1990) "Darwinian machines," or Edelman's (1989) "neural Darwinism." The basic move in these proposals is quite similar. First, start from the modular items of cognitive capacities (i.e., the "soft" problems). Second, construct a theoretical framework to put the items together so that their unity amounts to an account of experience. The strategy to bridge the emergent unity and experience itself varies, but typically the explanation is left vague because the proposals rely almost entirely on a third-person or externalistic approach to obtain data and to validate the theory. This position represents the work of an important segment of researchers in cognitive science. Its popularity rests on the acceptance of the reality of experience and mental life while keeping the methods and ideas within the known framework of empirical science.

Finally, to the left, is the sector that interests me most, the one that can be roughly described as giving an explicit and central role to first-person accounts and to the irreducible nature of experience while at the same time refusing both a dualistic concession or a pessimistic surrender. This sector has odd bedfellows such as Lakoff and Johnson's (1987) approach to cognitive semantics, Searle's (1994) ideas on ontological irreducibility, Globus's (1995) "post-modern" brain, and, at the edge, Flannagan's (1992) "reflective equilibrium" and Chalmers's (1996) formulation of the hard problem in the study of consciousness.

What is interesting about this diverse group, within which I place myself, is that even though we share a concern for first-hand experience as basic fact to incorporate in the future of the discipline, the differences are patent in the *manner* in which experience is taken into account. The phenomenological approach is grounded in the exploration of experience, which is the center of my proposal. This sufficiently clarifies, I hope, the context for my ideas within today's debate. Now I can move into the heart of the matter: the nature of the circulation between a first-person account and an external account of human experience, the phenomenological position in fertile dialogue with cognitive science.

A NEUROPHENOMENOLOGICAL APPROACH

Irreducibility: The Basic Ground

The phenomenological approach starts from the irreducible nature of conscious experience. Lived experience is where we start from. Most modern authors are either disinclined to focus on the distinction between mental life in a general sense and experience or they manifest some suspicion about the status of mental life.

From a phenomenological standpoint, conscious experience is at variance with that of mental content as it figures in the Anglo-American philosophy of mind. The tension between these two orientations appears in a rather dramatic fashion in Dennett's book, (1991) in which he concludes with little effort (15 lines in a 550-page book) that phenomenology has failed. He remarks:

Like other attempts to strip away interpretation and reveal the basic facts of consciousness to rigorous observation, such as the Impressionistic movements in the arts [*sic*] and the Introspectionist psychologists of Wundt, Titchener and others, Phenomenology has failed to find a single settled method that everyone could agree upon. (p.44)

This passage is revealing: Dennett mixes apples and oranges by putting impressionism and introspectionism into the same bag; he confuses introspectionism with phenomenology, which it is most definitely not (see later discussion), and he draws his conclusion from the absence of some idyllic universal agreement that would validate the whole. Surely we would not demand "that everyone could agree" on, say, Darwinism, to make it a remarkably useful research program. And certainly *some* people agree on the established possibility of disciplined examination of human experience. Similarly, although Flannagan (1992) claims to make phenomenology into an essential dimension of his inclusive position, one does not find a single reference to what this tradition has accomplished or to some of its main exponents! In books that are in many other respects savant and insightful, this display of ignorance concerning phenomenology is a symptom that says a lot about what is amiss in this field.

Method: Moving Ahead

We need to explore, beyond the spook of subjectivity, the concrete possibilities of a disciplined examination of experience that is at the very core of the phenomenological inspiration. As stated earlier, the rediscovery of the primacy of human experience and its direct, lived quality is phenomenology's foundational project. This is the sense within which Edmund Husserl inaugurated such thinking in the West and established a long tradition that is well and alive today not only in Europe but worldwide.

It is fair to say that phenomenology is, more than anything else, a *style of thinking* that was started in the West by Husserl but which does not exhaust his personal options and style. (I do not here want to engage in an account of the diversity and complexity of western phenomenology—see e.g., Spiegelberg 1962.) The contributions of individuals such as Eugen Fink, Maurice Merleau-Ponty, or Aaron Gurwitsch, to cite only a few, attest to the continuing development of phenomenology. More recently, various links with modern cognitive science have been explored (see, for instance, Dreyfus 1982; Varela, Thompson, and Rosch 1991; Petitot, Varela, Pachoud, and Roy et al. 1998; Thompson and Varela 1998).[3] My observation is that most people unfamiliar with the phenomenological movement automatically assume that phenomenology is some sort of old-fashioned, European school.

My position cannot be ascribed to any particular school but represents my own synthesis of phenomenology in the light of modern cognitive science and other traditions focusing on human experience. Phenomenology can also be described as a *special type of reflection* or attitude about our capacity for being conscious. All reflection reveals a variety of mental contents (mental acts) and their correlated orientation or intended contents. Natural or naive attitude takes for granted a number of received claims about both the nature of the experiencer and its intended objects. It was Husserl's hope (and the basic inspiration behind phenomenological research) that a true science of experience would gradually be established—one that could not only stand on equal footing with the natural sciences, but that could give them a needed ground, since knowledge necessarily emerges from our lived experience.

On the one hand, experience is suffused with spontaneous preunderstanding; thus, it might seem that any theory about experience is quite superfluous. On the other hand, preunderstanding itself must be examined since it is unclear what kind of knowledge it represents. Experience demands specific examination to free it from its status as habitual belief. Phenomenology aims its movement towards a fresh look at experience in a specific gesture of reflection or *phenomenological reduction* (PhR).[4]

This approach or gesture changes the habitual ways in which we relate to our lived world, which does not mean to consider a different world, but to consider the present one *otherwise*. This gesture transforms a naive or unexamined experience into a reflexive or second-order one. Phenomenology correctly insists on a shift from the natural to the phenomenological attitude because only then can the world and experience appear as open and in need of exploration. The meaning and pragmatics of PhR have taken several variants from this common trunk.[5]

The conscious gesture at the base of PhR can be decomposed into four intertwined moments or aspects:

Attitude: Reduction

The attitude of reduction is the necessary starting point. It can also be defined by its similarities to doubt: a sudden, transient suspension of beliefs about what is being examined, a putting in abeyance of habitual discourse about something, a bracketing of the preset structuring that constitutes the ubiquitous background of everyday life. Reduction is self-induced (it is an active gesture), and it seeks to be resolved (dissipating doubts) because it is here as a source of experience. A common mistake assumes that suspending habitual thinking means stopping the stream of thoughts, which is not possible. The point is to turn the direction of the movement of thinking from its habitual, content-oriented direction backwards toward the arising of thoughts themselves. This is no more than the very human capacity for reflexivity, and the lifeblood of reduction. To engage in reduction is to cultivate a systematic capacity for reflexiveness and thus open up new possibilities within one's habitual mind stream. For instance, right now you, the reader, are probably making some internal remarks concerning what reduction is, what it reminds you of, and so on. To mobilize an attitude of reduction begins by noticing those automatic thought patterns, taking a reflexive distance from them, and focusing reflection toward their source.

Intimacy: Intuition

The result of reduction is that a field of experience appears both less encumbered and more vividly present, as if the habitual distance separating the experiencer and the world has been dispelled. As William James saw, the immediacy of experience thus appears surrounded by a diversity of horizons to which we can turn our interest. The gain in intimacy with the phenomenon is crucial because it is the basis of the criteria of truth in phenomenological analysis, the nature of its evidence. Intimacy or immediacy is the beginning of the process, and it continues by cultivation of imaginary variations, in the virtual space of mind considers multiple possibilities of the phenomenon as it appears. These ideal variations are familiar to us from mathematics, but here they serve whatever becomes the focus of our analysis: perception of three-dimensional form, the structure of nowness, the manifestations of empathy, and so on. Through these multiple variations a new stage of understanding arises, an "Aha!" experience, which adds a new evidence that carries a force of conviction. This moving intimacy with our experience corresponds well to what is traditionally referred to as intuition, and represents, along with reflection, the two main human capacities that are mobilized and cultivated in PhR.

Description: Invariants

To stop at reduction followed by imaginary variations would be to condemn this method to private ascertainment. As crucial as the preceding ones is the next component. The gain in intuitive evidence must be inscribed or translated into communicable items, usually through language or other symbolic inscriptions (e.g., sketches or formulae). The materialities of these descriptions, however, are also a constitutive part of the PhR and shape our experience as much as the intuition that shapes them. In other words, we are not talking about an "encoding" into a public record but of an "embodiment" that incarnates and shapes what we experience. I refer to these public descriptions as invariants because through variations one finds broad conditions under which an observation can be communicable. This is not so different from what mathematicians have done for centuries—the novelty is its application to the contents of consciousness.

Training: Stability

As with any discipline, sustained training and steady learning are key. A casual inspection of consciousness is a far cry from the disciplined cultivation of PhR. This point is particularly relevant because the attitude of reduction is notoriously fragile. If one does not cultivate the skill to stabilize and deepen one's capacity for attentive bracketing and intuition along with the skill for illuminating descriptions, no systematic study can mature. This last aspect of the PhR is perhaps the greatest obstacle for the constitution of a research

Table 2.1 Aspects of Phenomenological Reduction

Aspect	Characteristics of Resulting Examination
Attitude	Bracketing, suspending beliefs
Intuition	Intimacy, immediate evidence
Invariants	Inscriptions, intersubjectivity
Training	Stability, pragmatics

program since it implies a disciplined commitment from a community of researchers. Table 2.1 summarizes the four aspects of phenomenological reduction.

AVOIDING STANDARD TRAPS

Previous presentations of these ideas have prompted a number of recurrent traps and misleading conclusions. Let me address a few of them in a preventive move.

Phenomenological Analysis Is Not Introspectionism

As many have remarked, introspection presupposes that we have access to our experience in the same manner that we have access to an inner visual field, as the etymology of the word suggests, by inspection. Such an internal examination is a normal cognitive ability of reflective doubling, a gesture in which we engage regularly.

In the days of prephenomenology (i.e., without reduction) introspection elicited a wave of interest in psychology, starting with the work of Wundt and followed by others such as Titchener in the United States and the Würzburg school. Despite an initial enthusiasm, the research program advanced by introspectionism did not take root. Among other problems, reports from different laboratories could not reach a common ground of validation. The historical account of Lyons (1986) was written as an obituary for introspection, but it was a hasty conclusion, as Howe (1991) reminded us. This manner of mobilizing reflexive capacities still falls into the natural attitude for a phenomenologist, for it rides on the wave of previous elaborations and assumptions.

Phenomenology does share with introspectionism an interest in the reflexive doubling as a key move of its approach to phenomena, but there the two attitudes part company. In PhR, the skill to be mobilized is called *bracketing* for good reasons, since it seeks precisely the opposite effect of an uncritical introspection—it cuts short our quick and fast elaborations and beliefs, in particular location, and puts in abeyance what we consider we think we should find, or some expected description. Thus, PhR is not a "seeing inside," but a tolerance concerning the suspension of conclusions that allows a new aspect or insight into the phenomenon to unfold. In consequence, this move does not sustain the basic subject–object duality but opens into a field of phenomena in which it becomes less obvious how to distinguish between subject and object (the "fundamental correlation" discussed by Husserl).

Intuition Is Not "Some Fluffy Stuff"

Many people react to the mention of intuition with suspicion. In this context, intuitive capacity does not refer here to some elusive, will-o'-wisp inspiration. It is, on the contrary, a basic human ability that operates constantly in daily life and that has been widely discussed in studies of creativity. In mathematics, for example, ultimately the weight of a proof is its convincing nature—the immediacy of the evidence imposed on us beyond the logical chains of symbolic reasoning. This is the nature of intuitive evidence: born not of argument but from the establishment of a clarity that is fully convincing. We take this capacity for granted and do little to cultivate it in a systematic manner. Obviously, there is no contradiction here with reasoning and inference—intuition without reasoning is blind, but ideas without intuition are empty.

Life Beyond the Objective–Subjective Duality

One of the originalities of the phenomenological attitude is that it does not seek to oppose the subjective to the objective but to move beyond the split into their fundamental correlation. PhR takes us quickly into the evidence that consciousness is inseparably linked to what goes beyond itself ("transcendental" in Husserlian terms).

Consciousness is not some private, internal event having, in the end, an existence of the same kind as the external, nonconscious world. Phenomenological investigation is not my "private trip" since it is destined for others through intersubjective validation. In this sense, what one is up to in phenomenological attitude is not radically different from other modes of inquiry.

Through PhR, consciousness appears as a foundation that sheds light on how derived notions such as objectivity and subjectivity can arise in the first place. Hence, consciousness in this style of examination is drastically different from that of Anglo-American empiricism. We are not concerned with a private inspection but with a realm of phenomena in which subjectivity and objectivity, as well as subject and others, emerge from the method applied and from its context. This is a point that reductionists and functionalists often miss. Experience is clearly a personal event, but that does not mean it is private in the sense that it is a kind of isolated subject parachuted down to a pregiven objective world. One of the most impressive discoveries of the phenomenological movement is to have quickly realized that an investigation of the structure of human experience inevitably induces a shift toward considering several levels of my consciousness as inextricably linked to those of others and to the phenomenal world in an empathic mesh (Depraz 1995).

Consequently, the usual opposition of first-person vs. third-person accounts is misleading. It makes us forget that so-called third-person, objective accounts are done by a community of people who are embodied in their social and natural worlds as much as are first-person accounts.

Better Pragmatics Are Needed

On the whole, my claim is that neurophenomenology is a natural solution that can allow us to move beyond the hard problem in the study of consciousness. It has little to do with some theoretical or conceptual "extra ingredient," to use Chalmers's (1996) formula. Instead, it acknowledges a realm of *practical* ignorance that can be remedied. It is also clear that, like all solutions in science that radically reframe an open problem instead of trying to solve it within its original setting, it has a revolutionary potential. In other words, instead of finding extra ingredients to account for how consciousness emerges from matter and brain, my proposal reframes the question to that of finding meaningful bridges between two irreducible phenomenal domains. In this specific sense, neurophenomenology is a potential solution to the hard problem by framing what "hard" means in an entirely different light.

Unfortunately, a pragmatics of what is available in published form about reduction are limited.[6] This situation is both a symptom and a cause for the relative paucity of recent work bearing on phenomenological approaches to mind. The reader cannot be blamed for not having had more than a passing whiff of what I mean by emphasizing the gesture of reduction, the core of the my methodological remedy. It is remarkable that this capacity for becoming aware has been paid so little attention as a human pragmatic. It is as if the exploration of rhythmic movement had led to no development of dance training. A phenomenologically inspired reflection requires strategies for its development, as cognitive practicians have known for some time (Vermersch 1994) and as attested in the mindfulness tradition of various Buddhist schools (Varela, Thompson, and Rosch 1991). My only comment concerning this relative poverty of pragmatical elaboration is that it represents an urgent call for research to fill this gaping need. (My contribution concerning the practice of reduction and its training will be presented in Depraz, Varela, and Vermersch 1998).

In the West we have not had a rich pantheon of individuals gifted for phenomenological expertise (with notable exceptions, such as Husserl or James), who have rendered their investigations to an attentive community. In consequence, this avenue of inquiry may appear foreign to many readers. But my contention is precisely that this absence is at the root of consciousness's opacity for science today. What is needed are precisely the connecting structures provided by PhR because they are both immediately pertinent for experience by their very nature and, at the same time, are sufficiently intersubjective to serve as constructive counterparts for external analysis.

From the standpoint of phenomenology, experimental psychology and modern cognitive science miss a fundamental dimension of mental phenomena by dismissing an analysis of immediate, direct experience. Husserl stated that even if it took time, some day the scientific community would "consider the instrument of phenomenological eidetic theory to be no less important, indeed at first probably very much more than mechanical instruments" (one could add, today, computers and electronics). In this context Husserl also raised an "analogy of proportionality" between mathematics and modern physics and between pure phenomenology and psychology. Clearly, this analogy has to be handled with care, but it is useful in this context because it highlights the inescapable need to seek a disciplined approach to include experience in our study of mind and toward a genuine science of consciousness.

A NEUROPHENOMENOLOGICAL CIRCULATION

In recent years, a number of different studies, although remaining well-grounded in the scientific tradition of cognitive neuroscience, have shown that the part played by lived experience is progressively more important to the extent that it begins to enter inescapably into the picture apart from any interest in first-person accounts (Picton and Stuss 1994). Clearly, as more sophisticated methods of brain imaging become available, we shall need subjects whose competence in making phenomenological discriminations and descriptions is developed. This is an important philosophical issue, but it is also a pragmatic, empirical need.

For instance, temporality is inseparable from all experience, at various horizons of duration from present nowness to an entire life span. One level of study is precisely the experience of immediate time, the structure of nowness as such (or in James's happy phrase, "the specious present"). This has been a traditional theme in phenomenological studies and describes a basic, three-part structure of the present with its constitutive threads into past and future horizons, the so-called protentions and retentions (Husserl 1966; McInerny 1991). In fact, these structural invariants are not compatible with the point-continuum representation of linear time we have inherited from physics. But they do link naturally to the body of conclusions in cognitive neuroscience that there is a minimal time required for the emergence of neural events that correlate to a cognitive event (Dennett and Kinsbourne 1992). This noncompressible time framework can be analyzed as a manifestation of long-range neuronal integration in the brain linked to a widespread synchrony (Varela 1995). The link illuminates both the nature of phenomenological invariants via a dynamical reconstruction that underlies them and gives to the process of synchrony a tangible experiential content. I have developed this neurophenomenological view of temporal nowness in detail elsewhere (Varela 1998).

The evocation of study cases such as this one is meant to provide a concrete background to discuss further the central concern of the neurophenomenological program. On one hand, we have a process of emergence with well defined neurobiological attributes; on the other, a phenomenological description that links directly to our lived experience. To make further progress we need cutting-edge techniques, analyses from science, and consistent development of phenomenological investigation for the purposes of the research itself.

Do I expect the list of structural invariants relevant to human experience to grow ad infinitum? Certainly not. I surmise that the horizon of fundamental topics can be expected to converge towards a corpus of well-integrated knowledge. When and how fast this happens depends on the pace at which a community of researchers committed to this mode of inquiry is constituted to create further standards of evidence.

THE WORKING HYPOTHESIS OF NEUROPHENOMENOLOGY

Only a balanced and disciplined account of both the external and experiential side of an issue can make us move closer to bridging the biological mind—experiential mind gap:

Phenomenological accounts of the structure of experience and their counterparts in cognitive science relate to each through reciprocal constraints.

The key point here is that by emphasizing a *codetermination* of both accounts one can explore the bridges, challenges, insights, and contradications between them. Both domains of phenomena have equal status in demanding full attention and respect for their specificity. It is quite easy to see how scientific accounts illuminate mental experience, but the reciprocal direction, from experience towards science, is what is typically ignored.

Phenomenological accounts provide at least two main aspects of the larger picture. First, without these accounts, the first-hand quality of experience vanishes or becomes a mysterious riddle. Thus, they provide scientific studies with a dimension of meaning that is otherwise lost. Second, structural accounts provide constraints on empirical observations. For instance, a computational, step-by-step interpretation of time is in fact excluded by the phenomenological evidence, whereas a dynamical account of resonance is strongly suggested (Varela 1998).

The study of experience is not a convenient stop on our way to a real explanation, but an active participant in its own right. Clearly, in this research program, a certain body of evidence is slowly accumulated; other aspects are more obscure and difficult to seize. The study cases mentioned above need substantially more development, but I hope it is clear how they begin to provide a stereoscopic perspective on the various large, local issues in which experience and cognitive science become active partners.

The demand for a disciplined circulation is both a more precise and a more demanding standard than the "reflective equilibrium" proposed by Flannagan (1992) or the "conscious projection" put forth by Velmans (1996). Although there is a similarity in intention to what I am proposing here, these authors have proposed no explicit or new methodological grounds for carrying out these intentions.

Still, is this not just a fleshed-up version of the well-known identity theory (or at least a homomorphism) between experience and cognitive neuro-scientific accounts? Not really, because I claim that the correlates are to be established, not just as a matter of philosophical commitment or physicalist assumption, but from a methodologically sound examination of experiential invariants. This is a question of pragmatics and learning of a method, not of a priori argumentation or theoretical completeness.

One obtains an intellectually coherent account of mind and consciousness at the point at which the experiential pole enters directly into the formulation of the complete account and thus makes direct reference to the nature of our lived experience. In all functionalistic accounts, what is missing is not the coherent nature of the explanation but its alienation from human life. Only putting human life back can erase that absence, not an extra ingredient or a theoretical fix.

CONCLUSION

One must take seriously the double challenge my proposal represents. First, it demands relearning and a mastery of the skill of phenomenological description. This should not be different from the acquisition of any other skill, like learning to play an instrument or to speak a new language. Anyone who engages in learning is bringing forth a change in everyday life. This is the meaning of the fourth item in PhR: sustained, disciplined learning *does* entail transformation just as does anything else one does in a sustained mode. One needs to reject the assumption (as I do) that there is a type of well-defined standard for what counts as real or normal experience. Experience appears to be inherently open ended and pliable; hence, there is no contradiction in saying that sustained training in a method can make available aspects of experience that were not available before. The point of PhR is to overcome the habit of automatic introspection; we need not mourn for what may be lost, but turn our interest to what can be learned.

The second challenge that my proposal represents is that of a call for transforming the style and values of the research community itself. Unless we accept that at this point in intellectual and scientific history radical relearning is necessary, we cannot hope to move forward in the compulsive history of the ambivalent rejection—fascination with consciousness in philosophy of mind and cognitive science. My proposal implies that every good student of cognitive science who is also interested in issues at the level of mental experience must inescapably attain a level of mastery in phenomenological examination to work seriously with first-person accounts.

This can only happen when the entire community adjusts itself to the corresponding acceptance of arguments, the refereeing standards and editorial policies in major scientific journals, which can make this added competence an important dimension of a young researcher. To the long-standing tradition of objectivist science this sounds like anathema, and it is. But it is not a betrayal of science; it is a necessary extension and complement. Science and experience constrain and modify each other as in a dance. This is where the potential for transformation lies. It is also the key for the difficulties this position has found within the scientific community because it requires us to leave behind a certain image of how science is done and to question a style of training in science which is part of the very fabric of our cultural identity.

In brief, then:

1. I take lived, first-hand experience as a proper field of phenomena, irreducible to anything else. My claim is that there is no theoretical fix or extra ingredient in nature that can possibly bridge this gap.

2. This field of phenomena requires a proper, rigorous method and pragmatics for its exploration and analysis.

3. The orientation for such method is inspired from the style of inquiry of phenomenology to constitute a widening research community and a research program.

4. The research program seeks articulations by mutual constraints between field of phenomena revealed by experience and the correlative field of phenomena established by the cognitive sciences. I call this point of view *neurophenomenology*.

ACKNOWLEDGMENTS

My thanks to all my phenomenological seekers–partners in Paris and elsewhere, especially Jean Petitot, Jean-Michel Roy, Natalie Depraz, Evan Thompson, and Pierre Vermersch.

NOTES

1. This paper is a modified version of Varela (1996), keeping the main ideas that were actually presented for my invited lecture at Tucson. I am grateful to the editors of the *Journal of Consciousness Studies* for letting me recycle my text for the present volume. Some ideas also appear in D. Aerts, ed. *Einstein Meets Magritte: An Interdisciplinary Conference*. Amsterdam: Kluwer Associated, 1997.

2. The usage of "neuro" should be taken here as a nom de guerre: It is chosen in explicit contrast to the current usage of "neurophilosophy," which identifies philosophy with the Anglo-American philosophy of mind. Further, "neuro" here refers to the entire array of scientific correlates that are relevant in cognitive science. But to speak of a neuropsychoevolutionary phenomenology is not very handy.

3. Cognitive scientists may have read the collection edited by Dreyfus (1982), which presents Husserl as some sort of protocomputationalist, and assume that this historical anecdote is all they need to know about phenomenology. As critics have made clear, however, Dreyfus's reading of Husserl is seriously flawed—see Langsdorf (1985), McIntyre (1986), and Roy (1995).

4. The reader should refrain from the temptation to assimilate this usage of the word "reduction" with that of "theoretical reduction" as it appears, for instance, in the neuroreductionist framework and as well-articulated in the writings of P. Churchland. The two meanings run completely opposite one another; it is convenient to append a qualifier.

5. For a recent discussion about the varieties of reduction see Bernet (1994), pp. 5–36. Husserl's first articulation can be found in his breakthrough lectures of 1910 (Husserl, 1970).

6. But see the early attempts of Don Ihde (1977) to remedy this situation as cited in Marbach (1988), p. 254.

REFERENCES

Baars, B. 1988. *A Cognitive Theory of Consciousness*. Cambridge: Cambridge University Press.

Bernet, R. 1994. *La Vie du Sujet*. Paris: Presses Universitaire de France.

Calvin W. 1990. *Cerebral Symphony: Seashore Reflections on the Structure of Consciousness*. New York: Bantam Books.

Chalmers, D. 1996. *The Conscious Mind: In Search of a Fundamental Theory*. New York: Oxford University Press.

Damasio, A. 1994. *Descartes' Error: Emotion, Reason and the Human Brain*. New York: Grosset/Putnam.

Dennett, D. 1991. *Consciousness Explained*. Boston: Little, Brown.

Depraz, N. 1996. *Transcendence et Incarnation*. Paris: J. Vrin.

Depraz, N., F. Varela, and P. Veermersch. 1998. *On Becoming Aware: Exploring Experience with a Method*. (forthcoming).

Dreyfus, H., ed. 1982. *Husserl: Intentionality and Cognitive Science*. Cambridge: MIT Press.

Edelman, G. 1989. *The Remembered Present: A Biological Theory of Consciousness*. New York: Basic Books.

Flannagan, O. 1992. *Consciousness Reconsidered*. Cambridge: MIT Press.

Globus, G. 1995. *The Post-Modern Brain*. New York: Benjamin.

Howe, R. B. 1991. Introspection: A reassessment. *New Ideas in Psychology* 9:24–44.

Husserl, H. 1970. *The Idea of Phenomenology*, The Hague: Martinus Nijhoff.

Husserl, E. 1966. *Zur Phänomenologie des Inneren Zeitbewusstseins (1893–1917)*. R. Bohm, Ed. The Hague: Martinus Nijhoff. (Partial English translation: *The Phenomenology of Internal Time Consciousness, Bloomington*, Indiana University Press. 1976).

Ihde, D. 1977. *Experimental Phenomenology*. New York: Open Court.

Jackendorff, R. 1987. *Consciousness and the Computational Mind*. Cambridge: MIT Press.

James, W. 1912. *The Principles of Psychology*. Reprinted 1996. Cambridge: Harvard University Press.

Langsdorf, L. 1985. Review of Husserl: Intentionality and cognitive science (1982). *Husserl Studies* 3:303–311.

Lyons, W. 1986. *The Disappearance of Introspection*. Cambridge: MIT Press.

Lyotard, J.-F. 1954. *La Phénoménologie*. Paris: Presses Universitaire de France.

Marbach, E. 1988. How to study consciousness phenomenologically or quite a lot comes to mind. *Journal of the British Society of Phenomenology* 19:252–264.

McIntyre, R. 1986. Husserl and the representational theory of mind, *Topoi* 5:101–113.

Merleau-Ponty, M. 1945. *La Phénoménologie de la Perception*. Paris: Gallimard.

McInerney, P. 1991. *Time and Experience*. Philadelphia: Temple University Press.

Petitot, J., F. Varela, B. Pachoud, and J. M. Roy, eds. 1998. *Naturalizing Phenomenology: Contemporary Issues on Phenomenology and Cognitive Science*. Stanford: Stanford University Press, (in press).

Picton, T., and D. Stuss. 1994. Neurobiology of conscious experience. *Current Biology* 4:256–265.

Roy, J. M. 1995. Le "Dreyfus bridge": Husserlism and Fodorism. *Archives de Philosophie* 58:533–549.

Spiegelberg, F. 1962. *The Phenomenological Movement*, 2nd ed. The Hague: Martinus Nihjoff.

Thompson, E., and F. Varela. 1998. *Why the Mind Is Not in the Head*. Cambridge: Harvard University Press, (forthcoming).

Varela, F. J., E. Thompson, and E. Rosch. 1991. *The Embodied Mind: Cognitive Science and Human Experience*. Cambridge: MIT Press.

Varela, F. 1995. Resonant cell assemblies: A new approach to cognitive functioning and neuronal synchrony. *Biological Research* 28:81–95.

Varela, F. 1996. Neurophenomenology: A methodological remedy for the hard problem, *Journal of Consciousness Studies* 3:330–349.

Varela, F. 1998. The specious present: The neurophenomenology of time consciousness. In J. Petitot et al. eds., *Naturalizing Phenomenology: Contemporary Issues on Phenomenology and Cognitive Science*. Stanford: Stanford University Press, (in press).

Velmans, M. 1996. *The Science of Consciousness*. London: Routledge.

Vermersch, P. 1994. *L'Entretien d'Explicitation*. Paris: ESF Editeurs.

3 Goodbye to Reductionism

Max Velmans

To understand consciousness we must first describe accurately what we experience. But oddly, current dualist versus reductionist debates characterize experience in ways that do not correspond to ordinary experience. Indeed, there is no other area of inquiry in which the phenomenon to be studied has been so systematically misdescribed. Thus, it is hardly surprising that progress toward understanding the nature of consciousness has been limited.

Our current world view is dominantly materialist and reductionist, an ontology that has served well in natural science. But for consciousness, materialist reductionism has not worked—for the simple reason, I believe, that it cannot be made to work. Although this limits the range of convenience for the materialist, reductionist program, it matters little for science. The investigation of consciousness can take place, unimpeded, within a more inclusive, nonreductionist science.

DUALIST AND REDUCTIONIST DESCRIPTIONS OF CONSCIOUSNESS

Within consciousness studies, the reductionist agenda has been set by that which it opposes, the classical dualism of Plato and Descartes. For Descartes, the universe was composed of two interacting substances: *res extensa*, the material stuff of the physical world, body, and brain, which has extension in space, and *res cogitans*, nonmaterial stuff that "thinks," which has no location or extension in space. The physical world affects consciousness through sensory perception; motions in the external world are transduced by the eye and nerves into motions in the pineal gland, which, in turn, produces conscious experiences in the soul. That is, events located in space cause experiences of those events which themselves have no spatial location or extension.

Modern studies of the visual system have revealed a very different and far more complex physiology than that envisaged by Descartes. Reductionists now claim that consciousness is nothing more than a state or function of the brain. But in one crucial respect in modern accounts, the causal sequence in perception remains the same. Events in the world still cause conscious experiences that are located in some quite different inner space—albeit in the brain, not in an inner, nonmaterial soul. In short, both dualist and reductionists agree that there is clear separation of the external physical world from the world of conscious experience.

MISDESCRIPTIONS OF EXPERIENCE

Given that we all have conscious experience, it is amazing that dualist and reductionist descriptions of this experience have persisted. For Descartes, thoughts were the prime exemplar of conscious experience, and it is true that, phenomenologically, thoughts seem to be like *res cogitans*, without clear location and extension in space (although thoughts might loosely be said to be located in the head or brain). But conscious thoughts (phonemic imagery or "inner speech") form only a very small part of conscious experience. While reading this page, for example, one might experience conscious thoughts but, at the same time, also experience print on paper that is attached to a book on a table or lap as well as a surrounding, physical world that extends in three-dimensional, phenomenal space. Thus, the bulk of what one experiences has an extended, phenomenal nature very different from that of *res cogitans*.

Reductionism provides a description of what consciousness is really like that is even further removed from its actual phenomenology. Even reductionists themselves do not claim that we experience our phenomenal worlds to be nothing more than states or functions of the brain. Phenomena as experienced do not even seem to be in the brain! The stubborn fact is that we experience our phenomenal heads (and the thoughts within them) to exist within surrounding phenomenal worlds, not the other way around. Given this, it seems sensible to develop a model of the way consciousness relates to the brain that is consistent with science *and* with what we experience.

This is the aim of the *reflexive model of perception* (Velmans 1990, 1993, 1996). This model adopts a conventional, scientific description of perceptual processing, which can only be determined by investigation of the brain, viewed from an external observer's third-person perspective. Unconventionally, the reflexive model also assumes that one cannot understand consciousness without an accurate phenomenological description of consciousness, which can only be undertaken from the subject's first-person perspective. If some conscious experiences are *not* like thoughts, so be it. If *no* conscious experiences seem to be like brain states, too bad for reductionism. The investigation of consciousness can proceed quite happily without reductionism by finding out how events perceived from the subject's first-person perspective actually relate to the events perceived from the external observer's third-person perspective.

Consider how the differences between the dualist, reductionist, and reflexive models work out in a simple example. Suppose I stamp on your foot, and you experience pain. Pain is universally assumed to be a mental event within philosophy of mind. But where *is* the pain? Is it nowhere, as dualists claim? Is it in the brain, as reductionists claim? Or is it in the foot? Readers in doubt on this issue may want to test this example with a friend.

The reflexive model adopts the common-sense position that the pain is in the foot (in spite of its being a mental event). That is, a stimulus in the foot is transmitted to the brain and the resulting phenomenal experience (produced by mental modeling) is subjectively projected[1] back to the foot (where the mind–brain judges the initiating stimulus to be). That is why the process is called reflexive. Similarly, events that originate in the external world are experienced to be in the world, and events that originate in the mind–brain are experienced to be in the mind–brain. In short, the modeling process that subjectively projects experienced events to the judged locations of the initiating stimuli is, under most circumstances, reasonably accurate.[2] Together, the experienced events (in the world, body, and mind–brain) form the content of our conscious, phenomenal worlds.

As noted above, such phenomenal worlds can be investigated from a first-person perspective, or be related to brain states viewed from a third-person perspective, without any need to reduce their phenomenology to anything else. There are also many consequences of the nonreductive approach for consciousness science and for philosophy of mind (Velmans 1990, 1993, 1996). Given the current dominance of reductionism, it is sufficient here to examine whether reductionism can cope with a more accurate description of everyday experience.

THE APPEARANCE–REALITY DISTINCTION

Given the dissimilarities between conscious experiences and brain states, reductionism has a problem. How can things that seem to be different be the same? This problem becomes acute once one accepts that conscious contents include not just ephemeral thoughts, but entire phenomenal worlds. To bridge the gap, reductionists mostly rely on the appearance–reality distinction. They accept that conscious experiences *appear* to have phenomenal qualities but argue that science will eventually show that the experiences are *really* states or functions of the brain. For this view to work, it must of course apply to all phenomenal qualities, including the apparent location and extension of perceived events (such as pains) in phenomenal space. John Searle (1992), for example, pointed out that:

Common sense tells us that our pains are located in physical space within our bodies, that for example, a pain in the foot is literally in the physical space of the foot. But we now know that is false. The brain forms a body image, and pains like all bodily sensations, are parts of the body image. The pain in the foot is literally in the physical space in the brain. (p. 63)

For reductionism to work, common sense must be wrong. If Searle is right, this demonstrates just how wrong common sense can be. So let us examine Searle's assertion carefully. It is true that science has discovered representations of the body in the brain, for example, a tactile mapping of the body surface distributed over the somatosensory cortex (SSC). The area of SSC devoted to different body regions is determined by the number of tactile receptors in those regions. In SSC, for example, the lips occupy more space that does the torso. Furthermore, body regions adjacent in phenomenal space may not be adjacent in SSC. For example, we feel the face to be connected to the head and neck, but in SSC, the tactile map of the face is spatially separated from the map of the head and neck by maps of the fingers, arm, and shoulder. That is, the topographical arrangement of the body image is very different from that of the body as perceived.

Given this, how does the body image relate to the body as perceived? According to Searle, science has discovered that tactile sensations in the body are, literally, in the brain. In truth, however, no scientist has discovered body sensations in the brain, and no scientist ever will—for the simple reason that, viewed from an external observer's perspective, the body as experienced by the subject cannot be perceived. Science has nevertheless investigated the relationship of the body image (in SSC) to tactile experiences. Penfield and Rassmussen (1950), for example, exposed areas of cortex preparatory to surgical removal of cortical lesions responsible for focal epilepsy. To avoid surgical damage to areas essential to normal functioning, the functions of these areas were explored by lightly stimulating them with a microelectrode and noting the subject's consequent experiences. As expected, stimulation of the somatosensory cortex produced reports of tactile experiences. However, feelings of numbness, tingling, and the like were subjectively located in different regions of the *body*, not in the brain.

In summary, science has discovered that neural excitation of somatosensory cortex causes tactile sensations that are subjectively located in different regions of the body—which is exactly what the reflexive model describes. But if tactile sensations cannot be found in the brain, viewed either from the experimenter's third-person perspective or from the subject's first-person perspective, how can one argue that the experiences are nothing more than brain states?

COMMON REDUCTIONIST ARGUMENTS AND FALLACIES

Reductionist arguments come in many forms, but they all claim that the phenomenology of consciousness is misleading and people's trust in it to be naive. Commonly, reductionists try to show that if one can find the neural causes or correlates of consciousness in the brain, this discovery will establish consciousness itself to be a brain state (see, for example, Place 1956; Churchland 1988; Crick 1994). Let us call these views the "causation argument" and the "correlation argument." I suggest that such arguments are based on a fairly obvious fallacy. To be nothing more than a brain state consciousness must be *ontologically identical* to a brain state. However, correlation and causation are very different from ontological identity.

Ontological identity is symmetrical. If A is ontologically identical to B, then B is ontologically identical to A. Ontological identity also obeys

Leibniz's law—if A is identical to B, then all the properties of A are also properties of B and vice versa (A and B must exist at the same time, occupy the same location in space, and so on). A classic example of apparently different entities shown by science to be the same entity are the "morning star" and the "evening star,"—both are the planet Venus (viewed in the morning and evening).

Correlation is symmetrical but does not obey Leibniz's law. If A correlates with B, then B correlates with A, but all the properties of A are not properties of B. For example, height in humans correlates with weight and vice versa, but height and weight do not have the same properties.

Causation is not symmetrical and does not obey Leibniz's law. If A causes B, it does not follow that B causes A. Nor are the properties of A the same as those of B. If one throws a stone in a pond, ripples form in the water, but it does not follow that the ripples in the water cause the stone to be thrown in the pond. Nor are the properties of thrown stones and water ripples identical.

Once the obvious differences between causation, correlation, and ontological identity are laid bare, the weakness of the causation argument and the correlation argument are clear. Under appropriate conditions, brain states may be shown to cause or correlate with conscious experiences, but it does not follow that conscious experiences are nothing more than states (or, for that matter, functions) of the brain.[3] To demonstrate this claim one would have to establish an ontological identity in which all the properties of a conscious experience and corresponding brain state were identical. Unfortunately for reductionism, few if any properties of experience (accurately described) and brain states appear to be identical. In the case of pains in the foot and other events as perceived in the phenomenal world, the brain states (observed by the experimenter) and associated conscious phenomena (observed by the subject) do not even seem to be in the same place!

Faced with this difficulty, reductionists usually turn to analogies from other areas in science in which a reductive, causal account of a phenomenon has led to an understanding of its ontology (very different from its phenomenology). Ullin Place (1956), for example, used the example of lightning, which we now understand to be nothing more than the motion of electrical charges through the atmosphere. This reduction, Place argued, is justified once we know that the motion of electrical charges through the atmosphere causes what we experience as lightning. Similarly, a conscious experience may be said to be a given state of the brain once we know that brain state to have caused the conscious experience.

The lightning analogy is seductive because it is half true. That is, for the purposes of physics it is true that lightning can be described as nothing more than the motion of electrical charges. But psychology is interested in how this physical stimulus interacts with a visual system to produce lightning as perceived—in the form of a jagged flash of light in the phenomenal world. This experience of lightning may be said to represent an event in the world that physics describes as a motion of electrical charges. But the *phenomenology itself* cannot be said to be nothing more than the motion of electrical charges. Prior to the emergence of life forms with visual systems on this planet, there presumably was no such phenomenology, although the electrical charges that now give rise to this experience did exist.

Patricia Churchland (1988) tried to achieve phenomenological reduction through theory reduction. She argued that psychological theory and neurophysiological theory continue to coevolve until, in some distant future, the higher level, psychological theory is reduced to a more fundamental, neurophysiological theory. When this happens, Churchland claimed, consciousness will have been shown to be nothing more than a state of the brain. Whether a complete, interlevel, theoretical reduction is possible is open to debate. But even if this were possible, fundamental problems remain. Theories *about* phenomena do not make phenomena go away. Furthermore, neurophysiological theories of consciousness deal with the neural causes and correlates of consciousness, not with its ontology, for the simple reason that causes and correlates are all one can observe in the brain. And, as shown above, even a complete understanding of neural causes and correlates would not suffice to reduce conscious phenomena to states of the brain.

John Searle (1987) agreed that causality should not be confused with ontology, and his case for physicalism appears to be one of the few that has addressed this distinction head-on. The gap between what *causes* consciousness and what conscious *is* can be bridged, Searle suggested, by an understanding of how microproperties relate to macroproperties. Liquidity of water is *caused* by the way H_2O molecules slide over each other, but it *is* nothing more than an emergent property of the combined effect of the molecular movements. Likewise, solidity is *caused* by the way molecules in crystal lattices bind to each other, but it *is* nothing more than the higher-order, emergent effect of such bindings. In similar fashion, consciousness is *caused* by neuronal activity in the brain, but it *is* nothing more than the higher-order, emergent effect of such activity. That is, consciousness is just a physical macroproperty of the brain.

This argument too, is seductive, but needs to be examined with care. The brain undoubtedly has physical macroproperties of many kinds. The one closest to liquidity and solidity is sponginess. But there are also more interesting, psychologically relevant macroproperties, for example, the mass action of large neuronal populations and electroencephalography. Some properties, no doubt, cause or correlate with conscious experiences. Unfortunately for physicalism, however, there is no reason to suppose that consciousness is ontologically identical to these properties or to any other known physical properties of the brain. As shown above, even simple experiences such as a pain in the foot pose a problem for reductionist theory. Searle disputes this idea, but he accepts that *subjectivity* and *intentionality* are defining characteristics of consciousness. Unlike physical phenomena, the phenomenology of consciousness cannot be observed from the outside; unlike physical phenomena, it is always *of* or *about* something. So, even if one accepts that consciousness in some sense is caused by or is emergent from the brain, why call it physical instead of mental or psychological? Merely *relabeling* consciousness does not solve the mind–body problem!

The absence of any completely persuasive reductionist case, in spite of the eloquence of its protagonists, suggests that reductionist accounts of consciousness attempt to do something that cannot be done. Examination of the brain from the outside can reveal only the physical causes and correlates of consciousness; it can never reveal consciousness itself. Many phenomenal properties of conscious experience appear very different from those of brain states. Consequently, it is difficult to imagine what science could discover to demonstrate that experiences are ontologically identical to states of the brain.

To put matters another way, once one abandons the atrophied descriptions of consciousness implicit in dualism and reductionism, any realistic hope of reducing its phenomenology to brain states disappears. As Searle (1992) noted:

... consciousness consists in the appearances themselves. Where appearance is concerned we cannot make the appearance–reality distinction because the appearance is the reality. (p. 121)

If so, reductionism is dead within philosophy of mind. Let us wave it goodbye without tears, and say hello to a nonreductionist science of consciousness, which takes phenomenology seriously and does not ignore common sense.

NOTES

1. Note that the perceptual projection is a subjective, psychological effect produced by unconscious cognitive processing. Nothing physical is projected from the brain. Extensive evidence for perceptual projection is given in Velmans (1990).

2. If the experienced world did not correspond reasonably well to the actual one, our survival would be threatened. Nevertheless, mismatches such as hallucinations and referred pains occur. At great distances, our distance judgments and consequent experiences bear little resemblance to actual distances—how far away does the moon look? Or a star?

3. It is worth keeping in mind that many nonreductionist positions also assume that there are neural causes and correlates of given conscious experiences, including the reflexive model, dualism, epiphenomenalism, emergent interactionism, and so on. The causes and correlates of conscious experience should not be confused with their ontology.

REFERENCES

Churchland, P. S. 1988. *Neurophilosophy: Toward a Unified Science of Mind and Brain.* Cambridge: MIT Press.

Crick, F. 1994. *The Astonishing Hypothesis: The Scientific Search for the Soul.* London: Simon & Schuster.

Penfield, W., and T. B. Rassmussen. 1950. *The Cerebral Cortex of Man.* Princeton: Princeton University Press.

Place, U. T. 1956. Is consciousness a brain process? *British Journal of Psychology* 47:42–51.

Searle, J. R. 1987. Minds and brains without programs. In C. Blakemore and S. Greenfield, eds. *Mindwaves: Thoughts on Intelligence, Identity,* and *Consciousness.* New York: Blackwell.

Searle, J. R. 1992. *The Rediscovery of the Mind*. Cambridge: MIT Press.

Velmans, M. 1990. Consciousness, brain and the physical world. *Philosophical Psychology* 3(1):77–99.

Velmans, M. 1993. A reflexive science of consciousness. In *Experimental and Theoretical Studies of Consciousness. Ciba Foundation Symposium 174*. Chichester: Wiley.

Velmans, M. 1996. What and where are conscious experiences? In M. Velmans, ed. *The Science of Consciousness: Psychological, Neuropsychological and Clinical Reviews*. London: Routledge.

4

What Can Mysticism Teach Us About Consciousness?

Robert K. C. Forman

I am honored to be included in this work with such eminent scientists and philosophers. It is a tribute to the scientific community as a whole and to the Tucson organizing committee that both have opened their doors to another source of knowledge about consciousness, and this much, this soon. After all, it was only in 1980 that Brian Josephson observed what was then correct:

mystical experience is not at the moment considered by the majority of scientists to be a matter worthy of scientific attention.... This is to some extent purely an arbitrary decision.[1]

Here it is, a mere 17 years later, and this volume now includes a study of mysticism.

WHY MYSTICISM?

I think it is right to look at some of the more responsible mystics for insights about consciousness. Why? When a biologist seeks to understand a complex phenomenon, one key strategy is to look at the phenomenon in its simplest form. For example, probably the most famous humble bacterium is *Escherichia coli*. Its simple gene structure has allowed biologists to understand much of the gene functioning of complex species. Similarly, many biologists have turned to the "memory" of the simple sea slug to understand humans' more kaleidoscopic memory. Freud and Durkheim both used totemism, which they construed as the simplest form, to understand the complexities of religious life. The methodological principle is: To understand something complex, turn to its simple forms.

Is there a simple expression of human consciousness? Usually our minds are an enormously complex stew of thoughts, feelings, sensations, wants, snatches of song, pains, drives, daydreams, and consciousness itself, more or less aware of it all. To understand consciousness *in itself*, the obvious thing would be to clear away as much of the internal clutter and noise as possible.

Mystics may be doing precisely that. The technique that most mystics use is some form of meditation or contemplation. These procedures systematically reduce mental activity. During meditation, one begins to slow down the thinking process to have fewer or less intense thoughts. One's thoughts become more distant, vague, or less preoccupying; one stops paying much attention to bodily sensations; one has fewer or less intense fantasies and daydreams. Finally, one may come to a time of inner stillness—one becomes utterly silent inside, analogous to a gap between thoughts. One neither thinks nor perceives any mental or sensory content. Yet, despite this suspension of content, one emerges from this event confident that one had remained awake, conscious.

This experience, which has been called the pure consciousness event (PCE) (Forman 1990), has been identified in virtually every tradition. Though PCEs typically happen to any single individual only occasionally, they are quite regular for some practitioners.[2] The pure consciousness event may be defined as a wakeful but contentless (nonintentional) consciousness. PCEs, encounters with consciousness devoid of intentional content, may be the least complex encounter with awareness per se that we students of conscious seek. The PCE may serve, in short, as the *E. coli* of consciousness studies.[3]

But the story does not stop here. Regular and long-term meditation, according to many traditions, leads to advanced experiences, known in general as "enlightenment." The discriminating feature of these experiences is a deep shift in epistemological structure—the relationship between the self and one's perceptual objects changes profoundly. In many persons, this new structure is permanent.[4]

Long-term shifts in mystical epistemological structure often take the form of two quantum leaps in experiences; typically, they develop sequentially.[5] The first is an experience of a permanent interior stillness, even while engaged in thought and activity—one remains aware of one's own awareness simultaneously with consciousness of thoughts, sensations, and actions. Because of its phenomenological dualism—a heightened cognizance of awareness plus consciousness of thoughts and objects—I call this experience the dualistic mystical state (DMS). The second shift is described as a perceived unity between one's own awareness per se with the objects around one, an immediate sense of a quasiphysical unity between self, objects, and other people. This experience I call the unitive mystical state, UMS.

Like the PCE, the latter two states may serve as fertile fields for students of consciousness to plow. To understand these states I introduce the idea of the relative intensity of a thought or desire. Some desires have a high relative intensity. Suppose I am walking across the street and I see a huge truck hurtling at me. Virtually all of my attention is taken up with the truck, the fear, and getting out of the way. It is virtually impossible for me to think about anything else at that time. I don't even consider keeping my suit clean, how my hair might look, the discomfort in my tummy, or the classes I will teach tomorrow. The fear and running are *utterly intense* and consume nearly 100 percent of my attention.

That evening, I come home feeling starved, and rush to the refrigerator. I may be civil to my wife and children, but I have very little patience because my desire for food is *very intense*; it preoccupies most of my consciousness but consumes less of my attention than did jumping away from the truck.

Some thoughts consume very little of my attention. For example, driving to work the next day, I might ruminate about my classes, remember the near miss with the truck, half hear the news on the radio, and think about getting some noise in the car fixed—nearly all at once. None of these thoughts or desires is very intense, for none has a strong emotional cathexis that draws me fully into it, and my attention can flow in and out of any of them or to the traffic ahead, effortlessly. In short, the intensity of a thought or desire is *directly* proportional to the amount of my consciousness that is taken up with the thought or feeling. Conversely, a thought's intensity is *inversely* proportional to the amount of attention I have for other issues and for my wider perspective. Roughly, cathexis is inversely proportional to available consciousness.

Now, as I understand them, advanced mystical experiences result from the combination of regular PCEs and minimization of the relative intensity of emotional and cognitive attachments. That is, over time, one decreases the compulsive or cathexis intensity of all of one's desires. The deintensifying of emotional attachments means that, over the years, one's attention is available to sense its own quiet interior character more fully, until eventually one is able to effortlessly maintain a subtle cognizance of one's own awareness simultaneously with thinking about and responding to the world.

The state of being cognizant of one's own inner awareness and simultaneously maintaining the ability to think and talk about that consciousness offers students of consciousness a unique situation. These subjects may be able to be both unusually cognizant of features or patterns of their own awareness and also describe that awareness to us—a kind of living microscope into human consciousness. In short, although not as phenomenologically simple as PCEs, these experiences may provide us with highly useful reports about the character of human awareness.

Using these reports will cause us to draw conclusions about human consciousness from the experiences of a very few people. Most of us have not had mystical experiences, and some may sound quite strange. Yet, we often generalize from the unusual to the general. We have concluded a lot about consciousness from epileptics, people with unusual skull accidents or brain injuries, the man who mistook his wife for a hat, and the like. From the pathology of a very few we have learned a great deal about the relationship of one side of the brain to the other, of two kinds of knowing, of information storage and retrieval, of impulse control, and so forth. Indeed, it is common practice to take data about a few unusual individuals and generalize that data to many persons. Many people who have had mystical experiences— Sakyamuni Buddha, Teresa of Avila, Ramana Maharishi—are not pathological but unusually self-actualized. Are we not as willing to learn from the experiences of the unusually healthy as we are to learn from the unusually diseased?

What do we mean by mysticism? What is generally known as mysticism is often said to have two strands, traditionally distinguished as *apophatic* and *kataphatic* mysticism, that is, oriented respectively toward "emptying" or toward imaginal experience. The two strands are generally described in terms of being either *without* or *with* sensory language. The psychologist Roland Fischer distinguished a similar pairing as *trophotropic* and *ergotropic*, experiences that phenomenologically involve either inactivity or activity. *Kataphatic* (imagistic) mysticism involves hallucinations, visions, auditions, or a sensory-like experience of smell or taste; it thus involves activity and is ergotropic. *Apophatic* mystical experiences are devoid of such sensory-like content, and are thus trophotropic. In using nonsensory, nonimagistic language,[6] authors such as Eckhart, Dogen, al-Hallaj, Bernadette Roberts, and Shankara are thus apophatic mystics.

Finally, phenomenology is *not* science. When we describe mystical experiences, we do not gain hard scientific proof or even theorems. There can be many ways to explain an unusual experience. One might say it was the result of what one ate for dinner, a faulty memory, psychosomatic processes, a quantum microtubule collapse, or as an experience of an ultimate truth. Without further argumentation, phenomenology cannot serve as the sole basis for any theory of reality; rather, it may be taken only as a finger pointing in some direction or as evidence for or against a particular thesis. In short, I see the mystics as the "Deep Throats" of consciousness studies, pointing towards a thesis. But it will take the hard-working Woodwards and Bernsteins in the trenches to verify or deny their suggestions. Because visions and other ergotropic experiences are not the simple experiences of consciousness that we require, I will focus here on the quieter, apophatic form.

THREE MYSTICAL PHENOMENA AND THEIR IMPLICATIONS

Pure Consciousness Events

There are several reports of the first of the mystical phenomena mentioned above, the PCE.[7] From Christian mystical literature, St. Teresa of Avila (James 1983) writes of the "orison of union":

During the short time the union lasts, she is deprived of every feeling, and even if she would, she could not think of any single thing ... She is utterly dead to the things of the world ... I do not even know whether in this state she has enough life left to breathe. It seems to me she has not; or at least that if she does breathe, she is unaware of it ... The natural action of all her faculties [are suspended]. She neither sees, hears, nor understands ... (p. 409)

Several key features of this experience are notable. First, Teresa tells us that one reaches orison of unity by gradually reducing thought and understanding to eventually become "utterly dead" to things, thus encountering neither sensation, thought, nor perceptions. One becomes as simple as possible. Eventually one stops thinking altogether—not able to "think of any single thing ... arresting the use of her understanding ... utterly dead to the things of the world."[8] And yet, she clearly implies, one remains awake.

Meister Eckhart (Walshe 1979) describes something similar as the *gezucken*, rapture, of St. Paul, Eckhart's archetype of a transient mystical experience:

... the more completely you are able to draw in your powers to a unity and forget all those things and their images which you have absorbed, and the further you can get from creatures and their images, the nearer you are to this and the readier to receive it. If only you could suddenly be unaware of all things, then you could pass into an oblivion of your own body as St Paul did, ... In this case ... memory no longer functioned, nor understanding, nor the senses, nor the powers that should function so as to govern and grace the body ... In this way a man should flee his senses, turn his powers inward and sink into an oblivion of all things and himself.

Like St. Teresa, Eckhart specifically asserts the absence of sensory content ("nor the senses"), as well as mental objects (devoid of memory, understanding, senses, etc.). One becomes oblivious of one's "own body" and "all things."

The absence of thought and sensation is repeated in the following passage from the Upanishads (Hume 1931) describing the state the early Hindu texts call *turiya*, the "fourth":

Verily when a knower has restrained his mind from the external, and the breathing spirit (prana) has put to rest objects of sense, thereupon let him continue void of conceptions. Since the living individual (jiva) who is named "breathing spirit" has arisen here from what is not breathing spirit, therefore, verily, let the breathing spirit restrain his breathing spirit in what is called the fourth condition (*turiya*).

Here, again, one is "putting to rest objects of sense," (i.e., gradually laying aside all sensations) and continuing "void of conceptions," (i.e., not thinking). Yet the Upanishads are insistent that one remains conscious, indeed becomes nothing but consciousness itself. The consciousness that one reaches in *turiya* is known in Samkhya philosophy as *purusha*, often translated as awareness or consciousness itself, that which "illuminates" or "witnesses" thoughts, feelings, and actions.[9] The purusha or consciousness that one reaches during this experience is described as "sheer contentless presence (*sasksitva*) ... that is nonintentional" (Larson 1979).

PCEs in Theravada Buddhism are called by several names: *nirodhasamapatti*, cessation meditation, *samjnavedayitanirodha*, the cessation of sensation and conceptualization, or, most famously, *samadhi*, meditation without content.[10] What is most fascinating about Buddhist reports is that, despite the fact that one is said to be utterly devoid of content, according to Vasumitra and to Yogacara Buddhist theorists, one's consciousness is said to persist as "some form of contentless and attributeless consciousness."[11]

A report from a 48-year-old male practitioner of Neo-Advaitan meditation[12] confirms the persistence of consciousness throughout these sorts of phenomena:

Sometimes during meditation my thoughts drift away entirely, and I gain a state I would describe as simply being awake. I'm not thinking about anything. I'm not particularly aware of any sensations, I'm not aware of being absorbed in anything in particular, and yet I am quite certain (after the fact) that I haven't been asleep. During it I am simply awake or simply present.

It is odd to describe such an event as being awake or being present, for those terms generally connote an awareness of something or other. But in this experience there is no particular or identifiable object of which I am aware. Yet I am driven to say I am awake for two reasons. First, I emerge with a quiet, intuited certainty that I was continually present, that there was an unbroken continuity of experience or of consciousness throughout the meditation period, even if there seemed to have been periods from which I had no particular memories. I just know that there was some sort of continuity of myself (however we can define that) throughout.

In sum, the PCE may be defined as a wakeful but contentless (nonintentional) experience. Though one remains awake and alert and emerges with the clear sense of having had "an unbroken continuity of experience," one neither thinks, perceives, nor acts.

What implications can we draw from the PCE about the nature of human consciousness?

1. This pattern has been seen across cultures and eras and, in combination with the reports offered in Forman (1990), suggests that these phenomena are not an artifact of any one culture but are closer to experiences that are reasonably common and available in a variety of cultural contexts.[13]

2. Thomas Clark and other recent theoreticians of consciousness have suggested that consciousness is *identical to* certain of our information-bearing, behavior-controlling functions; he even defines consciousness in these terms (Clark 1995). Others have suggested that consciousness is an artifact or an epiphenomenon of perception, action, and thought and that it arises *only* as a concomitant of these phenomena. Bruce Buchanan suggests, for example, that "consciousness is inherently evaluative and that's what it does. According to this view, unintentional consciousness would not be possible" (Buchanan 1996). Our accounts tend to disconfirm this view. Rather, they suggest that consciousness *can* persist even when one has *no* perception, thought, or evaluation. This suggests that consciousness should not be defined as merely an epiphenomenon of perception or perceptual functions, but as something that can exist *independently* of these functions.

3. Some have suggested that if we can understand how we can tie together perceptions and thoughts—the so-called binding problem—we will, ipso facto, understand consciousness.[14] How we bind together perceptions is a very interesting question for cognitive psychology, neurobiology, and philosophy of mind. But even if we understand how we tie together perceptions, we will not necessarily understand the phenomenon of consciousness because, according to the mystical accounts, consciousness is more fundamental than a mere binding function. These reports suggest that binding is something done *by* or *for* consciousness, not something that creates consciousness.[15]

4. Our evidence suggests that we should conceptually and linguistically differentiate merely being aware or awake from functional activities. If so, I

propose distinguishing between awareness itself and consciousness. Let us reserve the term *consciousness* for the feature of experience that is cognizant when we are *intentionally* aware of something and the term *awareness* for the facet of consciousness that is aware within itself and may persist even without intentional content. This distinction is in accord with Deikman's (1996) separation of awareness from the other senses of "I", and with Chalmers's (1995) distinction.[16]

5. Reports of pure awareness suggest that, despite the absence of mental content, these people were somehow aware *that* they remained aware throughout the period of the PCE. Apparently, they sensed a continuity of consciousness through past and present. If they did, even though there was no content, they must have somehow directly recalled that they had been aware despite the absence of remembered content. This implies that human awareness has the ability to tie itself together and to know intuitively that it has persisted.[17] Being conscious seems to entail this sort of direct self-recollection, a presence to oneself that is distinct from the kind of presence we have to perceptions and other intentional content. In this sense, the PCE tends to affirm Bernard Lonergan's distinction (McCarthy 1990) between our conscious presence to intentional objects and our consciousness of consciousness itself:

There is the presence of the object to the subject, of the spectacle to the spectator; there is also the presence of the subject to himself, and this is not the presence of another object dividing his attention, of another spectacle distracting the spectator; it is presence in, as it were, another dimension, presence concomitant and correlative and opposite to the presence of the object. Objects are present by being attended to but subjects are present as subjects, not by being attended to, but by attending. As the parade of objects marches by, spectators do not have to slip into the parade to be present to themselves; they have to be present to themselves for anything to be present to them.

The Dualistic Mystical State: The Peculiar Oceanic Feeling

The second mystical phenomenon bears a dualistic pattern. One report comes from the autobiography of a living American mystic, Bernadette Roberts (1984), a middle-aged former nun who became a mother, housewife, and author of *The Experience of No-Self*. Roberts had been in the practice of meditating in a nearby monastery, she tells us, and had often had the experience of complete silence described earlier. Previously, such experiences had sparked fear in her, a fear perhaps of never returning. But on one particular afternoon, as her meditation was ending

... once again there was a pervasive silence and once again I waited for the onset of fear to break it up. But this time the fear never came.... Within, all was still, silent and motionless. In the stillness, I was not aware of the moment when the fear and tension of waiting had left. Still I continued to wait for a movement not of myself and when no movement came, I simply remained in a great stillness.... Once outside, I fully expected to return to my ordinary energies and thinking mind, but this day I had a difficult time because I was continually falling back into the great silence. (p. 20)

Roberts became silent inside but, to her surprise, did not emerge from that silence. She stood up and walked out of her chapel, "like a feather floats in the wind," while her silence continued unabated. Not a temporary meditative experience, this was a permanent development of that quiet empty interior silence.[18] She "remained in a great stillness," as she drove down the road, talked on the phone, and cut carrots for dinner. In fact, the sense of a silent interiors was never again to leave her.

Roberts experienced her interior silence as her original "consciousness," by which she meant that she experienced it as devoid of the intellectual self-reflection that generally accompanies experiences. She describes this new state as a continuation of what she had encountered when she was in her meditative silence (PCE), only here she remained fully cognizant of her own silent awareness even while active.

A similar autobiographical report from the Neo-Advaitan practitioner cited earlier clearly associates a permanent interior silence with consciousness:

This happened in 1972. I had been practicing meditation for about 3 years, and had been on a meditation retreat for $3\frac{1}{2}$ months. Over several days something like a series of tubes running down the back of my neck became, one by one, dead quiet. This transformation started on the left side and moved to the right. As each one became silent, all the noise and activity inside these little tubes just ceased. There was a kind of a click or a sort of "zipping" sensation, as the nerve cells or whatever it was became quiet.[19] It was as if there had always been this very faint and unnoticed activity, a background of static so constant that I had never before noticed it. When each of these tubes became silent, all that noise just ceased entirely. I only recognized the interior noise or activity in these tubes in comparison to the silence that now descended. One by one these tubes became quiet, from left to right. It took a few days, maybe a week. Finally the last one on the right went *zip*, and that was it. It was over.

After the last tube had shifted to this new state, I discovered that a major though subtle shift had occurred. From that moment forward, I was silent inside. I don't mean I didn't think, but rather that the feeling inside of me was as if I was entirely empty, a perfect vacuum.[20] Since that time all of my thinking, my sensations, my emotions, etc., have seemed not quite connected to me inside. It was and is as if what was *me*, my consciousness itself, was now this emptiness. The *silence* was now me, and the thoughts that go on inside have not felt quite in contact with what is really "me," this empty awareness. "I" was now silent inside. My thinking has been as if on the outside of this silence without quite contacting it: When I see, feel or hear something, that perception or thought has been seen by this silent consciousness, but it is not quite connected to this interior silence.[21]

In this account, the silence is explicitly associated with awareness. The silence is experienced as "the I," "what was really me," "my consciousness itself." Somehow the area in the back of the head seems to be associated with being aware; as it became silent, the subject seemed to have a more articulated sense of the self within and experienced the self as silent. Like Roberts's experience, the shift to an interior silence was permanent.[22] Thus, we should call it a state, not a transient experience. I call it DMS.

This sort of experience is surprisingly common in the mystical literature. Teresa of Avila (1961) wrote of such a dualistic state. Speaking of herself in the third person:

However numerous were her trials and business worries, the essential part of her soul seemed never to move from [its] dwelling place. So in a sense she felt that her soul was divided ... Sometimes she would say that it was doing nothing but enjoy[ing] itself in that quietness, while she herself was left with all her trials and occupations so that she could not keep it company. (p. 211)

Thus, St. Teresa also described an experience in which, even while working and living, one maintains a clear sense of interior awareness, a persisting sense of an unmoving silence at one's core.

Meister Eckhart (Clark and Skinner 1958) described something similar and called it the "birth of the Word in the soul." One of Eckhart's clearest descriptions is from the treatise *On Detachment*, which analogized the two aspects of man with a door and its hinge pin. Like the outward boards of a door, the outward man moves, changes, and acts. The inward man, like the hinge pin, does not move. He—or it—remains uninvolved with activity and does not change at all. Eckhart concluded that this is the way one should really conduct a life—one should act yet remain inwardly uninvolved. Here is the passage:

And however much our Lady lamented and whatever other things she said, she was always in her inmost heart in immovable detachment. Let us take an analogy of this. A door opens and shuts on a hinge. Now if I compare the outer boards of the door with the outward man, I can compare the hinge with the inward man. When the door opens or closes the outer boards move to and fro, but the hinge remains immovable in one place and it is not changed at all as a result. So it is also here. (p. 167)

A hinge pin moves on the outside and remains unmoving at its center. To act and yet remain "in her inmost heart in immovable detachment" depicts precisely this dualistic life. One acts, yet at an unchanging level within is a sense of something unmoving. One lives a dichotomous existence. Inside, one experiences an interior silence, outside one acts. Eckhart described this experience:

When the detached heart has the highest aim, it must be towards the Nothing, because in this there is the greatest receptivity. Take a parable from nature: if I want to write on a wax tablet, then no matter how noble the thing is that is written on the tablet, I am none the less vexed because I cannot write on it. If I really want to write I must delete everything that is written on the tablet, and the tablet is never so suitable for writing as when absolutely nothing is written on it. (p. 168)

The emphasis in this passage is on the achievement of emptiness within. One has "deleted" everything inside; one comes to a "Nothing" inside; the tablet is "blank." When one is truly empty within, comes to "the Nothing," what goes on outside is of lesser significance. Only after the interior "Nothing" is established does one truly begin acting rightly. This is highly reminiscent of the empty interior silence achieved by other reporters.

In sum, this mystical phenomenon, the DMS, is marked by its dualism. The mystic has a sense, on a permanent or semipermanent basis, of being in touch with his or her own deepest awareness experienced as a silence at one's core, even while remaining conscious of the external sensate world. Awareness itself is experienced as silent and as separate from its intentional content.

This dualistic mystical state seems to evolve gradually into another state. Our Neo-Advaitan continues:[23]

Over the years, this interior silence has slowly changed. Gradually, imperceptibly, this sense of who I am, this silence inside, has grown as if quasiphysically larger. In the beginning it just seemed like I was silent inside. Then this sense of quietness has, as it were, *expanded* to permeate my whole body. Some years later, it came to seem no longer even limited to my own body, but even wider, larger than my body. It's such a peculiar thing to describe! It's as if who I am, my very consciousness itself, has become bigger, wider, less localized. By now it's as if I extend some distance beyond my body, as if I'm many feet wide. What is *me* is now this expanse, this silence that spreads out.

Although retaining something of the dualistic character, the subject's sense of the self or awareness itself seems to have become as if quasiphysically expanded, extending beyond the sensed borders of his usual physical frame. Freud called this a "peculiar oceanic feeling," which seems to communicate both the ineffability and the expanded quality of this perception.[24]

Being in the middle of an expanse is reminiscent of the well-known passage from Walt Whitman (James 1983). As if having a conversation with his soul, Whitman recalls,

I mind how once we lay, such a transparent summer
    morning,
Swiftly arose and *spread around me* the peace and
knowledge that pass all the
argument of the earth. (p. 396)

The sense seems to be that what one is, one's awareness itself, is experienced as oceanic, unbounded, expanded beyond the limits of the self. Here, I believe, a theist might plausibly associate the silence that seems to be both inside yet quasiphysically expansive in terms of God. If this is true, then St. Teresa's (1961) "Spiritual Marriage" is very much like this experience. In it, one is permanently "married" to the Lord,

... the Lord appears in the centre of the soul ... He has been pleased to unite Himself with His creature in such a way that they have become like two who cannot be separated from one another: even so He will not separate Himself from her. [In other words, this sense of union is permanent.] The soul remains all the time in [its] centre with its God.... When we empty ourselves of all that is creature and rid ourselves of it for the love of God, that same Lord will fill our souls with Himself. (pp. 213–216)

To be permanently filled within the soul with the Lord may be phenomenologically described as experiencing a sense of a silent but omnipresent
(i.e., expansive), "something" at one's core. If so, this experience becomes
remarkably like the descriptions of other experiences of expansiveness at
one's core.

The sense of an interiority that is also an expanse is reconfirmed by
St. Teresa's disciple, St. John of the Cross, who says,

the soul then feels as if placed in a *vast* and profound solitude, to which no
created thing has access, in an *immense* and *boundless* desert. (p. 123)

In sum, the interior silence at one's core sometimes comes to be experienced as expanded, as if being quasiphysically larger or more spacious than
one's body. What might this DMS be able to teach us? It offers several suggestions about consciousness.

1. Human capacity may include more epistemological modalities than is generally imagined. It is clear from these reports that one can be self-reflexively
cognizant of one's own awareness more immediately than usual. Mystics
apparently have the ability to become aware of their own awareness per se
on a permanent or semipermanent basis. This is not like taking on a new
awareness. None of our sources describes this experience as a sense of
becoming a different person, or of a discontinuity with what the person had
been; St. Teresa's descriptions seem to be that of becoming more *immediately*
cognizant of the awareness she had always enjoyed.

2. We suggested above that consciousness should not be defined in terms of
perceptions, content, or its other functions because awareness can continue
even when perceptions do not. Here awareness is not only not implicated
with thoughts and perceptions but is experienced as entirely different in
quality or character—unchanging, without intrinsic form—than is its content. It is different in quality and unconnected with all intentional content.
Even thoughts do "not quite contact it." Awareness itself is experienced as
still or silent, perceptions as active and changing. Instead of defining awareness in terms of its content, these reports suggest that we should think about
awareness and its mental and sensory functions as two independent phenomena that somehow interact, which tends to militate for a dualistic
approach to consciousness such as Popper and Eccles's "interactionism" or
John Beloff's (1994) "radical dualism."

3. The sense of being expanded beyond one's own body, what Freud called
"the peculiar oceanic feeling," is a very peculiar sense indeed. Yet, if we take
these widespread reports seriously, as I think every open-minded thinker
should, what do they suggest?

The experience, simply put, suggests that consciousness may be not limited
to the body. Consciousness is encountered as something more like a field
than like a localized point, a field that transcends the body and yet somehow
interacts with it.[25]

This mystical phenomenon tends to confirm William James's hypothesis in his monumental *Principles of Psychology* that awareness is like a field. This thought was picked up by Peter Fenwick and Cris Clarke in the Mind and Brain Symposium in 1994—the mind may be nonlocalized, like a field; experience arises from some sort of interplay between nonlocalized awareness and the localized brain. This idea is also seen in Pockett's (forthcoming) suggestion that awareness is some sort of field, akin to the four fields of physics and to Benjamin Libet's (1994) hypothesis of a "conscious mental field."[26] It is as if these mystical reporters had an *experience* of that sort of fieldlike, nonlocality of awareness (Freeman 1994).

The heretical suggestion is not that there is a ghost in the machine, but rather that there is a ghost in and *beyond* the machine. It is not a ghost that thinks, but a ghost *for which* there is thinking.

4. This phenomenon also tends to disconfirm the theory that consciousness is the product of the materialistic interactions of brain cells. The experience of awareness as some sort of field suggests, rather, that awareness may somehow transcend individual brain cells and perhaps the entire brain. This concept suggests a new way to think about the role of the physical body: Brain cells may receive, guide, arbitrate, or canalize an awareness that is somehow transcendental to them. The brain may be more like a receiver or transformer for the field of awareness than like its generator—less like a power plant than like a television receiver.

5. If consciousness is indeed a field, perhaps akin to the four fields of physics, a Pandora's box of basic and potentially revolutionary questions opens. What is that field, and how might it relate to the four established fields of physics? Is it a new field? An addition to the established four? If so, why have physicists not stumbled across it already?[27] Or might it relate to one or several of the other four fields? If so, how? If it is connected with only one field, the obvious question is: Why might this field be subjectively conscious while the others are not?[28] Many more questions are implicit in this tantalizing suggestion. To these questions we have no answers. But just because this concept generates unanswered questions, its suggestions are not necessarily false.

The Unitive Mystical State

Our last commonly reported mystical experience is a sense of becoming unified with external objects. It is nicely described by the German idealist Malwida von Meysenburg (James 1983):

I was alone upon the seashore ... I felt that I ... return[ed] from the solitude of individuation into the consciousness of unity with all that is, [that I knelt] down as one that passes away, and [rose] up as one imperishable. Earth, heaven, and sea *resounded as in one vast world* encircling harmony.... I *felt myself one* with them (p. 395, emphasis mine).

The keynote of Malwida's experience is that she sensed in some sort of immediate or intuitive manner that she was connected with the things of the world—she was a part of them and they part of her. It is as if the membranes of her experienced self became semipermeable, and she flowed in, with, or perhaps through her environment.

A similar experience is described in Starbuck's nineteenth-century collection of experience reports (quoted in James 1983, p. 394). Here again we see a sense of unity with the things of the world.

... something in myself made me feel *myself a part of something bigger* than I, that was controlling. I *felt myself one with* the grass, the trees, birds, insects, everything in nature. I exulted in the mere fact of existence, of being a part of it all, the drizzling rain, the shadows of the clouds, the tree-trunks and so on.

The author goes on to say that after this experience he constantly sought experiences of the unity between self and object again, but they occurred only periodically, which implies that for him they were temporary phenomena that lasted only a few minutes or hours.

The sense of the unity between self and object, the absence of the usual lines between things, is clearly reminiscent of Plotinus' First Ennead (8:1) (Otto 1930):

He who has allowed the beauty of that world to penetrate his soul goes away no longer a mere observer. For the object perceived and the perceiving soul are *no longer two* things separated from one another, but the perceiving soul has [now] within itself the perceived object.

It is not clear from this passage whether Plotinus is describing a transient or a permanent experience. Some reporters, however, clearly tell us that such an experience can be constant. Though it is often hard to distinguish biography from mythography, Buddhist descriptions of the Buddha's life clearly imply that his Nirvana was a *permanent* change in epistemological structure. The Hindu term for an enlightened one, *jivanmukti* (enlightened in active life), clearly suggests that this experience can be permanent.

But perhaps the most unmistakable assertion that these shifts can be permanent comes from Bernadette Roberts (1984). Sometime after her initial transformation, she had what is clearly a development of her earlier dualistic sense of an expanded consciousness. She wrote:

I was standing on [a] windy hillside looking down over the ocean when a seagull came into view, gliding, dipping, playing with the wind. I watched it as I'd never watched anything before in my life. I almost seemed to be mesmerized; it was as if I was watching myself flying, for there was not the usual division between us. Yet, something more was there than just a lack of separateness, "something" truly beautiful and unknowable. Finally I turned my eyes to the pine-covered hills behind the monastery and still, there was no division, only something "there" that was flowing with and through every vista and particular object of vision.... What I had [originally] taken as a trick of the mind was to become a permanent way of seeing and knowing. (p. 30)

Roberts described the "something there" that flowed with and through everything, including her own self, as a "that into which all separateness dissolves." She concluded with an emphatic assertion: "I was never to revert back to the usual relative way of seeing separateness or individuality." Again we have a state, not a transient episode.

We could multiply these examples endlessly. The UMS, either temporary or permanent, is a very common mystical phenomenon. It is clearly an evolution on the previous sense. First, one continues to sense that one's awareness is fieldlike. Second, we have a recurrence of the previous sense that the self is experienced as larger, expanded beyond the usual boundaries. One feels oneself "a part of something bigger," which is to say, one senses a lack of borders or a commonality between oneself and this "something." Indeed, in Bernadette Roberts's case, her sense of "something there" *followed* and was an evolution of her initial dualistic mystical state. Third, the perceived expansion of the self is experienced as none other than permeating with and through the things of the world. One's boundaries become permeable, connected with the objects of the world. The expanded self seems to be experienced as of the same metaphysical level, of the same "stuff," as the world. What I am *is* the seagull, and what the seagull is, *I* am.

From this phenomenon we may draw several implications about consciousness.

1. The perceived spaciousness of awareness suggests that consciousness is like a field. Unitive experiences reaffirm this implication and suggest that such a field may not only transcend one's bodily limits but somehow may interpenetrate both self and external objects. This is reminiscent of the physical energy fields and the quantum-vacuum field at the basis of matter because these fields are also both immanent within and transcendent to any particular expression—a parallel that Fritjof Capra, Lawrence Domash, and others have pointed out.

2. The perception of unity suggests that the field of awareness may be common to all objects and, however implausibly, to all human beings. This perception suggests that my own consciousness may be somehow connected to a tree, the stars, a drizzle, a blade of grass and to your experience. Thus, these unitive experiences point towards something like de Quincey's suggestion of a panexperiencialism—the experience or some sort of consciousness may be "an ingredient throughout the universe, permeating all levels of being" (de Quincey 1995). This concept opens up more fascinating but peculiar questions: What might the consciousness be of a dog, flower, or even a stone? Or does the claim of a perceived unity merely point to some type of ground of being and not to a consciousness that is in any sense self-reflective like our own consciousness?

3. Not everyone who meditates encounters these sorts of unitive experiences. This suggests that some persons may be genetically or temperamentally predisposed to mystical ability—borrowing from Weber, the "mystically musical."

One might want to object that the awareness these persons have is categorically different from that of other persons, that is, these persons are connected to the world in ontologically deep ways in which the rest of us are not. I find this unconvincing, since every mystic I have read says he or she began as an ordinary (i.e., nonmystical) person and only later realized something about what he or she had "always been." Reports do not suggest that awareness itself is experienced as having changed, but rather that these persons come to sense a state of affairs that had "always" been the case. Whichever explanation we opt for, however, it is clear that there is some ability the mystics have been able to develop—through meditation or whatever—that most of us have not developed.

CONCLUSION

The three modalities of mystical experiences point clearly toward a distinction between awareness per se and the ordinary functional processes of sensation and thought. The modalities suggest that awareness is not a side effect of the material processes of perception or, perhaps, by the brain. Rather, they suggest a dualism between consciousness and the brain. Furthermore, they suggest that awareness may have a nonlocalized, quasispatial character much like a field. Finally, they tend to suggest that this field may be transcendental to any one person or entity much like the energy fields of physics transcend any one atom or quark.

Phenomenology is not science. There can be many ways to explain any experience, mystical or otherwise, and we should explore them. But in the absence of compelling reasons to deny the suggestions of the reports of mystics, we would be wise to seriously examine the direction towards which the finger of mysticism points. If the validity of knowledge in the universities is indeed governed, as we like to claim, by the tests of evidence, openness, and clarity, we should not be too quick to dismiss the baby swimming in the bath water of mysticism.

NOTES

1. This quote was sent to me in a private communication from Roland Fischer.

2. See Section One of Forman (1990).

3. Mangan (1994) suggests this when he says that "mystic encounters ... would seem to manifest an extreme state of consciousness."

4. This piece of James's famous characterization of mysticism (James 1983) states that a defining feature of mysticism is "transiency" (p. 381). My evidence says this is simply wrong.

5. I say "typically" because sometimes one may either skip or not attain a particular stage. Wilber (1980) claims sequence. Barnard (1995), however, disputes this claim of sequence.

6. Cf. Smart (1965), p. 75.

7. Forman (1990) offers a rich compendium of reports of PCE. I have intentionally offered here several reports of this experience that are not included in that compendium.

8. The mystic apparently remains conscious throughout. Teresa does not explicitly say the mystic is not asleep, but I cannot imagine anyone spilling so much ink while merely sleeping or being blacked out or while being in a coma or comalike state.

9. These two are not quite equivalent. Atman, when seen in its fullest, according to the Upanishads and to Advanta Vedanta, merges with Brahman and thus is experienced as including the object or content of perception. Purusha, according to Samkhya philosophy, is more an independent monad. It thus remains forever separate from its content. But both represent the human awareness, however differently understood.

10. See P. Griffiths, Pure consciousness and Indian Buddhism in Forman (1990).

11. See P. Griffiths, in Forman (1990), p. 83.

12. This is an autobiographical report of the author, similar to one in Forman (forthcoming, 1997).

13. See especially Part I of Forman (1990).

14. See Hardcastle (1994). My apologies to Ms. Hardcastle—although throughout her essay she hints at this connection, she does not make the connection as baldly as I have suggested here.

15. Logically, awareness is a necessary but not sufficient condition for binding; binding is neither a necessary nor sufficient condition for awareness.

16. I have reversed Chalmers's terms. Chalmers calls awareness in itself "consciousness" and connects its various functional phenomena with the term "awareness." I believe that my usage is closer to ordinary usage. (My thanks to Jonathan Shear for pointing out this difference.)

17. Here language fails us. The awareness is not in any sense conscious *of* the passage of time; rather, I am suggesting that awareness ties itself together through what an external observer would note as the passage of time.

18. William James's belief that mysticism is "transient" (i.e., short-lived) clearly does not capture Bernadette Roberts's experience or many of the experiences documented here.

19. Here I am struck by the parallel with the rapid shifting of a physical system as it becomes coherent. Disorganized light "shifts" or "zips" into laser light nearly instantaneously.

20. I think of the parallel between this sense and Bernadette Roberts's sense of having lost the usual "unlocalized sense of herself."

21. Cf. Forman (forthcoming, 1997).

22. It is my impression that awareness of the specific locations within the body is not essential to this transformation.

23. Cf. Forman (forthcoming, 1997).

24. Freud was employing a phrase from his correspondence with Romain Rolland. See Parsons (forthcoming, 1998).

25. Of course, that implies that one has some sort of nonsensory sense—the ability to sense one's own expansive presence even though there are no visible mechanisms of sensation. But is that so strange? If we can sense our own awareness directly in the PCE, why should we not be able to sense something of its nonlimited character in a more permanent way?

26. See also Libet's talk "Solutions to the Hard Problem of Consciousness," delivered at Toward a Science of Consciousness, 1996.

27. Perhaps they have, in the well-known and little-understood interaction of consciousness with fine particles.

28. For the substance of this paragraph, I am indebted to a private communication from Jonathan Shear. He notes that Fritjof Capra and Laurence Domash long ago pointed out this parallel.

REFERENCES

Barnard, W. 1995. Response to Wilber. Unpublished paper delivered to the Mysticism Group of the American Academy of Religion.

Beloff, J. 1994. Minds and machines: A radical dualist perspective. *Journal of Consciousness Studies* 1:35.

Buchanan, B. March 9, 1996. *Journal of Consciousness Studies* online dialog.

Chalmers, D. 1995. Facing up to the problem of consciousness. *Journal of Consciousness Studies* 2:200–219.

Clark, T. W. 1995. Function and phenomenology: Closing the explanatory gap. *Journal of Consciousness Studies* 2:241.

Clark, J., and T. Skinner. 1958. *Meister Eckhart: Selected Treatises and Sermons*. London: Faber and Faber.

Deikman, A. 1996. The I of awareness. *Journal of Consciousness Studies* 3:350–356.

de Quincey, C. 1995. Consciousness all the way down? An analysis of McGinn's "Critique of Panexperientialism." *Journal of Consciousness Studies* 2:218.

Forman, R. K. C. ed. 1990. *The Problem of Pure Consciousness*. New York: Oxford University Press.

Forman, R. K. C. 1997. *Mysticism: Forgetting or Remembering?* Albany: State University of New York Press. (forthcoming).

Freeman, A., 1994. The science of consciousness: Non-locality of mind. *Journal of Consciousness Studies* 1:283–284.

Hardcastle, V. G. 1994. Psychology's binding problem and possible neurobiological solutions. *Journal of Consciousness Studies* 1:66–90.

Hume, R., trans. 1931. Maitri Upanishad 6:19. *The Thirteen Principal Upanishads*. London: Oxford University Press, p. 436.

James, W. 1983. *The Varieties of Religious Experience*. New York: Longmans, Green, 1902. Reprinted, New York: Penguin.

Larson, J. G. 1979. *Classical Samkhya: An Interpretation of Its History and Meaning*. Santa Barbara, CA: Ross/Erikson, p. 77.

Libet, B. 1994. A testable field theory of mind–brain interaction. *Journal of Consciousness Studies* 1:119–126.

Mangan, B. 1994. Language and experience in the cognitive study of mysticism—Commentary on Forman. *Journal of Consciousness Studies* 1:251.

McCarthy, M. H. 1990. *The Crisis in Philosophy*. Albany: State University of New York Press, p. 234.

Otto, R. 1930. *Mysticism East and West*, B. Bracey and R. Payne, trans. New York: Macmillan, p. 67.

Parsons, W. 1998. *The Enigma of the Oceanic Feeling*. New York: Oxford University Press (forthcoming).

Pockett, S. Physics and consciousness. *Journal of Consciousness Studies* (forthcoming).

Roberts, B. 1984. *The Experience of No-Self*. Boulder, CO: Shambala.

Smart, N. 1965. Interpretation and mystical experience. *Religious Studies* 1:75–84.

Teresa of Avila. 1961. *The Interior Castle*, E. A. Peers, trans. New York: Doubleday, p. 211.

Walshe, M. O'C., trans. 1979. *Meister Eckhart: German Sermons and Treatises*, vol. I. London: Watkins, p. 7.

Wilber, K. 1980. *The Atman Project: A Transpersonal View of Human Development*. Wheaton, IL: Theosophical Publishing House.

5 Reductionism Revisited

Alwyn C. Scott

On his more daring days, the reductive materialist claims that dynamics throughout the universe are governed by interactions between the fundamental fields and particles of physics. There is a basic mathematical law (or set of laws)—sometimes called a "theory of everything"—guiding the evolution of the universe and all that moves within it. In the words of Stephen Hawking, these laws embody "the mind of God." Although many practicing scientists disavow such an extreme view, the reductive attitude continues to guide our culture and influence its discourse in diverse and subtle ways. To sort things out, I suggest that we begin by thinking about the nature of reductive theories.

First of all, surely we can agree that the practice of reductive science has many positive aspects. Since reliable knowledge is potentially useful, efforts to understand the relationships between natural phenomena should be encouraged and further successes sincerely applauded. The reductionist program has worked well in several areas of science, for example, mechanics, electromagnetism, and the theory of gravity. That is the reason modern technology is so impressive, and why Andy Weil would check himself into the allopathic jungle of a modern emergency room if he were to be hit by a truck. To be properly motivated, persons searching for order must assume that order exists, because the practice of sound science requires years of dedicated concentration. Nonetheless, the belief that *all* intricate phenomena can be reduced to and explained in terms of more elementary aspects of nature requires examination. Exactly what intricate phenomena? Which simpler aspects? Let us consider three examples.

Isaac Newton showed that the falling of an apple and the coursing of the planets can be explained by the same simple ideas: his famous laws of motion and the equation for universal gravitation. This demonstration had a revolutionary effect on eighteenth-century thought and set the stage for the reductive paradigm to play a leading role in current affairs. But the motions of apples and planets are simple. What of more intricate dynamic systems?

A television set, most would agree, is a fairly intricate object, but it can be analyzed and understood in the language of James Clerk Maxwell's electromagnetic equations and some rather simple relations between electric voltage and current that engineers learn as undergraduates. For this particular gadget and level of fundamental description, the reductive perspective works well. Like a clock and the solar system, a television set is a mechanism. But suppose we tried to reduce the operation of a television set to a description in terms of string theory. The difficulties of such effort would be enormous and, arguably, not worth the effort. Thus, the level of description to which one attempts to reduce a problem is a key consideration in plotting a reductive strategy.

As an example of true intricacy, consider the current turmoil in Bosnia. Surely it would be useful to understand the dynamics of this situation in terms of simpler concepts, but is this possible? When a political scientist and historian as skilled and knowledgeable as George Kennan shakes his head slowly in despair, who would claim that the events of recent years are the mere working out of some cosmic equation, waiting to be discovered? Are not matters of love and hate and good and evil beyond the purview of reductionism? Surely they have little connection with the equations of quantum chemistry.

In considering such examples, one notices a fundamental difference between the education of scientists and that of humanists. As a fledgling physicist, I spent many days studying problems that can be quantified and reduced to simpler descriptions—atomic structure was derived from the properties of electrons, protons, and neutrons; chemistry was related to the atomic elements; and so on. From years of conditioning, we scientists unconsciously tend to believe that all problems can be reduced to simpler formulations, and many philosophers follow our lead. Humanists, on the other hand, often deal with questions that are impossible to quantify and remain enveloped in ambiguities, for example, ethics and esthetics. To humanists, the reductive attitude of traditional science appears both narrow and naive.

From the perspective of modern science, there are two widely discussed problems for which one can ask whether a reductive approach is appropriate. The first is a description of life in terms of genetic codes (genetic reductionism); the second is a description of human consciousness in terms of the switchings on and off of the brain's individual neurons (computer functionalism). Let us briefly consider the validity of the reductionist program in the two areas: life and consciousness.

What is life? This little question is the title of two books, the first of which, by Austrian physicist Erwin Schrödinger, appeared in 1944. At the time, Schrödinger was 57 years old and had completed the great work on quantum theory for which he had been awarded a Nobel Prize in physics. He had also written his famous "cat paper," which denied the applicability of quantum theory in the realms of biology, and had recently become the Founding Director of Dublin's Institute for Advanced Studies. From this position, Schrödinger encouraged his colleagues to turn their atention from linear problems of classic and quantum theory toward the vast domain of nonlinear science, in which the effects of different causes cannot be treated separately because the whole is characteristically more than the sum of its parts. Three decades later, the wisdom of Schrödinger's intuition has been confirmed by revolutionary developments in applied mathematics, the implications of which many scientists and most philosophers are not yet aware.

A year earlier, Schrödinger had realized that measurements of the mutation rates of fruit flies induced by gamma rays implied that corresponding genetic alterations must take place within the volume of a single molecule— a result, he soon learned, that had been anticipated by Max Delbrück in Germany. As a statutory requirement of his position (and because he thoroughly enjoyed it), Schrödinger presented a series of public lectures that first introduced to a general audience the idea of a genetic message written in a molecular code. At the end of the enormously influential book that followed (it sold more than 100,000 copies worldwide), Schrödinger launched the field of molecular biology by asking, "Is life based on the laws of physics?" His widely quoted conclusion was:

From all we have learned about the structure of living matter, we must be prepared to find it working in a manner that cannot be reduced to the ordinary laws of physics. And that is not on the ground that there is any new force directing the behavior of the single atoms within a living organism, or because the laws of chemistry do not apply, but because life at the cellular level is more ornate, more elaborate than anything we have yet attempted in physics.

A second book, *What is Life?*, written recently by Lynn Margulis and Dorion Sagan, attempts, in a tribute to Erwin Schrödinger, to show how intricate the biosphere really is and thereby to "put life back into biology." Steering skillfully between the Scylla of mechanism and the Charybdis of animism, the authors sketch life's development on Earth from the appearance of the first bacterial cells some 3,500 million years ago to the present day. The evolution of life was dominated for two billion years by bacterial cells that casually squirted DNA codes into each other (much as both they and the biotechnologists do today) until the earliest eukaryotic cells appeared, which introduced meiotic sex and programmed death. A mere 570 million years ago the animal kingdom emerged, followed closely by the plants and the fungi.

The myriad species of these five kingdoms interact today in an intricate and robust equilibrium; they maintain the level of Earth's atmospheric oxygen near 21 percent and perhaps also help to regulate Earth's temperature. Although competition for genetic advantage between members of a particular species is an important aspect of this story, there is more to tell. Biologists now agree that a symbiotic merging of bacteria led to the first eukaryotes, with their membrane-bound nuclei and mitochondria keeping track of genetic inheritance and processing energy.

Such is the story of life on Earth. Does the perspective of genetic reductionism suffice to comprehend it? With uncounted feedback loops of implication interwoven throughout many hierarchical levels of dynamic organization (some stabilizing, others self-limiting, and still others leading to happenstance events), where does cause end and effect begin? What can one predict about such an intricate system? How does one begin to understand the phenomenon of life? To what could one reduce it?

But perhaps this example is overly challenging. One might object that it is not necessary to consider the entire biosphere to characterize life. Its essence is embodied in a single organism. Thus, let us consider one humble bacterium. The little guy's DNA code specifies the primary amino acid sequences of hundreds of different protein molecules, and each molecule is an individual dynamic system whose intricate behavior is vital for certain aspects of the bacterium's life. Some proteins act as enzymes to promote cycles of biochemical activity; others mediate the flow of food and waste through the cell membranes, detect light, or induce his flagellum to wiggle appropriately, thereby avoiding danger or searching for food. Interwoven cycles of activity interact at higher levels of organization to regenerate the DNA code or direct energetic activities at lower levels. Again we discover a myriad of closed loops, many spanning several hierarchical levels of cellular organization and tangled in a densely interwoven tapestry of nonlinear dynamics. Amid all this activity, our little bacterium continues to produce himself, a property that Francisco Varela has termed "autopoietic," which is derived from the Greek words for self-maker and poet. We are entitled to a suspicion, at the very least, that proponents of genetic reductionism might miss some essential features of this intricate phenomenon.

Can genetic reductionism explain life? Is everything that transpires in the biosphere encoded in molecules of DNA? Not being trained as a biologist, I do not pretend to know the answer to such questions. Perhaps there is a way to sort out and understand the implications of all the interwoven layers and loops, but it is not obvious. That is my point. The method is *not* obvious. With respect to the phenomenon of life, genetic reductionism currently remains a theory, not a fact of nature. Nonetheless, I would not argue against ongoing efforts by molecular biologists to formulate and solve equations of life.

Along these lines, important progress was made in an interesting book, *The Hypercycle: A Principle of Natural Self-Organization* by Manfred Eigen and Peter Schuster, which appeared in 1979. In the view of these authors, life is organized as cycles within cycles within cycles to form hierarchical hypercycles of nonlinear dynamic activity. Each level of a hypercycle is governed by a set of integrodifferential equations and may interact with any of the other levels. Time and space averages of the dependent variables on the lower levels act as changing parameters on the higher levels, and dependent variables at higher levels act as changing boundary conditions at lower levels. Such descriptions of living systems are often dismissed as mere examples of complex system theory, but this misses the point. The dynamics of life are theoretical terra incognita and extremely difficult to study numerically because each level of the hierarchy evolves at a different rate, thus making the time and space scales of the highest level differ from those of the lowest by many orders of magnitude. Interacting dynamic hierarchies are just now entering the stage as a subject of research in applied mathematics; as yet there is little understanding of their global properties.

David Chalmers tells us that life is easier to understand than is consciousness, but from an evolutionary perspective, the two phenomena may have become deeply intertwined. Few would deny that conscious decisions taken by humans today can influence the character of tomorrow's biosphere, but how far back do such interactions between life and consciousness go?

An answer to this question was proposed by Schrödinger in another book, *Mind and Matter* (which today is published together with *What Is Life?*). Following suggestions by Julian Huxley, Schrödinger sketched ideas that help to dispel some of the gloom related to genetic reductionism. Why is the theory of genetic reductionism gloomy? Because it holds that the phenomena of life can be understood entirely in terms of a mechanistic struggle between DNA codes for survival. According to this view, making choices has no influence in the process of evolution; try as we may, life develops in its preordained way.

The notion that an individual's experiences can alter the genetic code that is passed to its immediate offspring formed the basis for an evolutionary theory proposed by French naturalist Jean Baptiste de Lamark early in the nineteenth century. Although Lamark's ideas mitigate the pessimism of genetic reductionism, the basis of his theory has been thoroughly discredited by modern scientific studies. There is absolutely no evidence that an individual's behavior can directly modify the structure of its own DNA—none whatsoever. Without violating this scientific principle, however, Schrödinger suggested a "feigned Lamarkism" that does permit changes in behavior patterns to alter the course of evolutionary development. How can this be so?

Schrödinger asked his readers to consider a species that is beset by unfavorable factors (several able predators, a harsh environment, no symbiotic arrangements for profit sharing, etc.) that are managed by producing very large numbers of offspring. As one considers the history of life on earth, this is not an unusual situation, merely one in which only a small fraction of the many offspring survive long enough to reproduce. We might say that such a species is ripe for rapid development. How can conscious choice play a role in this evolutionary progress?

If certain members of our stressed species elect a change in behavior that would be aided by a particular genetic mutation—for example, by changing their habitat by moving from the ocean to land or by climbing into trees to avoid ground-based predators—their descendants who subsequently experience supporting mutations are better off and more likely to select the new behavior. This is a quintessential example of a nonlinear process: the whole is more than the sum of its parts, and the ultimate outcome is difficult if not impossible to predict from its initial conditions. A change in behavior favors chance mutations that reinforce the original change in behavior, which greatly increases the survival chances of the mutation in their offspring. In Schrödinger's words:

> The most important point is to see that a new character, or modification of a character, acquired by variation, may easily arouse the organism in relation to its environment to an activity that tends to increase the usefulness of that

character and hence the "grip" of selection on it. By possessing the new or changed character, the individual may be caused to change its environment—either by actually transforming it or by migration—or it may be caused to change its behavior towards its environment, all of this in a fashion so as strongly to reinforce the usefulness of the new character and thus to speed up its further selective improvement in the same direction.

If one accepts the possibility that such nonlinear interactions between chance mutations and elective behaviors can significantly influence the course of life's history, the evolutionary role of consciousness becomes particularly important. Introduction of the ability to choose between different behaviors becomes a catalytic factor in development, and the rates of change in subsequent variations increase by orders of magnitude. In this manner, Schrödinger's feigned Lamarkism makes the evolutionary landscape appear less bleak. Margulis and Sagan wrote:

If we grant our ancestors even a tiny fraction of the free will, consciousness, and culture we humans experience, the increase in complexity on Earth over the last several thousand million years becomes easier to explain: life is the product not only of blind physical forces but also of selection in the sense that organisms choose. All autopoietic beings have two lives, as the country song goes, the life we are given and the life we make.

What, then, of computer functionalism? Many suggest that this perspective fails to capture essential aspects of our subjective experiences. Because this is not a new thought, why do some of us find it so surprising and disturbing? Is it not because we were born and raised in a culture that is dominated by the assumptions of reductive science? But computer functionalism is a mere theory of the mind, and our experiences of qualia and free will are widely observed facts of nature. What are we to believe—our own perceptions or a belief handed to us by tradition?

Upon consideration of the brain's many interacting levels of dynamic activity between the proteins of an active nerve membrane and the configurations of a human culture, I conclude that mere studies of the switchings on and off of the brain's individual neurons are not sufficient to describe the bewildering spectrum of phenomena displayed by human life. To remain relevant, computer functionalism must somehow be augmented to accommodate the evident facts of psychic reality. Although such modifications are unnecessary to describe the inanimate world, they may be needed for studies of life, and they seem surely to be required for an adequate understanding of human consciousness. How might we enlarge the reductive paradigm? How are we to sort out the many claims and counterclaims?

As we continue our investigations into the nature of consciousness, let us try to be less academically territorial and more open to unfamiliar morsels from the rich broth of ideas in which we are all swimming. We are making progress in this direction, but more effort is needed. Let us learn to listen to each other and learn from each other, for none of us carries the whole truth in his or her pocket, and, as we have learned from Lynn Margulis, the evolution of life has often made effective uses of symbiosis.

Instead of emphasizing the differences between our respective views, let us join hands in a search for areas of agreement. In this way, we may find our discussions evolving away from doctrinaire reductionism or dualism toward a collective understanding of consciousness as an interacting spectrum of phenomena that transcends the perspectives of traditional professional boundaries. It may reach from the biochemistry of protein molecules through the algorithmic jungle of neural network theory and the laboratories of experimental psychology to the configurations of culture and the ecstatic mysteries of the human spirit.

Is this too much to ask? Perhaps, but in my view it is no less than the task that lies before us.

II Ontology, the Hard Problem of Experience, Free Will, and Agency

OVERVIEW

David J. Chalmers

Foundational questions about consciousness fall into many classes, typified by the following four examples. There is the *conceptual* question: What do we mean by "consciousness"? There is the *epistemological* question: How can we come to know about consciousness? There is the *explanatory* question: How can we explain consciousness? And there is the *ontological* question: What is consciousness?

In addressing the conceptual question, philosophers and others have distinguished many different senses of the term consciousness. Block (1995) distinguishes "access consciousness" from "phenomenal consciousness." Chalmers (1995) distinguishes "awareness" from "experience." Nelkin (1993) distinguishes "phenomenality," "intentionality," and "introspectability." Tye (1996) distinguishes "higher-order," "discriminatory," "responsive," and "phenomenal" consciousness. The distinctions can be made in many different ways, but there is widespread agreement that the hardest questions about consciousness concern *phenomenal consciousness*, or *subjective experience*. It is with consciousness in this sense that most of the chapters in Part II are concerned.

The epistemological question about consciousness is discussed in the chapters in Part I. Many hold that our knowledge of consciousness is importantly different from knowledge in other domains. For example, where knowledge of the physical world is intersubjective, knowledge of phenomenal consciousness seems to be more purely subjective. Some of the most important data are gathered through first-person experience, and one person's experience is not straightforwardly accessible by someone else. Thus, in Part I, the chapters that attempt to establish a methodology for the rigorous study of consciousness have a particularly crucial role. Basic epistemological questions about neurobiological research on consciousness are also addressed in chapters by Block and Chalmers elsewhere in this book.

Most chapters in Part II deal with the explanatory and ontological questions. These questions are closely related. Once we give a satisfactory explanation of consciousness, we will presumably have a good idea of what consciousness is. But there is little agreement about what constitutes an appropriate explanation of consciousness and about the true nature of consciousness. Perhaps the most central area of disagreement concerns whether consciousness can be wholly explained in physical terms and whether consciousness is itself a physical phenomenon.

As noted above, it is widely believed that the hardest questions about consciousness concern phenomenal consciousness, or subjective experience. The problems raised by subjective experience have been discussed by many thinkers, notably Nagel (1974) and Levine (1983) in a paper that introduces the idea of an "explanatory gap." Chalmers (1995) distinguishes between the "easy" problems of explaining how various cognitive and behavioral functions (e.g., discrimination, integration, self-monitoring, verbal report) are performed, and the "hard" problem of explaining why these processes are accompanied by conscious experience. Unlike the easy problems, the hard problem does not appear to be a problem about how functions are performed, which suggests that different methods are needed for its solution.

Michael Lockwood provides a particularly vivid exposition of the explanatory problems associated with conscious experience. He argues that consciousness ("sentience") raises questions that are not dealt with by physical science in its current form and suggests that a solution may lie in a reconception of the nature of matter itself. Once we recognize that physics is as silent about the intrinsic nature of matter as it is about consciousness, we may find room for consciousness within the natural order.

Opposing viewpoints are provided by Daniel Dennett and Patricia Churchland. Dennett suggests that the view that there is a special problem of consciousness stems from embracing a faulty picture of the mind—a view in which perceptual stimuli are "transduced" twice, first into the cognitive system and then into consciousness. Once we rid ourselves of the idea that there is a "center" of consciousness in the brain, Dennett suggests, the problem loses its bite.

Churchland suggests that there may not be a distinction between the easy and hard problems. She suggests that the border between easy and hard phenomena may be fuzzy and that the distinction may arise more from our present ignorance than from any distinction in the phenomena themselves. She also criticizes other theories that she holds to be "nonneural": Searle's proposal that consciousness is an intrinsic property of the brain and Hameroff and Penrose's proposal that consciousness stems from quantum collapses in microtubules. (Hameroff replies in his chapter in this volume; Chalmers (1997) replies in his journal article).

A quite different and often-overlooked explanatory problem associated with consciousness is discussed by Rosenberg. This problem is the *boundary problem*, stemming from the striking fact that consciousness seems to have inherent boundaries at the midlevel of the physical world, but the physical world itself does not appear to have inherent boundaries at the same level. Rosenberg does not offer a definitive answer to this problem, but he discusses a number of interesting routes that we might follow in trying to address it.

One way of dealing with both the hard problem of experience and the boundary problem is to embrace a *panpsychist* ontology, in which experience is found at all levels of the physical world. This sort of view has often been unpopular, but it has been embraced with increasing frequency in recent years. The chapters by Farleigh and by Shepard and Hut explore ideas in this direction. The closely related ideas in these two chapters offer suggestions about how we can deal with consciousness while avoiding the standard options (and problems) of materialism, dualism, and functionalism. Farleigh discusses Whitehead's neglected "event ontology," which sees all events as constituted by "occasions of experience." Hut and Shepard suggest that we ought to turn the hard problem "upside down." They wonder how the physical world can emerge from experience, and they speculate that consciousness may be rooted in a fundamental dimension of nature much as motion is rooted in the dimension of time.

Mangan offers a different suggestion about the ontology of consciousness—that consciousness should be viewed as a "medium" in which information is carried and that questions about consciousness are medium specific (e.g., questions about DNA) and not medium neutral (e.g., questions about computation). The methods of functionalism are best suited for medium-neutral questions; Mangan uses his reasoning to suggest that functionalism provides an inadequate framework for the study of consciousness.

Antireductionists (e.g., Kirk 1974) have sometimes made their case by pointing to the logical possibility of a zombie: a being physically or functionally identical to a normal human, but who has no conscious experience. The hard problem can be expressed as the problem of why we are not zombies, for example. Thomas's paper tries to systematically counter this line of thought by arguing that the notion of a zombie is incoherent. He focuses on the intriguing fact that zombies seem to *say* that they are conscious and maintains that their claims must be interpreted either as lies, as mistakes, as true claims with a different meaning, or as meaningless. Thomas argues that each interpretation leads to disaster and that the best solution is to reject the very concept of a zombie.

Finally, Hodgson's chapter offers a defense of the ontology of "folk psychology." Hodgson argues that standard psychological concepts are indispensable in the law because one can make no sense of the crucial idea of guilt without standard concepts and that the importance of justice and human rights is undermined without these concepts. Hodgson also argues that contemporary scientific results provide no good reason to reject this conceptual scheme; thus it should be embraced and refined.

REFERENCES

Block, N. 1995. On a confusion about the function of consciousness. *Behavioral and Brain Sciences*.

Chalmers, D. J. 1995. Facing up to the problem of consciousness. *Journal of Consciousness Studies* 2(3):200–219.

Chalmers, D. J. 1997. Moving forward on the problem of consciousness. *Journal of Consciousness Studies* 4:3–47.

Levine, J. 1983. Materialism and qualia: The explanatory gap. *Pacific Philosophical Quarterly* 64:354–361.

Nagel, T. 1974. What is it like to be a bat? *Philosophical Review* 4:435–450.

Tye, M. 1996. The burning house. In T. Metzinger, ed, *Conscious Experience*. Paderborn: Ferdinand Schoningh.

6 The Enigma of Sentience

Michael Lockwood

In 1975 the Royal Society for The prevention of Cruelty to Animals (RSPCA) brought a prosecution against an assistant in a fish-and-chip shop who had been observed passing the time between customers by tossing live prawns onto a hotplate, where they writhed piteously before finally expiring. The RSPCA lost the case. But the incident subsequently inspired the inclusion, in the Moral and Political Philosophy paper of the Oxford PPE Final Honors School, of the question, "Is it possible to torture prawns?" When this chapter was first presented as a talk at the Tucson II Conference, I suggested to the audience that, in spite of their combined expertise on the subject of consciousness (probably exceeding that of any group of scholars previously assembled in one place), none of them was in a position to answer this question with any confidence, or even to offer a halfway decent idea as to how one might set about discovering the answer. No one seemed inclined to challenge my contention. That, then, is one measure of the problem which we face.

The terms "consciousness" and "sentience" are ones that I use as synonyms. But in speaking of the enigma of *sentience*, I wish to emphasize that what I have in mind is something very basic or primal—and something which, in all likelihood, is not remotely confined (on this planet) to higher mammals (regardless of whether it extends to prawns). The enigma of sentience, as I understand it, arises with the lowliest organism, which, when you prod it with a stick or toss it onto a hotplate, does not just react, but actually feels something.

It seems probable that sentience—albeit that its first appearance on Earth was presumably the result of a chance mutation—has spread and developed because sentience confers an adaptive advantage on the creatures that possess it. Specifically, I assume that there are some cognitive tasks which, given the operative biological constraints, can either not be performed at all, without sentience, or can be performed more efficiently with sentience. Nevertheless, the tasks whose performance, or efficient performance, was initially facilitated by sentience may have been tasks that it would be sheer child's play to program into any modern computer. Thus, if one succeeded in making a computer do what, in the living world, can be done only in the presence of sentience, it would not in the least follow that the computer, or its program, was *itself* sentient. And this would remain true even when the higher reaches of human intelligence were being successfully simulated. Maybe Mother Nature would not have needed to evolve sentience if she had had etched silicon to work with instead of organic carbon. That consideration seems to place a serious question mark over the much-vaunted Turing test, as a proposed criterion of sentience.

The real enigma of sentience—or of consciousness—is not *why* it evolved, given that it lay within the resources of nature to produce it. What is mysterious is the very fact that producing consciousness *does* lie within nature's repertoire. Absolutely nothing in our current, highly articulated theories of the material world allows for this fact. Great progress has been made in fundamental physics and in our appreciation of how chemistry and biology can be understood, ultimately, in terms of the underlying physical laws. The last few decades, in particular, have seen striking advances in our understanding of how ordered complexity can arise spontaneously in systems maintained (as are living organisms) far from thermodynamic equilibrium. But in this increasingly coherent and satisfying picture, consciousness sticks out like the proverbial sore thumb or like bacon at a bar mitzvah. Like a piece that is left over in the box after you have completed the jigsaw, it simply does not appear to belong.

This is not to deny, of course, that consciousness is a perfectly legitimate subject of empirical investigation in its own right. Indeed scientific study of consciousness has lately made huge strides on a number of fronts—to which the chapters in this volume bear eloquent testimony. One might cite, for example, the fascinating work done by Larry Weiskrantz and others on the phenomenon of blindsight, and its analogues with respect to other sensory modalities and memory (Weiskrantz, Warrington, Sanders, and Marshall 1974; Weiskrantz 1986). Blindsight, roughly speaking, is the ability to make correct visual judgments in the absence of visual experience.[1] Moreover, there has been a veritable breakthrough in relation to the perceptual binding problem with the discovery of synchronous firing among neurons in the visual system responding to what the subject appears to perceive as a single object (Gray, König, Engel, and Singer 1989; Stryker 1989). The establishment of such synchrony may turn out, more generally, to be central to our understanding of attention.

Another crucial advance is the recognition that consciousness is indissolubly bound up with short-term memory (Crick and Koch 1990). (I now have a picture in my mind, which some of the other contributors to this volume may deem questionable, of what happens when I drift off to sleep: my short-term memory span gradually shrinks to a point.)

I have high hopes, in fact, that in the coming decades neuroscience will progressively build up a psychophysical lexicon in which conscious states and processes can be systematically paired off with their neurophysiological correlates. Indeed, it may not be utterly fanciful to suppose that one day, a supercomputer hooked up to a brain scanner may, with unerring accuracy and in minute detail, describe what is going on in the conscious mind of the person whose brain is being scanned. Perhaps such methods will also yield new insights into the minds of nonhuman animals.

But we must ask how far such work can be seen as a steady progress in the direction of understanding what consciousness really *is*, in physical terms, or of *integrating* it into our physical worldview. Imagine having brought to completion the task of correlating conscious states and processes with neurophysiological states and processes as well as the task of understanding how the brain itself works as a physical device. This accomplishment would be rightly hailed as a momentous scientific achievement. But far from constituting a solution to the enigma of sentience, it would serve only to highlight it: to present the problem to the world in its starkest form. Consider, by contrast, the reaction if the attempt to understand, in conventional physical terms, the brain functions associated with sentience, had foundered at some point. Suppose that the project had encountered certain physical anomalies—apparent violations of the established laws of physics—that manifested themselves only when there was independent reason to think that sentience was involved. Such an encounter really *would* have concentrated minds; and the theorists could then have got to work on the idea of consciousness as some sort of force or field, hitherto unknown to science.

Assume however, (as seems to me distinctly more probable), that the project of identifying neurophysiological correlates for conscious processes and making sense of the physicochemical mechanisms involved roars ahead without encountering any such anomalies or unexpected impediments. Then the deep problem remains. We are left wondering why these particular physical events have subjective correlates when the majority of physical events (e.g., the swirl of organic molecules when I stir my tea) presumably do not. What is so special about the physics and chemistry of the brain—a lump of matter possessing (as Turing famously remarked) the consistency of cold porridge?

Here, it would seem, the neuroscientist has nothing useful to say. The psychophysical correlations that have been so laboriously established, present themselves, in the end, as brute facts—utterly incomprehensible in terms of our current understanding of the material world and serving only to mock the unifying ambitions of physical science. Specifically, does it not seem contrary to the very spirit of physics that such a fundamental divide within nature as that between sentient and nonsentient beings should depend, as it apparently does, on certain sorts of organic complexity? Whatever is truly fundamental, in nature, should be capable, one would think, of manifesting itself in very simple situations.[2]

Nor is that all. I also assume that, at this point, we would have come to understand the workings of the brain in physical terms. Presumably we could then, in principle, explain all behavior without ever having to refer to conscious states as such—which seems to leave consciousness in the cold, a causal irrelevance. How, then, could we prevent conscious states from becoming, in this manner, mere epiphenomena? The tempting thing to say is that conscious states have not genuinely been omitted in the physical explanation of our behavior; they are, in reality, just a subset of the neurophysiological states, albeit not described as such—which, indeed, is what I am strongly inclined to believe. (Philosophers call this view the *identity theory*.) But the question is: How can that be? For conscious states are known, from direct introspection, to have a number of features which it seems impossible to accommodate within our current scientific conception of the material world.

First, there are qualia, phenomenal qualities. Science has taught us that Democritus was right, two-and-a-half millennia ago, in denying that the color or the scent of a rose were intrinsic properties of the flower itself. In thinking of the rose in the common-sense way, we are, in effect, illicitly projecting onto external reality features of our own stream of consciousness— features that are merely the causal upshot of a complex chain of events that ultimately leads back to the rose's fine-grained physical structure. But for a would-be materialist, that insight seems only to postpone the problem of accounting for color and scent. If it is a mistake to seek intrinsic color and scent amidst the swarm of subatomic particles of which the rose is constituted, is it not equally a mistake to seek color and scent amidst the swarm of subatomic particles of which our brains are constituted? Where, then, are qualia to find a home? It will not do to suggest that qualia are simply an illusion, for illusoriness is an attribute of one thing considered as a (misleading) representation of something else. What we are talking about here is a feature of the perceptual representation of the rose considered in its own right, not *as* a representation.

A similar problem arises with respect to meaning or "aboutness"—what philosophers call *intentionality*. We are surrounded with things that have meaning, for example, words on paper. Considered in themselves, these are just patches of ink. As such, they are not intrinsically meaningful, but are meaningful only in virtue of the relations in which they stand, directly or indirectly, to things that have gone on in certain conscious minds. But if—as the identity theory claims—these processes are, in their turn, mere physical processes in the brain, should they not, likewise, be regarded as intrinsically meaningless? Ostensibly, yes. But they are patently *not* meaningless. Indeed, were it not that certain processes—our thoughts and so forth—had *intrinsic* meaning, nothing could have the kind of *extrinsic* or conventional meaning that is possessed by words, symbols, pictures, and the like. Consciousness, in short, is where the semantic buck ultimately stops.

I would go further. Consciousness—and here I include the consciousness of lower organisms—seems to me to be inherently suffused with meaning inasmuch as something's figuring in consciousness at all, requires it to be subject to conceptualization, interpretation, or identification, however minimal.

Finally, there is the problem of the unity of consciousness. Within the material world, the unity of a physical object is invariably a matter of degree—whether that be degree of cohesion, of spatial proximity, or of functional integration. But the unity of consciousness—at least, as it strikes us subjectively—seems to be an all-or-nothing affair. As Descartes (1964) in 1642 said in his *Sixth Meditation*:

When I consider the mind—that is, myself, in so far as I am merely a conscious being—I can distinguish no parts within myself; I understand myself to be a single and complete thing.... Nor can the faculties of will, feeling, understanding and so on be called its parts; for it is one and the same mind that wills, feels and understands. On the other hand, I cannot think of any corporeal or extended object without being readily able to divide it in thought. (p. 121)

So impressed was Descartes by this unity that he judged not only every mind to be a distinct thing ("substance") but also the entire material universe to be just a single thing ("substance") rather than a collection of separate ones.

What is the would-be materialist to make of all this? Such is the authority of physics, these days, that the material world is normally considered as the constant in the equation—that to which consciousness needs somehow to be reconciled. A host of philosophical strategies are designed for this purpose: central state materialism with topic neutrality (Smart 1959), functionalism (Putnam 1971), eliminative materialism (Rorty 1970), and Dennett's (1991) heterophenomenological approach, to name but four. I have discussed these strategies at length elsewhere (Lockwood 1989, 1993a, 1993b). They are all, in my view, ultimately futile exercises in intellectual contortionism—motivated by a commendable respect for the physical sciences, but strongly reminiscent of theological exercises such as attempting to steer a middle course between identity and distinctness in regard to the Persons of the Trinity, or to make simultaneous sense of God's omniscience and human free will. I think that we simply have to bite the bullet, at this point, and face the fact that there must be more to matter than meets the physicist's gaze or registers on laboratory instruments.

This is in line with a currently neglected philosophical tradition that casts a critical eye over our pretensions to know the physical world in the first place. The thought, here, is that the whole conceptual edifice that we bring to bear on the external world—from common-sense conceptions, at one end, to the dizzying heights of theoretical physics, at the other—is essentially formal. It is structure without explicit content: a lattice of abstract causal relations between postulated variables, which makes contact with direct experience only at the periphery, where conscious states and events are hypothetically linked into the structure.

The overtly algebraic character of modern physics makes this situation plain. It is clearly impossible to get an illuminating answer to the question of what, for example, the variables in Maxwell's equations *really* stand for. If one grasps the mathematics and uses it to generate predictions about what one will experience in various situations, that is all the understanding one can reasonably hope for.

But, in reality, our common-sense conception of the material world (including our own bodies) is in precisely the same boat. The only reason this is disguised from us is that we flesh out the formal structure in our mind's eye with features drawn from our perceptual and introspective awareness.

This is the projection that I mentioned earlier in connection with the scent and color of the rose; it exemplifies what David Hume (in his *Treatise of Human Nature*) referred to as the mind's "great propensity to spread itself on external objects, and to conjoin with them any internal impressions which they occasion". Consider Wittgenstein's example (*Tractatus Logico-Philosophicus*, 4.014) of the relation between the pattern of marks making up a printed musical score, the motions of a musician playing the music, the pattern of sound waves that results, and, finally, the pattern of undulating grooves on a bakelite disk (or, in contemporary terms, of pits on a compact disk). There is a sense in which these are all embodying the same information; yet, as concrete physical realities, they are utterly disparate. The point is that all we can really know about the nature of the external world on the strength of our conscious perceptions is that it is a *something-or-other* that stands to certain contents of consciousness in a formal relation of isomorphism analogous to the relation of, for instance, the grooves on the disk to the physical motions of the musician.

Do we therefore have no genuine knowledge of the intrinsic character of the physical world? So it might seem. But, according to the line of thought I am now pursuing, we do, in a very limited way, have access to *content* in the material world as opposed merely to abstract causal *structure*, since there is a corner of the physical world that we know, not merely by inference from the deliverances of our five senses, but because we *are* that corner. It is the bit within our skulls, which we know by introspection. In being aware, for example, of the qualia that seemed so troublesome for the materialist, we glimpse the intrinsic nature of what, concretely, realizes the formal structure that a correct physics would attribute to the matter of our brains. In awareness, we are, so to speak, getting an insider's look at our own brain activity.

This idea has appealed to me ever since I first encountered it in the writings of Bertrand Russell (1927); I shall therefore refer to it as *Russellian materialism*. The view antedates Russell, however. Its clearest nineteenth-century exponent was the mathematician William Clifford (1878), who influenced Sir Arthur Eddington (1928), among others. I am personally convinced that any satisfactory materialist resolution of the problem of sentience is going to have to incorporate this idea—or insight, as I prefer to describe it—in some form. But here we encounter a host of problems.

We can start with what the late Wilfrid Sellars (1965) called the *grain problem*: the problem of reconciling the structure and sheer riot of qualitative diversity that we encounter within our own subjective experience with what the physical sciences tell us about the matter that makes up our brains. This problem is nicely expressed by one of the characters in Carl Sagan's novel *Contact* (1985): "Think of what consciousness feels like, what it feels like at this moment. Does that feel like billions of tiny atoms wiggling in place?" (p. 255.)

The grain problem, as I see it, challenges the would-be materialist to find a way of construing conscious states in general, and qualia in particular, both as particular views or perspectives on the brain, and as being embedded in the corresponding brain states as parts or aspects of the latter. As a very rough analogy, think of the different patterns (whorls, concentric circles or ellipses, roughly parallel wavy lines) that are revealed when a block of wood is sawed along various different planes lying at different angles to the surface. Each pattern offers a different perspective on the underlying constitution of the block. But unlike a drawing or a photograph, which is merely a perspectival *depiction* of the object photographed, the pattern of whorls or lines is, from the outset, literally *present* in the block on the relevant cross section.

This analogy may point us in the direction of a subtle fallacy in the argument offered by Sagan's character. It is natural to think that there is—at least from a God's-eye view—a unique, canonical, scientific way of describing things: a form of description that as Plato put it in his *Politicus*, "slices reality at its joints." What more natural candidate, one then thinks, is there than a description in terms of atoms (or better yet, elementary particles)? But that is both to misunderstand how modern physics slices reality and to fail to appreciate that physics typically offers not just a single, "canonical" way of slicing reality, but, as with the block of wood, an infinity of equally valid ways related to each other by symmetry transformations.

The notion of a *physical system* will presumably be unfamiliar to most nonphysicists. But the concept is exceedingly useful, helping to wean us away from the rather restrictive categories of ordinary language description. When we are invited, as Descartes puts it, to "divide in thought" some chunk of reality, our visually driven imagination almost invariably gravitates toward a sort of *spatial* division. But a physicist considering that same chunk of reality thinks in terms of a partitioning of its degrees of freedom: the physically independent ways in which it can change state or store energy. For example, a rigid body able to move freely in space has six degrees of freedom corresponding to the three coordinates required to fix the position of its center of mass and the three angles required to fix its orientation.

One puzzle about the mind, quite aside from the problem of sentience, is that the mind seems to elude ordinary categories. It does not appear to be an object, in any ordinary sense, or a collection of objects. Nor is it merely an attribute of an object (or collection of objects) or a process that it undergoes. If we assume, however, that there is some subset of the brain's (or at least, the body's) vast number of degrees of freedom that are not just causally, but *constitutively* involved in mental processes, there is nothing counterintuitive, from a materialist perspective, in equating the mind with the physical system, presumably a subsystem of the brain, that is defined by the mentality-involving degrees of freedom.

Every physical system has its associated *state space*. This is an abstract space, the dimensionality of which depends on the number of degrees of freedom, and the elements of which—the points or vectors of which it is composed—denote possible states of the system. That there is, in physics,

Michael Lockwood: The Enigma of Sentience

no canonical, or uniquely authoritative, way of describing a physical system, then corresponds to the fact that there is no canonical choice of coordinates for the system's state space.

In quantum mechanics, the state space of a physical system goes by the name *Hilbert space*. We then have different so-called *representations* of a physical system, which correspond, in effect, to different choices of coordinate system for the system's Hilbert space (analogous to different choices of Lorentz frame, in special relativity).

My suggestion, very roughly, is that consciousness at any given time is associated with a specific representation of the relevant subsystem of the brain. To a first approximation, I am suggesting that this representation embodies the distinctive (and from the standpoint of neuroscience, highly unfamiliar) *perspective* from which this brain subsystem views its own states—a perspective, incidentally, in which atoms need not figure explicitly at all. What is presented to consciousness under such a representation is, I insist, a part or aspect of the underlying reality, not merely a depiction of that reality. Compare the way in which, in special relativity, different frames of reference define different ways of slicing space-time into successive simultaneity planes, which are themselves embedded in space-time.

At this point, a degree of technicality is unavoidable (some readers may prefer to pass rather lightly over this and the following paragraph). Representations in quantum mechanics correspond to *complete sets of compatible observables*. In other words, they correspond to sets of simultaneous measurements that an ideal observer could make on the relevant physical system, sets of measurements that yield maximal information about the system— information that could not be enhanced by the performance of any further measurements. For each observable in such a set, there is a range of possible results of measuring that observable known as the observable's *eigenvalues*. Here, I speculatively suggest, qualia may enter the picture.

My proposal is that a quale is the intrinsic reality corresponding to an occupied point within an n-dimensional quality space, points within which are defined by n-tuples of simultaneously realizable eigenvalues[3] of a set of n compatible observables on the relevant subsystem of the brain. More generally, I suggest that, at a given time, the total contents of consciousness should be regarded as the intrinsic reality corresponding to a set of simultaneous eigenvalues of some subset of a complete set of compatible observables, which serves to define the (current) consciousness representation of the relevant subsystem of the brain.

Although I am using the language of quantum mechanics, my proposal is intended to be neutral with regard to the question of whether there is anything distinctively quantum-mechanical about the brain, which would ultimately defeat any attempt to understand it classically. Likewise, I am not intending to prejudice the question of whether, or in what circumstances, the quantum-mechanical wave function collapses (which I discuss at length in Lockwood 1989). I use the language of quantum mechanics because, together with the language of general relativity, it provides the deepest and most scientifically authoritative way of conceptualizing nature. By analogy, it is not only valid, but preferable, for philosophical purposes, to conceptualize the motion of my pencil, after it has rolled off my desk, in terms of geodesics in curved space-time rather than in terms of a Newtonian gravitational force. The fact that classical mechanics is adequate, for all practical purposes, to predict the pencil's trajectory should not blind us to the fact that there is, in reality, no such force.

I may have succeeded in giving a partial solution to the qualia problem, but the proposal gives rise to obvious consequential difficulties: Why are only *some* representations of *some* physical systems associated with consciousness? For it is possible to go through the same formal motions with absolutely any representation of any physical system—for example, the transmission system of my car—and thereby come up with formal counterparts of qualia. Indeed, we can do so, in particular, for the relevant subsystem of the human brain when it is dreamlessly asleep or in coma. Should we, then, postulate the existence of *unsensed* qualia and think of consciousness as a kind of inner illumination that touches some representations of some favored systems, at some times, but not others? Perhaps so. But if we took this course, then this "illumination" would itself be something that the net of physical description had thus far failed to capture; we would appear, in consequence, to be no further forward in integrating consciousness into the physical scheme of things.

What about intrinsic meaning and unity? How might they fit into the picture just sketched? As regards meaning, I do not know. But, crude though it is in many ways, the image of consciousness as a kind of active light playing over an inner arena of qualia (active, in the sense that it can alter what it touches) has, I think, some explanatory advantages. It is tempting to associate meaning with the light itself. All inner sensing becomes, as Wittgenstein would say, sensing *as*. That is, some sort of conceptualization, interpretation, or identification should be thought of as being effectively built in. Something very like this conception (though with gratuitous theological accoutrements) was once standard fare in medieval Western and Islamic philosophy. Nevertheless, it is unclear how one might attempt to posit this plausibly, along Russellian lines, as the content of any structure that one could expect to find in a physical description of the working brain.

Finally, what about the unity of consciousness. One idea that has been going the rounds for some years is that certain sorts of *collective* states, such as arise in quantum mechanics (e.g., superconductivity or laser light) might be candidates for the kind of unity, within the physical world, that is required to ground consciousness, materialistically construed. These collective states exhibit a kind of spatiotemporally extended unity that is without precedent in classical physics; they are a particularly striking manifestation of so-called *quantum holism*. As Penrose (1987) said ten years ago:

Quantum mechanics involves many highly intriguing and mysterious kinds of behavior. Not the least of these are the *quantum correlations* ... which can occur over widely separated distances. It seems to me to be a definite possibility that such things could be playing an operative role over large regions of the brain. Might there be any relation between a "state of awareness" and a highly coherent quantum state in the brain? Is the "oneness" or "globality" that seems to be a feature of consciousness connected with this? It is somewhat tempting to believe so. (p. 274)

More recently Penrose has collaborated with Stuart Hameroff to develop a specific physical model involving microtubules, which might serve to implement this idea. To the best of my knowledge, however, the first person to speculate along these lines was Walker. Since his original article (Walker 1970), there have been a number of similar proposals. Indeed, a glance at the book of abstracts of papers presented to the Tucson II Conference suggests that the application of quantum mechanics to the brain, with the aim of shedding light on consciousness, has now become a major growth industry.

I have long been intrigued by Ian Marshall's (1989) idea of basing a physical model of consciousness on a pumped phonon system in the brain, such as Fröhlich (1968, 1986) suggested might exist within living organisms. Moreover, while I was writing *Mind, Brain and the Quantum* (1989), it occurred to me that if something like Marshall's proposal were viable, the brain might be utilizing quantum coherence for purposes of quantum computation. Anyone who puts forward a physical model of consciousness must have an eye to the adaptive value of what is being suggested. (There's no reason, after all, to think that nature is interested per se in giving us an inner life.) Quantum computation is potentially far more powerful than is classical computation because it can exploit the quantum-mechanical superposition of states to engage in a new kind of parallelism that, unlike its classic counterpart, is not limited by the number of separate processors one is able to string together.

On the other hand, there are severe limitations having to do with the strictures quantum measurement places on what information can subsequently be extracted. When I wrote my book, there were already some examples in the literature (notably, Deutsch 1985) of tasks that could be carried out much faster on a quantum computer than on a classical one. But these examples appeared to be of little practical interest. More recently, however, some far more impressive examples have emerged. Most dramatic is the discovery by Shor (1994) of a quantum-computational algorithm which could in principle enable one to factorize, in a relatively short time, numbers so large that no conceivable conventional computer could do this task in less than the age of the universe. Less spectacular, but probably of greater relevance to the present discussion, is the discovery of algorithms for determining, much faster than could any conventional computer, global properties of certain Boolean functions.[4] Though this sounds rather esoteric, it has a direct application to pattern recognition.

I do not deny the highly speculative character of these reflections. Even if Fröhlich were right in thinking that coherent states can be created and sustained at the high temperature of the brain, is it plausible that, in such an environment, the brain could exercise the fine control that would be required to put these states to worthwhile computational use? Most researchers in the field of quantum computation think not. In addition, would the coherence not have to extend over an implausibly large region of the brain to encompass the neural substrate of all the things that consciousness is capable of simultaneously encompassing?

So it would appear. But in fact this is far from clear. No doubt, as revealed in positron-emission tomography, (PET) large regions of the brain are simultaneously active when we engage in various conscious tasks. But how do we know that the cortical regions that light up in PET scans represent the actual *locus* of conscious activity, as opposed merely to regions whose processing is, inter alia, directed toward providing consciousness, wherever it may actually occur, with appropriate input?

During the conference, Jeffrey Gray and Joseph Bogen[5] invoked a distinction between the *stream* of consciousness and the *contents* of consciousness. Consider, for example (my analogy, not theirs) your television set. If you switch it on with the antenna disconnected and with no input from a video-cassette recorder (VCR), you receive no intelligible pictures or sound, just the characteristic "snow" and an auditory hiss. Content has to be supplied from outside the set. Perhaps consciousness is a bit like this—its contents may to a large degree be generated elsewhere. This is not to suggest that consciousness is merely a passive recipient of content. As you can select channels with the controls on your television set, so consciousness is presumably able, to a considerable extent, to engage in channel selection, and (going now beyond the analogy) is capable of performing exquisitely sophisticated information processing in its own right and of emitting signals that, in addition to controlling actions, help direct external processing. If such an analogy is broadly correct, the actual *locus* of consciousness might not, after all, have to occupy a large area of the brain.

Indeed, this is the line taken by Bogen. On the basis of such anatomical requirements as "widespread afference, widespread efference, direct and robust efference to motor systems, and sensitivity to small lesions," he argues that the best candidates for the anatomical locus of consciousness are the intralaminar nuclei of the thalamus. The idea that quantum coherence could be created and sustained within these small structures, or at least in a substantial part of them at any given time, is presumably going to be an easier case to make out, than that quantum coherence could be sustained over large regions of the cortex.

Although I remain cautiously skeptical about attempts to ground the unity of consciousness in quantum coherence, I am willing to be persuaded. For if something along these lines turns out to be true, it seems to me that—without, in itself, *solving* the mind–body problem—these ideas could be a key element in developing Russellian materialism into a research program that makes genuine inroads into the problem of finding a plausible niche for sentience within the physical world.

NOTES

1. Weiskrantz has recently attempted to locate in the brain visual systems that are active only when the subject has visual experience. He took subjects with matched performance on certain visual discrimination tasks, some associated visual awareness and some unassociated. Using positron-emission tomography to discover which regions of the brain were respectively active in the two cases, he used the familiar "subtraction" technique to determine which regions lit up only in the subjects for whom the discrimination was attended with visual awareness. The results (tantalizingly) were not available at the time of the Tucson conference, but can be found in Weiskrantz's contribution to this volume.

2. A caveat should perhaps be entered at this point. Sentience may be relatively simple in itself but a complex physical arrangement may be required to create, sustain and utilize it. Compare, for example, the complex apparatus required to produce a Bose–Einstein condensate, which in itself admits of a very simple physical description.

3. For the benefit of those who understand these things, I mean eigenvalues associated with *shared eigenstates* of the compatible observables.

4. See Bennett (1993) and references therein.

5. See their contributions to this volume.

REFERENCES

Bennett, C. H. 1993. Certainty from uncertainty. *Nature* 362:694–695.

Clifford, W. K. 1878. On the nature of things-in-themselves. Reprinted (in part) in G. N. A. Vesey, ed. 1964. *Body and Mind*. London: George Allen & Unwin, pp. 165–671.

Crick, F., and C. Koch. 1990. Towards a neurobiological theory of consciousness. *Seminars in the Neurosciences* 2:263–275.

Dennett, D. C. 1991. *Consciousness Explained*. Boston: Little, Brown.

Descartes, R. 1964. Meditations on First Philosophy (1st ed., 1642). In E. Anscombe and P. Geach, trans./eds., *Descartes: Philosophical Writings*. London: Nelson, pp. 59–124.

Deutsch, D. 1985. Quantum theory, the Church-Turing principle and the universal quantum computer. *Proceedings of the Royal Society of London, A.* 400:97–117.

Eddington, A. 1928. *The Nature of the Physical World*. Cambridge: Cambridge University Press.

Fröhlich, H. 1968. Long-range coherence in biological systems. *International Journal of Quantum Chemistry* 2:641–649.

Fröhlich, H. 1986. Coherent excitation in active biological systems. In F. Gutman and H. Keyzer, eds, *Modern Bioelectrochemistry*. New York: Plenum, pp. 241–261.

Gray, C. M., P. König, A. K. Engel, and W. Singer. 1989. Oscillatory responses in cat visual cortex exhibit inter-columnar synchronization which reflects global stimulus properties. *Nature* 338:334–337.

Lockwood, M. 1989. *Mind, Brain and the Quantum: The Compound "I."* Oxford: Blackwell.

Lockwood, M. 1993a. Dennett's mind. *Inquiry* 36:59–72.

Lockwood, M. 1993b. The grain problem. In H. Robinson, ed. *Objections to Physicalism*. Oxford: Clarendon Press, pp. 271–291.

Marshall, I. N. 1989. Consciousness and Bose-Einstein condensates. New Ideas in Psychology. 7:73–83.

Penrose, R. 1987. Minds, machines and mathematics. In C. Blakemore and S. Greenfield, eds. *Mindwaves*. Oxford: Basil Blackwell, pp. 259–276.

Putnam, H. 1971. The nature of mental states. In D. M. Rosenthal, ed., *Materialism and the Mind-Body Problem*. Englewood Cliffs, NJ: Prentice-Hall, pp. 150–161.

Rorty, R. 1970. In defense of eliminative materialism. *Review of Metaphysics* 24:112–121.

Rosenthal, D. M., ed. 1971. Materialism and the Mind-Body Problem. Englewood Cliffs, NJ: Prentice-Hall.

Russell, B. 1927. *The Analysis of Matter*. London: Kegan Paul.

Sagan, C. 1985. *Contact*. New York: Simon & Schuster.

Sellars, W. 1965. The identity approach to the mind-body problem. *Review of Metaphysics* 18: 430–451.

Shor, P. 1994. Algorithms for quantum computation: Discrete logarithms and factoring. In *Proceedings of the 35th Annual Symposium on the Foundations of Computer Science*, Santa Fe, NM, 20–22 November 1994. Los Alamitos, CA: IEEE Computer Society Press, pp. 124–134.

Smart, J. J. C. 1959. Sensations and brain processes, *Philosophical Review* 68:141–156.

Stryker, M. P. 1989. Is grandmother an oscillation? *Nature* 338:297–298.

Walker, E. H. 1970. The nature of consciousness. *Mathematical Biosciences* 7:131–178.

Weiskrantz. L., E. K. Warrington, M. D. Sanders, and J. Marshall. 1974. Visual capacity in the hemianopic field following a restricted occipital ablation. *Brain* 97:709–728.

Weiskrantz, L. 1986. *Blindsight: A Case Study and Implications*. Oxford Psychology Series. Oxford: Oxford University Press.

7   The Myth of Double Transduction

Daniel C. Dennett

Do you remember Woodstock? I now know what it was like to be a cop at Woodstock. Even at Woodstock there were good cops and bad cops and I would like to be remembered as a good cop—one of those who went around saying, "Smoke what you like and have a good time and just try not to hurt anybody; it'll all blow over after a while. It may take 20 years, but go and let a thousand desert flowers bloom." The Tucson Conference was a great opportunity to expose to the bright desert air a great variety of ideas—most of which will turn out to be wrong—but that is the way we make progress on this topic.

My own view is skeptical. All through my youth I considered myself a sort of radical, but now I see that I am actually a sort of conservative. I say we do not need scientific revolutions. We have all the materials we need at hand—ordinary normal science. The same science that can explain immunology and metabolism and volcanoes can explain consciousness. What I am seeing is what we might call the "heartbreak of premature revolution."

Consider the cartoonists' convention of the thought balloon or thought bubble, a fine metaphorical way of referring to somebody's stream of consciousness. It is vivid and maybe even accurate and precise, but it is a metaphor for what is actually going on *somewhere*—I say in the brain, but others may want to locate the activity elsewhere. The problem of consciousness, as I understand it, is this: If a thought balloon is the metaphorical truth, what is the literal truth? What is actually happening for which a thought balloon is such a fine metaphorical representation?

The temptation is to view conscious observation as a very special sort of transduction. Transduction is a good term because it cuts crisply across the artificial and the natural. We have artificial transducers, such as photocells, and natural transducers, such as the rods and cones in the retina. The transducers take information in one medium and, at a boundary surface, transduce it; the same information is sent on in some other physical medium—by turning photons into sound or by turning photons into spikes of electrochemical activity in a neuron's axon. There is a temptation to think that consciousness *is* a very special sort of transduction—the sort that we call observation.

Observation

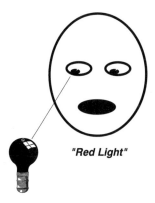

"Red Light"

Figure 7.1 A conscious observer reports awareness of a red light.

Figure 7.1 shows a conscious observer seeing a red light and letting us know that he's seen it by saying "Red light!" Some people think that consciousness is a fundamental division in nature, which divides things that are conscious from things that are unconscious. The things that are conscious (sentient) engage in this very special sort of transduction. Of course, just saying "Red light!" under this condition does not guarantee that a person is conscious. After all, we might have an experimental subject who stands all day saying "Red light, red light, red light, red light." The fact that after someone flashes a red light in the subject's eyes, the subject says "Red light!" is no indication that the subject is conscious of the red light.

The implication is just as dubious if we think about other things that the subject might do. Suppose a person is driving along the highway and a red stoplight appears. The person's foot descends on the brake pedal, but does that response give us evidence of the driver's consciousness? Jeffrey Gray (Chapter 25) talks about this sort of issue in his example of playing tennis. His view is clear: Reacting appropriately to such a stimulus would not show consciousness. We could readily design a simple AI gadget—not even near the cutting edge of AI—that could respond to a bright red stoplight by pressing on the brake pedal of an automobile or respond to a tennis ball in flight by swinging a racket. There certainly would not have to be conscious transduction; there would not have to be *any* special observation going on in such a case. That is the way we are inclined to think about consciousness— that it is a very special sort of transduction. Consider a diagram from Frisby (1979).

Figure 7.2 illustrates one of the ways people convince themselves that there is a special sort of late transduction event occurring in the brain, a transduction event which *is* consciousness. In the figure, light is transduced at the retinas and then (in the medium of neuronal pulses) the information

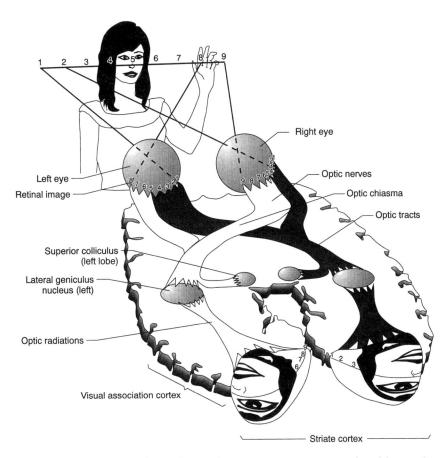

Figure 7.2 Transduction of a visual image from retina to striate cortex. (Adapted from Frisby 1979, by Dave Cantrell.)

works its way back via the lateral geniculate nucleus to the cortex. As Frisby's illustration vividly shows, by the time the information gets back to the occipital cortex, to visual area 1 (V1), the information seems distorted. Somebody who looked at your cortex while you were looking at the woman in the figure would not see the image depicted; nevertheless, the patterns of stimulation on the cortex would be approximately as shown—distorted, inverted, and twisted. A natural reaction is to say, "Well, that's interesting, but that's surely not how it seems to *me* when I look at the woman—so I guess the *seeming to me* must happen at some later point in the process. There must be some place in which *how it seems to me* is restored or put together in some later transduction."

The transduction at the retina, into neuronal pulses, seems to have taken us into an alien medium, not anything we recognize as the intimate medium with which we are familiar. "The activity in V1 is not in the *Me*dium," one might say. "It may be a medium of visual information in my brain, but it's not "moi." It's not the medium in which I experience consciousness." So the idea takes root that if the pattern of activity in V1 looks like *that* (and that is

Daniel C. Dennett: The Myth of Double Transduction

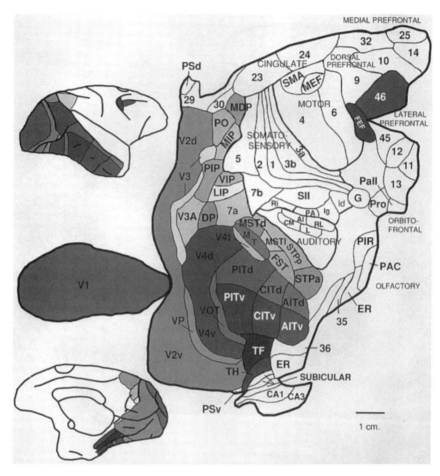

Figure 7.3 Visual areas in the cerebral cortex of the macaque monkey. (Adapted by Dave Cantrell with permission from D. C. van Essen.)

not what consciousness is like), a later, second transduction into the medium that *is* consciousness must occur.

Figure 7.3 is David van Essen's famous color-coded diagram of the visual areas in the brain of the macaque monkey. The big area on the left is V1. Another famous area is the motion-serving area (MT). V4 is where color is the main topic. Other areas deal primarily with shape and location. All the different aspects of vision are parceled out to specialist areas in the brain. Looking at a map like this, one is inclined to wonder whether there is some area on this map (or in some more covert area not yet drawn, deeper in the system) where "it all comes together" for consciousness—the place in which the soundtrack is put together with the color track, which is put together with the shape track, the location track, the motion track, the smell track—everything brought together into a single, multimedia representation: the representation of one's *conscious experience.*

If you are tempted to think that way (and if you are not, I think you are a very rare individual) you are making a fundamental mistake, the mistake I

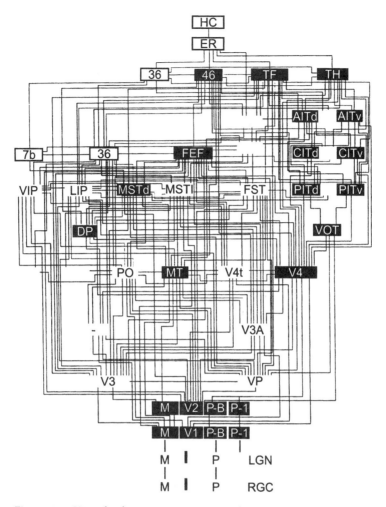

Figure 7.4 Hierarchical connections among visual areas in macaque cerebral cortex. (Adapted by Dave Cantrell with permission from D. C. van Essen.)

call *Cartesian Materialism*. This idea is that there is a second transduction somewhere in the brain (that is why this is a form of materialism). The idea is that a privileged medium exists in the brain where *and when* the consciousness happens, a place in which all the various features of a conscious experience become "bound"—and then, most importantly, are appreciated.

Figure 7.4 is another of van Essen's diagrams. It shows some of the connectivity between the areas in Figure 7.3, but there are no arrowheads on the connecting lines because arrowheads would be redundant—there would have to be arrowheads on both ends of nearly every connecting line. In the illustration at least as many pathways go down to V1 and down to V2 from "higher" regions as come up from the eyes. The very tempting idea that one can move up, up, up from the sense organs at the periphery to "the summit" or in, in, in to "the center" must be abandoned when you get to V1 because there you are already "home"! There is no more central headquarters toward which input moves in the brain.

There might have been. People ask whether my theory is an empirical theory or an a priori theory. It is both. It *might have been* the case that there was a little guy who sat in a little house in the middle of your brain, who looked at many screens, who listened to many speakers, and who pushed many buttons. There *might have been* what I call a "Cartesian Theater" in each of our heads. It is an empirical discovery that there is no such thing. If there were, however, we'd simply have to start our theory all over with the homunculus: What happened inside *his* brain (or whatever occupied that functional role in him)? The empirical side of my theory is quite uncontroversial, though not trivial because empirical researchers often stumble over it: there is no Cartesian Theater in the human brain. The conceptual point of my theory is that at some point, one must get rid of the Cartesian Theater, get rid of the little guy sitting in the control center. As soon as that happens, one must change the assumptions of the theory in a rather dramatic way.

Figure 7.5 is the Cartesian Theater (in an old spoof that first appeared in *Smithsonian* magazine many years ago). We can all laugh at this; we all know this picture is wrong. The tough question is: With what do we replace it? Exactly what is wrong? It is not that the little observers are wearing white coats or that they have arms and legs or that there are two of them. What is wrong is actually much subtler. We know what is wrong, but we have not yet come to grips with all the implications. Here is what is wrong:

The work done by the homunculus in the Cartesian Theater must be distributed in both space and time within the brain.

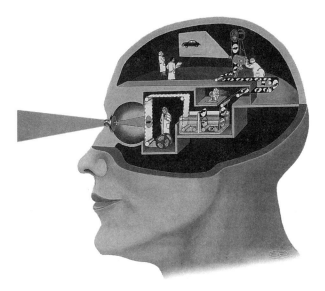

Figure 7.5 The "Cartesian Theater." (Adapted by Dave Cantrell with permission from Sally Bensussen. Originally published in *Smithsonian* 16, no. 1 (April 1985): 97.

Part II: Ontology, the Hard Problem of Experience, Free Will, and Agency

There is widescale agreement on this view. But there is also a lot of back-sliding; understanding this is no easy task.

I want to comment at this point on the word "work." David Chalmers might say:

Yes, the *work* done in the Cartesian Theater—all that *functional* work—that's all distributed around in various parts of the brain just as you insist. Getting clear about all that *work*—those are the Easy Problems. But after we've figured out how all that work is done (and distributed it around in the brain) we won't have touched the interesting, Hard Problem—which is the *play*, the fun, the qualia, the subjective experience itself (which of course we want to distinguish from all that *work*).

However, the work that must be distributed is not just pattern recognition, discrimination, locomotion, and the like. It is also the generation of feelings of disgust or delight; it is the appreciation of the scene. Getting the appropriate emotional reactions is just as much part of the work that has to be distributed within the brain as controlling the stroke of a tennis racket. If we recognize that the work done in the Cartesian Theater has to be distributed in space and time, we have an answer to Jeffrey Gray's problem about the tennis player. It is simply a mistake to suppose that first all the work is done in the brain and later comes the consciousness (ohmigosh, too late to matter!—as if consciousness itself were something that happened too late to control the tennis stroke.)

Consciousness itself is distributed in time, not just in space, and there is no good reason not to say that part of one's *conscious* reaction to the tennis stroke starts within 10, 15, 20, 50, or 100 milliseconds of the arrival of the visual information at your cortex. It is a mistake to suppose that one must wait 100, 200, or 500 milliseconds for a *finished product* to be created in your consciousness, a building process that takes too much time, so much that it will be too late for *you* to do anything about it. We fall into this error if we suppose that there is still a task to be performed in the Cartesian Theater—a task of conscious appreciation and decision in addition to the processes that have already begun to take effect thanks to the distributed activity in the brain.

The task of deciding when and how to hit the tennis ball has to be distributed in time. One should not make the mistake of withholding the honorific of consciousness until all the work is done. (This point has often come up in discussion of Benjamin Libet's results. All his evidence for how long it takes to become conscious of something—what he calls "rising time to consciousness"—could just as well be taken as evidence for what we might call "curing time in memory." There can be only arbitrary grounds for taking some point in that interval of several hundred milliseconds and declaring it to be the onset of consciousness. Consciousness does not *have to have* an onset measurable to the millisecond; it is much better to think of consciousness as distributed in both space and time.

Figure 7.6 is one of Vesalius' wonderful anatomical drawings of the brain. In the middle, marked L, is the pineal gland, the epiphysis. But for the

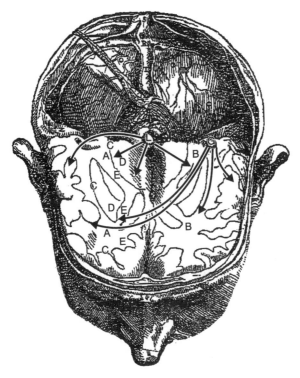

Figure 7.6 Anatomical drawing of the brain. (By Vesalius; adapted by Dave Cantrell.)

moment consider Figure 7.6 a picture of the globe, and let me use it to tell a rather different story—the story of the war of 1812 and the battle of New Orleans. The war officially ended on Christmas Eve, 1814, at Ghent (marked G in Vesalius' diagram!), when the British and American ambassadors signed a treaty. The news that the war was over traveled out from Ghent in all directions, at various rather slow speeds. The news arrived in London in hours or maybe even a day or two after the signing. It took weeks for the news to get across the Atlantic to New Orleans, where, in the meantime, British and American troops fought a battle in which several thousand British troops were killed. The battle was needless in one sense because the war was officially over; the truce had already been signed. But neither army knew that. It may have been even later when the people in Calcutta or Bombay or Moscow or Hong Kong learned about the signing of the truce.

Ask yourself a weird question: When did the British Empire learn about the signing of the truce? You may protest that the British Empire was not the sort of thing that could be said to *learn* anything. But that is not really true. In a certain important sense, the British Empire was a person, a legally responsible agent, a framer and executer of intentional actions, a promise maker, a contract signer. The Battle of New Orleans was a legitimate, intended activity of an arm (almost literally) of the British Empire, fighting under the British flag. It was not some sort of renegade action. The signing of the truce was another official action of the British Empire, executed by one of its proper parts.

Suppose historians could tell us the exact day or hour or minute when every official of the British Empire (every proper part of the Empire, one might say) learned of the signing of the truce. It is hard to imagine that any *further* facts could be relevant to the question of when the British Empire "itself" learned. But then we can readily see that we cannot date the onset of this recognition, the onset of consciousness *by the British Empire*, any more finely than by specifying a period of about 3 weeks. When did the British Empire learn? It learned during the period between Christmas Eve 1814 and several weeks into January, 1815. One might be tempted to disagree, saying that what mattered was when the news reached London (or Whitehall, or the ears of George III) (*L'Empire, c'est moi?*). After all, was not London the headquarters of the Empire? In this instance, that's particularly implausible because when George III learned anything was hardly decisive! (Not so many years ago many of us were going around chanting "What did he know and when did he know it?"—but that was Ronald Reagan, and in that case, too, the question was of merely ceremonial interest. It did not really matter much when either of these "rulers" learned things.)

The point is this: Unless one is prepared to identify some quite specific subregion of the brain as *headquarters*, the place where "moi" is, so that entry into that charmed precinct is what *counts*, one cannot, logically, make precise determinations about *when* consciousness of one item or another happens. (In a discussion of Jeffrey Gray's presentation, a number of questions brought out that his "subicular comparator," although perhaps a very important crossroads in the brain, would have to function by sending out appeals here and there. The system under discussion was not just the hippocampus and the subiculum. It is only in concert with other large and widespread parts of the brain, as Jeffrey eventually acknowledged, that the effects that matter could be produced. It follows from this that one can only arbitrarily point to *any* one stage in this process and say *that* is where the consciousness happens—or more important for present purposes—that is *when* the consciousness happens. (*When* various vehicles of information arrive at the hippocampus is an interesting fact, but it does not settle anything about the timing of consciousness.)

Here is the moral of my story so far:

Since *you* are nothing beyond the various subagencies and processes in your nervous system that compose you, the following question is always a trap: "Exactly when did *I* (as opposed to various parts of my brain) become informed, aware, conscious, of some event?"

It is easy to see reasons why people are tempted by the hypothesis of a second transduction. In some regards, the computer revolution has made this mistake easier. We now have many systems that are *media neutral*. Consider the steering system of a modern ship, in which the helm is attached to the distant rudder not by pulleys and wires or cables or chains but by a couple of little electric wires. Information is all that is carried by these wires—information about the position of the helm and feedback from the rudder. The wires could readily be replaced by any medium that carried the same information (glass fibers, radio waves, etc.). Such familiar examples give us a clear understanding of how one can have information transmission in, essentially, a media-neutral way between the "Boss"—the steerer, the governor, the cyberneticker—and the rudder. As long as the information is preserved, what the medium is does not matter.

However, when we think of information transmission in neurons, mere nerve impulses, it seems, just cannot be the medium of consciousness! It doesn't seem to be enough. Somehow, it seems, we have to put the helmsman back in there. It seems that we have to have a boss or an appreciator, some more central agent to be the audience for all that information. Otherwise, the nervous system seems to be a phone system with no subscribers. There is nobody home to answer the phone. There is a television cable network without any viewers. It certainly seems as if we need to posit an audience somewhere to appreciate all that information—to appreciate it in a second "transduction."

The alternative to this bad idea takes some getting used to. The alternative is the idea that the network *itself*—by virtue of its structure and the powers of transformation that it has, and hence its capacity for controlling the body—could assume all the roles of the inner Boss and thus harbor consciousness. That idea at first seems preposterous to many people. Both David Chalmers and Michael Lockwood remarked in their sessions in Tucson that although they acknowledge that there are people who maintain this view, they think it is simply a nonstarter. That "the subjective point of view" can somehow be captured in the third-person resources of the structure of this functional network strikes them as inconceivable. To me it is not. When people declare to me that they cannot conceive of consciousness as simply the activity of such a functional network, I tell them to try harder.

A common reaction to this suggestion is frank bewilderment, expressed more or less as follows:

OK. Suppose all these strange competitive processes are going on in my brain, and suppose that, as you say, the conscious processes are simply those that win the competitions. How does that make them conscious? What happens next to them that makes it true that *I* know about them? For after all, it is *my* consciousness, as I know it from the first-person point of view, that needs explaining!

That question, I think, betrays a deep confusion; it presupposes that what *you* are is something *else*, some Cartesian *res cogitans* in addition to all the brain-and-body activity. What you are, however, *is* this organization of all the competitive activity between a host of competences that your body has developed. You "automatically" know about these things going on in your body because, if you did not, it would not be your body! The acts and events you can tell us about, and the reasons for them, are yours because you made them—and they made you. What you *are* is that agent whose life you can tell about. For me the "hard problem" is getting people to see that once you have solved the "easy problems," you have solved them all—except for *my* hard problem, which I am continuing to work on as you can see!

REFERENCES

Frisby, J. P. 1979. *Seeing: Illusion, Brain and Mind.* Oxford: Oxford University Press.

8 Brainshy: Nonneural Theories of Conscious Experience

Patricia Smith Churchland

Understanding how the mind/brain works is difficult for many reasons. Some are conceptual or theoretical, some involve unavailability of suitable techniques, and some are rooted in practical difficulties involved in performing needed experiments even given available techniques (e.g. for ethical or financial reasons, or because of the sheer labor or man-hours required). Quite apart from these obstacles, the idea that conscious awareness is not at bottom a neural matter motivates some theorists to call for a nonneural approach. One variation on this theme suggests that consciousness is a fundamental property of the universe based in information (David Chalmers); another sees consciousness as unexplainable in terms of brain properties because it is an "intrinsic" property (John Searle); a third (Roger Penrose) adopts the hypothesis that consciousness is a property arising out of quantum-level phenomena, below the level of neurons. Otherwise discordant, the three share the conviction that understanding the brain will not yield an understanding of consciousness. In exploring each of these possibilities, I conclude that none is sufficiently appealing—empirically, theoretically, or logically—to merit serious research investment. At this stage, I believe the evidence strongly favors neuroscience and psychology as having the best shot at solving the problem.

CHALMERS' APPROACH

Conceptualizing a problem so we can ask the *right* questions and design *revealing experiments* is crucial to discovering a satisfactory solution to the problem.[1] Asking where animal spirits are concocted, for example, turns out not to be the right question to ask about the heart. When Harvey asked, "How much blood does the heart pump in an hour?" he conceptualized the problem of heart function very differently. Reconceptualization was pivotal in coming to understand that the heart is really a pump for circulating blood; there are no animal spirits to concoct. My strategy here, therefore, is to take the label, "The Hard Problem" in a constructive spirit—as an attempt to provide a useful conceptualization concerning the very nature of consciousness that could help steer us in the direction of a solution. My remarks will focus mainly on whether anything positive is to be gained from the "Hard Problem" characterization or whether that conceptualization is counter-productive.

I cannot hope to do full justice to the task in short compass, especially since the contemporary characterization of the problem of consciousness as *the* intractable problem has a rather large literature surrounding it. The watershed articulation of consciousness as "the most difficult problem" is Thomas Nagel's (1974) classic paper. Nagel comes straight to the point: "Consciousness is what makes the mind–body problem really intractable." Delineating a contrast between the problem of consciousness and all other mind–body problems, Nagel asserts: "While an account of the physical basis of mind must explain many things, this [conscious experience] appears to be the most difficult."

Following Nagel's lead, many other philosophers, including Frank Jackson, Saul Kripke, Colin McGinn, John Searle, and most recently, David Chalmers, have extended and developed Nagel's basic idea that consciousness is not tractable neuroscientifically.

Although I agree that consciousness is, certainly, a difficult problem, difficulty per se does not distinguish it from oodles of other neuroscientific problems. Such as how the brains of homeotherms keep a constant internal temperature despite varying external conditions. Such as the brain basis for schizophrenia and autism, and why we dream and sleep. Supposedly, something sets consciousness apart from all other macrofunction brain riddles so that consciousness stands alone as The Hard Problem. As I have tried to probe precisely what that is, I find my reservations multiplying.

Carving Up the Problem Space

The "Hard Problem" label invites us to adopt a principled empirical division between consciousness and problems on the "Easy" (or perhaps hard but not Hard?) side of the ledger. "Easy" presumably encompasses problems such as the nature of short-term memory, long-term memory, autobiographical memory, the nature of representation, the nature of sensory-motor integration, and top-down effects in perception—not to mention such capacities as attention, depth perception, intelligent eye movement, skill acquisition, planning, decision-making, and so forth. On the other side of the ledger, all on its own, stands consciousness—a uniquely Hard Problem.

My lead-off reservation arises from this question: What is the rationale for drawing the division exactly *there*? Might not say, attention, be as hard a problem as awareness? Does dividing consciousness from all the so-called easy problems imply that we could understand those phenomena and still not know … know what? How the "qualia light" goes on? Now that conceptualization is about as insightful as supposing babies are brought by storks.

What exactly is the evidence for the conviction that we could explain all the "Easy" phenomena and still not understand the neural mechanisms for consciousness? The "evidence" derives from a thought experiment, explained roughly as follows: We can conceive of a person like us in all the afore-mentioned, Easy-to-explain capacities (attention, short-term memory etc.), but lacking qualia. This person would be *exactly* like us, save that he would be a zombie—an anaqualiac, one might say. Since the scenario is conceivable supposedly that makes it possible; and if it is possible, then whatever con-sciousness is, it is explanatorily independent of those activities.[2] (Something akin to this was argued by Saul Kripke in the 1970s.)

I take this argument to be a demonstration of the feebleness of thought experiments. *Saying* something is possible does not thereby guarantee it *is* a real possibility. How do we know the anaqualiac idea is really possible? To insist that it *must* be possible is simply to beg the question at issue. That is, it is to insist that the neurobiology for attention, short-term memory, decision making, integration, and so forth could all be understood without our ever understanding consciousness. But that claim is what we want an argument *for*; it cannot be used to prove itself. As Francis Crick has observed, it might be like saying that one can imagine a possible world where gases do not get hot, even though their constituent molecules are moving at high velocity. As an argument against the empirical identification of temperature with mean molecular kinetic energy, the thermodynamic thought experiment is feebleness itself.[3]

Is consciousness—the problem on the Hard side of the ledger—sufficiently well-defined to sustain the Hard–Easy division as a fundamental *empirical* principle? Although it is easy enough to agree about the presence of qualia in certain prototypical cases, such as the pain felt after a brick has fallen on a bare foot or the blueness of the sky on a sunny summer after-noon, things are less clear cut once we move beyond the favored prototypes. Some of our perceptual capacities are rather subtle, as, for example, posi-tional sense is often claimed to be. Some philosophers, such as Elizabeth Anscombe, have actually opined that we can know the position of our limbs without any "limb-position" qualia. As for me, I am inclined to say I do have qualitative experiences of where my limbs are—it feels different to have my fingers clenched than unclenched, even when the fingers are not visible. The disagreement itself, however, betokens the lack of consensus once cases are at some remove from the central prototypes.

Vestibular-system qualia are yet another nonprototypical case. Is there something "vestibular-y" it feels like to have my head moving? To know which way is up? Whatever the answer, at least the answer is not glaringly obvious. Do eye movements have eye-movement qualia? Some maybe do, and some maybe do not. Are there "introspective qualia" or is introspection just paying attention to perceptual qualia and talking to yourself? Ditto for self-awareness. Thoughts are also a bit problematic in the qualia department. Some of my thoughts seem to me to be a bit like talking to myself and, hence, like auditory imagery; others come out of my mouth as I am talking to someone or affect decisions without ever surfacing as a bit of inner dia-logue. Do these cases belong on the "Hard" or the "Easy" side of the ledger?

None of this denies the pizzazz of qualia in the prototypical cases. Rather, the point is that prototypical cases give us only a *starting point* for further investigation, nothing like a full characterization of the class to which they belong.

My suspicion with respect to The Hard-Problem strategy is that it seems to take the class of conscious experiences to be much better defined than it is. The point is, if you are careful to restrict the focus to prototypical cases, you can easily be hornswoggled into assuming the class is well defined. As soon as you broaden the horizons, troublesome questions about fuzzy boundaries and the connections between attention, short-term memory, and awareness are present in full, "what-do-we-do-with-*that*" glory.[4]

Are the Easy Problems *known to be easier* than The Hard Problem? It is important to acknowledge that for none of the so-called "easy" problems, do we have an understanding of their solution. (See the partial list given p. 110.) It is just false that we have anything approximating a comprehensive theory of sensorimotor control or attention or short-term memory or long-term memory. Consider one example. My signature is recognizably mine whether signed with the dominant or nondominant hand, with the foot, with the mouth, with the pen strapped to my shoulder, or written in half-inch script or in 2-ft. graffiti. How is "my signature" represented in the nervous system? How can completely different muscle sets be invoked to do the task, even when the skill was not acquired using those muscles? We still do not understand the general nature of sensorimotor representation.

Notice that it is not merely that we are lacking details, albeit important details. The fact is, we are lacking important conceptual–theoretical ideas about how the nervous system performs fundamental functions such as time management, motor control, learning, or information retrieval. We do not understand how back projections work, or the degree to which processing is organized hierarchically. These are genuine and very deep puzzles, and it is unwise to "molehill" them in order to "mountain" up the problem of consciousness. Although quite a lot is known at the cellular level, how real neural networks work and how their output properties depend on cellular properties still abound with nontrivial mysteries. Naturally I do not wish to minimize the progress that has been made in neuroscience, but it is prudent to have a probative assessment of what we really do not yet understand.

Carving the explanatory space of mind–brain phenomena along the Hard and the Easy line, as Chalmers proposes, poses the danger of inventing an explanatory chasm where there really exists just a broad field of ignorance. It reminds me of the division, deep to medieval physics, between Sublunary physics (motion of things below the level of the moon) and Superlunary physics (motion of things above the level of the moon). The conviction was that sublunary physics is tractable, and is essentially based on Aristotelian physics. Heavy things fall because they have gravity, and they fall to their Natural Place, namely Earth, which, of course, is the center of the universe. Things like smoke have levity, and consequently they rise *up* being their Natural Place. Everything in the sublunary realm has a Natural Place, and that is the key to explaining the behavior of sublunary objects. Superlunary events, by contrast, can neither be explained nor understood—not, at least, in sublunary terms.

This old division was not without merit, and it did entail that events such as planetary motion and meteors were considered unexplainable in terrestrial terms, as those things were Divinely governed. Although I do not know that Chalmers's Easy–Hard distinction will ultimately prove to be as misdirected as the Sublunary–Superlunary distinction, neither do I know it is any more sound. What I do suspect, however, is that it is much too early in the science of nervous systems for this distinction to command much credence.

One danger inherent in embracing the distinction as a principled empirical distinction is that it provokes the intuition that only a real humdinger of a solution will suit The Hard Problem. The idea seems to go as follows: The answer, if it comes at all, is going to have to come from somewhere Really Deep—like quantum mechanics, or—Wow—perhaps it requires a whole new physics. As the lone enigma, consciousness surely cannot be only a matter of a complex dynamical system doing its thing. Yes, there are emergent properties from nervous systems, such as the coordinated movement when an owl catches a mouse, but consciousness must be an emergent property like unto no other. After all, it is "The Hard Problem!" Consequently, it will require a very deep, very radical solution. That much is sheerly evident from the hardness of The Hard Problem.

I confess I cannot actually see that. I do not know anywhere near enough to see how to solve either the problem of sensorimotor control or the problem of consciousness. I certainly cannot see enough to know that one problem does, and the other does not, require a "Humdinger" solution.

Using Ignorance as a Premise

In general, what substantive conclusions can be drawn when science has not advanced very far on a problem? Not much. One of the basic skills we teach philosophy students is how to recognize and diagnose the range of non-formal fallacies that masquerade as kosher arguments: what it is to beg the question, what a non sequitur is, and so on. A prominent item in the fallacy roster is *argumentum ad ignorantiam*—argument from ignorance. The canonical version of this fallacy uses ignorance as the key premise from which a substantive conclusion is drawn. The canonical version looks like this:

We really do not understand much about phenomenon P. (Science is largely ignorant about the nature of P.)

Therefore, we *do* know that:

(1) P can never be explained or
(2) Nothing science could ever discover would deepen our understanding of P or
(3) P can never be explained in terms of scientifically familiar properties of S.

Patricia Smith Churchland: Brainshy: Nonneural Theories of Conscious Experience

In its canonical version, the argument is obviously a fallacy. None of the tendered conclusions follow, not even a *little* bit. Surrounded with rhetorical flourish, brow-furrowing, and hand-wringing, however, versions of this argument can hornswoggle the unwary.

From the fact that we do not know something, nothing very interesting follows—we just do not know. Nevertheless, the temptation to suspect that our ignorance is telling us something positive, something deep, something metaphysical, even radical, is ever present. Perhaps we like to put our ignorance in a positive light by supposing that, but for the "profundity" of the phenomenon, we *would* have knowledge. But there are many reasons for not knowing, and the specialness of the phenomenon is, quite regularly, not the real reason. For instance, I am currently ignorant of what caused an unusual rapping noise in the woods last night. Can I conclude it must be something special, something unimaginable, something ... alien ... otherworldly? Evidently not. For all I can tell now, it might merely have been a raccoon gnawing on the compost bin. Lack of evidence for something is just that: lack of evidence. It is not positive evidence for something else, let alone something of a humdingerish sort. That conclusion is not very glamorous, perhaps, but when ignorance is a premise, that is about all one can grind out of it.

Now if neuroscience had progressed as far on the problems of brain function as molecular biology has progressed on transmission of hereditary traits, we would be in a different position. But it has not. The only thing one can conclude from the fact that attention is mysterious, or that sensorimotor integration is mysterious, or that consciousness is mysterious, is that we do not yet understand the mechanisms.

Moreover, the mysteriousness of a problem is not a fact about the phenomenon; it is not a metaphysical feature of the universe—it is an epistemological fact about *us*. It is about where we are in current science, it is about what we can and cannot understand. It is about what, given the rest of our understanding, we can and cannot imagine. It is not a property of the problem itself.

It is sometimes assumed that there can be a valid inference from "we cannot now explain" to "we can never explain," so long as we have the help of a subsidiary premise, namely, "I cannot *imagine* how we could ever explain ..." But it does not help, and this inference is nothing but an application of argument from ignorance. Adding "I cannot imagine explaining P" merely adds a psychological fact about the speaker, from which again, nothing significant follows about the nature of the phenomenon in question.

Whether we can or cannot imagine a phenomenon being explained in a certain way is a psychological fact about us, not an objective fact about the nature of the phenomenon itself. To repeat, it is an epistemological fact about what, given our current knowledge, we can and cannot understand. It is not a metaphysical fact about the nature of the reality of the universe.

Typical of vitalists generally, my high school biology teacher argued for vitalism thus: "I cannot imagine how you could get living things out of dead molecules—out of bits of proteins, fats, sugars—how could life itself emerge?" He thought it was obvious from the sheer mysteriousness of the matter that it could have no solution in biology or chemistry. He assumed he could tell that it would require a humdinger solution. Typical of lone survivors, a passenger of a crashed plane may say:"I cannot imagine how I alone could have survived the crash when all other passengers died instantly. Therefore, God must have plucked me from the jaws of death."

Given that neuroscience is still very much in its early stages, it is actually not a very interesting fact that someone or other cannot imagine a certain kind of explanation of some brain phenomenon. Aristotle could not imagine how a complex organism could come from a fertilized egg. That, of course, was a fact about Aristotle, not a fact about embryogenesis. Given the early days of science (circa 350 B.C.), it is no surprise that he could not imagine what it took scientists hundreds of years to discover. I cannot imagine how ravens can solve a multistep problem in one trial, or how temporal integration is achieved, or how thermoregulation is managed. But this is a (not very interesting) psychological fact about me. One could, of course, use various rhetorical devices to make it seem like an interesting fact about me, perhaps by emphasizing that it is a really, *really* hard problem. If, however, we are going to be sensible about this, it is clear that my inability to imagine how thermoregulation works is *au fond*, pretty boring.

The "I-cannot-imagine" gambit suffers in another way. Being able to imagine an explanation for P is a highly open-ended and under-specified business. Given the poverty of delimiting conditions of the operation, you can pretty much rig the conclusions to go whichever way your heart desires. Logically, however, that flexibility is the kiss of death.

Suppose someone claims that she *can* imagine the mechanisms for sensorimotor integration in the human brain but *cannot* imagine the mechanisms for consciousness. What exactly does this difference amount to? Can she imagine the former in detail? No, because the details are not known. What is it, precisely, that she can imagine? Suppose she answers that in a very general way she imagines that sensory neurons interact with interneurons that interact with motor neurons, and that via these interactions, sensorimotor integration is achieved. If that is all "being able to imagine" takes, one might as well say one can imagine the mechanisms underlying consciousness. Thus, "The interneurons do it." The point is this: If you want to contrast being *able* to imagine brain mechanisms for attention, short-term memory, planning, and the like, with being *unable* to imagine mechanisms for consciousness, you must do more that say you can imagine neurons doing one but cannot imagine neurons doing the other. Otherwise, you simply beg the question.

To fill out the point, consider several telling examples from the history of science. Before the turn of the twentieth century, people thought that the problem of the precession of the perihelion of Mercury was essentially trivial. The problem was annoying, but ultimately it would sort itself out as more data came in. With the advantage of hindsight, we can see that assessing this as an easy problem was quite wrong—it took the Einsteinian revolution in physics to solve the problem of the precession of the perihelion of Mercury. By contrast, a really hard problem was thought to be the composition of the stars. How could a sample ever be obtained? With the advent of spectral analysis, that problem turned out to be readily solvable. When heated, the elements turn out to have a kind of fingerprint that is easily seen when light emitted from a source is passed through a prism.

Consider now a biological example. Before 1953, many people believed, on rather good grounds actually, that to address the copying problem (transmission of traits from parents to offspring), one would first have to solve the problem of how proteins fold. The former was deemed a much harder problem than the latter, and many scientists believed it was foolhardy to attack the copying problem directly. As we all know now, the basic answer to the copying problem lay in the base pairing of DNA; the copying problem was solved first. Humbling it is to realize that the problem of protein folding (secondary and tertiary) is *still* not solved. *That*, given the lot we now know, does seem to be a hard problem.

These stories reinforce the message of the argument from ignorance: From the vantage point of ignorance, it is often very difficult to tell which problem is harder, which will fall first, what problem will turn out to be more tractable than some other. Consequently, our judgments about relative difficulty or ultimate tractability should be appropriately qualified and tentative. Guesswork has a useful place, but let us distinguish between blind guesswork and educated guesswork and between guesswork and confirmed fact. The philosophical lesson I learned from my biology teacher is that when not much is known about a topic, don't take terribly seriously someone else's heartfelt conviction about what problems are scientifically tractable. Learn the science, do the science, and see what happens.

SEARLE'S APPROACH

Rather different neural-naysayers are John Searle and Roger Penrose. Each has a distinct but articulated mistrust of the prospects for success of the neurobiological project, though neither rejects the value of neuroscience in contributing to our understanding of consciousness. Rather, both believe that a fundamental change in science is needed to do justice to the phenomenon of conscious experience. I shall focus first on Searle's views, and in the next section, on those of Penrose and his collaborator, Stuart Hameroff.

Searle's view is that the brain *causes* conscious states, but that conscious states are *not explainable* in terms of states of the brain. Why not? According to Searle, being aware of the smell of cinnamon, for example, is *ontologically* distinct from any physical state of the brain. His basic point is that consciousness is an intrinsic property. What does this mean? To a first approximation, that it has no hidden structure, no aspects not immediately available to introspection; crudely, it is what it is and not another thing. Taking Searle at his word that he is no dualist, what does "ontological distinctness" mean? Since Searle says that ontology has to do with "what real features exist in the world," what does the brain inexplicability of mental states mean as a matter of ontology?

Here Chalmers might chime in bravely: "It means that conscious experience is a fundamental feature of the universe, along with mass, charge, and spin." Searle does not say precisely that, though he does seem to rub shoulders with it when he suggests that science as it currently exists is not equipped to cope with the ontological distinctness of conscious awareness. Moreover, he seems to suggest that he is indifferent to going the "fundamental-feature-of-reality" route and going the property dualism route, according to which, mental states are nonphysical states of the brain. Searle (1992) says,

Whether we treat the irreducibility from the materialist or the [property] dualist point of view, we are left with a universe that contains an irreducibly subjective physical component as a component of reality. (p. 117)

In this respect then, Chalmers and Searle are like minded.[6]

What is it about mental states that makes them inexplicable in terms of brain states, even though they *are* brain states? Is it that the subjectivity of mental states is owed to the fact that we *know* something about them from the inside by having them? Apparently not, for Searle (1992) emphasizes repeatedly that his point is *ontological*, not *epistemological*; it is ".... not, except derivatively, about how we know about those features" (p. 117).

Searle gets to his radical, irreducible-to-brain-states conclusion on the back of a premise he takes to be obviously true: Although science might find the reality behind the appearance for objective phenomena—fire, light, life, and so forth—in the case of consciousness, the appearance *is* the reality. And if the appearance—seeing blue, feeling pain—is the reality, nothing neuroscience can discover will ever show me anything about the pain that is more real than feeling it. Feeling the pain is all the reality there is to pain.

Searle's premise has an obviously true bit and a probably false bit, and the second slips in under the skirts of the first. What is obviously true is that sensations are real. My pains are quite as real as Searle's. What is troublesome is the idea that all the reality there is to a sensation is available through sheerly having it. How could you possibly know that? I suggest, instead, a rather simple alternative: A sensation of pain is real, but not *everything* about the nature of pain is revealed in introspection—its neural substrate, for example, is not so revealed.

Commonly, science discovers ways of taking us beyond the manifest or superficial properties of some phenomenon. Light is refracted in water—that is observable. Light turns out to be electromagnetic radiation, a property not straightforwardly observable. Does the observable property—refraction—

cease to be real or reputable or in good standing when we discover one of light's unobservable properties? No. If a property seems by common sense to be "structureless," is that a guarantee that it *is* structureless? No.

Perhaps Searle has been led to his "irreducible-property-of-the-brain" idea as a result of his assumption that reductionism implies "go-away-ism." Applying this extreme characterization of reductionism to the case of conscious experience, he is misled in these ways: (1) if we get an explanation of conscious states in neurobiological terms, that means that means we have a reduction; (2) If we have a reduction, conscious states are not to be considered real—they are eliminated; (3) but conscious states *are* real—anyone knows that. Therefore, we cannot explain conscious states neurobiologically.

The undoing of this argument is the falsity of its second premise. Reductions are *explanations*—of macrophenomena in terms of microphenomena. When physics explains, for example, that temperature *is* mean molecular kinetic energy or that electricity *is* movement of electrons, or that light *is* electromagnetic radiation, science does not *thereby* say there is no such thing as temperature, electricity, or light. Just as when we discovered that Kim Philby was in fact the Russian mole, K5, it did not imply that Kim Philby did not exist. It is just that where we thought there were two distinct men, there is in fact just one, conceived in different ways under distinct circumstances.

Eliminative discoveries, such as the explanation of burning in terms of oxygen rather than phlogiston, do imply the nonexistence of phlogiston, but only because oxygen and phlogiston provide mutually *incompatible* explanations. Only *some* scientific developments are eliminativist, however. Whether a theory about some macrophenomenon is smoothly reduced to a microlevel theory, or whether there is a kind of conceptual revolution, depends on the facts of the case. It does not depend on what sounds funny to time-honored intuitions.

The main difference between Searle's (1992) view and my view as articulated in *Neurophilosophy* (1986a), as well as in many articles—concerns whether it is reasonable to try to explain consciousness in neurobiological terms (e.g., Churchland 1983, 1988, 1990, 1994, 1995). I think it is worth trying. Searle does not. If, however, you took Searle's rendition of my view, you would conclude I was a blithering idiot. He repeatedly claims that I hold a "ludicrous and insane view"—to wit, that consciousness is to be eliminated from science, that consciousness does not really exist, that there is no such thing as awareness.[7]

Do I hold this view? Is the Pope Presbyterian? In print and in conversation with Searle, I have consistently argued that, of course, the *phenomenon* is real. I have no inclination whatever to deny the existence of awareness. I do think science may discover some surprising things about it, that scientific discoveries may prompt us to redraw some categorical boundaries, perhaps to introduce some new words and to discover a more insightful vocabulary. Whether that actually happens depends on the nature of the empirical discoveries.

The not-very-subtle distinction Searle ignores is the distinction between reconfiguration of a concept and denial of a phenomenon. I envisage the possibility of lots of conceptual reconfiguration as the brain and behavioral sciences develop. Never have I come even close to denying the reality of my experiences of pain, cold, and so forth. In a reply to critics (1986b), I wrote a section called "Eliminative Materialism: What Gets Eliminated?" in which I said,

Now, to put not too fine a point on it, the world is as it is; theories come and go, and the world keeps on doing whatever it is doing. So theory modification does not entail that the nature of the world is *ipso facto* modified, though our understanding of the nature of the world is modified. So if anyone thought eliminativism means that some part of the *ding an sich*—say, whatever it is that we now think of as "qualia"—is eliminated by a mere tinkering with theory, then with Campbell, I agree he is certainly confused. (p. 247)

This was written four years before the publication of Searle's book.

There may be another badger to be flushed from the woodpile. A few philosophers (I do not know whether this includes Searle) expect that the difference between *my* feeling a pain and *your* feeling a pain would somehow be unreal or nonexistent on the hypothesis that pain is actually a neurobiological state. As supportive illustration, the naysayer imagines a scenario in which the neural reality behind the felt reality of pain was known to be a pattern of activity in neurons. Further in the scenario, it transpires that when I see that pattern right now in your brain, so I too have that pain. The scenario is really silly; ergo, the hypothesis is really silly.

Not so fast. The scenario is silly, but does it follow from the hypothesis in question? Not at all. Suppose the hypothesis is true—pains are physical states of the brain. Then I would expect that *you* will feel a pain only if the appropriate pattern of neuronal activity exists in *your* brain, and *I* will feel it only if the activity exists in *my* brain, and so on. Why ever assume that my seeing your neuronal activity would produce that very pattern of activity in my brain? After all, I can see the pattern of neuronal activity that produces a knee jerk in you, without my own knee jerking.

Subjectivity is a matter of whose brain is in the relevant physical state such that the person feels something or sees something or hears something. As I see it, pain is a real, *physical* state of the brain—felt as painful by the person whose brain is appropriately configured, though detectable as a pattern of activity by a neuroscientist, given a sufficiently powerful non-invasive imaging technique to make it visible.

Adopting Searle's hypothesis that my feeling a pain is either an irreducible state of the universe (unexplainability) or a nonphysical state of the universe (property dualism) is to take a grand leap in the dark. The more sensible course would be to leap only when it is tolerably clear that the data demand it. And the data, so far anyway, do not demand it–they do not even make it moderately tempting. This is not to say Searle's hypothesis is definitely wrong, but only that adopting it is very costly in pragmatic terms, since no one has the slightest, testable idea how to make it fit with what we know about physics, chemistry, evolutionary biology, molecular biology, and the rest of neuroscience.

PENROSE AND HAMEROFF'S APPROACH

Roger Penrose and Stuart Hameroff also harbor reservations about explaining awareness neurobiologically, but they are moved by rather different reasons (Penrose and Hameroff 1995). They believe the dynamical properties at the level of neurons and networks to be incapable of generating consciousness, regardless of the complexity. For Penrose and Hameroff, the key to consciousness lies in quantum events in tiny protein structures—microtubules—within neurons. Why *there*? And why *quantum-level* phenomena? Because the nature of mathematical understanding, Penrose believes, transcends the kind of computation that could conceivably be done by neurons and networks.

As a demonstration of neuronal inadequacy, Penrose cites the Gödel Incompleteness Result, which concerns limitations of provability in axiom systems for arithmetic. What is needed to transcend these limitations, according to Penrose, are unique operations at the quantum level. Quantum gravity, were it to exist, could do the trick. Granting that no adequate theory of quantum gravity exists, Penrose and Hameroff argue that microtubules are about the right size to support the envisioned quantum events, and they have the right sort of sensitivity to anesthetics to suggest they do sustain consciousness.

The details of the Penrose–Hameroff theory are highly technical and draw on mathematics, physics, biochemistry, and neuroscience. Before investing time in mastering the details, most people want a measure of the theory's "figures of merit," as an engineer might put it.[8] Specifically, is there any hard evidence in support of the theory, is the theory testable, and if true, would the theory give a clear and cogent explanation of what it is supposed to explain? After all, there is no dearth of crackpot theories about everything from consciousness to sunspots. Making theories divulge their figures of merit is a minimal condition for further investment.

First, a brief interlude to glimpse the positive views Penrose has concerning the question of how humans understand mathematics. In 1989 he suggested as unblushing a Platonic solution as Plato himself proposed circa 400 B.C.:

Mathematical ideas have an existence of their own, and inhabit an ideal Platonic world, which is accessible via the intellect only. When one "sees" a mathematical truth, one's consciousness breaks through into this world of ideas, and makes direct contact with it.... mathematicians communicate ... by each one having *a direct route to truth* [Penrose's italics.] (p. 428)

As a solution to questions in the epistemology of mathematics, Platonism is not remotely satisfactory (for recent discussions, see Benacerraf and Putnam 1983; Kitcher 1984). Knowing what we now know in biology, psychology, physics, and chemistry, the Platonic story of mathematical understanding is as much a fairy tale as the idea that Eve was created from Adam's rib. Far better to admit we have no satisfactory solution than to adopt a "And-God-said—Lo!" solution.

Let us return now to evaluating the quantum-gravity-microtubule theory of conscious experience. The figures of merit are not encouraging. First, mathematical logicians generally disagree with Penrose on what the Gödel result implies for brain function (Feferman 1996; Putnam 1994). In addition, the link between conscious experiences, such as smelling cinnamon, and the Gödel result is, at best, obscure.

Is there any significant evidential link between microtubules and awareness? Hameroff believes microtubules are affected by hydrophobic anesthetics in such a way as to cause loss of consciousness. But there is no evidence that loss of consciousness under anesthesia depends on the envisaged changes in microtubules, and only indirect evidence that anesthetics do in fact (as opposed to "could conceivably") have *any* effect on microtubules. On the other hand, plenty of evidence points to proteins in the neuron membrane as the principal locus of action of hydrophobic anesthetics (Franks and Lieb 1994; Bowdle, Horita, and Kharasch 1994; Franks and Lieb in Chapter 38 of this volume).

Is there any hard evidence that quantum coherence happens in microtubules? *Only that it might happen.* But surely the presence of cytoplasmic ions in the microtubule pore would disrupt these effects? *They might not.* Surely the effects of quantum coherence would be swamped by the millivolt signaling activity in the neuronal membrane? *They might not.* Can the existence of quantum coherence in microtubules be tested experimentally? *For technical reasons, experiments on microtubules are performed in a dish, not in the animal.* If tests under these conditions failed to show quantum coherence, would that be significant? *No, because microtubules might behave differently in the animal, in which we cannot test for the effects.* Does any of this, supposing it to be true, help us explain such things as recall of past events, filling in of the blindspot, hallucinations, and attentional effects on sensory awareness? *Somehow, it might.*

The want of directly relevant data is frustrating enough, but the explanatory vacuum is catastrophic. Pixie dust in the synapses is about as explanatorily powerful as quantum coherence in the microtubules. Without at least a blueprint, an outline, a prospectus, or *something* showing how, if true, the theory could explain the various phenomena of conscious experience, Penrose and Hameroff are offering a make-believe pig in a fantasy poke. None of this shows that Penrose and Hameroff are wrong—only that the theory needs work.

Conceptual innovation is needed for a host of problems quite apart from sensory awareness. To be sure, most new ideas are bound to go the way of the three-legged trout. The idea-climate should not, of course, be so harsh as to snuff out any contender that looks outlandish. For this reason, I applaud the boldness of Penrose and Hameroff. Having looked closely at the details of their proposal, however, I find I am inclined to look elsewhere for ideas that have figures of merit strong enough to invite serious investment.

CONCLUSION

1. Consciousness is a difficult problem, but for all we can tell now, it may turn out to be more tractable than other problems about neural function, such as how the brain manages to get timing right. We shall have to do the science and see.

2. Thought experiments are typically too under-described to give real credence to the conclusions they are asked to bear. Too often they are merely a heartfelt intuition dressed up to look like a scientifically grounded argument.

3. Consciousness might turn out to be a fundamental property of the universe, but so far there is no moderately convincing reason to believe it is. Insofar as most information processing in brains and machines is nonconscious, it is not plausible to assume that an information-based physics *per se* is the key to consciousness.

4. Consciousness might turn out to be produced by quantum coherence in microtubules, but so far there is no moderately convincing reason to believe that it is.

5. Let's keep plugging away at experimental psychology and neuroscience, trying to invent revealing experiments that will help us make progress on the problem. We need to continue developing both direct strategies (that have the neural substrate for awareness as their immediate target) and indirect strategies (that focus on perception, motor control, attention, learning and memory, emotions, etc.) with the hope that, along the way, much will be revealed about awareness in those functions. We need to continue to address theoretical as well as experimental questions and to foster new ideas targeting how the brain solves problems such as sensory-motor integration, time-management, and using back projections in sensory systems to bias the perception, to fill in, and to "see as."

NOTES

1. The first sections of this chapter are drawn from my 1996 article, "The Hornswoggle Problem" in the *Journal of Consciousness Studies*, and they are republished here with permission. In preparing that article and this chapter, I am greatly indebted to Paul Churchland, Francis Crick, Joe Bogen, David Rosenthal, Rodolfo Llinas, Michael Stack, Clark Glymour, Dan Dennett, Ilya Farber, and Joe Ramsay for advice and ideas.

Part II: Ontology, the Hard Problem of Experience, Free Will, and Agency

2. As I lacked time in my talk at Tucson to address the "Mary problem" first formulated by Frank Jackson in 1982, let me make several brief remarks about it here. In sum, Jackson's idea was that someone, call her Mary, could exist, who knew everything there was to know about how the brain works but still did not know what it was to see the color green (she lacked "green cones," to put it crudely). Jackson believed that this possibility showed that qualia are therefore not explainable by science.

The main problem with Jackson's argument is that for Mary to experience green qualia, certain wiring has to be in place in Mary's brain, and certain patterns of activity have to be obtained. Since, by Jackson's own hypothesis, Mary does not have that wiring, presumably the relevant activity patterns in visual cortex are not caused and she does not experience green. Who would expect her visual cortex (e.g., V4) would be set a-humming just by virtue of her propositional (linguistic) knowledge about activity patterns in V4? Not me. Mary can have propositional knowledge via other channels, of course, including the knowledge of what her own brain lacks vis-à-vis green qualia. Nothing whatever follows about whether science can or cannot explain qualia.

3. In *Neurophilosophy* I suggested that a typical weakness with philosophers' thought experiments is that there is too much thought and not enough experiment.

4. As I understand Dennett, these considerations loom large in his approach—see, for example, his *Consciousness Explained* (1994).

5. In *Matter and Consciousness*, Paul Churchland (1988) raises this possibility and evaluates it as being, at best, highly remote. Searle appears indifferent to Churchland's evaluation and its rationale.

6. For an earlier and quite detailed discussion of this approach, see Bennett, Hoffman, and Prakash (1989).

7. In *The Rediscovery of the Mind* Searle (1992) claims that my reply to McGinn shows that I hold insane views about the elimination of consciousness. I enclose my entire reply to McGinn as an appendix to this chapter. I am at a loss to understand what Searle has in mind. In my first paper on consciousness (1983), I am talking about the transmutation of a concept. Moreover, in that paper I suggest how we might make progress in studying the phenomenon: "In addition to the research already discussed, studies to determine the neurophysiological differences between conscious and nonconscious states, to find out what goes on in the brain during REM sleep and during non-REM sleep, to determine the order and nature of events during the various facets of attention, and how this fits into a broader scheme of intelligent brain activity, would surely contribute to a deeper understanding of what sort of business consciousness is" (p. 93). Does this sound like I want to eliminate consciousness? Where is Searle getting his claim?

Is the insane idea perhaps in *Neurophilosophy*? There I say, "This research [on sleep and dreaming] raises questions about whether there are different kinds of conscious states, and different ways or different levels of being aware that we have yet to understand" (p. 208). Rather mild, I think. I also say, "The brain undoubtedly has a number of mechanisms for monitoring brain processes, and the folk psychological categories of 'awareness' and 'consciousness' indifferently lump together an assortment of mechanisms. As neurobiology and neuropsychology probe the mechanisms and functions of the brain, a reconfiguring of categories can be predicted" (p. 322). This obviously concerns reconfiguration of the categories, it does not deny the existence of the phenomenon. See also P. S. Churchland (1988). Where is the evidence that I want to eliminate the phenomenon of consciousness?

8. For details behind my reservations, see Grush and Churchland (1995) and the reply by Penrose and Hameroff (1995). See also Putnam (1994, 1995), Feferman (1995), Benacerraf and Putnam (1983), and Kitcher (1984). Pat Hayes and Ken Ford found Penrose's mathematical argument so outlandish that they awarded him the Simon Newcombe Award in 1995 (Hayes and Ford 1995). They explain that Simon Newcombe (1835–1909) was a celebrated astronomer who insisted that manned flight was physically impossible.

REFERENCES

Benacerraf, P., and H. Putnam, eds. 1983. *Philosophy of Mathematics: Selected Readings.* Englewood Cliffs, NJ: Prentice-Hall.

Bennett, B. M., D. D. Hoffman, and C. Prakash. 1989. *Observer Mechanics.* San Diego: Academic Press.

Bowdle, T. A., A. Horita, and E. D. Kharasch. 1994. *The Pharmacological Basis of Anesthesiology.* New York: Churchill Livingstone.

Chalmers, D. 1996. *The Conscious Mind.* Oxford: Oxford University Press.

Chalmers, D. 1995. The puzzle of conscious experience. *Scientific American* 273:80–86.

Churchland, P. M. 1988. *Matter and Consciousness.* Cambridge: MIT Press.

Churchland, P. M. 1995. *The Engine of Reason: The Seat of the Soul.* Cambridge: MIT Press.

Churchland, P. M. 1996. The rediscovery of light. *Journal of Philosophy* 93:211–228.

Churchland, P. M., and P. S. Churchland. 1991. Intertheoretic reduction: A neuroscientist's field guide. *Seminars in the Neurosciences* 2:249–256.

Churchland, P. S. 1983. Consciousness: The transmutation of a concept. *Pacific Philosophical Quarterly* 64:80–95.

Churchland, P. S. 1986a. *Neurophilosophy: Toward a Unified Science of the Mind-Brain.* Cambridge: MIT Press.

Churchland, P. S. 1986b. Replies to commentaries on *Neurophilosophy. Inquiry* 29:241–272.

Churchland, P. S. 1988. Reductionism and the neurobiological basis of consciousness. In *Consciousness in Contemporary Science.* A. M. Marcel and E. Bisiach, eds., Oxford: Oxford University Press, pp. 273–304.

Crick, F. H. C. 1994. *The Astonishing Hypothesis.* New York: Scribner.

Feferman, S. 1995. Penrose's Gödelian argument. *Psyche* 2:23.

Franks N. P., and W. R. Lieb. 1994. Molecular and cellular mechanisms of general anesthesia. *Nature* 367:607–614.

Grush, R., and P. S. Churchland. 1995. Gaps in Penrose's toilings. *Journal of Consciousness Studies* 2:10–29.

Hayes, P., and K. Ford. 1995. The Simon Newcombe Awards. *AI Magazine* 16:11–13.

Jackson, F. 1982. Epiphenomenal qualia. *Philosophical Quarterly.* 32:127–36.

Kitcher, P. 1984. *The Nature of Mathematical Knowledge.* Oxford: Oxford University Press.

Nagel, T. 1974. What is it like to be a bat? *Philosophical Review* 83:435–50.

Penrose, R. 1989. *The Emperor's New Mind.* Oxford: Oxford University Press.

Penrose, R. 1994a. Interview with Jane Clark. *Journal of Consciousness Studies* 1:17–24.

Penrose, R. 1994b. *Shadows of the Mind.* Oxford: Oxford University Press.

Penrose, R., and S. Hameroff. 1995. What gaps? *Journal of Consciousness Studies* 2:99–112.

Putnam, H. 1994. The best of all possible brains? Review of *Shadows of the Mind. New York Times Book Review,* November, 3.

Searle, J. 1992. *The Rediscovery of the Mind.* Cambridge: MIT Press.

Searle, J. 1995. The mystery of consciousness: Part II. *New York Review of Books* 42:58–64.

APPENDIX TO CHAPTER 8

This letter was published March 13, 1987, in *The Times Literary Supplement*:

Sir,

Galileo's telescope, and experimental evidence generally, were scorned by the cardinals as irrelevant and unnecessary. They knew that the celestial order was revealed as a matter of faith, pure reason, and sacred text. The very idea of moons revolving around Jupiter was an affront to all three. Observation of denormalizing data in the form of sun spots and Jovian satellites was therefore impossible. In his review (February 6, 1987) of my book, *Neurophilosophy*, Colin McGinn displays a general reaction to neuroscience that bears a chilling resemblance to that of the cardinals. For McGinn, the very idea that our intuitive convictions concerning the nature of the mind might be reassessed is "virtually inconceivable." Intuitive (folk) psychology, insists McGinn, is an "autonomous mode of person understanding" [*sic*], and the autonomy he claims for it keeps it sacred, shielding it from whatever might be discovered by empirical investigation. But to call an explanatory framework "autonomous" is just to cobble up a polite label for digging in and refusing to allow the relevance of empirical data. This is no more acceptable for psychology than it was for folk physics, folk astronomy, creationism vitalism or alchemy.

The main theme of the book is that if we want to understand the mind, research in neuroscience will have an essential role, as will research in psychology, ethology, computer modeling *and* philosophy. Very briefly, the reason is this: the brain is what sees, thinks, feels, and so forth, and if we want to know how it performs these jobs, we will have to look at its components and organization. Psychology is essential, because it provides constraints at a higher level, and helps the neurobiologist specify the functions to be explained by neural networks. Modeling is essential because there are properties at the level of circuits that cannot be determined at the level of single cell analysis. Co-evolution of theories at all levels, where each level informs, correct and inspires the others, is therefore the research ideology that looks most productive. At the same time, there is the empirical possibility that the result of a substantial period of co-evolution will yield a psychology and a neurobiology that look quite different from what we now work with. Some evidence in this direction is already available, as I show in several chapters of my book. Beyond the normal apprehension of things new, this prospect should not alarm McGinn, for it represents a deepening of our understanding of human nature.

What then is the role of philosophy? My view here is that philosophy is also essential to the wider project of understanding how the mind-brain works. It is, as always, the synoptic discipline: it attempts to synthesize the existing sciences into a unified and coherent account of reality. And it is, as always, a seminal discipline: in addressing the limits of common-sense

Patricia Smith Churchland: Brainshy: Nonneural Theories of Conscious Experience understanding, it attempts to found new sciences where none existed before. I think this role is very much in keeping with the long tradition in philosophy, as exemplified by Aristotle, Hume, Kant, James and Pierce. But I also say, "this sort of philosophy is not an *a priori* discipline pontificating grandly to the rest of science; it is in the swim with the rest of science, and hence stands to be corrected as empirical discovery proceeds." (p. 482)

McGinn, however, finds this conception of philosophy "absurd." He apparently wants to keep philosophy free from the taint of empirical science, pure to undertake that most subtle of tasks, the analysis of concepts. Whose concepts? The concepts of the scientifically uninformed. The trouble is, *know-nothing philosophy is dead-end philosophy*, and the divination of *a priori* truths is a delusion. Without bridges to the relevant disciplines, philosophy becomes insular, in-grown, and wanting in vigor. Such observations motivated Kenneth Craik's call in 1943 (!) for an "experimental philosophy" of mind.

The real absurdity is to make a virtue out of ignorance and to scoff at informed research as "scientism." The doctrine of keeping philosophy pure makes the discipline look silly, and it is philosophy pursued under the banner of purity that quite naturally provokes the impatience and incredulity of the wider intellectual community. Moreover, the very best research by contemporary philosophers is richly cross-disciplinary, as can be seen in the work of Ned Block, Dan Dennett, John Earman, Arthur Fine, Jerry Fodor, Clark Glymour, Adolf Grunbaum, John Haugeland, Philip Kitcher, Michael Redhead, Elliott Sober and Stephen Stich, to name a few. A willingness to cooperate across boundaries and an acute sense of the value of such exchanges is increasingly visible in this decade. This is surely a healthy development as we collectively get on with the question of how to make sense of our universe—and ourselves.

Whitehead's *Even More* Dangerous Idea

Peter Farleigh

... any doctrine which refuses to place human experience outside nature, must find in descriptions of human experience factors which also enter into the descriptions of less specialized natural occurrences. If there can be no such factors, then the doctrine of human experience as a fact within nature is mere bluff, founded upon vague phrases whose sole merit is a comforting familiarity. We should either admit dualism, at least as a provisional doctrine, or we should point out the identical elements connecting human experience with physical science.

—Alfred North Whitehead (1933)

"Old habits die hard" Daniel Dennett (1996) wrote in a short newspaper article that was part of a prelude to the Tucson II conference. He continued:

... especially habits of thinking, and our "intuitive" ways of thinking about consciousness are infected with leftover Cartesian images, an underestimated legacy of the dualist past.

Materialists and functionalists pride themselves on how much they have rejected Cartesian dualism with its bifurcation of nature into two separate entities—mind things and substance things. They attempt to explain how mind arises either from raw matter, or from some sort of information processing. Others, who think that mind is "mere bluff," choose a third option—the eliminativist one. Consciousness for the third group does not really exist as we might imagine, but is a construction based on our "old habits" of folk psychology.

Materialists, functionalists, and eliminativists may have critically rejected the Cartesian images of consciousness from their schemes, but, for whatever reason, they have uncritically accepted the Cartesian image of matter—an existent thing that requires nothing but itself to exist, matter as "simply located." In sharing this much with the dualists, should they more properly claim to have rejected just *half* the dualist doctrine?

Cartesian substance provides the ground for the classic mechanistic paradigm, Newton's "world-machine"—the "billiard-ball" universe—a powerful metaphor still very much with us today (e.g., Dawkins 1995). Although some contemporary forms of materialism have a less deterministic view of substance, modified in the light of modern physics and biology (e.g., Searle

1992), the functionalists have gallantly upheld the very traditional, mechanistic concept of matter in motion. Their prime model is the computational metaphor for the mind.

In rejecting folk psychology concepts, we could equally make a case for rejecting "folk physics" concepts, too (i.e., the billiard-ball variety). But if we were to throw out the machine along with the ghost, what would our starting point be? If it is not substance and not information processing, what then? Are we to exclude these concepts altogether, or are they part of a much larger scheme?

WHITEHEAD'S DANGEROUS IDEA

Darwin is rightly said to have had a "dangerous" idea with his theory of natural selection (Dennett 1995). With respect to the nature of mind and matter, Alfred North Whitehead had an *even more dangerous* idea. He investigated his idea in enormous detail, particularly in his major philosophical work, *Process and Reality*, written in 1929. His idea rejected Cartesian dualism *fully*, and in "point[ing] out the identical elements connecting human experience with physical science," constructed a scientific worldview in terms of events and their relations, rather than in terms of matter in motion. Certain sorts of events and temporal series of events (processes), then held the status as the fundamental units ("primitives") of the universe—a position traditionally the domain of Cartesian substance. These events provided a unity between the observer and the observed, subject and object. Rejecting dualism fully meant, for Whitehead, that epistemology had no priority over ontology—any inquiry into knowing was simultaneously an inquiry into being (Cobb 1981).

Whitehead's process cosmology has dangerous implications in many areas of science and philosophy, and not primarily because Whitehead offered us new answers to old problems. Rather, it is dangerous because we are offered another perspective, one that includes the observer in the observing. Dangerous, particularly for dualists, materialists, functionalists, and eliminativists, because his view displaces the concept of machine as the primary metaphor for our understanding the world, a position now given to the concept of organism. In this short chapter, I briefly introduce Whitehead's event ontology with respect to the philosophy of mind.

FROM SUBSTANCE THINKING TO EVENT THINKING

Events, as we commonly refer to them, are happenings in certain places, at certain times, for particular durations—everything from the fall of an autumn leaf, to the fall of the Roman Empire. We can discuss such events by starting with concepts of matter in motion, but such an approach is a limited case of a more general view that regards matter itself as aggregates of subatomic events, as modern physics has shown. Subatomic events are instances of the fundamental types of events that Whitehead used as the basis for his ontology.

Bertrand Russell felt the force of Whitehead's idea. In 1914 Whitehead convinced him "to abandon Newtonian absolute time and space, and also particles of matter, substituting systems of events," and this "fitted in well with Einstein" (Ushenko 1949). Russell (1969) further elucidated the Whiteheadian concept of matter when he wrote:

An event does not persist and move, like the traditional piece of matter; it merely exists for its little moment and then ceases. A piece of matter will thus be resolved into a series of events. Just as, in the old view, an extended body was composed of a number of particles, so, now each particle, being extended in time, must be regarded as composed of what we may call "event-particles." The whole series of these events makes up the whole history of the particle, and the particle is regarded as being its history, not some metaphysical entity to which the events happen.

WHITEHEAD'S "ACTUAL OCCASIONS"

Whitehead did not confine his fundamental unit events to the subatomic level; his was not a quantum-mechanics theory of mind per se. Rather, his speculation was that universal principles operate at all levels in nature—quantum-mechanical phenomena are instances of these principles at one extreme, and psychological phenomena are instances at another. Not only low-grade, subatomic events, but also atomic, molecular, and cellular events count as fundamental Whiteheadian "actual occasions." The most complex high-grade events are the most familiar ones—moments of human perception, or percipient events. All these occasions have, to some degree, a subjective or psychophysical nature. For Whitehead, an occasion, technically, was an "occasion of experience," though not necessarily a conscious experience.

Although Whitehead was quite the opposite of an eliminativist, he nevertheless did not write extensively about consciousness itself, preferring to talk in more general terms about experience and feeling. He wrote (1938):

We experience more than we can analyze. For we experience the universe, and we analyze in our consciousness a minute selection of its details.

For instance, we are conscious of the person we are talking to at a party while we simultaneously experience the ambiance of the crowd. Whitehead saw the major role of consciousness as the explicit awareness that a present situation *could be other* than it is, and so one is conscious of *what* it is; that is, we *could be* talking to anyone at the party, but we *are* talking to *this* person.

Broadening the concept of experience beyond the familiar human realm to include the lowest levels of nature may be unsettling, but it is not completely unreasonable. The fact that many of day-to-day activities are performed without thinking and that decisions and judgments are often colored by forgotten or suppressed memories indicates that a continuity exists between conscious and unconscious experience. Ethologists such as Donald Griffin (1992) and Susan Armstrong-Buck (1989) provide evidence for such experience in animals. Others provide evidence for it in single-celled organisms

(Agar 1951). Evidence that even for subatomic particles have a very primitive subjective nature is given by McDaniel (1983).

The word panpsychism is often used to describe Whitehead's position, even though he did not use the word himself. The word can be problematic. For some, "psyche," which usually pertains to the human mind, suggests that this position holds that low-grade "individuals" such as bacteria, or even electrons, are conscious, but this certainly is not the case. David Ray Griffin (1988) suggests that "panexperientialism" is a more appropriate term. One should not expect all the characteristics of mentality we observe at the macroscale to be evident at the microscale, just as we no longer expect physicality to be the same at both levels. For instance, the atoms in a sponge are not themselves expected to be spongy.

The word "pan" should also not be misconstrued. Meaning "all," pan can imply that *everything* has some mentality, which again is certainly not true. Things such as tables, teapots, thermostats, and tetra-flop computers, are regarded as uncoordinated aggregates of low-grade occasions; they have no mental properties in themselves.

Whitehead (1933) distinguished these types of things from things such as cells and organisms:

... in bodies that are obviously living, a coordination has been achieved that raises into prominence some functions inherent in the ultimate occasions. For lifeless matter these functionings thwart each other, and average out so as to produce a negligible total effect. In the case of living bodies the coordination intervenes, and the average effect of these intimate functionings has to be taken into account.

In other words, in ordinary matter, neighboring occasions are "incoherent" and there is a "smoothing-out" effect of the tiny freedoms and unpredictabilities that can be found in those occasions in isolation. The causal chains are constant and predictable; thus, the descriptions of matter by traditional physical theory are therefore statistically very accurate. Hence, mechanistic analogies are most useful and appropriate.

In contrast, things such as molecules and organisms are temporal chains of high-grade occasions and are characterized by their part–whole relations. The organization of their parts depends on the mutual action of the parts on each other, with the consequence that the whole acts as a causal unit both on its own parts and on its environment. A molecule or an organism acts as a causal unit in a way other than the summed causal actions of the lower-grade occasions taken in isolation. For instance, the properties of a molecule are different from the sum of the properties of its constituent atoms, even though both the properties and synthesis of the molecule are *entirely* dependent on the intrinsic properties of those atoms. This does not occur because of some miraculous addition, but because the activity of all actual occasions, including mental and percipient events, is fundamentally relational from the start.

There has, of course, been a lot of study of the self-organization of living things with computer models using artificial life and artificial neural network techniques. No doubt these sorts of research programs provide us with new insights to understanding some of the nature of part–whole relations in actual organisms. On the other hand, the very fact that any modeling of the real world involves abstractions inevitably imposes limitations on the sort of results we should expect. It is sometimes easy to confuse the *abstract* with the *concrete*. For instance, if we were to believe that a computer virus is alive in the biological sense, we would be committing what Whitehead famously called the "fallacy of misplaced concreteness." A fallacy, by the way, that the biologist Waddington (1977) warns "is *dangerous* to forget!"

THE NATURE OF EVENTS AND THEIR RELATIONS

Having established in general what Whitehead meant by "actual occasions," some explanation of their nature needs to be made. One might expect to find the explanation by starting at the bottom and working up. In fact, the place to start (and the place that Whitehead wanted us to start) is at the level of human experience, for two reasons. First, because human experience at any moment is itself an actual occasion; it is the occasion we know better than any other, and we know it from the *inside*. Second, because high-level occasions are themselves highly coordinated societies of low-level occasions, certain features of human experiential events can be generically applied to more primitive occasions.

Consider the act of perception. By perception, which involves cognition, intentionality, and affective tone, we take account of our environment. I look at a pencil in front of me, for example. I have an immediate sense of its overall look—its shape, its length, its color. The pencil is set against a background of my desk and other things in my field of vision, but not things that I am acutely aware of at that moment. I am only vaguely aware of my body and its relation to the desk and pen. In seeing the pencil, a whole stream of associative memories are also stirred. All these perceptions and memories are gathered together into the unity that is this single, percipient event—a "specious present"—and the focal point or center of this event is my body. The pencil, the background, and the memories are all internal constituents of my experience and are therefore causally efficacious of that experiential event. They are *internally related* to this event. The objects at that moment are unaffected by my act of perception and so are *externally related* to the event.

The act of perception, then, establishes the causal relation of a subject to the external world at that moment. For Whitehead, perception and memory were high-level instances of a more general concept, which he called *prehension*. Most simply, for a subject to prehend an object, it is to experience it, perceive it, feel it, or "take it into account," though not necessarily in a conscious or reflective way. An object can be a physical object, such as a pencil, or a conceptual object such as a memory. Prehension is also a feature at lower levels of nature. According to this view, single cells "feel" because they take account of their environment (which is often other cells); within a series of subatomic

Peter Farleigh: Whitehead's *Even More* Dangerous Idea

events, each event prehends its antecedent event and is almost entirely determined by it.

The concept of prehension sounds like the more familiar concept of intentionality. Indeed, Nicholas Gier has examined in depth the relations between the two concepts. Gier (1976) pointed out their similarities:

Both prehension and intentionality describe the relationship of a subject and an object in such a way as to overcome this subject–object split. In the same way that intentionality is always "consciousness of an object," prehension is always "feeling of" some datum. This means that any prehensive unification or intentional act is codetermined by the respective data.

One major difference in the two concepts is that intentionality is discussed only in terms of human consciousness, but prehension is extended far beyond the human realm. Both concepts affirm a doctrine of internal relations in that consciousness is never simply "there," without content or object; however, with phenomenology, the relationship of consciousness and its object is not considered causal. Whitehead solved the problem of causation with his doctrine of asymmetrical relations between a present event and its past. Lewis Ford (Gier 1976) summed up the comparison by stating:

Rather than being simply identical with intentionality, prehension generalizes *both* intentionality *and* causality, thus unifying both phenomenology and science.

Although I am affected by the object I see, my experience is not completely determined by it. The present moment is tinged with the possibilities for what the next occasion might be, and this requires a certain creative response or choice by me that may or may not be a conscious choice. I have a fairly conscious anticipation about what I want to do with the pencil, (if anything at all, I may want a pen) and a much less conscious anticipation about how I am to pick up the pencil. A future event cannot be the *physical* cause of a present event—there is no backward causation. But a present event can be partly determined by the anticipation of the *conceptual* possibilities for what the succeeding event could be. This concept is known as the *subjective aim* of the occasion.

The breadth of possibilities for an event to occur is a measure of the amount of freedom within any particular causal chain—an extremely small degree at the subatomic level and a large degree of freedom at the human level. If the degree of freedom is zero, the causal chain is completely deterministic. Thus, Whitehead had a general theory of causation that was well adapted for explaining the nature of organic processes and mental events. Also, if taken to one extreme, his theory explains the more specific nature of mechanistic events.

CONCLUSION

It is dangerous to change our mode of thinking—from looking at the world in terms of substances to thinking of it in terms of events. All, not just some, of our old Cartesian images have to go. Mind and matter are not separate. Mind is not rejected in preference to matter, and mind does not arise from matter that initially has no mind because *both* concepts undergo a radical change within Whitehead's philosophy of organism and are replaced by the single concept of relational events. These events have characteristics that can be considered matterlike in some respects and mindlike in others.

As an approach that avoids many of the pitfalls of dualism, materialism, and functionalism, I believe Whitehead's theory is equally a solid candidate, worthy of serious consideration and discussion within the contemporary debate.

REFERENCES

Agar, W. E. 1951. *A Contribution to the Theory of the Living Organism,* 2nd ed. Melbourne: University of Melbourne Press.

Armstrong-Buck, S. 1989. Nonhuman experience: A Whiteheadian analysis. *Process Studies* 18:1–18.

Cobb, J. B. 1981. Whitehead and natural philosophy. In H. Holz and E. Wolf-Gazo, eds, *Whitehead and the Idea of Process.* Freiburg and Munich: Karl Alber.

Dawkins, R. 1995. *River Out of Eden: A Darwinian View of Life.* New York: Basic Books.

Dennett, D. C. 1995. *Darwin's Dangerous Idea.* New York: Simon & Schuster.

Dennett, D. C. 1996. Hume's internal bundle grows a few extra knots. In *The Times Higher Education Supplement,* London, April 5.

Gier, N. 1976. Intentionality and prehension. *Process Studies* 6:197–213.

Griffin, David R. 1988. Of minds and molecules. In D. R. Griffin, ed., *The Reenchantment of Science.* Albany: State University of New York Press.

Griffin, Donald R. 1992. *Animal Minds.* Chicago: The University of Chicago Press.

McDaniel, J. 1983. Physical matter as creative and sentient. *Environmental Ethics* 5:291–317.

Russell, B. 1969. *The ABC of Relativity,* 3rd ed. London: George Allen and Unwin Ltd.

Searle, J. R. 1992. *The Rediscovery of the Mind.* Cambridge: MIT Press.

Ushenko, A. P. 1949. Einstein's influence on philosophy. In P. A. Schilpp, ed., *Albert Einstein: Philosopher-Scientist.* New York: Open Court.

Waddington, C. H. 1977. *Tools for Thought.* London: Jonathan Cape Ltd.

Whitehead, A. N. 1926. *Science and the Modern World,* 2nd ed. Cambridge: Cambridge University Press.

Whitehead, A. N. 1933. *Adventures of Ideas.* Reprinted 1967, New York: Free Press.

Whitehead, A. N. 1938. *Modes of Thought.* Cambridge: Cambridge University Press.

Whitehead, A. N. 1978. *Process and Reality,* 1929. (corrected). Reprinted, New York: Free Press.

10 Against Functionalism: Consciousness as an Information-Bearing Medium

Bruce Mangan

GENUS AND SPECIES

In general, the scientific analysis of a biological information-bearing medium (e.g., DNA, neurons, the fluid in the cochlea) aims to answer two related but different questions: (1) What information does the medium bear? (2) In what specific *way* does the medium bear its information? The "information" in the first question can be realized without loss in a great many other information-bearing media, whether the media are natural or man-made. But this freedom of instantiation is quite beside the point for the second question, which asks about the *specific* characteristics of a given medium that allow it to bear information in a particular way.

To extend biological usage slightly, the answer to the first question tells us that something belongs to the genus known as information-bearing media; the answer to the second question tells us how to characterize a given information-bearing medium as a distinct species. Full scientific understanding of cognitive activity in our organism normally demands that we explore both questions.

It strikes me as odd that something like this kind of straightforward, biologically informed distinction has not been applied to consciousness, but as far as I know, it has not. Is consciousness simply one more species of information-bearing medium at work in our organism? There are various reasons to think so, some of them more or less conceptual, some quite empirical. For now, I want to concentrate on the conceptual issues, particularly the issues that contrast with the contemporary functionalist analysis of consciousness, especially that by Dennett.

Functionalism is an excellent foil for developing an information-bearing account of consciousness, in part because the medium formulation looks so powerful by comparison—it seems able to handle a whole range of scientific possibilities that functionalism cannot address in principle.

Both approaches can deal equally well with the general properties of the genus (information-bearing media), but functionalism cannot treat consciousness as a distinct species belonging to this genus because the defining assertion of functionalism is that consciousness necessarily instantiates in *any* medium when that medium is able to bear information that has a certain kind of abstract structure. As Dennett (1993) says,

the hallmark of functionalism [is] its commitment, at some level, to multiple realizability.

But an information-bearing medium is clearly not the sort of thing that can be fully realized by a different medium. Media instantiate information, not other media; media that bear the same information do not transmogrify into one another. Thus, if consciousness is a species of information-bearing media, it looks like a very poor candidate for multiple realizability.

Any argument that supports the consciousness-as-medium hypothesis is, at the same time, an argument against the functionalist theory of consciousness. Currently, the functionalist–antifunctionalist debate is quite abstract, generally argued at the level of thought experiments. But because the medium hypothesis is supported in part by experimental evidence (discussed below), the medium hypothesis is able to mount a direct challenge to functionalism solely on scientific grounds.

In any case, the medium hypothesis gives us a new, more precise way to state the crux of the dispute between functionalism and some of its opponents; even Dennett agrees that the hypothesis brings new clarity to the issue. But beyond this, the hypothesis lets us frame a basic, common-sense objection to functionalism in terms that do not go beyond the most conservative scientific notions already used to analyze cognition. The medium hypothesis does not need to make any appeal to so-called first-person experience or to qualia (though it is certainly compatible with and strengthened by such appeals).

Functionalism often tries to advertise itself as the only true scientific option for dealing with consciousness. Dennett's rhetoric, in particular, suggests that his opponents are simply unable to give up their vague, prescientific, common-sense intuitions. I do not think there is anything unscientific about appeals to direct experience. But the medium hypothesis can avoid the complications raised by qualia and still bring out a very serious problem with functionalism.

MEDIUM-SPECIFIC AND MEDIUM-INDEPENDENT RESEARCH

Consider a relatively unproblematic distinction between scientific concerns that are medium specific, and those that are medium independent. Medium-specific research works to understand a given information-bearing medium. Medium-independent research looks for findings that can be fully realized in various media. Medium-independent research can also be directed toward a specific medium but is only concerned with findings that can be *completely* reproduced in other media.

An entity is medium independent if all its properties can be understood without necessary reference to any given instantiating medium. Science studies many medium-independent entities—an air-foil, for example. The air-foil in a bird's wing is instantiated by bone and feathers; in an airplane wing, it is instantiated by metal, canvas, or plastic. "Vision," as used in cognitive science, is arguably a medium-independent concept because it can apply to any process that performs the visual function of converting photons into useful information about an environment. The paradigm case of a medium-independent entity is a computer program.

Obviously, science does more than investigate medium-independent entities or look for medium-independent features in specific media. How do the rods in the human eye detect photons? This question does *not* ask about vision in the functional sense. It is *not* a question about the common structural features found in all systems that can (or in theory could) "see" in black and white. The question asks about the *particular* makeup and activity of the rods in our eyes. In answering this particular question, part of medium-specific research is the finding that the rods are photosensitive because they contain rhodopsin. Rhodopsin is the specific medium that (first) bears the information that electromagnetic radiation has struck the rods of a human eye. To answer by naming any other chemical functionally equivalent to, but distinct from, rhodopsin would not only be misleading, it would be false. *No complete functional substitution or instantiation or realization is possible for the answer to a medium-specific question.*

Of course, medium-specific and medium-independent concerns usually work together for full scientific understanding. For example, consider the ear when someone shouts "FIRE!" Medium-independent information flows through a series of distinct information-bearing media, each of which instantiates the information in its own unique way: first the ear drum, then the middle ear, cochlea, basilar membrane, cilia, cells on which the cilia attach, and, finally, the auditory nerve.

The medium-independent question—What information does the auditory system bear?—has an inherently abstract answer, one that could apply to all functionally equivalent systems, however wildly different their makeup. But the medium-specific question—How does the human ear bear information?—always stays absolutely particular: a taut membrane of skin bears information at the ear drum; tiny jointed bones bear information in the middle ear; minute wisps of hair bear information in the inner ear.

Or consider genetics. In theory, a computer can store all the genetic information now stored by our genes (and if the Genome Project succeeds, it will store this information). This information is medium independent because it can be instantiated without loss by many different media (e.g., by DNA, RNA, a computer, a very thick book, a very long abacus). But science must also give us a precise account of the specific reality of genetic media; for example, that DNA and RNA differ in both their structure and evolutionary history or that they transmit information through complementary pairing, and so forth.

We can now state the gist of the functionalist–antifunctionalist dispute in terms that are neutral, scientifically grounded, and make no necessary reference to qualia. Functionalists tacitly assume that consciousness is a medium-independent entity. Many antifunctionalists tacitly assume that consciousness is a specific medium.

To establish this point, we need look no further than to Dan Dennett. I first proposed the idea that consciousness is an information-bearing medium in a critical review (Mangan 1993a) of Dennett's 1991 book, *Consciousness Explained*. To establish at least one point of agreement, I tried to rework the common-sense intuition about consciousness by putting it in straightforward, cognitive terms.

In response, Dennett (1993) agreed that my version indeed captured the point at issue:

What a fine expression of Cartesian materialism! I wish I had thought of it myself.... Now we can see why Mangan, Searle, and others are so exercised by the zombie question: they think of consciousness as a "distinct medium," not a distinct system of content that could be realized in many different media.

Dennett continued:

Is consciousness—could conscious be—a distinct medium? Notice that although *light* is a distinct medium, *vision* is not; it is a distinct content system (a distinct information system) that could in principle be realized in different media.

Dennett continues in this vein, arguing the point (not at issue) that distinct information systems such as vision or audition can be multiply instantiated. But he says nothing further about the logic of instantiation for a distinct medium such as light; he certainly seems to grant that light, as a distinct medium, cannot itself be fully realized in some other, nonluminous, medium. (The reader is encouraged to look at the full discussion.)

Thus we already have some significant agreement about the core intuition at issue, and on how we can make it explicit in scientific terms. But for some reason Dennett never directly set out clear reasons against the consciousness-as-medium thesis. He asked the central question "Is consciousness—could consciousness be—a distinct medium?" but what may look like his answer really just restates the uncontested fact that distinct information systems can be multiply realized. Dennett did not explain *why* consciousness is supposed to be like vision, not like light.

The same shift occurs as Dennett proceeds:

But someone might want to object that this leaves out something crucial: there is not any vision or audition at all—not any *conscious* vision or audition—until the information that moves through the fungible [multiply realizable] peripheral media eventually gets put into the "distinct medium" of consciousness. This is the essence of Cartesianism: Cartesian materialism if you think that there is something special about a particular part of the brain (so special that it is not fungible, not even in principle), and Cartesian dualism if you think the medium is not one more physical medium. The alternative hypothesis, which looks pretty good, I think, once these implications are brought out, is that, first appearances to the contrary, consciousness *itself* is a content system, and *not* a medium

It is not possible here to go over Dennett's arguments against the so-called Cartesian Theater (see Mangan, 1993a). But the above passage shows why Dennett's arguments against the Cartesian Theater are misdrawn if they are intended to work against the medium hypothesis. Dennett's argument pivots on the assumption that the medium hypothesis treats consciousness as something "special." But it is the "special" status of consciousness that the medium hypothesis denies. Dennett is absolutely right that we should be able to derive a medium-independent (functional) analysis for *all* the particular media that happen to make up our cognitive apparatus (including, I believe, consciousness). We can instantiate medium-independent findings in any medium able to bear information.

But Dennett forgets that the reverse is also true. *All* functionally equivalent systems are open to media-distinct analysis if they use distinct media. In other words, *all information bearing media are fungible from the standpoint of medium-independent research; no information-bearing medium is fungible from the standpoint of medium-specific research.* Just because we can ask medium-independent questions about consciousness, it hardly follows that consciousness is a medium-independent entity.

Functionalism must deny that consciousness is a distinct information-bearing medium or else functionalism fails. But, so far as I can see, no argument has been put forward to show why a medium-specific analysis of consciousness is a mistake (except that it would contradict functionalism). At the least, the consciousness-as-medium hypothesis is a logically possible alternative and is one that also gives us a new way to frame the functionalist–antifunctionalist debate.

CONSCIOUSNESS AS AN INFORMATION-BEARING MEDIUM

The medium hypothesis can appeal to much more than logical possibility. There are three reasons to think the medium hypothesis is, prima facie, scientifically plausible, not just logically possible. For a much more extensive discussion of these and related points, see Mangan (forthcoming).

1. Many people already suspect that something is wrong with functionalism. Probably the most serious problem is the account it must give of subjective experience. People not committed to functionalism find it hard to swallow the very wide range of entities (from thermostats to robots) that this or that functionalists insist are "conscious." For many of the uncommitted, the alternative looks unsavory because it seems to require a move away from scientific thinking, perhaps toward spiritual intuitions.

The medium hypothesis is able to explain, on purely scientific grounds, why so many people would feel uneasy about functionalism—functionalism ignores the entire domain of medium-specific research. Once we understand this, we can naturally extend the medium-specific stance and treat consciousness as just one more information-bearing medium along with neurons, rhodopsin, and the cochlea. The study of consciousness on the basis of this assumption is at least as scientifically plausible as is functionalism and does not have to pay functionalism's high, counterintuitive taxes in the bargain.

2. One of the most solid findings in consciousness research is that consciousness is extremely "narrow.' Psychologists of various stripes (e.g., James, Freud, Miller, Neisser) have looked at this feature of consciousness and have often equated it with the limits on attention. Baars (1988) has an excellent treatment of the limits on consciousness from a cognitive perspective.

One way to discuss this limitation is in terms of bandwidth. Bandwidth can be treated as a purely objective concept, as can the limited capacity of attention. All else equal, any physical or biological medium has its own characteristic bandwidth.

The study of attention can be carried out without any direct reference to subjective experience or qualia. Even a conservative behaviorist can study attention (see Berlyne 1971) and not fall from grace. It is clear that attention operates on a very narrow bandwidth; it is equally clear that neural structures of the brain enjoy a remarkably wide bandwidth (Baars 1988). Although difficult to quantify precisely, the difference between the bandwidth capacity of even relatively limited parts of the brain, on the one hand, and of attention on the other, is something like the difference in capacity between a good fiberoptic cable and the string on a tin-can telephone.

So we can point to a strong, *objective* correlation between a certain subset of cognitive functions and a peculiarly narrow bandwidth. These functions have been discussed by many people and cluster around behaviorally specifiable notions such as access, reporting, monitoring, novelty evaluation, and executive function.

One plausible scientific explanation for the observed correlation of a certain subset of cognitive functions with a narrow bandwidth is that these functions all load heavily *on a narrow bandwidth medium that is quite distinct from the neural medium's very wide bandwidth.* (Great bandwidth disparity between two operations is one indication they are carried out by two distinct media.) We have, then, some purely objective empirical evidence supporting the possibility that cognition involves an information-bearing medium distinct from the observed character of neurons.

This argument makes no direct appeal to qualia to justify the possibility that some "higher" cognitive activity in our organism is based on a medium distinct from neurons. This view is useful because it lets us frame an *empirical argument* against functionalism without having to complicate matters further with the vexed question of qualia.

3. Nevertheless, the medium hypothesis is certainly able to offer an account of qualia, an account that links qualia quite naturally with the genus–species distinction as applied to information-bearing media.

We have converging evidence that a peculiar medium (distinct from neurons as currently understood) is associated with both the limited bandwidth character of attention *and* with the remarkably narrow phenomenology of experience (Mangan, 1993b). This suggests (but does not prove) that the objectively observed narrow bandwidth medium of attention reflects the subjectively experienced fact of conscious experience or qualia. The subjective–objective limitation correspondence is further reason to think consciousness is a distinct medium and that the objective bandwidth findings do not simply reflect an unrelated neural bottleneck. Otherwise, we would have to assume that pure coincidence accounts for two different but correlated bandwidth anomalies.

It is possible to have good evidence that a medium of some sort is at work in our organism and yet have no specific idea about the particular constitution of that medium. For instance, people realized that some kind of medium bore genetic information long before they knew anything about DNA.

The medium hypothesis lets us place consciousness within a purely biological perspective. The answer to the genus question—What is consciousness?—is that consciousness is a distinct, information-bearing medium. But what about the species question—How does consciousness bear information? The natural answer is that *consciousness bears its information as experience.* The fact of experience distinguishes consciousness from all other media.

REFERENCES

Baars, B. 1989. *A Cognitive Theory of Consciousness.* Cambridge: Cambridge University Press.

Berlyne, D. E. 1971. *Aesthetics and Psychobiology.* New York: Appleton-Century-Crofts.

Dennett, D. 1993. Caveat emptor. *Consciousness and Cognition* 2:48–57.

Mangan, B. 1993a. Dennett, consciousness, and the sorrows of functionalism. *Consciousness and Cognition* 2:1–17.

Mangan, B. 1993b. Taking phenomenology seriously: The "fringe" and its implications for cognitive research. *Consciousness and Cognition* 2:2.

Mangan, B. (forthcoming) Consciousness as an information-bearing medium. *Psyche* http://psyche.cs.monash.au/

11 My Experience, Your Experience, and the World We Experience: Turning the Hard Problem Upside Down

Roger N. Shepard and Piet Hut

THE HARD PROBLEM OF CONSCIOUSNESS

We take the "hard problem" (Chalmers, 1995) as the first-person problem of understanding how the subjective quality of experience (including the seemingly nonphysical qualia of pains, colors, odors, etc.) can be explained as arising from a physical system described in terms of objective physical processes (whether at the level of neurons, atoms, subatomic particles, waves, strings, vacuum fluctuations, or whatever). No advance in understanding these physical processes has shown any promise of bridging the explanatory gap between physical description and subjective quality (Hut and Shepard 1996; Shepard 1993).

Nor does any such advance promise to explain how consciousness acts on the physical world. Yet, (as proposed by epiphenomenalists and often assumed by physical scientists) if conscious processes do not causally affect physical processes, why does it seem that one can control physical actions (free will)? How do some physical bodies perform the physical acts of speaking or writing, which express the hard problem of consciousness? (See Shepard 1993.)

TURNING THE HARD PROBLEM UPSIDE DOWN

Most approaches to the problem of consciousness (and of free will) build on an epistemologically weak foundation. They begin with the physical brain as described by physical science in terms of atoms, molecules, ions, electric fields, and the like. Yet the independent existence of such a physical system is an *inference* that one bases on regularities and correlations in the qualia that one directly experiences. The shakiness of the physicalist starting point is evident to those of us who experience vivid dreams populated with what we believe are independently existing physical objects (until we awaken).

The never-directly-experienced atoms, molecules, and fields that, according to the standard scientific view, constitute the material basis of any object, including a brain, are abstractions. These abstractions can be referred to only by words, diagrams, or equations, which, from the objective standpoint, are themselves but constellations of molecules or, from the subjective stand-point, only qualia in the scientist's own conscious experience. From the subjective standpoint, what the scientist means by "the physical world" can only be explained in terms of the scientist's expectations about what future experiences will ensue from the performance of particular operations. This view has been argued in various forms by physicists such as Bohr, Heisenberg, and (particularly forcefully) Bridgeman (1940).

Some expectations concern the behavior of objects that we denominate "other persons." Thus (to put the example, most appropriately, in the first person), from the experience of reading of Galileo's discovery of the moons of Jupiter, I infer that if I were to build and look through a telescope in a particular direction, I would have visual experiences similar to those described by Galileo.

Although this does not eliminate the hard problem, it may soften it. Everything is now grounded in my own indubitable immediate experience and not in a hypothesized "noumenal" world (Kant's term) of unexperienced atoms, particles, or waves. The problem of the existence of other minds is also softened in that by starting with my own subjective experience instead of with an independent "objective reality," I begin with something closer to other subjective experiences (such as yours).

Inverting the standard approach in this way, however, calls for radical changes in the way we think and talk about mind and matter. We should not point to our surrounding environment to indicate the objective physical world and to our head to indicate the locus of our subjective experience. Everything we experience (whether "out there" or "in here") is a part of our experience. The supposition that one's experience takes place somewhere else than in one's own head does not seem to have any implications for that experience. We should also resist the temptation to invoke the complexity of the brain as somehow crucial for an explanation of the quality of conscious experience. There is surely nothing complex about a momentary flash of red or twinge of pain.

The "given" from which we propose to start is not, however, pointillistic "sense data." In contrast with the British empiricists and more in line with Edmund Husserl, William James, or James Gibson, we find that what is given in our experience is a three-dimensional arrangement of objects that evoke expectations about what further experience will follow from various actions we might take (Hut and Shepard 1996). What is given is not confined to the concrete colors, shapes, sounds, tastes, odors, feels, and the like presented by any particular sensory modality. Rather, we are directly aware of relations, affordances, and meanings—including the "abstract ideas" denied by Berkeley, such as the idea of a general triangle that was neither acute nor obtuse, equilateral nor scalene.

Moreover, we do not exclude (as Berkeley did) the possible existence of a noumenal world behind the phenomena we directly experience. As a practical matter, we treat any notions about such a world as hypotheses that may be useful to the extent that they predict and explain the regularities in phenomenal experience.

CONSCIOUS EXPERIENCES BEYOND ONE'S OWN

Although we may view certain kinds of experienced regularities and surprises as manifestations of something behind the phenomena we experience, we may also view certain other kinds of experienced regularities and surprises as manifestations of other conscious minds. Thus (speaking again in the first person), I may experience another person's presenting an extended argument that leads to an unexpected conclusion. I may then convince myself of the validity of the conclusion by thinking through the argument or, perhaps, by performing an experiment. Such confirmations seem to provide compelling evidence for the occurrence of mental understandings independent of my own.

Granted, such manifestations of independent intelligences do not in themselves definitively answer the hard question of whether such intelligences experience the same qualia I do or, indeed, experience any qualia. It would, however, seem a strange and inexplicable violation of symmetry if other intelligences that express the same arguments and feelings that I do differed so radically from me as to be without consciousness.

In dreams we may also believe in the independent existence both of the physical world and of other minds. Yet, on awakening, that physical world and the other minds apparently vanish. Their apparent evanescence does not, however, preclude a dependence of their manifestations in one's consciousness on something beyond themselves. (In fact, the prevailing scientific view is that both the order and the surprises within the dream arise from ongoing activity of our own physical brains.) In short, there may be some justification in both waking and dreaming consciousness for hypothesizing the existence of something behind what we experience as an explanation for both the predictable and the creative aspects of these types of consciousness.

Even if we start with experience, then, we still have the problem of where to draw a line between the physical systems in our experience that are thus accompanied by "their own" conscious experiences and the systems that are not accompanied by conscious experiences. We even have the problem of distinguishing between processes within the *same* physical system that are or are not conscious. If a particular neurophysiological activity is necessary and sufficient for a particular experience (of one's own) or a report of an experience (in another person), what distinguishes that activity from the electrochemically identical kind of activity that is usually supposed not to have such an experiential accompaniment?

Would it not be less arbitrary and more symmetrical to suppose that every so-called physical event has a corresponding conscious manifestation, just as every conscious manifestation has been supposed to have a corresponding physical event?

THE CASE OF THE JOKE IN A DREAM

Although we may believe that regularity and, hence, predictability is especially indicative of an independently existing physical world, we may believe that novel and surprising events are especially indicative of an independently functioning mind. Particularly suggestive in this connection are instances in which a dream leads to an unexpected event or punch line, which the dreamer considers in retrospect to have required premeditation, cleverness, or humor. Such examples (perhaps even more than the well-known "split-brain" and "blindsight" phenomena) suggest that another mind, of which "I" am not conscious, is operating within "my" own brain. Could it be that all neural activities are accompanied by conscious experiences, but that only the activities with direct access to the speech centers of the brain are ordinarily considered as conscious?

We have kept dream journals for many years. The journals contain examples of the phenomenon in which we are surprised by a joke seemingly contrived by some agency outside our own consciousness. Following are three examples, two recorded by Shepard and one by Hut.

1. Shepard's dream of the early morning of February 12, 1972:

On a coffee table in front of me I notice a large-format hardcover book on dining out around the world. I pick up the book and it falls open to what appears to be the title page for a chapter: "Tips on Dining Out in Central Africa." With curiosity aroused, I turn the page. Across the following two-page spread, there is printed only the huge bold-face admonition, "DON'T EAT THE FOOD!" (Shepard 1990, p. 35.)

2. Shepard's dream of the early morning of January 17, 1979:

I am with my wife, who is consulting with her physician. My wife has expressed concern about how much her teaching job is cutting into her time with our children. Then, at the end of the consultation, she asks, "Do you think I should have a *mammogram*?"

The doctor replies, "No, I don't think that's necessary," and then, with an impish smile slowly spreading across his face, he adds, "But, given the professional demands on your time, your kids could use a *gramma, ma'm!*"

Doing a double take, I am greatly amused to realize that relative to "mammogram," "gramma, ma'm" is a phonetically perfect *anagram*.

3. Hut's dream of March 11, 1981 (a *lucid* dream, i.e., a dream in which Hut has become aware that he is dreaming):

I walked into a bar, where I found a group of people sitting, who looked at me when I entered, and immediately started singing in unison:

"This is Piet's dream,
We are all here,
And that is why
We get free beer."

As we already noted, evidence that intelligent thought has gone on outside one's own consciousness may not in itself entail that such intelligent thought was *conscious* thought. But, to the extent that one believes the evidence for intelligent thought as evidence for an independent consciousness when the evidence comes from another person in one's waking experience, on what grounds should one reject such an inference to an independent consciousness when the evidence arises in one's dream? If we assume, as most researchers do, that intelligent thought depends on neural activity, the principal difference between the two cases may merely be whether that neural activity occurs in another person's brain or in one's own brain.

ANOTHER "DIMENSION" COEXTENSIVE WITH SPACE AND TIME

When we try to make sense of the relation between subjective consciousness and the organizational structure of the brain as an objective physical entity, we are baffled by a seemingly unbridgeable gap. In our detailed understanding of the functioning of the human brain, great progress has been made since Descartes struggled with this problem, and now we certainly understand the correlations between physical processes and reports of conscious experiences much better. It is not clear, however, that our quantitative progress has translated into anything that can begin to bridge the gap.

It may be significant that we use spatial metaphors in talking about our bafflement (e.g., "gap"), or about anything to do with deeply felt meaning (e.g., the "depth" of meaning, the "height" of experience). In any given situation, even after specifying the configuration of the material elements in a region around a point in space and time, we still seem to have extra degrees of freedom. We can still move to a different level of interpretation and appreciation. The whole notion of "emergent properties" (another spatial metaphor, that is often presented as an explanation but so far is no more than a label for an as yet ill-understood though ubiquitous phenomenon) rests on this freedom.

Our conjecture is that it would make sense to investigate the structure of reality by positing a "metadimension" that gives room for consciousness, much as time gives room for motion. We illustrated this notion with an analogy (Hut and Shepard 1996). Start with space only and try to explain the presence of time. Yes, time is everywhere, like space. But, no, time is not draped over space, like a sauce or fluid or ether. Neither is time an epiphenomenon, a nonessential additive, or add-on. Rather, time and space are equiprimordial, not reducible to each other, although to some extent they are transformable into each other according to classic relativity theory. Similarly, perhaps all existence partakes in another, equally primordial metadimension, the presence of which allows conscious experience to arise analogously to the way in which the presence of time allows motion to occur.

CONCLUSION

1. The only epistemologically justifiable starting point is what I experience. I adopt the notion of an enduring physical world behind what I experience to

the degree that it explains and predicts regularities and correlations within my experience. Brains are part of what arises within my experience. I admit the existence of other minds (i.e., conscious experiences other than my own) to the extent that this helps me to understand why other bodies similar to my own behave in ways similar to the behavior that I consciously initiate.

2. Particularly compelling, among the kinds of evidence for other minds, are the instances in which I experience another person's presenting a line of thought that ends with a conclusion that surprises me but which I later accept as valid, ingenious, or humorous. Instances in which such evidence arises from individuals in my dreams suggest that other minds are associated with what I have called "my own" brain.

3. Possibly, reality includes, in addition to dimensions of space and time, a dimension that provides for consciousness in much the way that space provides for configuration and time provides for motion.

ACKNOWLEDGMENTS

Preparation of this work was supported by a grant to Hut and Shepard from the Sloan Foundation. This chapter is an abbreviated version of our paper as it was presented by Shepard at the Tucson II conference. A longer version, which develops some of the ideas more fully (but omits the case of the joke in a dream), was subsequently prepared (Hut and Shepard 1996).

REFERENCES

Bridgman, P. W. 1940. Science: Public or private? *Philosophy of Science* 7:36–48.

Chalmers, D. 1995. Facing up to the problem of consciousness. *Journal of Consciousness Studies* 2:200–219.

Shepard, R. N. 1990. *Mind Sights*. New York: W. H. Freeman.

Shepard, R. N. 1993. On the physical basis, linguistic representation, and conscious experience of colors. In G. Harman, ed., *Conceptions of the Mind*. Hillsdale, NJ: Erlbaum, pp. 217–245.

Hut, P., and R. N. Shepard. 1996. Turning "the hard problem" upside down and sideways. *Journal of Consciousness Studies* 3:313–329.

12 The Boundary Problem for Phenomenal Individuals

Gregg H. Rosenberg

The consciousness of an individual has inherent boundaries. Only some experiences are part of *my* consciousness; most experiences in the world are not. Arguably, these boundaries are what individuate *me* as a phenomenal individual in the world. This view immediately poses a problem that any theory of consciousness must answer. How *can* consciousness have boundaries? What element of the natural world dictates the way that these boundaries are drawn? On the face of it, the physical world does not have inherent boundary makers at the midlevel where consciousness exists, but consciousness has boundaries, nevertheless.

The boundary problem can be difficult to see at first. To begin, reflect on the fact that phenomenal individuals come in discrete tokens. I am one such token, so are you, and so is Bill Clinton. These tokens, the individuated phenomenal fields of experiencing subjects, contain coevolving elements. In an elusive sense of "unified," nature unifies the coevolving elements into a subject of experience. Together, the unity and boundedness of the phenomenal field are at the core of the concept of a phenomenal individual.

The possibility of these kinds of boundaries is essential to the possibility that the world could have human consciousness. The boundary problem comes from appreciating that the boundaries are primitive relative to our physical image of the world. Through such appreciation, one can begin to become aware that nature must have intrinsic structure that we do not yet fully appreciate.

The problem starts with observations that help define for us what it is to be a phenomenal individual. First, human consciousness is only a *species* of phenomenal individual. Other kinds of phenomenal individualities may exist in other kinds of beings. A phenomenal individual is a manifold of qualitative entities. We only roughly name these entities for ourselves with words like feeling, sensation, and appearance.

Second, for a given individual, not every feeling, sensation, or appearance that occurs in the world happens within the scope of the individual's phenomenal field. Clearly, phenomenal individuals *have* boundaries because feelings can be divided into those that occur within an individual's experience and those that do not. These events help to create subjects of experience, and these subjects are the phenomenal individuals to which I refer.

Third, in humans, the phenomenal individual is associated with a human body and its cognitive processing. Humans and the activity of human cognitive systems are individuated at a midlevel of the physical world. Typically, individuation of objects at this midlevel of nature is fluid, sensitive to context, and relative to interest. This kind of individuation is highly conceptual and hinges on facts about the abstract organization and causal cohesion of lower-level activity. Thus, levels of abstract organization and causal cohesion exist between microphysics and human cognition and between human cognition and the universe as a whole.

These observations should be obvious. The hard part is realizing that the phenomenal individuals could have been different individuals than they are and could have been different in ways that would prohibit human consciousness. Therefore, we need to explain why, in the first place, phenomenal individuals can be associated with specific, midlevel patterns of interaction and organization.

Here is a pointer to orient the imagination. Internally, the midlevel patterns consist of other patterns of interaction and organization. The phenomenal field of the subject stretches across the boundaries of these interactions. Yet, one's cognitive systems are also part of even larger patterns than our individual patterns. Somehow, the boundaries of the phenomenal individual do not continue to overflow and enlarge into these patterns.

Why do the boundaries exist *here* rather than *there*? This is not a question about why *my* (or *your*) consciousness is as large or as small as it is. It is a question about why a phenomenal individual that is me, or you, exists, rather than one phenomenal subject that is both of us, or many phenomenal subjects that are parts of us. What is special about some patterns to allow them to provide boundaries for phenomenal individuals? Unfortunately, the very obviousness of our own existence as midlevel phenomenal individuals is an obstacle to appreciating the question. Following are several thought experiments designed to loosen our intuitive grip on the inevitability of the boundaries that actually exist.

THE BRAIN AND ITS SUBSYSTEMS

The boundaries of our phenomenal consciousness correspond to the boundaries of certain kinds of activity in our brains. For instance, some evidence suggests that specially synchronized activity in and around the cortex is the boundary maker for human phenomenal individuals. To clarify the problem, consider whether any of the subsystems oscillating within the whole might also support a phenomenal individual. For example, certain patterns of synchronized activity carry and organize auditory information from our ears.

Is there a phenomenal individual associated solely with this activity? If yes, the picture should be that within ourselves as fully human phenomenal individuals, as experiencing subjects, there exist other phenomenal individuals. The others are perfectly complete subjects of experience, but are much simpler.

Thus, like Russian dolls, there are individuals within individuals within individuals, all of them phenomenal subjects.

An answer to our question should exist. The very definiteness of what it means to be a phenomenal individual seems to require an answer, and extension by analogy should allow us to make sense of the question. Recall the physical image of the world—we have a multitude of interacting microphysical entities at different places and times, the multitude congealing into a macroscopic whirlwind of finely layered patterns of organization. Imagine looking at these patterns from the perspective of a third-person observer. Note the coherence of causal and abstract organization at the many levels, and the many kinds that exist. We know that a set of these patterns supports boundaries that allow for the existence of us, within which boundaries we are one kind of phenomenal individual.

The present question is whether nature supports other kinds of feeling subjects, other kinds of phenomenal individuals. We are asking whether, analogous to *us* as phenomenal individuals, there might exist simpler, experiencing subjects. These subjects would have boundaries given by *subsets* of the activity that determines our experience as a whole. The subsets we are considering are like the complete set in many ways. They share common biology with the larger set of events; they carry information and are processing it; they process it in a very similar way; they are internally synchronized and coherent. Is any one of these subsets, itself, a phenomenal individual?

After reflecting on the physical situation, both yes and no answers seem possible. This point is merely conceptual, a point about how our intuitive understanding of what it is to be a phenomenal individual leaves the question open. Why *couldn't* phenomenal individuals at many levels of processing exist, associated with subsets of the cognitive activity that corresponds to our own phenomenal individuality? On the other hand, why *would* they exist?

Because such brain activity, taken as a whole, can correspond to the existence of phenomenal individuals, us, the point seems to support a mild claim. Our intuitive concept of what it is to be a phenomenal individual allows the possibility of simpler phenomenal individuals. These individuals would possess manifolds of much less rich and less cognitive experience. Therefore, the physical activity corresponding to the existence of one phenomenal individual might support other, simpler phenomenal individuals via the simpler patterns of organization it contains. Of course, it might not.

Traditional panpsychism takes advantage of the looseness in the concept to make its position intelligible. Process philosophies, such as that of Whitehead, typically take advantage of the looseness by making feeling and phenomenal individuality precognitive primitives. I want to parlay the looseness, in stages, into the full-blown boundary problem for phenomenal individuals.

FROM HUMAN CONSCIOUSNESS TO THE BOUNDARY PROBLEM

The first scenario we need to consider is a variant on Ned Block's well-known fiction of the Chinese nation simulating the functionality of a human brain. To make the case a little less fantastic, we can imagine the simulation of another, simpler kind of organism's brain—a fish. (Very likely, a fish is a phenomenal individual.)

Imagine building a robot fish. Imagine also that we have designed its nervous system to be functionally isomorphic to the nervous system of a naturally occurring fish. Furthermore, we have made the processing remote in the usual way, with inputs and outputs to the fish's central nervous system employing relays. The relays send signals to remote stations manned by human beings. The humans monitor the signals as they come in and relay an output to other destinations. Some signals are sent between remote stations and some are relayed back to the fish as motor outputs. In this way, we imagine that the relay system is functionally isomorphic to an actual fish's brain.

Does this system support the existence of a phenomenal individual? Block urges, plausibly, that our concept of phenomenal consciousness does not necessitate a positive answer. Nevertheless, the argument fails to show that the system could not, in fact, support the existence of a phenomenal individual. As functionalists sometimes point out, it seems just as surprising that our brains support consciousness, but, nevertheless, we know that they do.

The fact that the system has parts that are phenomenal homunculi should not make a difference. In the previous section I argued for the consistency of the idea of phenomenal individuals whose physical organization supported other phenomenal individuals. Because the human relay system is functionally like the fish's brain, it is conceivable that this system supports a phenomenal individual. In fact, both ideas seem to be possibilities:

1. Each homunculus is a phenomenal individual, but the whole system is not.

2. Each homunculus is a phenomenal individual, and so is the whole system.

These possibilities are not so innocent. We can redirect the principles that make them plausible back to a local system for the fish. The homunculi system is functionally isomorphic to the fish's cognitive system. Each homunculus maps onto some important part of the organizational structure of a naturally occurring fish. Imagine the mapping being made with one of the homunculi (Edna) mapped onto some functional part of the fish (the E-system). The first possibility seems to ground the possibility that the fish's E-system, the part corresponding to Edna, could be a phenomenal individual although the fish as a whole would not be.

By admitting the first possibility, we are admitting the coherence of a world in which (1) a system may contain phenomenal individuals; (2) the system may be functionally isomorphic to the fish's system; and yet (3) the system may not be a phenomenal individual. In the previous section, I argued that it seemed coherent that ordinary cognitive subsystems could be phenomenal individuals themselves. To imagine the E-system as a phenomenal individual, but not the fish, all one must do is combine the points.

To combine them, conceptually shift the boundaries that make phenomenal individuals. Shift the view of nature so that the phenomenal boundaries stretch through the E-system to encompass all the activity within it but do not overflow the boundaries of the E-system. The larger individual is abolished. Instead, the fish is a collection of simpler phenomenal individuals in interaction and cooperation. The experience of the E-system would be simpler and vastly different from the experiences of Edna. Nevertheless, one can coherently change the intuitively assigned boundaries and thereby rob the fish as a whole of its status as a phenomenal individual. Lacking clear criteria for natural boundaries, one can conceptually rearrange the boundaries and force individuality down to the E-system level.

Once we have seen the essential analogy between Edna and the E-system, we can begin to engage in other conceptual shifts. For instance, it certainly seems possible that the E-system might *not* be a phenomenal individual. It seems perfectly coherent that the only phenomenal individual associated with the fish's brain is the one existing at the global fish level. The coherence of the idea that natural fish do not have phenomenal E-systems seems to support a third possibility:

3. The homunculi system is a phenomenal individual, but *none* of the homunculi are phenomenal individuals.

Certainly, we all are confident that, *in fact*, Edna would be a phenomenal individual. We still need to explain why the third possibility is not true of our world. For instance, people are often inclined to think that phenomenal individuals emerge at a certain level of complexity. That might not be correct, but it seems like an empirical possibility. If it is possible, imagining the third possibility merely requires imagining such a world, dictating an appropriate kind of complexity, and moving the starting point upwards past Edna. The complexity point at which phenomenal individuals emerge would be higher than that possessed by the homunculi, but not the homunculi fish. The analog is that Edna could be a zombie and a component in a system supporting a phenomenal individual. What stops phenomenal individuality right *there*, between Edna's ears?

This reconception of boundaries is just the flip side of my earlier suggestion in which reconception was a movement of the phenomenal boundaries to lower levels of organization, which robbed wholes of their phenomenal individuality. Here, the reconception is to a higher level of organization, which robs *parts* of the phenomenal individuality. Such a world would be one in which the eddies of coherent causation that are human beings would not support phenomenal individuality. No human phenomenal consciousness would exist. Instead, the phenomenal individuals exist at a higher level. As humans move and swirl and interact with other eddies, the phenomenal individuals arises only for the supersystem. The possibility is analogous to the way we (or many of us) normally imagine that our cognitive subsystems contribute to our conscious lives without themselves being phenomenal individuals.

These science fiction tales are meant to make a vivid point. Our intuitive understanding of phenomenal individuality leaves boundary conditions very flexible. Once we have appreciated the basic point, we do not need to use thought experiments to make it. Even actual systems like economies, political systems, and nation states bring it out.

An economy is an extremely complex system of interacting components. In its own way, it processes and reacts to information and self-organizes. As a physical system, it stores information and seems to have a kind of memory, a synchrony between its parts, massive parallel communication, and so forth. The scale at which this process takes place is much larger than in an individual brain and much different in detail, but most basic kinds of activity exist. Suggesting that an economy might represent some kind of group mind is nothing new. The question is not just a philosopher's question; it is a legitimate question of fact about something that exists in the real world.

Once we see the possibility that *both* the economy and our bodies might support phenomenal individuals, we are only a short step from seeing another possibility. Perhaps *only* the economy was a phenomenal individual because we are analogous to it as neurons are to us. The boundaries of phenomenal individuality, once loosened, can begin to shift radically. Why could our bodies not be local, nonphenomenal causal eddies within a larger phenomenal individual? What grounds the bruteness of the boundaries?

THE BOUNDARY PROBLEM

The boundary shifting that occurs in these thought experiments is enabled because information about pattern and organization alone does not fix the boundaries. At higher levels of organization in the physical world, we individuate most objects via an act of abstraction, a process that involves extracting a significant pattern from the flux of microphysical interaction.

Merely adding these facts about pattern or abstract organization to the causation between the microphysical entities does not seem to go far enough in determining the proper sense of "inherent" in the idea that a phenomenal individual enjoys a kind of inherent individuality. One can coherently hypothesize almost as many ways of determining boundaries for phenomenal individuals as there are of abstractly organizing the patterns of microphysical interaction. The resulting scenarios are intuitively bizarre, but bizarreness is not inconsistency. That the boundaries can be drawn as they are, can be drawn in a way that allows for human consciousness, stands out as a brute fact.

At this point we are faced with the need to understand more deeply what it is to be an inherent individual in the natural world. We need a natural criterion for individuation, one that illuminates the specialness of some patterns compared with others as supporters of phenomenal individuality. A good set of candidates are the fields of the most primitive particles (or strings or whatnot). Each has a natural dynamic unity, one that seems inherent. A phenomenal individual might be associated with each of these particles.

This suggestion threatens human consciousness. If the fields of the primitive individuals of physics are the only natural individuals, the rest of us are mere abstractions from the pattern of their interaction. Each may be a simple phenomenal individual, supporting brief, firefly flicks of feeling buzzing at the lowest levels of spacetime, but above them the world is dark. This world is the panpsychist's world painted surreally: feeling, feeling everywhere, but none of it can think. This world does not include a mechanism to allow the creation of higher-level individuals. No mechanism can bootstrap us to human consciousness.

Perhaps by flowing through the lines of interactions, the phenomenal individuals could outrun the boundaries of the primitive individuals of physics. Here the trap concerns stopping the flow of interaction. It can seem that the flow of interaction in the universe is inherently unbounded, that no merely abstract pattern presents a natural condition for containing it. The patterns merely direct the flow from one area to another, orchestrate it, and move it along through the continuity of the universe. According to this view, phenomenal individuality must follow the boundaries to their limits along the lines of interaction, which creates the possibility of a universal phenomenal individual, perhaps some kind of cosmic consciousness. Unfortunately, no room exists for the more mundane, midlevel boundaries necessary for human consciousness to exist. Like the first view, this view banishes midlevel individuals from existence.

Thus, one view pushes us inward, past the point of midlevel individuation, to the realm of the subatomic. There, and only there, do we find natural, inherent individuals. Another view pushes us outward, past the boundaries of the subatomic individuals, ever outward along the lines of interaction, racing past the midlevel to the continuous unfolding of the cosmos. Only there, at the level of the universe, do we find an inherent individual.

Neither view allows for human beings. To navigate the middle ground, we must find a principle that allows us to push the boundaries outward, but only *just so far*. We must be able to go only "so far" past the microphysical level, but no further. *That* is the boundary problem for phenomenal individuals.

13 Folk Psychology, Science, and the Criminal Law

David Hodgson

On June 13, 1994, two residents of a youth refuge in suburban Sydney, girls aged 15 and 17, dragged Mrs. B, a worker at the refuge, into the refuge office, strangled her, and took turns stabbing her to death. The girls had originally planned to tie up Mrs. B and steal money and the refuge's van, but they became angry when Mrs. B was not cooperative. At the trial, psychiatrists gave evidence that each girl suffered from a personality disorder caused by a long history of abuse, violence, and deprivation. Both girls were convicted of murder.

Cases such as this often reignite debate about how and why innocent children develop into persons who commit terrible crimes—is it *nature* (something in their genetic makeup) or is it *nurture* (something in their environment, such as child abuse). However, I believe an even more fundamental question, which is less frequently the subject of community debate (perhaps because it is considered unanswerable), is whether anything *more* than nature and nurture is operating, whether any room exists in the etiology of such a crime for common-sense ideas of free will and responsibiity. If there is no room, what sense can be made of the notions of criminal responsibility that are routinely applied by courts dealing with criminal cases?

Our criminal law makes absolutely crucial the distinction between acts that involve a guilty mind and acts that do not—a distinction meaningful in terms of common-sense beliefs about free will and about how people behave generally (these beliefs have been called folk psychology) but which does not at present have any fundamental scientific explanation. This situation raises stark questions about the appropriateness of the legal categories relevant to the distinction and to the place of expert scientific and medical evidence about the categories.

In this chapter, I suggest that, in dealing with questions of criminal responsibility, we should assume that, except to the extent that the contrary is proved, common-sense beliefs about how people behave, including beliefs about free will and responsibility, are valid and respectable. First, I look at the fundamental distinction that our criminal law draws between acts that involve a guilty mind and acts that do not. Next, I outline some theoretical problems of the distinction. I then argue that the distinction is fundamental to widely held and strengthening views about justice and human rights. I conclude by suggesting that because theoretical attacks on the distinction are inconclusive, it would be worthwhile to make explicit and to refine a theoretical framework that makes sense of the operation of individual responsibility, together with nature and nurture, in the commission of crimes.

FOLK PSYCHOLOGY IN THE CRIMINAL LAW

A key principle of civilized criminal law is the principle of *mens rea*: that, generally, no person can be convicted of a crime unless the prosecution proves not only a guilty act but also a guilty mind. The action said to be in breach of the law must be *conscious* and *voluntary*. In relation to particular offenses, further folk-psychological concepts of *belief* and *intention* may be necessary for *mens rea*. For example, in theft of property, it has to be proved that the accused *did not believe* that he or she had a legal right to take the property and that the accused *did intend* to deprive the owner of the property.

The crime of rape is an interesting example, because the folk psychology of both the victim and the accused is particularly important. It has to be proved that sexual intercourse took place *without the consent* of the woman and that the accused *did not believe* there was consent. Whether one regards consent as being *subjective willingness* or *communication of willingness*, it irreducibly involves the folk-psychological concept of a willingness or voluntariness that is not vitiated by coercion, mistake, or lack of understanding. (This raises a hard question for persons who attack folk psychology: If folk-psychological notions were to go the way of discredited notions such as the heat substance caloric, what do the critics see as replacing the *consent of the woman* as the crucial factor in determining whether a particular act of sexual intercourse is to be regarded as unlawful and subject to criminal sanctions?)

The questions of *mens rea* and criminal responsibility are usually decided by the court (generally, by a jury) without the aid of any expert scientific or medical evidence; juries are requested by judges to use common sense and experience of the world and of how people behave in deciding these questions. Accordingly, in these cases, there is generally no explicit conflict in the court between the common-sense, folk-psychological categories that the law uses and scientific accounts of causation of human behavior, which might tend to discredit these categories.

In some cases, however, particularly in relation to defenses of insanity and sane automatism, these categories and other folk-psychological categories may become the subject of expert scientific and medical evidence (usually from psychiatrists or psychologists, but occasionally from neuroscientists). Thus, there is the potential for conflict between the folk-psychological categories and scientific accounts of causation of behavior. These defenses involve folk-psychological concepts such as defect of reason from a disease of the mind, knowing what one is doing, knowing that what one is doing is wrong, willed or voluntary action, and ability to control one's actions. Scientific and medical evidence touching on these categories tends to raise problems because, once one deals with human behavior in terms of scientific cause and effect, there appears to be no room left for folk-psychological concepts, which presuppose that persons are normally autonomous agents.

THEORETICAL PROBLEMS OF FOLK PSYCHOLOGY

All the categories I have identified, including the ones about which expert evidence may be given, are prescientific, folk-psychological concepts. The language that describes them is nonscientific, and, except in the clearest cases, the existence of the psychological state that they describe is not susceptible to scientific proof.

The fundamental reason that there is no scientific proof is that consciousness itself has no scientific explanation. For example, no scientific answer exists for the question whether computers could be made to be conscious (e.g., to feel pain); if an answer did exist, what would distinguish a conscious computer from a nonconscious one? Because there is no scientific account of what it is to be a conscious subject with experiences and the feeling of freedom and control, it is not surprising that no scientific explanation exists for what is acting voluntarily, knowing what one is doing (much less, knowing whether the action is wrong), having control over one's actions, and so on. Yet, these concepts are absolutely central to important issues of criminal responsibility—indeed, they are also central to our view of ourselves, our relationships, and our concepts of fairness and proper behavior (Strawson 1962).

Not only does no systematic scientific explanation of these concepts and categories exist, mainstream science and philosophy often seem to suggest that these concepts and categories, particularly concepts involving ideas of freedom and responsibility, are not intellectually respectable. Three broad trends can be identified in this view.

First, there is the recognition, which has come to the fore at least since the time of Freud, that a substantial part of our motivation is unconscious. More recently, psychological experiments have shown that our common-sense view of our behavior is often misconceived, partly because of a capacity we have for (unconsciously) fabricating and accepting plausible but untrue stories to explain our experiences and actions (Dennett 1991). Given that unconscious processes contribute to our actions, what is there about *us* beyond these unconscious processes, that determines how our conscious processes develop and that can make some mental processes guilty or blameworthy but others not so?

Second, and more broadly, there is the tendency to consider human beings as the products of nature and nurture, that is, purely the outcome of genes and environment. Whatever human beings become and do is understood as having causes in their heredity and in the circumstances in which they have been placed from time to time. Cases such as that of the girls at the Sydney youth refuge suggest that early home environment can predispose individuals to criminal behavior; much evidence supports this view.

Genetic and congenital factors may also be important. For example, according to Peter Fenwick (Clift 1993), a British forensic psychiatrist, there is evidence that

abnormal brain development during the fifth month of pregnancy can result in the absence of conscience in the child and hence an inability to empathize with others. High testosterone and low five-hydroxytryptamine levels in the brain result in a tendency to violence. Hence violent behavior is much more common in men than in women and especially amongst men with low 5-HT levels.

The evidence for links between the brain's physiology and criminal behavior is explored at length in Moir and Jessell (1995).

Thus, in the case of the girls in Sydney, it may not be reasonable to regard the murder as involving freely willed choices for which the killers were responsible—the murder was simply the outcome of the kind of persons the girls had become, by reason of nature and nurture, genes and environment. And if the girls' own previous choices and actions contributed to making the girls what they were, the previous choices and actions were themselves the outcome of genes and environment.

Third, and even more generally, the scientific view of the world assumes the universality of causal laws. This view regards all systems as developing over time in accordance with universal laws of nature, possibly with some randomness. That scientific view appears to leave no room for our common-sense view of choice and of intentional or voluntary action, much less for any notion of responsibility or a guilty mind.

An example of the scientific view of human beings is provided by Colin Blakemore in *The Mind Machine* (1988). In the final chapter Blakemore begins with three sentences that he says encapsulate the central thesis of his book:

The human brain is a machine, which alone accounts for all our actions, our most private thoughts, our beliefs. It creates the state of consciousness and the sense of self. It makes the mind.

Blakemore then sets out a number of cases in which criminal acts were committed under various mental conditions: hypoglycemia, a sublethal dose of chlorpyrifos from handling insecticide, premenstrual tension, epilepsy, manic depression, and deprivation and abuse in early life. Blakemore's main conclusions are stated as follows:

All our actions are products of the activity of our brains. It seems to me to make no sense (in scientific terms) to try to distinguish sharply between acts that result from conscious intention and those that are pure reflexes or that are caused by disease or damage to the brain. We *feel* ourselves, usually, to be in control of our actions, but that feeling is itself a product of the brain, whose machinery has been designed, on the basis of its functional utility, by means of natural selection. (p. 270)

Somewhat similar views can be found in the work of philosophers such as Daniel Dennett (1984, 1991), Patricia and Paul Churchland (1986, 1990), and in the work of other neuroscientists, such as Francis Crick (1994). The total abandonment of any element of desert and retribution in punishment is advocated by philosopher Ted Honderich (1993).

FOLK PSYCHOLOGY AND HUMAN RIGHTS

Judges are not unaware of the tension between the categories that the law uses and the views of mainstream scientists and philosophers. However, there is no sign that the law will move away from using such categories, and although the law's use of these categories can undoubtedly be very much improved, I contend (contrary to Blakemore) that there is good reason to continue to use these or similar categories, in particular to continue to insist on the fundamental distinction between acts that are voluntary and acts that are not.

Such categories have not been refuted by science or philosophy, and they are not merely entrenched in common sense; they are also presupposed in deeply held principles of justice and human rights, which are regarded as essential prerequisites for civilized societies. Indeed, these principles are increasingly recognized and, where possible, promoted by international law.

These principles give great weight to the autonomy of people and require respect for that autonomy. Accordingly, a citizen is generally entitled to freedom from interference from the coercive processes of the State unless he or she voluntarily breaches a fair rule of law publicly promulgated by the State. Thus, a citizen has a choice about whether to be liable to coercion; in this regard, folk-psychological categories such as belief, will, and voluntariness of action are of central importance.

This is not to suggest that criminals should be punished as retribution simply because that is what they deserve. On the contrary, what I am saying is entirely consistent with the view that the coercive system that is the criminal law is justified solely by its utility, because of the need to protect the majority of citizens from dangerous and antisocial activities of others. But, given that society needs such a system, the question is how the system should identify the persons to whom the coercion should be applied, and how it should determine how much coercion should be applied to these people.

The solution that has been adopted by civilized societies that have respect for justice and human rights is what I call the *human rights qualification* to the power of the State to coerce its citizens. As a general principle, the system should allow coercion to be applied only to people who have been proved, by due process of law, to have voluntarily acted in breach of a public law, and no more coercion should be applied than is proportional to the criminality involved.

It could be argued that there are good utilitarian or consequentialist reasons for the human rights qualification, reasons that do not require acknowledgment of the validity of any idea of criminal responsibility that legitimizes punishment or any basic distinction between acts that involve a guilty mind and acts that do not (see Hart 1968). For example, a good consequentialist argument is that there should be parsimony in threatening and applying coercion. Because, generally, only voluntary actions are susceptible to deterrence by threat of punishment, it makes sense to threaten and apply coercion only in respect to voluntary actions. But even this argument presupposes a fundamental distinction between actions that are voluntary and actions that are not.[1]

However, this view does not do away with the need to be able to rely on appeals to justice and human rights, and thereby on the basic distinction between acts that are voluntary and acts that are not—particularly because consequentialist arguments are irredeemably inconclusive. Governments that do not recognize the human rights qualification to the application of the coercive processes of the State generally assert that the good of society overrides human rights considerations; thus, for example, the detention without trial for political opponents is justified. The strengthening consensus of reasonable opinion throughout the world is that such an approach can be justified only in cases of real emergency, and then only as a temporary measure pending resolution of the emergency and as a part of the process of establishing or returning to a normality in which the human rights qualification does apply.

If one is limited to arguments about consequences, it is impossible to make a case that would convince anyone who wished not to be convinced; it is impossible to prove what all the consequences of the alternatives would be, let alone to prove which of the totalities of consequences would be "better." For example, imagine trying to prove to a previous Soviet government (or to Russians who now hanker for the "good old days") that there would have been better consequences if dissidents had not been confined in mental asylums, or trying to prove to the present Chinese government that the recognition of human rights qualification to the use of the coercive powers of the State would have had better consequences than not recognizing them (see "Three Mile Island Effect" in Dennett 1995).

Acceptance of the independent force of the considerations of fairness that justify the human rights qualification would mean that positive justification, in terms of real emergency, clear and present danger, and the like, would be needed to override the qualification. If justice and human rights are given independent weight, quite a heavy onus can be placed on governments that seek to deny human rights to their citizens.

Views about human rights are being increasingly recognized and promoted in international law and in the domestic law of many countries. For example, the Canadian Charter of Rights and Freedom requires that the criminal law respect "the principles of fundamental justice." The Canadian Supreme Court, in 1990, decided that those principles required that a person not be convicted of murder unless he or she actually intended that death would result from his or her conduct; the Court held invalid a law to the contrary: *R. v Martineau*, 2 5CR 633 (1990). My point is not that the Court was necessarily correct in its views of fundamental justice; rather, that this case illustrates how the importance of human rights and justice is being recognized.

A COMMON FRAMEWORK OF UNDERSTANDING

I contend that ideas of human rights, which are widely and increasingly accepted, depend crucially on discriminating between persons whose conduct makes it fair and permissible that their freedom be curtailed and persons whose conduct does not make it fair and permissible that their freedom be curtailed. If conduct is to make curtailment of freedom fair and permissible, it must at least involve voluntary action in breach of a public law.

If the notion of a guilty mind—and the crucial distinction between acts that are voluntary and acts that are not—is discredited, human rights will be damaged; there will appear to be no rational basis for saying that it is fair, and thus permissible, to curtail the freedom of a person who has had the bad luck to be caused by genes and environment to become a person who acts in breach of the law, but unfair, and thus impermissible, to curtail the freedom of a person who, without breaching any law, has had the bad luck to be regarded by the government as a danger to society.[2]

This approach does not mean that the folk-psychological categories and distinctions of the type I have discussed must be intellectually respectable. I think they probably are (Hodgson, 1991, 1994a, 1994b, 1995, 1996a, 1996b), but many scientists and philosophers argue that they are not. I suggest, however, that it does mean that, at least in relation to questions of criminal responsibility, the reasonable course for all of us, including scientists and philosophers, is to proceed on the assumption that categories of this type are valid and important and to continue to proceed on this assumption *unless and until* scientists, philosophers, or both (1) come up with a model of human behavior, without these categories, on which a workable system of justice and human rights can be based or (2) prove that the categories have no validity.

Scientists and philosophers are nowhere near doing either thing. Such a model of behavior has hardly been attempted, and I do not think that many scientists or philosophers would be sufficiently arrogant and blinkered to suggest that they are near to disproving the validity of the categories. So long as consciousness remains unexplained, the mechanistic view of the mind can, as Crick (1994) concedes, be no more than a hypothesis. In our everyday lives we all proceed on an assumption that the categories are valid (Strawson 1962), and even Dennett admits that we cannot maintain a mechanistic stance in relation to our own actions (Dennett 1978).

It is entirely appropriate for scientists to hypothesize a mechanistic view of the brain–mind, to explore the implications of the hypothesis, and to see how much of the brain–mind operation can be explained in terms of the hypothesis. Enormous advances have been achieved in our understanding of the brain–mind in this way. What I think is unfortunate is (1) that the hypothesis is often treated by scientists and philosophers as if it were established fact—indeed, one which (according to persons such as Blakemore) should be accepted in the application of criminal law; (2) that hardly any of the elite of neuroscience, cognitive science, and philosophy seem to recognize the possibility of an alternative hypothesis that makes sense of folk psychology, much less attempt to explore and refine such an alternative hypothesis; and (3) that much effort of the elite seems to be directed towards discrediting folk psychology and, thereby, the fundamental distinction between actions for which a person is responsible and actions for which a person is not responsible. Thus, we find assertions that folk-psychological explanations are like the prescientific explanations of heat by the heat substance caloric (Churchland 1986; Churchland 1990), that conscious experiences are fictions (Dennett 1991), that free will is an illusion (Crick 1993), and that free will is impossible (Strawson 1986).

The time has come for attention to be given by the elite to making explicit and to refining, as a tentative working framework, an alternative hypothesis in which the central distinction of folk psychology has a respectable place alongside the concepts of neuroscience and cognitive science. My suggestions for a theoretical framework follow. They represent a general approach to the relationship between the brain and the mind (which I have been suggesting for some time), but they are presented here as a provisional working hypothesis for application to criminal responsibility.

1. The human brain–mind is to be considered as a physical and mental whole; it has a *physical aspect*, in relation to which a purely objective, third-person approach is appropriate, and a *mental aspect*, which presupposes the existence of a conscious subject or agent and which can be understood only in terms of the first-person experiences and actions of such a subject.

2. The development over time of this system can be considered in terms of either the physical or the mental aspect:

(a) In terms of the physical aspect, development is regarded as occurring automatically in accordance with universal laws of nature (with or without randomness).

(b) In terms of the mental aspect, some development over time is by way of actions by the conscious subject; the actions are themselves choices between genuinely open alternatives and are made by the subject on the basis of nonconclusive reasons.

Neither aspect, on its own, can provide a complete account of how the system develops.

3. For normal persons, a choice is generally a *free choice*, for which the conscious subject is responsible, for these reasons:

(a) The choice is between alternatives that are left open by the physical aspect of the person and the universal laws of nature (this is one relevance of quantum theory, and possibly chaos theory, in suggesting that such alternatives may indeed be left open).

(b) The reasons for and against the choice are immeasurable, incommensurable, and nonconclusive; they are resolved for the first time by the choice, which is a unique efficacious event rather than merely a working out of universal laws.

(c) Accordingly, although history limits the alternatives, it does not determine which will be selected.

(d) To the extent that the person making the choice is the product of genes and environment, he or she is not responsible for his or her character, but this does not mean he or she is not responsible for the choice. The person's character and circumstances will determine the alternatives that are available, how the alternatives appear to the person, and how the reasons for and against the alternatives appear to the person. However, nothing in history, including the person's character, predetermines which choice is made. To that extent, there is free will. Further, a person's character is to some extent the outcome of previous free choices as well as genes and environment; to that extent, there is responsibility for character.

4. The choice will be influenced by unconscious factors of motivation and the physiology of the brain; unless and until the threshold of insanity or automatism[3] is crossed, freedom and responsibility are merely qualified, not eliminated. Abuse in early childhood, low serotonin levels, and so on affect the alternatives that are open for choice and, perhaps, make the right choice more difficult. For example, a person who is moderately dependent on a drug has a choice not to take the drug but has difficulty maintaining the choice. Similarly, it may be hard for a person abused in childhood to refrain from abusing others, or for a man with high testosterone and low serotonin levels to refrain from violence; in each case, until some appropriate threshold is crossed, the person can fairly be regarded as responsible, to a degree affected by those factors.

One important feature of this framework is that it stresses that reasons are not like physical forces. Physical forces are measurable, commensurable, and conclusive in that they act automatically and inevitably. Reasons are immeasurable, incommensurable, and nonconclusive; they presuppose the existence of a conscious subject who is able to choose whether to follow them. For instance, if I have money to spend and I dearly want to replace the ailing amplifier of my sound system, I have reasons to do so, but whether I use the money for this purpose requires me to choose. If, at the same time, there is an appeal for famine relief in Africa, I may feel strongly that I should donate the money to that cause; again, a choice is required. If I decide that I will do one or the other and have to choose between them, the opposing reasons are immeasurable and incommensurable, and they can be resolved only by choice (Hodgson 1994a).

One important advantage of this framework is that it has an answer to the basic dilemma about responsibility, which is strongly expressed by Galen Strawson (1986).

1. There is a clear and fundamental sense in which no being can be truly self-determining in respect of its character and motivation in such a way as to be truly responsible for how it is in respect of character and motivation.
2. When we act, at a given time, the way we act is, in some quite straightforward sense, a function of the way we then are, in respect of character and motivation. We act as we act because of how we then are, in respect of character and motivation.
3. It follows that there is a fundamental sense in which we cannot possibly be truly responsible for our actions. For we cannot be truly responsible for the way we are, and we act as we act because of the way we are.

According to the suggested framework, even if a person had no responsibility for character at a particular time, that character, together with the circumstances, would predetermine alternatives—how they appear to the person, and how the reasons for and against the alternatives appear—but not the choice. The person would not be responsible for having the capacity to choose but would be responsible for the choice, with degrees of responsibility and, thus, moral blameworthiness affected by how hard it was for the person in those circumstances to avoid making the "wrong" choice.[4] If those premises are accepted, insofar as character is the result of previous choices, the person also has some responsibility for character.

A second advantage is that the framework is flexible enough to allow the law to adjust to increasing knowledge of the etiology of crime and thus throw out the bathwater of outmoded attitudes of vengeance and disregard of the role of physiology in crime without also throwing out the baby of responsibility and human rights. Moir and Jessel (1995) strongly advocate that we recognize the role of physiology in crime and adjust our response to crime accordingly, but they are not prepared to entirely reject notions of free will and criminal responsibility. Thus, they talk about people with brain malfunctions having "to exercise far greater efforts to inhibit their behavior than do normal people" and about "seeking to identify and treat the damaged sex offender, while properly punishing the man who rapes for mere pleasure, revenge or sense of entitlement."

Some may see these passages as indicating lack of rigor and consistency— I think this is suggested by Hans Eysenck (1995) in his review of Moir and Jessel's book—but I see Moir and Jessel pointing toward the sort of framework that I advocate. My framework would make sense of the fundamental distinction drawn by the law between actions that are voluntary and actions that are not, as well as regarding factors such as abuse in childhood and physiological abnormalities as mitigating factors relevant to the amount and type of coercion that would be fair and appropriate.

I believe this framework is likely to be closer to the truth than is the orthodox mechanistic hypothesis, but, whether or not it is ultimately true, I contend the framework would be a useful working model for application to criminal responsibility, social and educational areas, and the practice of psychiatry. I think this framework would be useful for helping people who have problems, by explicitly recognizing that although they may be disadvantaged by nature and nurture, they themselves, through their past choices, bear some responsibility for what they have done and what they have become, and, more importantly, they have the ability and the responsibility to take charge of their lives and to make better choices in future.

NOTES

1. Braithwaite and Pettit (1990), in their powerful (and basically consequentialist) attack on retributive theories of justice, assumed that sense can and should be given to concepts such as morally culpable, blameworthy, fault, blameless, intend, and culpability. Indeed, this is a necessary concomitant of their "republican" theory of criminal justice.

2. There is an argument that the criminal law, by singling out for opprobrium and punishment only persons who have voluntarily breached a public law, exacerbates inequalities in society. It was noted last century how the law in its impartial majesty made it a crime, equally for the rich and the poor, to steal a loaf of bread. The tendency of the criminal law to exacerbate inequalities is illustrated by the disproportionate numbers of Aboriginals in Australian jails and of African Americans in American jails. However, the answer is not to do away with the notion that it is fair to punish persons who have voluntarily broken a public law but unfair to punish persons who have not. Rather, the answer is (1) to attack the inequalities by means of social programs, (2) to make the law, as far as possible, not weigh more heavily on disadvantaged minorities; (3) to ensure that law enforcement agencies do not target minorities; (4) to use powers to refrain from recording convictions in trivial cases; and (5) to find, on conviction, alternatives to jail for disadvantaged minorities if possible.

3. Increases in our understanding suggest that the present definitions of insanity and automatism need to be changed. The essential question is whether the person really *chose* to do the prohibited act; we may come to the view that circumstances exist, outside these present definitions, in which a person does not in substance have the capacity to make a choice. If the lack of capacity is caused by a physical or mental condition that could lead to a repetition of the prohibited act, regardless of whether this condition is called insanity, it seems reasonable that the authorities have power to protect society by treatment of the condition, detention, or both measures.

4. Lesser moral responsibility for doing an act prohibited by the law will not necessarily mean lesser punishment. If a person does a prohibited act in circumstances in which the threshold of insanity is approached but not crossed, considerations of deterrence and protection of society (coupled perhaps with the person's own partial responsibility for character) may make no reduction of sentence appropriate because of the person's limited responsibility for that particular act.

Euan Squires suggested that my approach means that a very selfish person A who steals $1,000 should be punished less than an unselfish person B who does likewise because it would have been easier for B to refrain from stealing. I accept that my approach means that B's act, considered in isolation, may indeed be judged morally worse than A's act, but, for the purposes of punishment, it is not considered in isolation and other factors are likely to justify greater punishment for A. A standard approach to punishment would first, look at the objective criminality (the nature of the act and the harm caused to the victim and to society) and, having regard to the maximal penalty, decide what penalty seems proportionate. Then, decisions would be made about whether some reduction is justified, having regard to such matters as:

(a) Factors outside the person's control that made the person more likely to commit crimes (congenital mental abnormality, child abuse, etc.). These factors mitigate responsibility, but they may not always greatly reduce punishment because they may be offset by a greater need to deter this person and similar persons from the criminal activity.

(b) Mitigating circumstances, for example, that the crime was prompted by genuine deprivation and hardship.

(c) Previous good character and remorse.

(d) Prospects for rehabilitation.

(e) Effect of disgrace and punishment on the offender.

Person B may not do too well under (a) and (b), but may do extremely well under (c), (d), and (e). A single act that is deemed "out of character," for which the offender is genuinely remorseful, and that is most unlikely to be repeated may itself be morally quite reprehensible but not call for heavy punishment, particularly if the disgrace will heavily affect the offender.

Person A, on the other hand, may be considered as answerable for his own selfishness (presumably contributed to by many selfish choices in the past) unless he can point to factors under (a) that reduce his responsibility; even then, this may be offset by the need for deterrence. Genuine remorse is unlikely with A, the prospects for rehabilitation may be small, and disgrace may be inconsequential. Thus, it is likely that greater punishment for A than for B would be justified.

REFERENCES

Blakemore, C. 1988. *The Mind Machine*. London: BBC Books.

Blakemore, C., and S. Greenfield, eds. 1987. *Mindwaves*. Oxford: Blackwell.

Braithwaite, J., and P. Pettit. 1990. *Not Just Deserts*. Oxford: Oxford University Press.

Churchland, P. M. 1990. Eliminative materialism and propositional attitudes. In W. S. Lycan, ed., *Mind and Cognition*. Oxford: Blackwell, pp. 206–223.

Churchland, P. S. 1986. *Neurophilosophy: Toward a Unified Science of the Mind-Brain*. Cambridge: MIT Press.

Clift, D. 1993. Mind, behavior and the law. *Network* 53:14–15.

Crick, F. 1994. *The Astonishing Hypothesis: The Scientific Search for the Soul*. London: Simon & Schuster.

Dennett, D. 1978. *Brainstorms*. Brighton, U.K. Harvester Press.

Dennett, D. 1984. *Elbow Room*. Oxford: Oxford University Press.

Dennett, D. 1991. *Consciousness Explained*. Boston: Little, Brown.

Dennett, D. 1995. *Darwin's Dangerous Idea*. New York: Simon & Schuster.

Eysenck, H. 1995. Review of *A Mind to Crime*. *New Scientist* 148:51.

Hart, H. L. A. 1968. *Punishment and Responsibility*. Oxford: Oxford University Press.

Hodgson, D. H. 1991. *The Mind Matters*. Oxford: Oxford University Press.

Hodgon, D. H. 1994a. Neuroscience and folk psychology—An overview. *Journal of Consciousness Studies* 1:205–216.

Hodgon, D. H. 1994b. Why Searle hasn't rediscovered the mind. *Journal of Consciousness Studies* 1:264–274.

Hodgson, D. H. 1995. Probability: the logic of the law—a response. *Oxford Journal of Legal Studies* 14:51–68.

Hodgson, D. H. 1996a. The easy problems ain't so easy. *Journal of Consciousness Studies* 3:69–75.

Hodgson, D. H. 1996b. Nonlocality, local indeterminism, and consciousness. *Ratio* 9:1–22.

Honderich, T. 1993. *How Free Are You?* Oxford: Oxford University Press. '

Lycan, W. S., ed. 1990. *Mind and Cognition*. Oxford: Blackwell.

Moir, A., and D. Jessel. 1995. *A Mind to Crime*. London: Michael Joseph.

Strawson, G. 1986. *Freedom and Belief*. Oxford: Oxford University Press.

Strawson, P. 1962. Freedom and resentment. *Proceedings of the British Academy* 48:1–25.

14 Zombie Killer

Nigel J. T. Thomas

Philosophers' zombies are hypothetical beings that are behaviorally and functionally (or perhaps even physically) equivalent to (and thus indistinguishable from) human beings, but that differ from humans in not having conscious (or, at least, qualitatively conscious) mental states. Zombies have the same information-processing capacities that we humans have, and, because of this, a similar capacity to form cognitive representations and perhaps even to enter into intentional states, but they are not conscious because they do not have sensations, or *qualia* as the jargon has it. Thus, a zombie can tell you that the rose before it is red, and it will wince and hastily withdraw its hand if it touches a hot stove; however, unlike us, it never experiences the quintessential redness, the "raw feel" of red, or the awfulness and misery of burning pain.

The zombie concept is significant because it seems to be inconsistent with certain widely assumed doctrines about the mind. Most cognitivists assume the truth of *functionalism*, the view that all mental states may be identified with functional states, which are usually understood as (connectionist or symbolic) computational states of a cognitive system. More generally, nearly everyone who hopes for a scientific account of the mind assumes the truth of *physicalism*, the view that the mind can be explained entirely within the terms of ordinary physical science, either in its present state or after some anticipated future advance. But if zombies functionally equivalent to conscious humans are a real conceptual possibility (they do not have to actually exist), then functionalism must be false because we are admitting that two functionally indiscernible beings could be mentally different—one conscious and the other not conscious. Thus, there must be more to mentality than cognitive functioning. Likewise, if zombies that are physically equivalent to conscious humans are a possibility, physicalism must be false.

In this chapter, I shall refer to persons who are inclined to argue this way as "zombiphiles," and to argue this argument as "the zombiphile argument" (some versions are also known as the "absent qualia" argument).

Many thinkers seem to accept, gleefully or grudgingly, that zombies really are conceptually possible and that the zombiphile argument is thus probably sound. However, I shall argue that when certain implications of the zombie concept are carefully examined, zombies are revealed as either failing to support the zombiphile argument or as being simply impossible, that is, conceptually contradictory. In this chapter, I shall concentrate on functionally equivalent zombies (i.e., equivalent in causal structure). Because we may safely take it that physically equivalent systems are also functionally equivalent (although not vice versa), any conceptual problems with functional zombiphilia also afflicts the physical version. Physicalism will be vindicated along with functionalism.

STRICT EQUIVALENCE

The concept of functional equivalence, however, is troublesome. In an important sense, it is extremely unlikely that any actual person could be entirely functionally equivalent to any other. After all, mental skills and propensities (even brain topography) differ markedly from one person to another. Furthermore, as there is no uncontroversial, principled and objective distinction to be drawn between program and data (Winograd 1975), functional architecture and mental content, or even brain structure and the neural embodiment of particular memories, people can be said to differ functionally one from another just in virtue of the fact that they have, inevitably, had different experiences and thus have different memories and attitudes. But if the zombiphile argument is to work, it would seem necessary to construe equivalence very strictly. If there is *any* functional difference between a zombie and a conscious human, it will always be open to the functionalist to argue that it is precisely that difference that makes the difference. If it should be discovered that there really *are* such beings living in our universe—and Moody (1994) argues persuasively that, under certain circumstances, characteristic and systematic behavioral differences between such zombies and conscious humans would inevitably appear—functionalists would surely be justified in treating this discovery as an exciting research opportunity rather than a disaster; any such discovery would greatly facilitate the discovery of the *actual* functional basis of consciousness.

Thus, Chalmers's (1996) way of setting up the zombiphile argument seems the least problematic. He asks us to consider a "zombie possible world," a parallel universe that remains at all times indiscernible from our universe in every "external" respect and that contains a physical (and functional and behavioral) "zombie twin" of every conscious person in this world, that is, a being who looks, functions, and lives exactly the same life as each of us but who does these things without consciousness.

In Chalmers's zombie world, some zombies inevitably *claim* to be conscious. (After all, my zombie twin behaves just like I do, and I make such a claim.) *My* claim is true, but what of the zombie's claim? Is it false, or is there some way of interpreting it as true? Or has it no truth value at all? We shall see that any line that zombiphiles take on these questions will get them into serious trouble.

FALSITY

If someone speaks falsely, they are either lying (i.e., intentionally stating things they disbelieve) or they are mistaken. However, because, *ex hypothesis*, my zombie twin is cognitively indiscernible from me, it cannot be lying when it claims to be conscious. Lying, after all, presupposes having an intention to lie, and if I do not have such an intention, neither does my cognitive doppelgänger.

Furthermore, telling a lie surely involves cognitive mechanisms different from those involved in speaking sincerely. If, for example, speaking sincerely involves a mechanism whereby inner belief representations are converted into articulate form, lying, at a minimum, must either involve an extra or alternative mechanism whereby the inner belief representations are, also, negated; or else it must apply the articulation mechanism to representations of certain *disbelieved* propositions (something I am certainly not doing when *I* claim to be conscious). In any case, my zombie twin cannot be both lying about being conscious *and* be cognitively indistinguishable from me.

But suppose the zombie genuinely but mistakenly *believes* that it is conscious. Its claims will then not be lies, and articulating them will involve exactly the same intentions and cognitive mechanisms that I employ in expressing my unmistaken belief. As before, the issue is whether there can be a coherent interpretation of such a circumstance. Let us consider the mechanisms of belief formation. Do I and my zombie twin *infer* that we are conscious from our mutual observation of something that is reliably correlated with (or even sufficient for) consciousness in this world but that is not so correlated in the zombie world? Sometimes perhaps—but this had better not be the only way we know about our consciousness, because we could not then discover the correlation (or sufficiency).

Conceivably, consciousness (and the correlation) might gain its place in our conceptual repertoire as a nonobservational term of some *folk theory*, but the zombiphile must surely reject this suggestion because it leaves the door wide open to standard eliminativist moves (Churchland 1979), that is, to the possibility that consciousness, like phlogiston, just does not exist, that *we* might be zombies. Furthermore, given the notorious difficulty of integrating it into our scientific world view, consciousness would make an unusually appropriate target for such elimination. But if consciousness does not (or even might not) exist (i.e., if *we* might be zombies), the zombiphile argument fails to show that functionalism might not fully explain us.

Thus, zombiphiles normally (and plausibly) insist that we know of our own consciousness directly, noninferentially. Even so, there must be some sort of cognitive process that takes me from the *fact* of my consciousness to my (true) *belief* that I am conscious. Because my zombie twin is cognitively indiscernible from me, an indiscernible process, functioning in just the same way, must lead the zombie from the fact of its nonconsciousness to the equivalent mistaken belief. Given either consciousness *or* nonconsciousness (and the same contextual circumstances—*ex hypothesis, ceteris* is entirely *paribus*), the process leads one to believe that one is conscious. It is like a stuck fuel gauge that reads FULL or not whether there is any gas in the tank.

Such a process, like such a gauge, is worse than useless; it can be positively misleading. If the process by which we come to believe that we are conscious can be like this, we can have no grounds for confidence that we ourselves are not zombies (unlike the empty car, there will be no behavioral evidence to indicate otherwise). But (as before) if we might be zombies, the zombiphile argument has no bite. If mistaken zombies are possible, the whole motive for ever considering such beings is undermined.

TRUTH

But perhaps there is a way of construing the zombie's claims as true. Although they sound like claims to be conscious like us, perhaps they are not. Perhaps zombies and humans attach different meanings to the relevant words. Moody (1994) suggests that zombies should be thought of as discussing not consciousness, but rather consciousness^z, and likewise for other mental words. However, we are now entitled to ask whether we can give any coherent interpretation to the notion of consciousness^z and to the zombie's use of it.

At first sight, it might seem that we can. The plausibility of Moody's move surely stems from the same presupposition that makes zombies themselves seem conceivable, that is, the widely accepted view that the aspects of mental life to do with the processing of information and the control of behavior are conceptually (and perhaps, in principle, actually) separable from the subjective, experiential, qualitative aspects. Zombies are supposed to have the former, but not the latter. Thus, Moody tells us, "conscious^z" ("conscious" as used by a zombie) means simply "responsive to the environment." By contrast, "conscious" as humans use it is *also* supposed to indicate the presence of the qualia that normally accompany such responsiveness in humans.

However, the very fact that we can explain the putative difference between consciousness and consciousness^z carries the seeds of incoherence. If *we* can express the difference, so can zombies; the zombie twin of anyone who explicitly claims to be conscious in the full sense, to be more than just environmentally responsive, will also make such a claim. It is not possible to construe this claim as true just by strewing around more superscripts. I can see no hope of motivating a distinction between qualia^z, for example, and qualia in the "ordinary" sense—qualia are meant to be precisely those aspects of consciousness that are subjective and experiential and *not* informational and behavioral. Even if we *did* find a way to draw some such distinction, the problem would simply iterate—zombies would always be as ready as their human counterparts to lay claim to qualitative consciousness in its fullest, least attenuated sense, but they could not be telling the truth because then they would not be zombies.

Part II: Ontology, the Hard Problem of Experience, Free Will, and Agency

MEANINGLESSNESS

Perhaps, however, a zombie's claims to be conscious are neither true nor false. Despite their indicative form, perhaps their claims have no truth value being, in effect, claims without meaning. This may initially seem quite plausible because, after all, the relevant referents for words such as qualia, "consciousness," and their cognates do not exist anywhere in the zombie's universe; thus, the words as the zombie uses them do not refer to anything.

However, mere nonreferring terms will not get us meaninglessness, at least not the right kind. It is controversial whether the fact that there are no jabberwocks makes an assertion such as "I have a jabberwock in my pocket" meaningless or just plain false; nevertheless, it seems clear that if I *do* assert it, I am either lying or mistaken. It is not like saying, "Blieble blieble blieble," or "I have a blieble in my pocket." After all, "jabberwock," despite having no referent, is not truly meaningless—it does have a sense of sorts (if we know our *Alice*, we "know" that jabberwocks are fearsome beasts, they can be slain with vorpal swords, they are fictional, and so forth), and it is our grasp of this sense allows us to reject the truth of the claim.

Surely "consciousness" is similarly going to have sense for a zombie (if anything does). My zombie twin hears, reads, and utters far more about consciousness than I (or it) ever do about jabberwocks, and most of this at least appears to be a good deal more intelligible than *Jabberwocky*. If a zombie can know or assert things at all, its claims to be conscious are meaningful enough to run us into the sorts of problems already discussed.

Perhaps a zombie *cannot* know or assert things at all. Perhaps *nothing* that it says, or even thinks, is meaningful. After all, Searle (1992) argued, on quite independent grounds, that intrinsic intentionality, the meaningfulness, of our thought (on which he takes the meaningfulness of our linguistic behavior to depend) itself depends on our consciousness. If we accept this "connection principle," or something like it, (and I think there is a lot to be said for doing so), it would seem that we not only can, but indeed *must*, acknowledge that zombie speech acts in general, and, in particular, zombie claims to be conscious, are without meaning. This would, finally, seem to provide a coherent account of the truth value of zombie claims to consciousness.

However, the zombiphile is now committed to saying that although many of the sounds and inscriptions that I make are meaningful, when my zombie twin makes exactly the same sounds or inscriptions in identical circumstances and with exactly the same effects on its fellows zombies, these noises and marks have no meaning whatsoever. This seems to conflict with basic notions about what it is for language to be meaningful. The zombie concept (and the epiphenomenalism which it bolsters) has a prima facie plausibility inasmuch as we think of consciousness as something that occurs entirely privately, completely "inside our heads," and is, thereby, causally inefficacious.

Regardless of whether this is the right way to think about consciousness, it is certainly not the right way to think about language. The meaningfulness of my utterances may depend in part on what happens inside my head, but it also depends just as crucially on what goes on in other people's heads and what goes on between people—on both the causes and the effects of utterances. Epiphenomenalism about language should have no appeal at all. The meaningfulness of language is a social, not a purely internal, mental matter.

Consider, after all, my zombie twin in its social world, which is, *ex hypothesis*, just like mine. If the zombie is greeted, it will reply politely (at least, it is as likely to do so as I am); if it is asked a question, it will generally make an appropriate reply; if it is asked to do something, it will frequently either seem to comply or else give reasons why it will not comply; if it is told a fact, its future behavior will (*ceteris paribus*) be appropriately adjusted. Likewise, the utterances produced by the zombie will have the same sorts of effects on its fellows. Language apparently serves exactly the same social functions in the zombie world as it does in ours. How, then, can we say that it is not meaningful for them? Chalmers (1993) seems to agree.

More importantly, it would seem perverse to deny truth values wholesale to zombie assertions. Suppose you ask how many people are in my house and I say, "Five." I could, for some reason, be lying or I could be mistaken (someone is hiding), but, unless you have good reason to think that such thing is happening, you will likely assume that the information I have conveyed is accurate, that I am speaking the truth, and plan accordingly (bring five gifts, say). Surely our zombie twins are in an exactly equivalent position. My twin would lie where I would (from cognitively equivalent motives and employing equivalent mechanisms) and would be mistaken in the same circumstances as I would. Your twin would catch the lie whenever you would catch me, and on the same basis. However, normally (and justifiably) your twin would respond as if reliable information had been conveyed, that is, as if my twin had told the truth. Can the zombiphile reasonably deny that it is right to do so? If not, the case for zombies is lost.

CONSCIOUSNESS, INTENTIONALITY, AND SCIENCE

If zombies are impossible, it is open to us to take the perfectly plausible position that complex social and linguistic interactions are impossible without consciousness. Thus, giving up zombies need not mean giving up Searle's principle of connection between consciousness and the intrinsic intentionality that underpins linguistic meaning. Indeed, we might go further than Searle and say that qualitative consciousness and intentionality (the *aboutness* or *directedness* of our thoughts, linguistic or otherwise) are best seen as different aspects of the same thing. "Intentionality" is essentially a term of art introduced to differentiate one key aspect of the complex pretheoretical notion of consciousness.

But consciousness certainly remains very puzzling. The flip side of zombiphile mysterianism is the quite unfounded confidence of most cognitive scientists that intrinsic intentionality need not concern them. Either they think there is no such thing or they assume there is no problem (or, at worst, a mere "tricky", technical problem) in understanding how brain states or functional states of machines could be inherently meaningful. In fact, it is hard to understand how *any* physical or functional state could be inherently *about* anything, but it is also quite clear that our thoughts *are* about things. The problem of intentionality is *hard*. Nonetheless, unlike Chalmers's "hard problem"—the problem of qualia in the context of zombiphilia—it is not deliberately constructed so as to be insoluble in ordinary scientific terms. A scientific understanding of consciousness is much more likely to follow from a serious engagement with intentionality than from the fascinated contemplation of "raw feels."

ACKNOWLEDGMENTS

This chapter was written while I was a participant in the 1996 NEH Summer Seminar, Metaphysics of Mind. I am grateful for comments and discussion from Dave Chalmers; Jessica Wilson; the seminar director, John Heil; and the other seminar participants, especially Eric Saidel, Jim Garson, Tony Dardis, David Pitt, and Steve Schwartz.

REFERENCES

Chalmers, D. J. 1993. Self-ascription without qualia: A case study. *Behavioral and Brain Sciences* 16:635–636.

Chalmers, D. J. 1996. *The Conscious Mind.* New York: Oxford University Press.

Churchland, P. M. 1979. *Scientific Realism and the Plasticity of Mind.* Cambridge: Cambridge University Press.

Moody, T. C. 1994. Conversations with zombies. *Journal of Consciousness Studies* 1:196–200.

Searle, J. R. 1992. *The Rediscovery of the Mind.* Cambridge: MIT Press.

Winograd, T. 1975. Frame representations and the declarative/procedural controversy. In D. G. Bobrow and A. Collins, eds., *Representation and Understanding.* New York: Academic Press.

III Discussions and Debates

OVERVIEW

Direct exchange of ideas and informed, logical debate are helpful in any field, particularly an interdisciplinary one. The Tucson conferences and the *Journal of Consciousness Studies* have encouraged such activity, as have electronic media like JCS-Online and PSYCHE-D. In that spirit Part III includes four chapters that are, in a way, dialogues.

The first two chapters grew out of a panel discussion at Tucson II on "Can machines be conscious?" Artificial-intelligence proponent Danny Hillis argues that, yes, machines can be conscious, but the skeptical Jaron Lanier doesn't think so.

To state his case, Hillis uses the increasingly standard *gedanken* or thought experiment, replacing one brain neuron with a computer device, then proceeding neuron by neuron to replace the entire brain. At some time, and surely at the end, consciousness will have been transferred to—and exist within—the computer. After recognizing one possible flaw (that it may not be possible to replace single neurons with computer devices), Lanier takes Hillis's argument *ad absurdum*, describing how consciousness could then be transferred to other simulatable dynamical systems.

The second pair of chapters are both responses to philosopher Patricia Churchland. Physicist Giuseppe Vitiello was so moved by her talk at Tucson II that he has written a soulful letter. Vitiello realizes that Churchland's objection to quantum effects in consciousness is based on mistaken identity—she rejects quantum mechanics—but the relevant paradigm should be quantum field theory. He patiently explains collective modes in crystals and the interplay between symmetry and order that can rescue her, he claims, from the mechanistic view of neurons as "eighteenth-century puppets."

Stuart Hameroff also responds to Patricia Churchland (Chapter 8) where she criticizes views expressed by Searle, Chalmers, and Penrose–Hameroff as "nonneural." He replies that the latter view of quantum effects in microtubules is decidedly neural, and takes the bait on Churchland's suggested comparison to "pixie dust in the synapses."

It is hoped that lively and good-natured exchange will continue in consciousness studies.

15 Can a Machine Be Conscious?

Danny Hillis

We human beings have always favored theories that seem to put us comfortably apart from and above the rest of the natural world. Historically, we liked the idea that our earth was at the center of the universe. The problem with tying our sense of self-importance to such theories is that we feel diminished when they turn out to be wrong. Galileo's telescope seemed to make us less special. So too did Darwin's version of our family tree.

Fortunately, our ability to reason seemed to make us unique. We could deal with Darwin's message by assuring ourselves that our noble rationality separated us from the beasts. Today we feel threatened, not by the beasts, but by the machines. Already, computers can keep track of details better than we can. They can prove theorems that we cannot. They usually beat us at chess. They are not yet as clever as we are, but they are getting smarter and they are getting smarter faster than we. Our unique position as rational beings is in peril and it is time to move our sense of self-worth to a higher perch.

And so, if reason is no longer a uniquely human attribute, how do we separate ourselves from machines? Many are placing their hopes on consciousness. According to this latest version of human-superiority theory, machines may become intelligent, but they will never feel; they will never be conscious. Other popular theories of human transcendence turned out to be wrong, but that does not necessarily mean this latest one is wrong also. It could be that this time the theory people want to believe will turn out to be correct. Maybe consciousness really is a uniquely human feature. If so, we have a convenient distinction to justify our intuition that we are a cut above machines.

People want to believe they are better than machines because the machines they are familiar with are stupid and simple. Most people do not even like to be compared to monkeys; current computers are much less intelligent. I do not think today's computers are conscious, and if they are it is not a form of consciousness that I find particularly interesting. To me, the question of consciousness becomes interesting only for much, much more intelligent machines. This view raises a problem with language. I paraphrase Alan Turing: the answer to the question, "Can a machine be conscious?" will depend on what we decide to mean by "conscious" and what we decide to mean by "machine." A world in which machines are complicated enough to be conscious is a world sufficiently far from our present one that it is hard to guess how current language should apply. For instance, if we constructed a device as complex as a brain, would we call it a machine? What if the builders did not understand the design? Such a machine would be so different from what we have today that we might well choose to call it something else.

We have similar problems with the word "consciousness." As long as human beings are the only conscious creatures on the planet, we do not need a special word for human consciousness, as opposed to other consciousness-like phenomena. What if we find out that the mental life of something else is as rich as, but very different from, our own? Do we call this state consciousness? Isolated tribes usually have one word that means both "humanity" and "a member of our tribe." When they meet other people they need a new word. When reality changes, vocabulary adapts.

When I ask, "Can a machine be conscious?" here is what I mean. By "machine," I mean something artificially constructed, although not necessarily something designed by current methods. When I talk about "machine consciousness," I am describing what I think it would feel like to be the machine. A conscious machine would have sensations and feelings. It would feel as if it were conscious. By those definitions, my guess is that the answer is, "Yes, a machine can be conscious"; that is, it would be possible to construct an artificial device that felt as if it were conscious. In fact, I suspect it would be difficult to construct a generally intelligent device that was not conscious.

This gedanken experiment is helpful in explaining what I mean. Imagine that with some future technology it becomes possible to build a device that mimics the function of a biological neuron. (You are free to assume that the device uses computers, microtubules, or any other component you feel is necessary to simulate a real neuron. My own guess is that the microtubules-as-source-of-consciousness theories will look pretty silly in a few years, but that assumption is not important to the argument.) Imagine that we can build a life-size neuron simulator with microscopic proportions. Such a machine could have electrical and chemical sensors allowing it to measure the same inputs as a biological neuron can. It could also use signaling systems to produce the same types of electrical and chemical outputs. The miniature mechanism would calculate an output response based on the inputs that would mimic a real neuron's response.

Such a neuron simulator could be used as a prosthesis. A human being paralyzed by a damaged spinal cord could have mobility restored by replacing the neurons in the spinal cord with neuron simulators, much as an artificial cornea can replace the damaged lens in a human eye. Such neuron simulators would restore feeling and control to the legs, because the artificial neurons would transmit exactly the same signals as their real counterparts. I expect that a person using such a prosthesis would perceive exactly the same sensations as anyone else. Such an artificial neuron could also be used to replace a specific neuron in the brain that had been damaged by a stroke. Again, the patient would perceive no difference as long as the neuron simulator accurately produced the same outputs as the neurons it replaced.

Imagine that a neural repair of the sort described above was repeated one neuron at a time for every neuron in your brain. At every stage your thinking could proceed normally. Every memory would remain intact, as would every prejudice and quirk of personality. Every sensation would feel the same. I believe the resulting machine would be conscious. I believe it would feel as if it were you.

People who do not believe that machines can be conscious usually disagree with my description of the experiment and its results, but they disagree in different ways. The first type of skeptic says, "Yes, it would feel, but it wouldn't be a machine," or "It would feel like me, but it wouldn't be conscious." I have no fundamental disagreement with these people; they are just choosing to use words differently than I. A second type of skeptic says, "The machine might *say* it felt conscious, but it would not really *feel* anything." Such people are just guessing (as am I), but I suspect that their guesses are based on the prejudices mentioned above. In other words, I suspect they do not *want* to believe that the machine would feel. The fourth type of skeptic questions the premise that a functional simulation of a neuron can be built. These are the skeptics whom I like best because they have an experimentally testable theory—science can prove them wrong.

The gedanken experiment does not prove anything; it is just a way to describe what I think, and to sort out ways in which others disagree. I do not believe such a human-imitated consciousness is the only type of machine consciousness that is possible, nor do I believe it is the most likely, but it will do for discussing the issue because it is relatively easy to define. Once the question is defined in this way it becomes obvious that no one has any strong evidence one way or the other about whether or not a machine can be conscious.

How can we ever determine for certain if even a fellow human being is conscious, much less a machine? We are reduced to arguing about plausibility. To me, it is most plausible that human attributes are manifestations of the physical world. I therefore expect that they can be artificially produced.

Not everyone accepts the premise that this matter needs to be resolved by experiment. Some people believe they can determine by pure thought whether or not machines can be conscious. I am suspicious, for philosophical arguments about the limits of technology have a very poor record of success. I am especially suspicious of arguments that deny consciousness to machines, because in today's climate any well-explicated theory that seems to elevate people above machines will be popular, irrespective of its scientific merit.

Today, the two most popular arguments against machine consciousness are Penrose's objection to Gödel's theorem, and Searle's "Chinese box." I cannot do justice to these well-crafted arguments in this short forum, but I will explain briefly why I believe they are wrong. The primary flaw in

Penrose's argument is a confusion between two senses of the word "algorithm." Penrose uses it to mean both "an effective procedure" and "a well-specified computation." Once these two senses of the word are separated, the argument falls apart. The difficulty in Searle's argument is subtler and tells us more about the nature of consciousness; it lies in the assumption that a change in scale cannot lead to a qualitative change. In Searle's argument he asks us to extrapolate from a simple, understandable situation to one that is unimaginably complex, and we are asked to assume that, in spite of this change in scale, nothing really changes in what is going on. This claim is similar to arguing that a large number of lifeless chemical interactions cannot possibly produce life. Consciousness and life are both emergent properties of very complicated systems. The property of the whole is not simply inherited from the properties of the parts.

My guess is that the most important progress on this issue will come not from abstract arguments but from building smarter and more complicated machines. I suspect that the question, "Can a machine be conscious?" will turn out to be more of a moral than a scientific question. It will be translated to, "Do machines feel sufficiently like us that we must respect them as fellow beings?" or more concisely, "Should we do unto them as we would have them do unto us?" When it comes to the moral question, I am inclined to give anything that acts as if it is conscious the benefit of the doubt.

16 Mindless Thought Experiments: A Critique of Machine Intelligence

Jaron Lanier

PART 1: YOUR BRAIN IN SILICON

Because no computer seems conscious at this time, the idea of machine consciousness is supported by thought experiments. Here is one old chestnut: "What if you replaced your neurons one by one with neuron-sized and -shaped substitutes made of silicon chips that perfectly mimicked the originals' chemical and electric functions? If you replaced just one neuron, surely you would feel the same. As you proceeded, as more and more neurons were replaced, you would stay conscious. Why would you not still be conscious at the end of the exchange, when you would reside in a brain-shaped glob of silicon? And why could not the resulting replacement brain have been manufactured by some other means?"

Let us take this thought experiment even further. Instead of physical neuron replacements, what if you used software? Every time you plucked a neuron out of your brain you would put in a radio transceiver that talked to a nearby computer running neuron simulations. When enough neurons had been transferred to software they could start talking to each other directly in the computer and you could start throwing away the radio links. When you were done your brain would be entirely on the computer.

If you think consciousness does not travel into software you have a problem. What is so special about physical neuron-replacement parts? After all, the computer is made of matter too, and it is performing the same computation. If you think software lacks some needed essence, you may as well believe that authentic, original, brand-name human neurons from your very own head are the only source of that essence. In that case, you have made up your mind: You do not believe in artificial intelligence (AI). But let us assume that software is a legitimate medium for consciousness and move on.

Now your consciousness exists as a series of numbers in a computer; that is all a computer program is, after all. Let us go a little further with this scheme. Let us suppose you have a marvelous new sensor that can read the positions of every raindrop in a storm. Gather all those raindrop positions as a list of numbers and pretend those numbers are a computer program. Now, start searching through all the possible computers that could exist up to a specified very large size until you find one that treats the raindrop positions as a program exactly equivalent to your brain. Yes, it can be done: The list of possible computers of any one size is large but finite, and so too is your brain—according to the earlier steps in the thought experiment, anyway.

Is the rainstorm, then, conscious? Is it conscious as being specifically you, because it implements you? Or are you going to bring up an essence argument again? You say the rainstorm is not really doing computation—it is just sitting there as a passive program—and so it does not count? Fine, then we'll measure a larger rainstorm and search for a new computer that treats a larger collection of raindrops as implementing *both* the computer we found before that runs your brain as raindrops *as well as* your brain in raindrops. Now the raindrops are doing the computing. Maybe you are still not happy with this description because it seems the raindrops are equivalent only to a computer that is never turned on.

We can go further. The thought-experiment supply store can ship us an even better sensor that can measure the motions, not merely the instant positions, of all the raindrops in a storm over a specified period. Let us look for a computer that treats the numerical readings of those motions as an implementation of your brain changing in time. Once we have found it, we can say that the raindrops are doing the same work of computing as your brain for at least a specified time. The rainstorm computer has been turned on. The raindrops will not cohere forever, but no computer lasts forever. Every computer is gradually straying into entropy, just like our thunderstorm. During a few minutes, a rainstorm might implement millions of minds; a whole civilization might rise and fall before the water hits the dirt.

And further still, you might object that the raindrops are not influencing each other, and so they are still passive, as far as computing your brain goes. Let us switch instead, then, to a large swarm of asteroids hurtling through space. They all exert gravitational pull on one another. Now we shall use a sensor for asteroid-swarm internal motion and with it get data that will be matched to an appropriate computer to implement your brain. Now you have a physical system whose internal interactions perform your mind's computation.

But we are not done. You should realize by now that your brain is simultaneously implemented everywhere. It is in a thunderstorm, it is in the birthrate statistics, it is in the dimples of gummy bears.

Enough! I hope you can see that my game can be played ad infinitum. I can always make up a new kind of sensor from the supply store that will give me data from some part of the physical universe that are related to themselves in the same way as your neurons are related to each other by a given AI proponent.

Artificial-intelligence proponents usually seize on some specific stage in my *reductio ad absurdum* to locate the point at which I have gone too far. But the chosen stage varies widely from proponent to proponent. Some concoct finicky rules for what matter has to do to be conscious, such as, it must be the minimum physical system isomorphic to a conscious algorithm. The problem with such rules is that they have to race ahead of my absurdifying thought experiments, and so they become so stringent that they no longer allow the brain itself to be conscious. For example, the brain is almost certainly not the minimal physical system isomorphic to its thought processes.

A few *do* take the bait and choose to believe in myriad consciousnesses everywhere. This has to be the least elegant position ever taken on any subject in the history of science. It would mean that there is a vast superset of consciousnesses rather like you, such as the one that includes both your brain and the plate of pasta you are eating.

Some others object that an asteroid swarm does not *do* anything, but a mind acts in the world in a way that we can understand. I respond that, to the right alien, it might appear that people do nothing, and asteroid swarms are acting consciously. Even on Earth we can see enough variation in organisms to doubt the universality of the human perspective. How easy would it be for an intelligent bacterium to notice people as integral entities? We might appear more as slow storms moving into the bacterial environment. If we are relying solely on the human perspective to validate machine consciousness, we are really just putting humanness on an even higher pedestal than it might have been at the start of our thought experiment.

We should take the variation among responses from AI proponents as the meaningful product of my flight of fancy. I do not claim to know for certain where consciousness is or is not, but I hope I have at least shown that we have a real problem.

Sometimes the idea of machine intelligence is framed as a moral question: Would you deny equal rights to a machine that seemed conscious? This question introduces the mother of all AI thought experiments, the Turing Test. Before I go on, here is a note on terminology: In this discussion, I will let the qualifiers "smart" and "conscious" blur together, even though I profoundly disagree that they are interchangeable. This is the claim made for machine intelligence, however: consciousness "emerges" from intelligence. To constantly point out my objection would make the tale too tedious to tell. That is a danger in thought experiments: You may find yourself adopting some of the preliminary thoughts while you are distracted by the rest of the experiment.

At any rate, Alan Turing proposed a test in which a computer and a person are placed in isolation booths and are allowed to communicate only via media that conceal their identities, such as typed e-mail. A human subject is then asked to determine which isolation booth holds a fellow human being and which holds a machine. Turing's interpretation was that if the test subject cannot tell human being and machine apart, then it will be improper to impose a distinction between them when the true identities are revealed. It will be time to give the computer equal rights.

I have long proposed that Turing misinterpreted his thought experiment. If a person cannot tell which is machine and which is human being, it does not necessarily mean that the computer has become more humanlike. The other possibility is that the human being has become more computerlike. This is not just a hypothetical point of argument, but a serious consideration in software engineering.

PART 2: PRAGMATIC OPPOSITION TO MACHINE INTELLIGENCE

As Turing pointed out, when a piece of software is deemed somewhat autonomous, the only test of the assertion is whether or not users believe it. Artificial-intelligence developers would certainly agree that human beings are more mentally agile than any software today, and so today it is more likely than not that a person is changing to make the software seem smart. Ironically, the harder a problem is, the easier it can be for human beings to believe that a computer is smart at it.

An AI program that attempts to make decisions about something we understand easily, such as basic home finance, is booted out the door immediately because it is perceived as ridiculous, or even dangerous. Microsoft's "Bob" program was an example of the ridiculous. But an AI program that teaches children is acceptable because we know little about how children learn, or how teachers teach, Furthermore, children will adapt to the program, making it seem successful. Such programs are already in many homes and schools. The less we understand a problem, the readier we are to suspend disbelief.

No functional gain can come from making a program "intelligent." Exactly the same capabilities found in an "intelligent" or "autonomous" program (such as ability to recognize a face) could just as well be inclusively packaged in a "nonautonomous" user interface. The only real difference between the two approaches is that if users are told a computer is autonomous, then they are more likely to change themselves to adapt to the computer.

Thus, software packaged as "nonintelligent" is more likely to improve because the designers will receive better critical feedback from users. The idea of intelligence removes some of the evolutionary pressure from software by subtly indicating to users that it is they, rather than the software, who should be changing.

As it happens, machine decision making is already running our household finances to a scary degree, but it is doing so with a Wizard of Oz-like remote authority that keeps us from questioning it. I refer to the machines that calculate our credit ratings. Most of us have decided to change our habits so as to appeal to these machines. We have simplified ourselves to be comprehensible for simplistic databases, making them look smart and authoritative. Our demonstrated willingness to accommodate machines in this way is ample reason to adopt a standing bias against the idea of AI.

Inserting a judgment-making machine into a system allows individuals to avoid responsibility. If a trustworthy, gainfully employed person is denied a loan, it is because of the algorithm, not because of another specific person.

The loss of personal responsibility can be seen most clearly in the military's continued fascination with intelligent machines. Artificial intelligence has been one of the most heavily funded and least bountiful areas of scientific inquiry in the second half of the twentieth century. It keeps on failing and bouncing back with a different name, only to be overfunded once again. The most recent marketing moniker was Intelligent Agents. Before that, it was Expert Systems. The lemminglike funding charge is always led by the defense establishment. Artificial intelligence is perfect research for the military to fund. It lets strategists imagine less gruesome warfare and avoid personal responsibility at the same time.

Artificial-intelligence proponents object that a Turing Test–passing computer would be spectacularly, obviously intelligent and conscious, and that my arguments apply only to present, crude computers. The argument I present relates to the way in which computers change, however. The AI fantasy causes people to change more than computers do; therefore it impedes the progress of computers. If there *is* a potential for conscious computers, I would ńot be surprised if the idea of AI turns out to be the thing that prevents them from appearing.

Artificial-intelligence boosters believe computers are getting better so quickly that we will inevitably see qualitative changes in them, including consciousness, before we know it. I am bothered by the attitude implied in this position: that machines are essentially improving on their own. This is a trickled-down version of the retreat from responsibility implied by AI. I think we in the computer-science community need to take more responsibility than that. Even though we are used to seeing spectacular progress in the hardware capabilities of computers, software improves much more slowly, and sometimes not at all. I heard a novice user the other day complain that she missed her old text-only computer because it felt faster at word processing than her new Pentium machine. Software awkwardness will always be able to outpace gains in hardware speed and capacity, however spectacular they may be. Once again, emphasizing human responsibility instead of machine capability is much more likely to create better machines.

Even strong AI enthusiasts worry that human beings may not agree on whether a future machine has passed the Turing Test. Some of them bring up the moral equal-rights argument for the machine's benefit. After the thought experiments fail to turn in definitive results, the machine is favored anyway, and its rights are defended.

This stage is where AI crosses a boundary and turns into a religion. A new form of mysterious essence is being proposed for the benefit of machines. When I say religion, I mean it. The culture of machine-consciousness enthusiasts often includes the express hope that human death will be avoidable by actually enacting the first thought experiment above, transferring the human brain into a machine. Hans Moravec (1987) is one researcher who explicitly hopes for this eventuality. If we can become machines we do not have to die, but only if we believe in machine consciousness. I do not think it is productive to argue about religion in the same way as we argue about

Jaron Lanier: Mindless Thought Experiments

philosophy or science, but it is important to understand when religion is what we are talking about.

I will not argue religion here, but I will restate the heart of my objection to the idea of machine intelligence. The attraction and the danger of the idea is that it lets us avoid admitting how little we understand certain hard problems. By creating an umbrella category for everything brains do, it is possible to feel we are making progress on problems we still do not even know how to frame.

Even though the question of machine consciousness is both undecidable and lacking in consequence until some hypothesized future time when an artificial intelligence appears, attitudes toward the question today have a tangible effect. We are vulnerable to making ourselves stupid just to make possibly smart machines seem smart.

Artificial-intelligence enthusiasts like to characterize their opponents as inventing a problem of consciousness where there need not be one so as to preserve a special place for people in the universe. They often invoke the shameful history of hostile receptions to Galileo and Darwin to dramatize their plight as shunned visionaries. In their view, AI is resisted only because it threatens humanity's desire to be special in the same way as these hallowed scientists' ideas once did. This spin on opponents was first invented, with heroic immodesty, by Freud. Although Freud was undeniably a decisive, original thinker, his ideas have not held up as well as Darwin's or Galileo's. In retrospect, he does not seem to have been a particularly objective scientist, if he was a scientist at all. It is hard not to wonder if his self-inflation contributed to his failings.

Machine-consciousness believers should take Freud's case as a cautionary tale. Believing in Freud profoundly changed generations of doctors, educators, artists, and parents. Similarly, belief in the possibility of AI is beginning to change present practices both in subjects I have touched on—software engineering, education, and military planning—and in many other fields, including aspects of biology, economics, and social policy. The idea of AI is already changing the world, and it is important for everyone who is influenced by it to realize that its foundations are every bit as subjective and elusive as those of nonbelievers.

17 Structure and Function

Giuseppe Vitiello

AN OPEN LETTER TO PATRICIA CHURCHLAND

Dear Patricia:

After your talk in Tucson I said to myself, "I must meet Patricia Churchland and discuss with her the role of quantum mechanics (QM) and quantum formalisms in consciousness studies." The conference was very dense, however, you were very busy, and I was not so sure ... how to start a discussion with you. And at the end I decided to write you this letter.

In your talk, which I enjoyed very much, you kept saying, "I am not so sure ...," "I am not so sure...." You explained very well why one should have real doubts about hard (and easy) problems (which I will not discuss in this letter) and especially about using QM in studying consciousness.

From what you were saying I realized that you were completely right: *If* QM is what you were describing, and *if* its use and purpose are the ones you were discussing, *then* your doubts are really sound and, furthermore, I confirm to you that QM is completely useless in consciousness studies; the popular expression, "a mystery cannot solve another mystery" is fitting.

As a physicist, however, I want to tell you that one should not talk much about QM. Physicists, chemists, engineers, and other scientists use QM in many practical applications in solid-state physics, electronics, chemistry, and so on with extraordinary success: Undeniably our everyday (real) life strongly depends on those successful applications of QM. Everything around us (including ourselves) is made of atoms and the periodic table of the elements is clearly understood in terms of QM (recall, e.g., the Pauli principle in building up electron shells in atoms). From this perspective, QM is not a mystery. The photoelectric cell on elevators or compact-disc players and computers is not counterintuitive. Of course I do not say that the success of QM by itself justifies using QM in consciousness studies. I will come back to this point later on.

I want to stress here that QM is *not* the *object* of our discussion. Certainly many problems remain open in the interpretation of aspects of QM that are of great epistemological and philosophical interest. These problems, however absolutely do not interfere with or diminish QM's great successes in practical applications. It is interesting to study these interpretative problems, *but* they are *not* our object in this discussion.

And please notice that here I am not defending QM, for, as I have clearly stated many times in my papers, QM does not provide the proper mathematical formalism for studying living-matter physics. Indeed, the proper mathematical formalism in such a study turns out to be quantum field theory (QFT). But this is too strong a statement at this moment in our discussion. Let me proceed by small steps, instead.

I confess that I am not prepared to discuss how to approach the study of consciousness. As a physicist, I start by considering some more material object, such as the brain itself, or, more generally, living matter, such as the living cell. Here I need to explain myself because the word "material" may be misleading.

In physics it is not enough to know what things are made of. Listing elementary components is a crucial step, but it is only one step. We want to know not only what things are made of but *also* how it all works: we are interested in the dynamics. In short, we are interested in structure *and* in function. We physicists are attached to our fixations in such a narcissistic way that we even so thoroughly mix up structure and function that we often blur the distinction between them. Thus to us, having a detailed list of components teaches us little about the system we are studying. Moreover, it is not even possible to make a complete list of components without knowing how they all work together in the system. The same component concept is meaningless outside a dynamical knowledge of the system. Thus when I say "material" I refer also to dynamical laws, not to the mere collection of components.

Quite simply, studying the Tucson phone book does not help us understand the city of Tucson. Let me give one more specific physical example: the crystal. As is well known, when some kind of atoms (or molecules) sits in some lattice sites we have a crystal. The lattice is a specific geometric arrangement with a characteristic length between sites (I am thinking of a very simple situation, which is enough for what I want to say). A crystal may be broken in many ways, say, by melting at high temperature. Once the crystal is broken, one is left with the constituent atoms. Thus the atoms may be in the crystal phase or (e.g., after melting) in the gaseous phase. We can think of these phases as the functions of our structure (the atoms): the crystal function, the gaseous function. In the crystal phase one may experimentally study, say, how neutrons are scattered on the crystal's phonons. Phonons are the quanta of the elastic waves propagating in the crystal. They are true particles living in the crystal. We observe them in their scattering with neutrons. In fact, from the complementarity principle, they are the same as the elastic waves: they propagate over the whole system as the elastic waves do (for this reason they are also called "collective modes"). The phonons (or the elastic waves) are in fact messengers exchanged by the atoms and are responsible for holding the atoms in their lattice sites. Therefore the list of the crystal components includes not only the atoms but also the phonons. If it includes only the atoms, our list is not complete. When you destroy the crystal, however, you do not find the phonons—they disappear. On the other hand, if you want to reconstruct your crystal after you have broken it, the atoms you were left with are not enough: you must supplement the information that tells them how to sit in the special lattice you want (cubic, hexagonal, fivefold symmetry, etc.). You need to supply the ordering information that was lost when the crystal was destroyed. Exactly this ordering information is dynamically realized in the phonon particles. Thus, the phonon particles exist only (but really exist) as long as the crystal exists, and vice versa. The function of being crystal is identified with the particle structure. As you see, there is a great deal to the quantum theory of matter, and please notice: the description of a crystal in terms of phonons has nothing to do with interpretative problems. It is a well-understood, experimentally well-tested physical description.

Such a situation happens many times in physics; other familiar examples are ferromagnets, superconductors, and so on. It is a general feature that occurs when the symmetry of the dynamics is not the symmetry of the system's states (symmetry is spontaneously broken, technically speaking). Let me explain what this statement means. Consider the crystal: the symmetry of the dynamics is the continuous-space translational symmetry (the atoms may move around, occupying any position in the available space). In the crystal state, however, such symmetry is lost (broken) as the atoms are ordered in the lattice sites. For example, they can no longer sit between two lattice corners: order is lack of symmetry. A general theorem states that when continuous symmetry is spontaneously broken (equivalently, as we have just seen, an ordered pattern is generated), a massless particle is dynamically created. This particle (the Nambu-Goldstone boson) is the phonon in the crystal case. Please notice that this particle is massless, which means that it can span the whole system volume without inertia. This condition in turn guarantees that the ordering information will be carried around without losses and that the ordered pattern is a stable one. The presence (or, as we say, the condensation) of the Goldstone particles of lowest momentum adds no energy to the state (it is enough to consider the lowest energy state, namely the ground state). Finally, the ordered ground-state crystal has the same energy as the symmetric, unordered gaseous one (we call this the normal ground state): they are degenerate states of equal energy. The crystal therefore does exist as a stable phase of the matter. Actually, ground states, and therefore the phases the system may assume, are classified by their ordering degree (the order parameter), which depends on the condensate density of Goldstone quanta. Thus we see that by tuning the condensate density (e.g., by changing the temperature) we can drive the system through the various phases it can assume. Because the system phases are macroscopically characterized (the order parameter is in fact a macroscopic observable), we have a bridge between the microscopic quantum scale and our everyday macroscopic scale.

All these conditions of course are possible only if the mathematical formalism provides us with many degenerate but physically nonequivalent ground states needed to represent the system phases, which in fact do have different physical properties, explaining why we have to use QFT and not QM, as I said earlier. In QM, all possible ground states are physically equivalent (the von Neumann theorem); on the contrary, QFT is much richer—it is equipped with infinitely many physically nonequivalent ground states. We must use QFT to study systems with many phases.

All I have said has been based on theorems, but I stress that these are fitted perfectly by real experiments and are the only available quantum theory (QFT indeed) on which the reliable working of any sort of technological gadget around us is based. This limitation applies in spite of the many unsolved epistemological and philosophical questions that quantum theories may stir up.

Now perhaps you understand why I need to start by considering actual material. The problem of consciousness is not simply a list of constituents, specific information from punctual observations, or a lot of real data and statistics. Rather, it is also the dynamics. Otherwise, the study of consciousness would be like one of those extremely patient and skillful Swiss watchmakers who in past centuries mechanically assembled a lot of wheels, levers, and hooks to build beautiful puppets able to simulate many human movements. But ... the puppets were not conscious, and the phone book is not enough if we want to know the city. None of these can be complete without the dynamics. We cannot hope to build up a crystal without long-range correlations mediated by phonons. Experiments tell us that to build a crystal hook by hook, placing atom by atom into their lattice sites, the coherent orchestra of vibrating atoms playing the crystal function does not occur.

For every new or more refined movement added to eighteenth-century puppets, more and more specialized units and wheels were needed. And certainly the brain, and living matter in general, present a lot of very specialized units, which need to be sought out. But our list of components will still be incomplete if we do not think of a dynamical scheme also. Properties of living matter, such as self-ordering, behavior far from equilibrium, nondissipative energy transfer on protein molecular chains in an overall context of extremely high chemical efficiency and at the same time extremely numerous chemical species, and so on, point to the existence of a nontrivial dynamical background from which arises the rich phenomenology of molecular biology. As with chemistry before the birth of QM, we are challenged to search for a unifying dynamical scheme that may help us understand those (collective) properties.

The problem is *not* why we should *expect* a quantum dynamical level in living matter (and in the brain). Even in its inert (or dead) phase the components of matter include atoms, molecules, and, as we have seen, other dynamically generated units (e.g., the phonon), all of which are ruled by quantum laws. The world would be really crazy if the same atoms, molecules, and dynamically generated units were not ruled by the same quantum laws in the living phase of matter.

Sometimes people get confused trying to distinguish between classical level and quantum level. Although we speak about a classical limit of quantum physics, we *never* mean that, for example, the Planck constant becomes (or goes to) zero in the classical limit (even when we do say that sloppily—sorry!). The Planck constant has a well-defined value that *never* is zero. By "classical" we mean only that some properties of the system are acceptably well described, from the observational point of view, in the approximation in which we neglect certain ratios between the Planck constant and some other quantity (of the same physical dimensions). Not that one puts the Planck constant equal to zero, because other behaviors (which the same system shows simultaneously with the classical ones), can be described only by keeping the nonzero value of the Planck constant in its full glory. An example: Our friend the crystal behaves as a classical object in many respects—without a doubt. The phonon, however, *is* a quantum particle (it *is* a quantum) and therefore the macroscopic function of being a crystal *is* a quantum feature of our system. It is indeed such a quantum behavior, that of being a crystal, which manifests the classical behavior of the component atoms as a whole. Therefore, a diamond is a classically behaving macroscopic quantum system when one gives it as a gift to his or her fiancé(e) (and let us hope they will not argue about the phonon, Schrödinger's cat, their love being classical or quantum, and all that; it would be not at all romantic).

In the same way, systemic features of living matter, such as ordered patterns, sequentially interlocked chemical reactions, nondissipative energy transfer, and nonlocal simultaneous response to external stimuli do, as macroscopic quantum features, support the rich phenomenology of molecular biology. In the QFT approach to living matter, the idea is to supplement the phenomenological random kinematics of biochemistry with a basic dynamics.

The problem then is not *if* a quantum dynamics exists in living matter (how could it not exist?), but which are its observable manifestations, if any, and how does the biochemistry show up? Of course, it is more and more urgent that we know all we can about the components, their kinematics, their engineering, and so on; we need working models to solve immediate problems (floating boats were used well before Archimedes' law was known). We even need patient assembly of cells hook by hook to form a tissue, but we cannot howl at the sky if a cancer develops. The hook strategy involves only random kinematics but no dynamics involved in tissue formation; as a consequence the same list of component cells has no reason for behaving as a tissue instead of as a cancer. (Sometimes the eighteenth-century puppets fell apart.) Therefore, it might be worthwhile to apply what we have learned about collective modes holding atoms in their lattice sites (the crystal is a "tissue"), spontaneous symmetry breakdown, coherence, boson condensation, and so on, to study (together with biochemists and biologists), the normal (or symmetric) state of cancer and the ordered state of tissue, as we say in QFT language.

The task is not at all simple. Living matter is not an inert crystal. And we should expect many surprises. For example, in the quantum model of the brain by Ricciardi and Umezawa (Brain and physics of many-body problems, *Kibernetic* 4:44, 1967.) the problem of memory capacity seems to be solved by seriously considering the brain's dissipative character. That dissipation comes into play can be naively understood by observing that information recording breaks the symmetry under time reversal; that is, it introduces the arrow of time: *"Now* you know it ... !" is the warning that after receiving information, one can no longer behave as before receiving it. Thus memorizing breaks time-reversal symmetry. Brain dynamics are therefore intrinsically irreversible. In more familiar words, the brain, like other biological systems, has a history—in this respect the brain is a clock. Well, to treat dissipative brain dynamics in QFT, one has to introduce the time-reversed image of the system's degrees of freedom. Thus one finds oneself dealing with a system made by the brain and by its mirror-in-time image, because of the mathematical scheme's internal consistency (if you want to know more about that subject, see my paper in *Internationed Journal Modern Physics B* (1995) 9:973). Perhaps consciousness mechanisms are macroscopic manifestations of the mirror brain dynamics. Does conscious experience of the flow of time arise from the brain's dissipative dynamics? The mirror modes are related to brain–environment coupling and at the same time to brain self-interaction, which may lead to the conscious sense of self.

I realize this is a long letter and I will not talk any longer about brain and living matter, consciousness and QFT. I hope we can resume our discussion on a future occasion to join our efforts in studying the brain.

Arrivederci a presto,
Giuseppe

18 "More Neural Than Thou"

Stuart R. Hameroff

In "Brainshy: Nonneural Theories of Conscious Experience" (this volume), Patricia Churchland considers three "nonneural" approaches to the puzzle of consciousness: (1) Chalmers's fundamental information, (2) Searle's "intrinsic" property of brain, and (3) Penrose-Hameroff quantum phenomena in microtubules. In rejecting these ideas, Churchland flies the flag of "neuralism." She claims that conscious experience will be totally and completely explained by the dynamical complexity of properties at the level of neurons and neural networks. As far as consciousness goes, neural-network firing patterns triggered by axon-to-dendrite synaptic chemical transmissions are the fundamental correlates of consciousness. We need not look elsewhere.

Churchland's "neuralism" and allegiance to the brain-as-computer doctrine obscure inconvenient details, however. For example:

1. Neurotransmitter vesicle release is probabilistic (and possibly noncomputable). Only about 15 percent of axonal action potentials reaching presynaptic terminals result in actual release of neurotransmitter vesicles. Beck and Eccles (1992) suggested that quantum indeterminacy acts here.

2. Apart from chemical synapses, primitive electrotonic gap junctions may be important in consciousness. For example, gap junctions may mediate coherent 40-Hz activity implicated in binding in vision and "self" (Jibu 1990, Hameroff 1996).

3. It is quite possible that consciousness occurs primarily in dendritic–dendritic processing and that axonal firings support primarily automatic, nonconscious activities (e.g., Pribram 1991, Jibu, Pribram, and Yasue 1996, Alkon 1989).

4. Glial cells (80 percent of the brain) are ignored in neuralism.

5. Neuralism ignores the cytoskeleton (Figures 18.1 and 18.2). Perhaps the most egregious oversight, neuronal microtubules and other cytoskeletal structures organizing the cell interior are *known* to establish, maintain, and regulate neuronal architecture and synapses, to service ion channels and synaptic receptors, to provide for neurotransmitter vesicle transport and release, and to be involved in "second-messenger" postsynaptic signaling. They are also *theorized* to integrate postsynaptic receptor activation, process information,

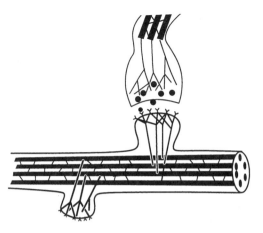

Figure 18.1 Neural synapse, showing cytoskeletal structures within two neurons. (top) Presynaptic axon terminal releases neurotransmitter vesicles (black spheres) into synaptic cleft. Thick black rodlike structures at top indicate microtubules; thinner filaments (e.g., synapsin) facilitate vesicle release. (bottom) Dendrite on postsynaptic neuron with two dendritic spines. Microtubules in main dendrite are interconnected by microtubule-associated proteins. Other cytoskeletal structures (fodrin, actin filaments, etc.) connect membrane receptors to microtubules. Based on Hirokawa (1991).

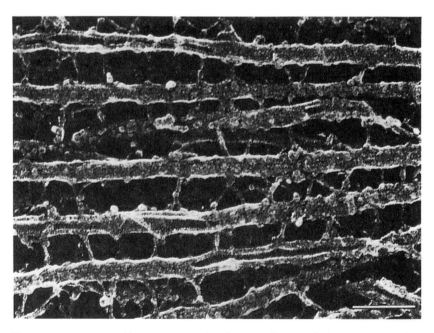

Figure 18.2 Immuno-electron micrograph of neuronal microtubules interconnected by microtubule-associated proteins. Scale bar: 100 nm. Reprinted with permission from Hirokawa (1991).

and communicate and compute both classically and by quantum-coherent superposition. Churchland's neuron *sans* cytoskeleton simulates a real neuron as an inflatable doll simulates a real person.

Shorn of these details, Churchland's neuralism remains convenient for computer analogy, but inadequate for consciousness. I begin by addressing some of Churchland's comments about Penrose–Hameroff quantum phenomena in microtubules.

PLATO AND THE PLANCK SCALE

Churchland derides Roger Penrose for resorting to Platonism, for believing "ideas have an existence … an ideal Platonic world … accessible by the intellect only … a direct route to truth …" (Plato 400 B.C.). In *Shadows of the Mind*, Penrose (1994) describes three worlds: the physical, the mental, and the Platonic. The physical and mental worlds are familiar and agreed upon as actual realities—clearly, the physical world exists and thoughts exist. Penrose's Platonic world includes mathematical truths, laws, and relationships, as well as aesthetics and ethics—our senses of beauty and morality. The Platonic world appears to be purely abstract. Could it simply exist in the empty space of the universe? If truth and beauty are indeed fundamental, perhaps the Platonic world is engrained at the most basic level of reality.

The same may be said of qualia. A line of panexperiential philosophy suggests that protoconscious experience is fundamental. Leibniz (e.g., 1768) saw the universe as an infinite number of fundamental units (*monads*)—each having a primitive psychological being. Whitehead (e.g., 1929) described dynamic monads with greater spontaneity and creativity, interpreting them as mindlike entities of limited duration ("occasions of experience"—each bearing a quality akin to "feeling"). More recently, Wheeler (e.g., 1990) described a "pre-geometry" of fundamental reality comprising information. Chalmers (1996a, 1996b) contends that fundamental information includes "experiential aspects" leading to consciousness.

If mathematical truth, aesthetics, ethics, and experience are actual and fundamental entities, a plausible location for them is the most basic level of reality.

What is fundamental reality? The Planck scale (10^{-33} cm, 10^{-43} sec) is the scale at which space-time is no longer smooth. At that scale, the vacuum of empty space actually "seethes with subtle activities" (e.g., Browne 1997). Branches of quantum theory known as quantum electrodynamics (QED) and quantum field theory predict that at the Planck scale particles and waves ("virtual photons") continuously wink into and out of existence (e.g, Jibu and Yasue 1995, Seife 1997), and that the churning quantum fluctuations (the "quantum foam"—Figure 18.3) imparts dynamic structure and measurable energy ("zero-point fluctuations").

This picture of the quantum vacuum had been developed by Max Planck and Werner Heisenberg in the 1920s. In 1948, the Dutch scientist Hendrick

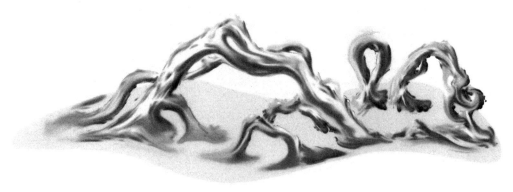

Figure 18.3 Quantum electrodynamics (QED) predicts that, at the Planck scale in the vacuum of empty space, quantum fluctuations produce a foam of erupting and collapsing virtual particles that may be visualized as topographic distortions in the fabric of space-time. Adapted from Thorne (1994) by Dave Cantrell.

Casimir predicted that the all-pervading zero-point energy could be measured using parallel surfaces separated by a tiny gap. Some (longer-wavelength) virtual photons would be excluded from the gap region, Casimir reasoned, and the surplus photons outside the gap would exert pressure, forcing the surfaces together. Recently this "Casimir force" was quantitatively verified quite precisely (Lamoreaux 1997), confirming the zero-point energy. Lamoreaux's experimental surfaces were separated by a distance d ranging from 0.6 to 6μ, and the measured force was extremely weak (Figure 18.4A). At the Tucson II conference, physicist George Hall (Hall 1996) presented calculations of the Casimir force on model microtubule cylinders. Hall considered the microtubule hollow inner core of 15 nm diameter as the Casimir gap d. Because the force is proportional to d^{-4}, Hall's models predict significant pressure (0.5 to 20 atm) exerted by the quantum vacuum on microtubules of sufficient length (Figure 18.4B). Microtubules actually *are* under compression in cells, a factor thought to enhance vibrational signaling and tensegrity structure (e.g., Ingber 1993). In the well-known "pressure reversal of anesthesia," unconscious, anesthetized experimental subjects wake up when ambient pressure is increased on the order of 10 atm. This phenomenon implies that a baseline ambient pressure such as the Casimir force acting on microtubules, as suggested by Hall, may be required for consciousness.

To provide a description of the quantum-mechanical geometry of space at the Planck scale, Penrose (1971) introduced "quantum-spin networks" (Rovelli and Smolin 1995a, 1995b), in which spectra of discrete Planck-scale volumes and configurations are obtained (Figure 18.3). These fundamental space-time volumes and configurations may qualify as philosophical (quantum) monads. Perhaps Planck-scale spin networks encode protoconscious experience and Platonic values.

The panexperiential view most consistent with modern physics is that of Alfred North Whitehead: (1) consciousness is a process of events occurring in a wider, basic field of raw protoconscious experience; (2) Whitehead's

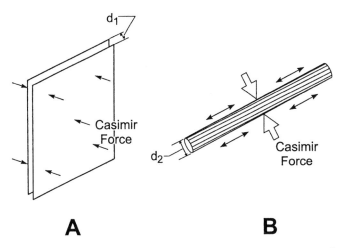

A **B**

Figure 18.4 (A) The Casimir force of the quantum-vacuum zero-point fluctuation energy may be measured by placing two macroscopic surfaces separated by a small gap d. As some virtual photons are excluded in the gap, the net "quantum foam" exerts pressure, forcing the surfaces together. In Lamoreaux's (1997) experiment, d_1 was in the range 0.6 to 6.0 μ ($\sim$1500 nm). (B) Hall (1996) calculated the Casimir force on microtubules. Because the force is proportional to d^{-4}, and d_2 for microtubules is 15 nm, the predicted Casimir force is roughly 10^6 greater on microtubules (per equivalent surface area) than that measured by Lamoreaux. Hall calculates a range of Casimir forces on microtubules (length-dependent) from 0.5 to 20 atm.

events (discrete occasions of experience) are comparable to quantum-state reductions (Shimony 1993).

This interpretation suggests that consciousness may involve a self-organizing quantum-state reduction occurring at the Planck scale. In a pan-experiential Platonic view consistent with modern physics, quantum-spin networks encode protoconscious "funda-mental" experience and Platonic values. In this view, various configurations of quantum-spin geometry represent varieties of experience and values. A self-organizing process capable of collapsing quantum-wave functions at Planck-scale geometry while somehow coupling to neural action is a candidate for consciousness. Is there such a process?

Objective reduction (OR) is Penrose's proposed quantum-gravity solution to the problem of wave-function collapse in quantum mechanics (Penrose 1989, 1994, 1996). In Penrose's OR, quantum superposition—actual separation, or displacement of mass from itself—also causes underlying space-time (spin networks) to separate (simultaneous curvatures in opposite directions). Such separations are unstable and a critical degree of separation results in instantaneous self-collapse—objective reduction. Superposed (separated) mass and space-time geometry select particular "unseparated" states. An event occurs. A choice is made.

The critical degree of space-time separation causing Penrose's OR reduction is related to quantum gravity and given by the uncertainty principle $E = \hbar/T$, where E is the gravitational self-energy of the superposed mass (displaced from itself by the diameter of its atomic nuclei), $\hbar$ is Planck's

Stuart R. Hameroff: "More Neural Than Thou"

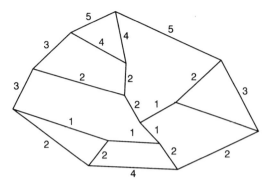

Figure 18.5 A spin network. Introduced by Roger Penrose (1971) as a quantum-mechanical description of the geometry of space, spin networks describe spectra of discrete Planck-scale volumes and configurations. Average length of each link: Planck length (10^{-33} cm, 10^{-25} nm). Reprinted by permission from Rovelli and Smolin (1995a).

constant over 2π, and T is the coherence time until self-collapse. (Without an objective criterion for reduction, space-time separation could presumably continue and result in separate, multiple space-time universes, as described in the Everett "multi-worlds" or "multi-minds" view of quantum theory.)

If isolated from environmental decoherence, a quantum-superposed mass E will self-collapse after time T to definite mass locations and space-time geometry. The postreduction mass locations and space-time geometry are chosen noncomputably—but only if the quantum collapse occurs by the OR process, rather than by environmental interaction causing decoherence (in which case the states are chosen randomly). The noncomputable influence in OR may be a Platonic grain in Planck-scale geometry.

"... one's consciousness breaks through into this world of ideas ...." (Plato 400 B.C.)

Could an OR process be occurring in our brains? How could biology "break through" to "funda-mental" space-time? The Penrose-Hameroff Orch OR model describes a biological OR occurring in microtubules (MTs) in the brain's neurons (Penrose and Hameroff 1995, Hameroff and Penrose 1996a, 1996b, Figures 18.6–18.8). Quantum reductions in MTs are consistent with Whitehead "occasions of experience" and coherent 40-Hz neural-level "cognitive quanta" (e.g., Crick and Koch 1990, Llinas, e.g., Joliot, Ribary, and Llinas 1994). Such events could link Platonism, biology, and funda-mental experience at the Planck scale.

ANESTHESIA

Churchland raises an interesting issue: the mechanism of anesthesia. Many types of molecules, including inhaled gases and intravenous drugs, can inhibit consciousness and be safely administered and eliminated from the body (see Franks and Lieb, Chapter 38, this volume). Even in the presence of significant doses of these anesthetics, some brain neural activities persist in unconscious patients (electroencephalograms [EEG], evoked potentials, autonomic drives, etc.). Thus, although anesthetics have other effects not directly related to consciousness (e.g., blood pressure, heart rate, muscle tone), anesthetic mechanisms may distinguish brain sites essential for consciousness. Churchland correctly remarks that "evidence points to proteins in the neuron membrane as the principal locus of hydrophobic anesthetics."

We have no consensus on anatomical sites of anesthetic effect. During anesthesia with volatile gases like halothane or isoflurane, the anesthetic molecules are widely distributed in most brain areas (although recent brain imaging has localized some effects of such intravenous anesthetics as propofol. See Alkire et al. this volume). The sites of anesthetic action at cellular and molecular levels have been studied extensively, however, particularly in the past two decades, by Franks and Lieb (e.g., 1982, 1985, Chapter 38, this volume, cf. Halsey 1989).

Their work shows that: (1) anesthetics act directly on proteins, rather than on membrane lipids; (2) relatively few brain proteins are anesthetic target sites; (3) anesthetics act in hydrophobic ("lipidlike") regions within target proteins; (4) anesthetics bind in these hydrophobic "pockets" by weak van der Waals forces.

Franks and Lieb (Chapter 38, this volume) suggest that the predominant anesthetic targets are postsynaptic membrane proteins belonging to the acetylcholine receptor genetic "superfamily." Strangely, some of these receptors are excitatory (serotonin, nicotinic) and others are inhibitory (GABA, glycine), and so anesthetics appear to potentiate some proteins and inhibit others. (Interestingly, GABA and glycine receptors are regulated by cytoskeletal microtubules—Franks and Lieb, Chapter 38, this volume, Delon and Legendre 1995).

Conspicuous by their relative insensitivity to inhaled-gas anesthetics are receptors for glutamate, the principal excitatory neurotransmitter in the mammalian central nervous system. Glutamate receptors (e.g., "NMDA": n-methyl-d-aspartate receptors), however, are sensitive to such "dissociative" anesthetics as ketamine, and the street-drug/animal anesthetic phencyclidine (PCP). In low-dose receptor occupancy these drugs induce sensory illusions, visual and auditory hallucinations, distortions of body image, and disorganized thought (see Flohr, Chapter 39, this volume). In high doses they cause general anesthesia.

Other neural proteins are just slightly anesthetic-sensitive, but widely distributed and heavily prevalent throughout the brain. These include voltage-gated ion channels, presynaptic vesicle-release proteins, and microtubules. As Franks and Lieb (this volume) point out, slight anesthetic effects on many sites could be important, particularly if those sites are essential for consciousness.

Like consciousness, anesthesia appears to be a global, collective phenomenon involving multiple sites. At anesthetic concentrations just sufficient for loss of consciousness, hydrophobic pockets in a class of neural proteins (ion channels, receptors, second messengers, enzymes, microtubule tubulin, actin, etc.) are likely to bind and mediate anesthetic effect.

ANESTHESIA AND MICROTUBULES

Tubulin, the component protein of microtubules, has a hydrophobic region comprising aromatic and other hydrophobic amino acids (e.g., Andreu 1986). The first studies of anesthetic effects on microtubules were performed by Allison and Nunn (1968, Allison et al. 1970). They studied the heliozoan *actinosphaerium*, a tiny urchin with hundreds of delicate spines (axonemes, or axopodia). The internal structure of each spine axoneme is a parallel array of microtubules interconnected in a double spiral (Figure 37.6). Allison and Nunn found that adding an anesthetic like halothane to the medium caused the spines to withdraw as the microtubules disassembled. When the anesthetic was removed, the spines reassembled. The amount of anesthetic required for complete axoneme disassembly was equivalent to about four times that required for clinical anesthesia, although axoneme shortening began at only twice the clinical dose. The esteemed authors suggested that anesthesia might be caused by reversible disassembly of brain microtubules. Subsequent studies in nerve preparations, however, failed to show effects of clinically relevant doses of anesthetic on microtubule assembly (Hinkley and Green 1970, Saubermann and Gallager 1973) and axoplasmic transport (Kennedy, Fink, and Byers 1972), and the "microtubule hypothesis" fell on hard times.

Refined techniques led to further studies. Hinkley and Samson (1972, Hinkley 1978) clearly demonstrated that halothane caused microtubules in vitro to reassemble into "macrotubules"—larger (48-nm vs. 25-nm diameter) with more protofilaments (24 vs. 15). In myelinated axons, Livingston and Vergara (1979) showed significant decrease in microtubule numbers and density after 20 millimolar (mM) halothane. Vergara and Livingston (1981) later studied binding of halothane to tubulin from rat brain. They found that 28 mM halothane displaced tubulin-bound colchicine. Hinkley and Telser (1974) and Uemura and Levin (1992) showed that very low concentrations of halothane cause disruption of actin gelation. Concentrations of gas anesthetics within cells are difficult to determine due to poor solubility in the aqueous phase, but it appears that at clinical concentrations anesthetics do bind to tubulin (without causing microtubule disassembly) and to actin in addition to membrane proteins.

The most intriguing question is why protein hydrophobic pockets are essential to consciousness.

CONSCIOUSNESS AND QUANTUM EFFECTS IN HYDROPHOBIC POCKETS

The collective locus of anesthetic effect is an array of hydrophobic sites in various types of proteins throughout the brain. They have a common hydrophobic solubility parameter that can best be described as similar to that of olive oil. The "cutoff effect" (e.g., Franks and Lieb this volume) tells us that anesthetic sites are smaller than a cubic nanometer. Thus we have an ordered array of discrete, tiny olive-oil pockets in strategic neural sites throughout the brain. The components of these pockets (e.g., aromatic amino-acid rings) utilize van der Waals interactions, couplings of electron quantum fluctuations. This condition requires delocalization: electrons must be mobile and relatively free to roam within the pocket among resonance orbitals of nonpolar amino acid groups (e.g., leucine, phenylalanine, etc.). Isolated from water, hydrophobic pockets are ideal settings for electron quantum effects. According to Fröhlich's (1968) suggestion, electron localizations in hydrophobic pockets cause the entire protein to assume one specific conformation; electron localizations in different intrapocket areas result in the protein's assuming a different conformation. In quantum theory, however, individual electrons (or electron pairs) can also be in a state of quantum "superposition" in which both positions are occupied (and the protein assumes both conformations—e.g., Figure 18.6). Anesthetics bind in hydrophobic pockets by weak van der Waals forces that are attractive couplings among quantum fluctuations in the electron clouds of anesthetic and pocket. (Van der Waals attractions are closely related to the Casimir force—Lamoreaux 1997.) Anesthetics are known to inhibit electron mobility (Hameroff and Watt 1983) and (by computer simulation) reduce hydrophobic-pocket van der Waals energy in an anesthetic-sensitive protein (Louria and Hameroff 1996). Quantum fluctuations in hydrophobic pockets may be necessary for consciousness.

It may be concluded that anesthetics act by preventing quantum-coherent superposition in hydrophobic pockets of (1) membrane proteins, (2) tubulins, or (3) both. Another possibility is that anesthetics disrupt actin gelation required for quantum-state isolation.

Drugs like the hallucinogenic ("psychedelic") tryptamine and phenylethylamine derivatives bind in a class of hydrophobic pockets, but obviously exert quite different effects than anesthetics. Composed of aromatic rings with polar "tails," these drugs are known to bind to serotonin and NMDA receptors, but their psychedelic mechanism is basically unknown (e.g., Weil 1996). Nichols, Shulgin, and Dyer (1977, Nichols 1986) showed that psychedelic drugs bind in hydrophobic pockets in serotonin receptors of less than 6 angstroms (Å) (0.6 nm) length. Kang and Green (1970) and Snyder and Merril (1965) showed correlation between hallucinogenic potency and the drug molecules' ability to donate electron orbital resonance energy (comparable to increase in van der Waals energy). In Louria and Hameroff (1996) we speculated that by such a mechanism psychedelic drugs promote quantum-coherent superposition in receptors and other proteins, including cytoskeleton. In Hameroff and Penrose (1996a) it is suggested that such a quantum-enhanced state increases intensity and frequency of conscious events and merges normally pre- and subconscious processes with consciousness by a baseline shift in quantum coherence. Psychedelic perceptions and

205   Stuart R. Hameroff: "More Neural Than Thou"

hallucinations may be glimpses into a preconscious–subconscious quantum-superposed world.

PIXIE DUST VS. ORCH OR

Churchland asserts that "pixie dust in the synapses" is as explanatory as the Penrose-Hameroff Orch OR model. Let us compare explanatory power of Orch OR with her synaptic pixie dust (I assume she is referring to her "neuralism," as described in the Introduction to this chapter). Let us see how each handles five enigmatic features of consciousness: (1) the nature of experience (hard problem), (2) binding, (3) free will, (4) noncomputability, and (5) transition from preconscious processes to consciousness.

Feature 1: Experience, Hard Problem (e.g., Chalmers 1996a, 1996b)

Pixie dust (neuralism): Postulate conscious experience emerging from unspecified critical level of neuronal computational complexity.

Orch OR: Philosophically ascribe to panexperientialism, following, for example, Spinoza, Leibniz, Whitehead, Wheeler, and Chalmers. Experience, qualia are deemed fundamental, a basic property of the universe such as matter or charge. If so, experience must be represented at the most basic level of reality—namely the 10^{-33} cm Planck scale at which space-time is no longer smooth. Penrose's (1971) quantum-spin networks (Rovelli and Smolin 1995) are possible descriptions of fundamental space-time geometry capable of experiential qualities. Orch OR is a self-organizing process in the Planck-scale medium that selects particular configurations of fundamental geometry (Figures 18.6–18.8). Thus, Orch OR postulates experience as a "fundamental" feature of reality, and provides a mechanism for accessing and selecting particular configurations of experience. The "smell of cinnamon" is self-selection of a particular funda-mental geometry.

Feature 2: Binding

Pixie dust (neuralism): Coherent neural-membrane activities (e.g., coherent 40 Hz) bind in vision, and in "self" by temporal correlation of neural firing.

Orch OR: Macroscopic quantum states (e.g., Bose-Einstein condensates) *are* single entities, not just temporally correlated separate entities.

Feature 3: Free Will

Pixie dust (neuralism):?

Orch OR: The problem in understanding free will is that our actions seem neither deterministic nor random (probabilistic). What else is there in nature? Penrose's objective reduction ("OR") is a possible solution. In OR, quantum superposed systems evolve (if isolated) until their energy–time product

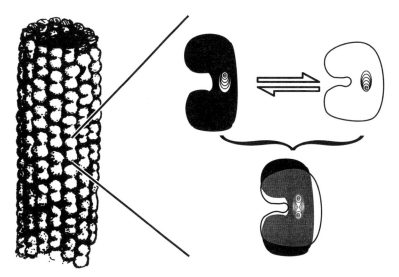

Figure 18.6 (left) Microtubule (MT) structure: a hollow tube of 25-nm diameter, consisting of 13 columns of tubulin dimers arranged in hexagonal lattice (Penrose 1994). (right, top) Each tubulin molecule can switch between two (or more) conformations, coupled to a quantum event such as electron location in tubulin hydrophobic pocket. (right, bottom) Each tubulin can also exist in quantum superposition of both conformational states. Hameroff and Penrose (1996).

reaches a barrier related to quantum gravity, at which instant they reduce, or collapse to definite states. The collapse "choices" are neither deterministic nor probabilistic, but rather are "noncomputable"—possibly reflecting influence by some hidden quantum-mathematical logic.

In Orch OR, the microtubule quantum superposition evolves (analogous to a quantum computer) so that it may be influenced at the instant of collapse by hidden nonlocal variables, or quantum-mathematical logic. The possible outcomes are limited, or probabilities set ("orchestrated"), by the neurobiological self-organizing process (in particular, microtubule-associated proteins—MAPs). The precise outcome is chosen by the effect of the hidden logic on the poised system.

Perhaps a sailboat analogy will be helpful. A sailor sets the sail in a specific way; the boat's direction is then determined by the action of the wind on the sail. Let us pretend the sailor is a nonconscious robot zombie trained and programmed to sail a boat across a lake. Setting and adjusting the sail, sensing the wind and position, and so on are algorithmic and deterministic, and may be analogous to the preconscious, quantum-computing phase of Orch OR. The direction of the wind (seemingly capricious) may be analogous to hidden nonlocal variables (e.g., "Platonic" quantum-mathematical logic inherent in space-time) that provide noncomputability. The choice, or outcome (the direction in which the boat sails, the point on shore where it lands) depends on the deterministic sail settings acted on repeatedly by the unpredictable wind. Our actions could be the net result of deterministic processes acted on by hidden quantum logic at each Orch OR event.

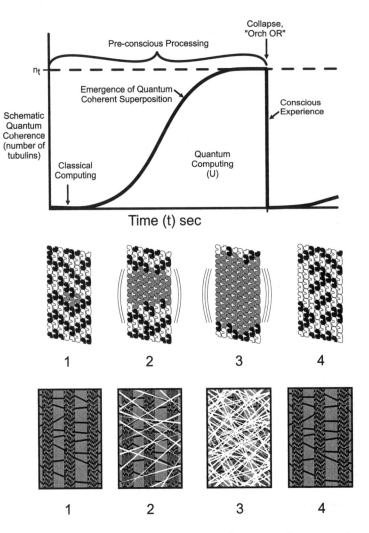

Figure 18.7 Steps in an Orch OR event. (top) Schematic graph of proposed quantum coherence (number of tubulins) emerging vs. time in microtubules. Area under curve connects mass–energy differences with collapse time in accordance with gravitational OR ($E = \hbar/T$). n_t is the number of tubulins whose mass separation (and separation of underlying space-time) for time T will self-collapse. For example, for time $T = 25$ msec (e.g., 40-Hz oscillations), $T = 2 \times 10^{10}$ tubulins. (middle) Microtubule simulation in which classical computing (step 1) leads to emergence of quantum-coherent superposition (and quantum computing—steps 2–3) in certain (gray) tubulins. Step 3 (in coherence with other microtubule tubulins) meets critical threshold related to quantum gravity for self-collapse (Orch OR). A conscious event (Orch OR) occurs in the step 3–4 transition. Tubulin states in step 4 are noncomputably chosen in the collapse, and evolve by classical computing to regulate neural function. (bottom) Schematic sequence of phases of actin gelation (quantum isolation) and solution (environmental communication) around MTs.

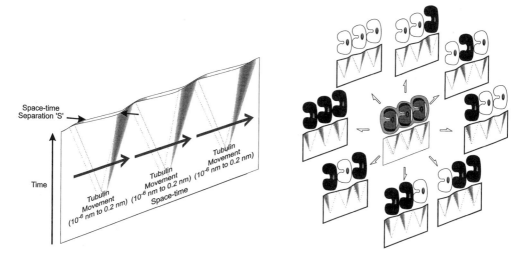

Figure 18.8 Space-time representations of tubulin superpositions (left) Schematic space-time separation illustration of three superposed tubulins. The Planck-scale space-time separations S are very tiny by ordinary standards, but relatively large mass movements (e.g., hundreds of tubulin conformations, each moving from 10^{-6} nm to 0.2 nm) indeed have such very tiny effects on the space-time curvature. A critical degree of separation causes an abrupt selection of one curvature or the other. (right center) Three superposed tubulins with corresponding schematic space-time separation illustrations. Surrounding the superposed tubulins are the eight possible postreduction "eigenstates" for tubulin conformation, and corresponding space-time geometry. The postreduction state is chosen noncomputably in Orch OR events.

Feature 4: Noncomputability

Pixie dust (neuralism): *What* noncomputability? Penrose's argument from Gödel's theorem that human thought requires noncomputability provoked a torrent of critical papers, mainly from defendants of and dependents on artificial intelligence (AI). (The overreaction reached the point of Penrose's being awarded a sarcastic prize from AI henchmen. [See Churchland, Chapter 8, this volume.]) However, most harped-on issues had been already answered (but apparently unnoticed) in *The Emperor's New Mind* and *Shadows of the Mind*, and Penrose responded point by point to a collection of critics ("Beyond the doubting of a shadow"—Penrose 1996b). For Penrose, the key to noncomputability is the nature of mathematical understanding, but noncomputability may also be evident in creativity (Casti 1996), and as favorable unpredictability in predator–prey interactions important in evolution (Barinaga 1996).

Orch OR: Self-organized quantum-gravity collapse of the wave function, Penrose's "objective reduction" is predicted to be noncomputable (Penrose 1989, 1994, 1996). The specific postcollapse states are neither random nor chosen algorithmically, but rather are influenced by unknown (nonlocal hidden variable) quantum logic inherent in fundamental space-time geometry.

Feature 5: Transition from Preconscious Processes to Consciousness

Pixie dust (neuralism): Conscious experience emerges at an unspecified critical threshold of neural activity.

Orch OR: The prereduction tubulin superposition ("quantum-computing") phase is equated with preconscious processes. When the quantum gravity threshold is reached according to $E = \hbar/T$, self-collapse (objective reduction) abruptly occurs. The tubulin superposition is a separation in underlying space-time geometry in which "funda-mental" experience presumably is contained. With each self-collapse a new geometry of experience is selected—each Orch OR is a conscious event.

Although I may be biased, it appears that when we consider difficult issues related to consciousness, Orch OR is far more explanatory than synaptic pixie dust (Churchland's neuralism).

CONCLUSION: NEURALISM

I applaud Professor Churchland's devotion to neurobiology and thank her for her interest, criticism, and kind comments and for the honor of being grouped with John Searle, David Chalmers, and Roger Penrose. I am obliged to inform her, however, that there is much more to neurons than meets her eye. Dendritic processing, gap junctions, probabilistic vesicle release, glial processing, and classical cytoskeletal dynamics clearly indicate that the neuron-as-switch concept is hopelessly naive. Add to this complexity the possibilities of quantum coherence in microtubules, actin gelation cycles, gap-junction quantum tunneling, and quantum-gravity self-collapse rearranging funda-mental space-time. And add one more certainty: neurons are alive! Until proven otherwise, consciousness is a process peculiar to living systems. We can not sweep the question of life under the carpet.

Churchland's neuralism may stem from reaction to her high-school biology teacher—an avowed vitalist! She explains that he could not imagine how living things issued from dead molecules, how life arose from bits of proteins, fats, and sugars. Surely, he thought, there was something else. Perhaps the rebellious position for a resolute teenager was to imagine that life did indeed arise directly from its material constituents. No mystery, just fact. What you see is what you get.

But sometimes you get more than you see. Take life, for example. With all we have learned about molecular biology in the past decades, are we any closer to understanding what life is? Pat's biology teacher was right—something is missing. Could it be that, like consciousness, life is a quantum process?

REFERENCES

Alkon, D. L. 1989. Memory storage and neural systems. *Scientific American* 261(1):42–50.

Allison, A. C, G. H. Hulands, J. F. Nunn, J. A. Kitching, and A. C. MacDonald. 1970. The effects of inhalational anaesthetics on the microtubular system in Actinosphaerium nucleofilm. *Journal of Cell Science* 7:483–499.

Allison, A. C., and J. F. Nunn. 1968. Effects of general anesthetics on microtubules. A possible mechanism of anesthesia. *Lancet* 2:1326–1329.

Andreu, J. M. 1986. Hydrophobic interactions of tubulin. *Annals of New York Academy of Sciences* 466:626–630.

Barinaga, M. 1996. Neurons put the uncertainty into reaction times. *Science* 274:344.

Beck, F., and J. C. Eccles. 1992. Quantum aspects of brain activity and the role of consciousness. *Proceedings of the National Academy of Sciences, U.S.A.* 89(23):11,357–11,361.

Browne, M. W. 1997. Physicists confirm power of nothing, measuring force of universal flux. *The New York Times*, January 21, 1997.

Casti, J. L. 1996. Confronting science's logical limits. *Scientific American* 275(4):102–105.

Chalmers, D. J. 1996a. The *Conscious Mind—In Search of a Fundamental Theory*. New York: Oxford University Press.

Chalmers, D. J. 1996b. Facing up to the problem of consciousness. In S. R. Hameroff, A. Kaszniak, and A. C. Scott, eds., *Toward a Science of Consciousness—The First Tucson Discussions and Debates*, Cambridge, MA.: MIT Press, pp. 5–28.

Crick, F., and C. Koch. 1990. Towards a neurobiological theory of consciousness. *Seminars in the Neurosciences* 2:263–275

Delon, J., and P. Legendre. 1995. Effects of nocodazole and taxol on glycine evoked currents on rat spinal-cord neurons in culture. *Neuroreport* 6:1932–1936.

Fröhlich, H. 1968. Long-range coherence and energy storage in biological systems. *International Journal of Quantum Chemistry* 2:641–649.

Franks, N. P., and W. R. Lieb. 1982. Molecular mechanisms of general anaesthesia. *Nature* 300:487–493.

Franks, N. P., and W. R. Lieb. 1985. Mapping of general anaesthetic target sites provides a molecular basis for cut-off effects. *Nature* 316:349–351.

Hall, G. L. 1996. Quantum electrodynamic (QED) fluctuations in various models of neuronal microtubules. *Consciousness Research Abstracts—Tucson II (Journal of Consciousness Studies)*, Abstract 145.

Halsey, M. J. 1989. Molecular mechanisms of anaesthesia. In J. F. Nunn, J. E. Utting, and B. R. Brown, Jr., eds., *General Anaesthesia*, 5th ed. London: Butterworth, pp. 19–29.

Hameroff, S. 1996. Cytoplasmic gel states and ordered water: Possible roles in biological quantum coherence. *Proceedings of the second advanced water symposium*, Dallas, Texas, October 4–6, 1996. http://www.u.arizona.edu/~hameroff/water2.html.

Hameroff, S. 1997. Funda-mental geometry: The Penrose-Hameroff Orch OR model of consciousness. In S. Huggett, L. J. Mason, K. P. Tod, S. T. Tsou, N. M. J. Woodhouse, eds., *Geometrical Issues in the Foundations of Science*. Oxford: Oxford University Press. (in press)

Hameroff, S. R., and R. Penrose. 1996a. Orchestrated reduction of quantum coherence in brain microtubules: A model for consciousness. In S. R. Hameroff, A. Kaszniak, and A. C. Scott, eds., *Toward a Science of Consciousness—The First Tucson Discussions and Debates*, Cambridge: MIT Press. Also pub. in *Mathematics and Computers in Simulation* 40:453–480. http://www.u.arizona.edu/~hameroff/penrose1.

Hameroff, S. R., and R. Penrose. 1996b. Conscious events as orchestrated spacetime selections. *Journal of Consciousness Studies* 3(1):36–53. http://www.u.arizona.edu/~hameroff/penrose2

Hameroff, S. R., and R. C. Watt. 1983. Do anesthetics act by altering electron mobility? *Anesthesia and Analgesia* 62:936–940.

Hinkley, R. E., Jr. 1978. Macrotubules induced by halothane: In vitro assembly. *Journal of Cell Science* 32:99–108.

Hinkley, R. E., and L. S. Green. 1970. Effects of general anesthetics on microtubules. *Lancet* 1(645):525.

Hinkley, R. E., and F. E. Samson. 1972. Anesthetic induced transformation of axonal microtubules. *Journal of Cell Biology* 53(1):258–263.

Hinkley, R. E., and A. G. Telser. 1974. The effects of halothane on cultured mouse neuroblastoma cells. I. Inhibition of morphological differentiation. *Journal of Cell Biology* 63:531–540.

Hirokawa, N. 1991. Molecular architecture and dynamics of the neuronal cytoskeleton. In R. D. Burgoyne, ed., *The Neuronal Cytoskeleton*. New York: Wiley-Liss, pp. 5–74.

Ingber, D. E. 1993. Cellular tensegrity: Defining new roles of biological design that govern the cytoskeleton. *Journal of Cell Science* 104(3):613-627.

Jibu, M. 1990. On a heuristic model of the coherent mechanism of the global reaction process of a group of cells. *Bussei Kenkyuu (Material Physics Research)* 53(4):431–436 (in Japanese).

Jibu, M., and K. Yasue. 1995. *Quantum Brain Dynamics: An Introduction*. Amsterdam: John Benjamins.

Jibu, M., K. H. Pribram, and K. Yasue. 1996. From conscious experience to memory storage and retrieval: The role of quantum brain dynamics and boson condensation of evanescent photons. *International Journal of Modern Physics B* 10 (13&14):1735–1754.

Joliot, M., U. Ribary, and R. Llinas. 1994. Human oscillatory brain activity near 40 Hz coexists with cognitive temporal binding. *Proceedings of the National Academy of Sciences U.S.A.* 91(24):11,748–11,751.

Kang, S., and J. P. Green. 1970. Steric and electronic relationships among some hallucinogenic compounds. *Proceedings of the National Academy of Sciences U.S.A.* 67(1):62–67.

Kennedy, R. D, B. R. Fink, and M. R. Byers. 1972. The effect of halothane on rapid axonal transport in the vagus nerve. *Anesthesiology* 36(5):433–443.

Lamoreaux, S. K. 1997. Demonstration of the Casimir force in the 0.6 to 6 micron range. *Physical Review Letters* 78(1):5–8.

Leibniz, G. W. 1768. *Opera Omnia*, 6 vols, ed. Louis Dutens. Geneva.

Libet, B., E. W. Wright, Jr., B. Feinstein, and D. K. Pearl. 1979. Subjective referral of the timing for a conscious sensory experience. *Brain* 102:193–224.

Livingston, A., and G. A. Vergara. 1979. Effects of halothane on microtubules in the sciatic nerve of the rat. *Cell Tissue Research* 198:137–144.

Louria, D., and S. Hameroff. 1996. Computer simulation of anesthetic binding in protein hydrophobic pockets. In S. R. Hameroff, A. Kaszniak, and A. C. Scott, eds., *Toward a Science of Consciousness—The First Tucson Discussions and Debates*. Cambridge: MIT Press, pp. 425–434.

Nichols, D. E. 1986. Studies of the relationship between molecular structure and hallucinogenic activity. *Pharmacology, Biochemistry and Behavior* 24:335–340.

Nichols, D. E., A. T. Shulgin, and D. C. Dyer. 1977. Directional lipophilic character in a series of psychotomimetic phenylethylamine derivatives. *Life Sciences* 21(4):569–576.

Penrose, R. 1996a. On gravity's role in quantum state reduction. *General Relativity and Gravitation* 28(5):581–600.

Penrose, R. 1996b. Beyond the doubting of a shadow: A reply to commentaries on *Shadows of the mind*. http://psyche.cs.monash.edu.au/volume 2-1/psyche-96-2-23-shadows-10-penrose.

Penrose, R. 1971. In E. A. Bastin, ed., *Quantum Theory and Beyond*, ed. Cambridge: Cambridge University Press.

Penrose, R. 1989. *The Emperor's New Mind*. Oxford: Oxford University Press.

Penrose, R. 1994. *Shadows of the Mind*. Oxford: Oxford University Press.

Penrose, R., and S. R. Hameroff. 1995. What gaps? Reply to Grush and Churchland. *Journal of Consciousness Studies* 2(2):99–112.

Pribram, K. H. 1991. *Brain and Perception*. Hillsdale, NJ: Lawrence Erlbaum.

Rovelli, C., and L. Smolin. 1995a. Discreteness of area and volume in quantum gravity. *Nuclear Physics B* 442:593–619.

Rovelli, C., and L. Smolin. 1995b. Spin networks in quantum gravity. *Physical Review D* 52(10)5743–5759.

Saubermann, A. J., and M. L. Gallagher. 1973. Mechanisms of general anesthesia: Failure of pentobarbital and halothane to depolymerize microtubules in mouse optic nerve. *Anesthesiology* 38:25–29.

Seife, C. 1997. Quantum mechanics: The subtle pull of emptiness. *Science* 275:158.

Shimony, A. 1993. *Search for a Naturalistic World View, vol. II. Natural Science and Metaphysics*. Cambridge: Cambridge University Press.

Snyder, S. H., and C. R. Merril. 1965. A relationship between the hallucinogenic activity of drugs and their electronic configuration. *Proceedings of the Natioal Academy of Sciences U.S.A.* 54:258–266.

Spinoza, B. 1677. Ethica in Opera quotque reperta sunt, 3rd ed., J. van Vloten and J. P. N. Land, eds. Den Haag, Netherlands.

Uemura, E., and E. D. Levin. 1992. The effect of halothane on cultured fibroblasts and neuroblastoma cells. *Neuroscience Letters* 145:33–36.

Vergara, G. A., and A. Livingston. 1981. Halothane modifies colchicine binding to tubulin. *Pharmacology* 23(5):264–270.

Weil, A. 1996. Pharmacology of consciousness: A narrative of subjective experience. In S. R. Hameroff, A. Kaszniak, and A. C. Scott, eds., *Toward a Science of Consciousness—The First Tucson Discussions and Debates*, Cambridge: MIT Press, pp. 677–689.

Wheeler, J. A. 1957. Assessment of Everett's "relative state" formulation of quantum theory. *Reviews of Modern Physics* 29:463–465.

Wheeler, J. A. 1990. Information, physics, quantum: The search for links. In W. Zurek, ed., *Complexity, Entropy, and the Physics of Information*. Reading, MA: Addison-Wesley.

Whitehead, A. N. 1929. *Process and Reality*. New York: Macmillan.

IV Neural Correlates of Consciousness

OVERVIEW

"Wouldst there were a meter to monitor the mind!"

But there is not. As David Chalmers emphasizes in the opening chapter in Part IV, a main task for neuroscience in consciousness studies is identifying the neural system or systems primarily associated with conscious experience—the neural correlate of consciousness (NCC). This is a vital task, and a score of NCC candidate models—listed here by Chalmers—have been put forward. But how, he asks, can we find the NCC when consciousness itself cannot be directly observed? Chalmers suggests that the search would be much simpler if we had a device that could detect consciousness as a Geiger counter detects radioactivity. Unfortunately, we have no such device. (During his talk at Tucson II, however, Chalmers demonstrated a prototype consciousness meter. This instrument was said to have been developed by combining "neuromorphic engineering, transpersonal psychology, and quantum gravity," although it strikingly resembled a hair dryer. The detector appeared to function well. It lit up appropriately when pointed at most audience members, with occasional exceptions.)

Chalmers's well-made point is that we are stuck with external analysis in interpreting neuroscientific results. "Preexperimental" assumptions are required to identify a process as conscious and thus to isolate the NCC. Such principles are implicit in all NCC research, but Chalmers tries to make them explicit, focusing on the function served by oral reports and "direct availability for global control." He applies this analysis to draw conclusions about several NCC candidate models.

As Chalmers also observes, the degree to which various NCC models are mutually compatible is interesting and perhaps significant. The problem of consciousness is so complex and multidimensional that explanations are necessary at many levels.

p. 231 In Chapter 20, Susan Greenfield attempts to devise a Rosetta stone of consciousness that will describe both neurophysiology and phenomenology. She argues against a specialized brain region responsible for consciousness, and against consciousness being either entirely present or entirely absent in any one organism or at any one time. Rather, Greenfield proposes that the degree of consciousness correlates with brain connectivity as an emergent property of nonspecialized, divergent neuronal networks. These always entail, according to Greenfield, a stimulus focus or epicenter that can be spatially multiple yet temporally unitary (single at any one time). The size of the neuronal assembly (and the degree of consciousness) depends upon the arousal and the epicenter's recruiting power. This power, in turn, depends on the associative neuronal connectivity and strength of stimulus. Greenfield relates her theory to such diverse data as electroencephalograph (EEG) recordings from premature babies, content of dreams, and psychopharmacological treatment of schizophrenia—showing how the intensity of subjective experience may correlate with size of neuronal assembly.

For a number of years, patients with intractable seizure disorders were treated surgically by severing the corpus callosum—the major connection between left and right cerebral hemispheres. A side effect of this procedure is apparent dual experience and behavior in these so-called split-brain patients (see Chapters 12–14 in the Tucson I book). The neurosurgeon known for pioneering this technique is Joseph Bogen, author of Chapter 21. Bogen attributes subjectivity to neuronal activity in and immediately around the intralaminar nuclei of the thalamus. Characteristics of the intralaminar nuclei that make them likely loci for the entity that Kinsbourne (1995) calls the subjectivity pump include widespread access to cortical and other brain regions, and evidence linking these structures to coordination of both attention and action. Bogen points out that whereas large lesions elsewhere in the brain may deprive the subject of conscious content, small bilateral areas of damage within the intralaminar nuclei can cause immediate unresponsiveness and apparent unconsciousness. Following the suggestion by other investigators (e.g., Crick and Koch 1990, Llinas and Ribary 1993), Bogen speculates that the "appropriate interaction" required for subjective experience occurs between the intralaminar nuclei and the cortical neuronal representation of any content, and involves synchronization of neuronal activity at 40 Hz.

In Chapter 22, Richard Lane and colleagues describe neural correlates of the conscious experience of emotion. They outline "levels of emotional awareness" (differing abilities to recognize and describe emotion in oneself and others), and approaches to the measurement of this construct. The authors use positron emission tomography (PET) to correlate levels of emotional awareness with blood flow in the anterior cingulate cortex (a bilateral structure in the medial, posterior region of the frontal lobes). Lane and coworkers point out consistency with previously published data indicating a function for the anterior cingulate cortex in conscious awareness of perceptual stimuli, as well as with clinical reports of decreased emotional response following surgical lesioning of this region to treat intractable pain. They close by speculating about how the anterior cingulate cortex affects emotional awareness and disregulation theory (Schwartz 1983), which holds that conscious awareness of emotions promotes both physiological and psychological health.

In Chapter 23 Michael Alkire, Richard J. Haier, and J. H. Fallon use PET's functional brain imaging capabilities to assess regional brain metabolism during alterations in state and level of consciousness induced by general anesthesia. Their studies demonstrate that PET measurement of regional metabolic activity (assumed to reflect underlying neuronal activity) is dramatically lower in an anesthetized, unconscious brain than in an awake brain. Studies with the inhalational gas anesthetic isoflurane and the intravenous drug propofol indicate that the cerebral cortex is more metabolically depressed during anesthesia than subcortical gray matter. Additional studies in which the anesthetic dose is titrated are interpreted as showing—at the present level of PET resolution—that anesthetic loss of consciousness is caused by a uniform reduction in neuronal functioning rather than by changes in any specific "consciousness circuit." On the other hand, Alkire and colleagues find localization of aspects of consciousness in further studies of conscious and unconscious memory ("implicit memory during anesthesia"). Metabolic activity of encoding differed most between conscious and unconscious memory in the mediodorsal thalamic nucleus. The authors speculate that the thalamus may play a critical part in subjective awareness by continually comparing the present moment with the past.

Additional theoretical arguments for the thalamocortical system's function in consciousness are provided in Chapter 24. Here Bernard Baars, James Newman, and John Taylor outline a theory of neuronal mechanisms of consciousness that integrates Taylor's mathematical development of a competitive neural network with the Newman and Baars position that the thalamocortical system provides a brain mechanism capable of supporting the global-workspace architecture of Baars's (1988) cognitive theory of consciousness. The merger results in a "relational global workspace" framework that claims: (1) Consciousness is an architectural aspect of brain organization with global influences and effects. (2) A number of brain mechanisms could support such functions. (3) Conscious experience involves continuing interaction between sensory input and memory. (4) Cortical foci of activity provide consciousness with its content. (5) The brain stem–thalamocortical axis supports the state but not the content of consciousness. (6) A selective attention system, including the nucleus reticularis of the thalamus, selects among many possible conscious contents. (7) Posterior cortex provides sensory conscious content, and anterior cortex is involved in active, voluntary control (both are required for normal conscious experience and volition). The authors extend their theory to vision and a function for consciousness in a stable contextual self-system with predictability in varied situations.

In Chapter 25, Jeffrey Gray describes "creeping up on the hard question of consciousness." Drawing from previous work on the neuropsychology of anxiety (Dray 1982), and observations on symptoms of schizophrenia, Gray proposes a neuropsychological hypothesis for generating the content of consciousness. He posits that conscious content corresponds to the output from a "comparator," identified with the subiculum of the hippocampal complex within the medial temporal lobe. The current state of the organism's perceptual world is continually compared with a predicted state. Although this hypothesis may account for key features of consciousness, Gray concludes that neither this nor any other hypothesis is yet able to explain why the brain should generate conscious experience (i.e., Chalmers's "hard problem"). To creep up on the hard problem, Gray proposes brain-imaging experiments in word-color synaesthetes (those who experience a sensation in one sensory modality triggered involuntarily and automatically by a sensation in a different sensory modality) and control subjects. The aim of this research program would be to determine whether synaesthetes' special sensory experiences are due to hard wiring or an idiosyncratic history of associative learning. Should such research provide evidence consistent with hard wiring, Gray asserts, this condition would imply that specific conscious experiences depend upon neuronal events, and not on informational transactions that could go on in non-neuronal systems such as computers.

Common threads are evident among these models—anatomically, certain regions in the thalamus direct the spotlight of awareness toward various cortical epicenters in which content resides. Another recurrent theme is that consciousness involves continuing temporal feedback between the present moment and both the immediate past and predicted future. This interpretation touches on the relationship between time and consciousness taken up in Part XII.

REFERENCES

Baars, B. J. 1988. *A Cognitive Theory of Consciousness*. New York: Cambridge University Press.

Chalmers, D. J. 1996. *The Conscious Mind*. Oxford: Oxford University Press.

Crick, F., and C. Koch. 1990. Towards a neurobiological theory of consciousness. *Seminars in the Neurosciences* 2:263–275.

Gray, J. A. 1982. *The Neuropsychology of Anxiety*. Oxford: Oxford University Press.

Kinsbourne, M. 1995. The intralaminar thalamic nuclei: Subjectivity pumps or attention-action coordinators? *Consciousness and Cognition* 4:167–171.

Llinas, R., and U. Ribary. 1993. Coherent 40-Hz oscillation characterizes dream state in humans. *Proceedings of the National Academy of Sciences U.S.A.* 90:2078–2081.

Schwartz, G. E. 1983. Disregulation theory and disease: Applications to the repression/cerebral disconnection/cardiovascular disorder hypothesis. *International Review of Applied Psychology* 32:95–118.

19 On the Search for the Neural Correlate of Consciousness

David J. Chalmers

I will discuss one aspect of the role neuroscience plays in the search for a theory of consciousness. Whether or not neuroscience can solve all the problems of consciousness singlehandedly, it undoubtedly has a major role to play. Recent years have seen striking progress in neurobiological research bearing on the problems of consciousness. The conceptual foundations of this sort of research, however, are only beginning to be laid. I will look at some of the things that are going on, from a philosopher's perspective, and will try to say something helpful about these foundations.

We have all been hearing a lot about the "neural correlate of consciousness." This phrase is intended to refer to the neural system or systems primarily associated with conscious experience. The acronym of the day is "NCC." We all have an NCC inside our head; we just have to find out what it is. In recent years we have seen quite a few proposals about the identity of the NCC, one of the best known being Crick and Koch's suggestion about 40-Hertz oscillations. That proposal has since faded away a little, but all sorts of other suggestions are out there. The picture is almost reminiscent of particle physics, where they have something like 236 particles and people talk about the "particle zoo." In studying consciousness, one might talk about the "neural-correlate zoo."

A brief list of suggestions that have been put forward includes:

- 40-Hz oscillations in the cerebral cortex (Crick and Koch 1990).
- Intralaminar nucleus in the thalamus (Bogen 1995).   *p. 237*
- Reentrant loops in thalamocortical systems (Edelman 1989).
- 40-Hz rhythmic activity in thalamocortical systems (Llinas et al. 1994).
- Nucleus reticularis (Taylor and Alavi 1995).
- Extended reticular-thalamic activation system (Newman and Baars 1993).
- Anterior cingulate system (Cotterill 1994).
- Neural assemblies bound by NMDA (Flohr 1995).
- Temporally extended neural activity (Libet 1994).
- Back-projections to lower cortical areas (Cauller and Kulics 1991).
- Visual processing within the ventral stream (Milner and Goodale 1995).

- Neurons in visual cortex projecting to prefrontal areas (Crick and Koch 1995).
- Neural activity in V5 (Tootell et al. 1995).
- Certain neurons in the superior temporal sulcus and inferior temporal cortex (Logothetis and Schall 1989; Sheinberg and Logothetis 1997).
- Neuronal gestalts in an epicenter (Greenfield 1995).
- Outputs of a comparator system in the hippocampus (Gray 1995).
- Quantum coherence in microtubules (Hameroff 1994).
- Global workspace (Baars 1988).
- High-quality representations (Farah 1994).
- Selector inputs to action systems (Shallice 1988).

This list includes a few "cognitive correlates" of consciousness (CCC?), but the general idea is similar. We find some intriguing commonalities among the proposals in this list. A number of them give a major role to interactions between the thalamus and the cortex, for example. All the same, the great number and diversity of the proposals can be overwhelming. I propose to step back and try to make sense of all this activity by asking some foundational questions.

A primary question is this: How *can* one search for the neural correlate of consciousness? As we all know, measuring consciousness is problematic. The phenomenon is not directly and straightforwardly observable. It would be much easier if we had a way of getting at consciousness directly—if we had, for example, a consciousness meter.

If we had such an instrument, searching for the NCC would be straightforward. We would wave the consciousness meter and measure a subject's consciousness directly. At the same time, we would monitor the underlying brain processes. After a number of trials, we would say such-and-such brain processes are correlated with experiences of various kinds, so there is the neural correlate of consciousness.

Alas, we have no consciousness meter, and for principled reasons it seems we cannot have one. Consciousness just is not the sort of thing that can be measured directly. What, then, do we do without a consciousness meter? How can the search go forward? How does all this experimental research proceed?

I think the answer is this: we get there with principles of *interpretation*, by which we interpret physical systems to judge the presence of consciousness. We might call these *preexperimental bridging principles*. They are the criteria that we bring to bear in looking at systems to say (1) whether or not they are conscious now, and (2) which information they are conscious of, and which they are not. We can not reach in directly and grab those experiences, so we rely on external criteria instead.

That is a perfectly reasonable thing to do. But something interesting is going on. These principles of interpretation are not themselves experimentally determined or experimentally tested. In a sense they are preexperimental assumptions. Experimental research gives us a lot of information about processing; then we bring in the bridging principles to interpret the experimental results, whatever those results may be. They are the principles by which we make *inferences* from facts about processing to facts about consciousness, and so they are conceptually prior to the experiments themselves. We cannot actually refine them experimentally (except perhaps by first-person experimentation!), because we have no independent access to the independent variable. Instead, these principles will be based on some combination of (1) conceptual judgments about what counts as a conscious process, and (2) information gleaned from our first-person perspective on our own consciousness.

I think we are all stuck in this boat. The point applies whether one is a reductionist or an antireductionist about consciousness. A hard-line reductionist might put some of these points a little differently, but either way the experimental work will require preexperimental reasoning to determine the criteria for ascribing consciousness. Of course such principles are usually left implicit in empirical research. We do not usually see papers saying, "Here is the bridging principle, here are the data, and here is what follows." But it is useful to make them explicit. The very presence of these principles has strong and interesting consequences in the search for the NCC.

In a sense, in relying on these principles we are taking a leap into the epistemological unknown. Because we do not measure consciousness directly, we have to make something of a leap of faith. It may not be a big leap, but nevertheless it suggests that everyone doing this work is engaged in philosophical reasoning. Of course one can always choose to stay on solid ground, talking about the empirical results in a neutral way, but the price of doing so is that one gains no particular insight into consciousness. Conversely, as soon as we draw any conclusions about consciousness, we have gone beyond the information given. So we need to pay careful attention to the reasoning involved.

What are these principles of interpretation? The first and by far the most prevalent is the principle of verbal report. When someone says, "Yes, I see that table now," we infer that they are conscious of the table. When someone says, "Yes, I see red now," we infer that they are having an experience of red. Of course one might always say, "How do you know?"—a philosopher might suggest that we may be faced with a fully functioning zombie—but in fact most of us do not believe the people around us are zombies, and in practice we are quite prepared to rely on this principle. As preexperimental assumptions go, this one is relatively safe—it does not require a huge leap of faith—and it is very widely used.

The principle here is that when information is verbally reported, it is conscious. One can extend this principle slightly, for no one believes an *actual* verbal report is required for consciousness; we are conscious of much more than we report on any given occasion. Thus an extended principle might say that when information is directly *available* for verbal report, it is conscious.

Experimental researchers do not rely only on these principles of verbal report and reportability. The principles can be somewhat limiting when we want to do broader experiments. In particular, we do not want to restrict our studies of consciousness to subjects that have language. In fact, at this conference we saw a beautiful example of research on consciousness in language-free creatures. I refer to the work by Nikos Logothetis and his colleagues (e.g., Logothetis and Schall 1989, Leopold and Logothetis 1996, Sheinberg and Logothetis 1997). This work uses experiments on monkeys to draw conclusions about the neural processes associated with consciousness. How do Logothetis et al. manage to draw conclusions about a monkey's consciousness without getting any verbal reports? They rely on the monkey's pressing bars: if the monkey can be made to press a bar in an appropriate way in response to a stimulus, we can say that the stimulus was consciously perceived.

The criterion at play seems to require that the information be available for an arbitrary response. If it turned out that the monkey could press a bar in response to a red light but could do nothing else, we would be tempted to say that it was not a case of consciousness at all, but some sort of subconscious connection. If on the other hand we find information that is available for response in all sorts of ways, then we will say that it is conscious.

The underlying general principle is something like this: When information is *directly available for global control* in a cognitive system, then it is conscious. If information is available for response in many motor modalities, we will say it is conscious, at least in a range of relatively familiar systems such as humans, other primates and so on. This principle squares well with the preceding one, when the capacity for verbal report is present: availability for verbal report and availability for global control seem to go together in such cases (report is one of the key aspects of control, after all, and it is rare to find information that is reportable but not available more widely). But this principle is also applicable when language is not present.

A correlation between consciousness and global availability (for short) seems to fit the first-person evidence—that gleaned from our own conscious experience—quite well. When information is present in my consciousness, it is generally reportable, and it can generally be brought to bear in controlling behavior in all sorts of ways. I can talk about it, I can point in the general direction of a stimulus, I can press bars, and so on. Conversely, when we find information that is directly available in this way for report and other aspects of control, it is generally conscious information. One can bear out this idea by considering cases.

There are some tricky puzzle cases to consider, such as blindsight, where one has *some* availability for control but arguably no conscious experience. Those cases might best be handled by invoking the directness criterion: insofar as the information here is available for report and other control processes at all, the availability is indirect by comparison to the direct and automatic availability in standard cases. One might also stipulate that it is availability for *voluntary* control that is relevant, to deal with cases of involuntary unconscious response, although that is a complex issue. I discuss a number of puzzle cases in more detail elsewhere (Chalmers 1997), where I also give a much more detailed defense of the idea that something like global availability is the key preempirical criterion for the ascription of consciousness.

But this principle remains at best a first-order approximation of the functional criteria that come into play. I am less interested today in getting all the fine details right than in exploring the consequences of the idea that some such functional criterion is required and is implicit in all the empirical research on the neural correlate of consciousness. If you disagree with the criterion I have suggested—presumably because you can think of counterexamples—you may want to use those examples to refine it or to come up with a better criterion of your own. The crucial point is that in the very act of experimentally distinguishing conscious from unconscious processes, *some* such criterion is always at play.

My question is: if something like this is right, then what follows? That is, if some such bridging principles are implicit in the methodology for the search for the NCC, then what are the consequences? I will use global availability as my main functional criterion in this discussion, but many of the points should generalize.

The first thing one can do is produce what philosophers call a *rational reconstruction* of the search for the neural correlate of consciousness. With a rational reconstruction we can say: Maybe things do not work exactly like this in practice, but the rational underpinnings of the procedure have something like this form. That is, if one were to try to *justify* the conclusions one has reached as well as possible, one's justification would follow the shape set by the rational reconstruction. In this case, a rational reconstruction might look something like this:

1. Consciousness ↔ global availability (bridging principle)

2. Global availability ↔ neural process N (empirical work), and so

3. Consciousness ↔ neural process N (conclusion).

According to this reconstruction, one implicitly embraces some sort of preexperimental bridging principle that one finds plausible on independent grounds, such as conceptual or phenomenological grounds. Then one does the empirical research. Instead of measuring consciousness directly, we detect the functional property. We see that when this functional property (e.g., global availability) is present, it is correlated with a specific neural process (e.g., 40-Hz oscillations). Combining the preempirical premise and the empirical result, we arrive at the conclusion that this neural process is a candidate for the NCC.

Of course it does not work nearly so simply in practice. The two stages are highly intertwined; our preexperimental principles may themselves be refined as experimental research goes along. Nevertheless I think one can make a separation into preempirical and experimental components for the

David J. Chalmers: On the Search for the Neural Correlate of Consciousness sake of analysis. With this rational reconstruction in hand, what sort of conclusions follow? I want to draw out about six consequences here.

1. The first conclusion is a characterization of the neural correlates of consciousness. If the NCC is arrived at via this methodology, then whatever it turns out to be, it will be a *mechanism of global availability*. The presence of the NCC wherever global availability is present suggests that it is a mechanism that *subserves* global availability in the brain. The only alternative is that it might be a *symptom* rather than a *mechanism* of global availability; but in principle that possibility ought to be addressable by dissociation studies, lesioning, and so on. If a process is a mere symptom of availability, we ought to be able to empirically dissociate it from global availability while leaving the latter intact. The resulting data would suggest to us that consciousness can be present even when the neural process in question is not, thus indicating that it was not a perfect correlate of consciousness after all.

(A related line of reasoning supports the idea that a true NCC must be a mechanism of *direct* availability for global control. In principle, mechanisms of indirect availability will be dissociable from the empirical evidence for consciousness, for example by directly stimulating the mechanisms of direct availability. The indirect mechanisms will be "screened off" by the direct mechanisms in much the same way as the retina is screened off as an NCC by the visual cortex.)

In fact, if one looks at the various proposals, this template seems to fit them pretty well. For example, the 40-Hz oscillations discussed by Crick and Koch were put forward precisely because of the role they might have in binding and integrating information into working memory, and working memory is of course a major mechanism whereby information is made available for global control in a cognitive system. Similarly, it is plausible that Libet's extended neural activity is relevant precisely because the temporal extendedness of activity gives certain information the capacity to dominate later processes that lead to control. Baars's global workspace is a particularly explicit example of such a mechanism; it is put forward explicitly as a mechanism whereby information can be globally disseminated. All these mechanisms and many of the others seem to be candidates for mechanisms of global availability in the brain.

2. This reconstruction suggests that a full story about the neural processes associated with consciousness will do two things. First, it will *explain* global availability in the brain. Once we know all about the relevant neural processes, we will know precisely how information is made directly available for global control in the brain, and this will be an explanation in the full sense. Global availability is a functional property, and as always the problem of explaining a function's performance is a problem to which mechanistic explanation is well suited. So we can be confident that in a century or two global availability will be straightforwardly explained. Second, this explanation of availability will do something else: it will isolate the processes that

underlie consciousness itself. If the bridging principle is granted, then mechanisms of availability will automatically be correlates of phenomenology in the full sense.

Now, I don't think this is a full *explanation* for consciousness. One can always ask why these processes of availability should give rise to consciousness in the first place. As yet we cannot explain why they do so, and it may well be that full details about the processes of availability still fail to answer this question. Certainly, nothing in the standard methodology I have outlined answers the question; that methodology *assumes* a relation between availability and consciousness, and therefore does nothing to *explain* it. The relationship between the two is instead taken as something of a primitive. So the hard problem remains. But who knows: Somewhere along the line we may be led to the relevant insights that show why the link is there, and the hard problem may then be solved. In the meantime, whether or not we have solved the hard problem, we may nevertheless have isolated the *basis* for consciousness in the brain. We just have to keep in mind the distinction between correlation and explanation.

3. Given this paradigm, it is likely that there will be many neural correlates of consciousness. This suggestion is unsurprising, but the rational reconstruction illustrates just why such a multiplicity of correlates should exist. There will be many neural correlates of consciousness because there may well be many mechanisms of global availability. There will be mechanisms in different modalities: the mechanisms of visual availability may be quite different from the mechanisms of auditory availability, for example. (Of course they *may* be the same, in that we could find a later area that would integrate and disseminate all this information, but that is an open question.) There will also be mechanisms at different stages in the processing path whereby information is made globally available: early mechanisms and later ones. All these may be candidates for the NCC. And we will find mechanisms at many levels of description: for example, 40-Hz oscillations may well be redescribed as high-quality representations, or as part of a global workspace, at a different level of description. It may therefore turn out that a number of the animals in the zoo, so to speak, can coexist because they are compatible in one of these ways.

I will not speculate much further on just what the neural correlates of consciousness *are*. No doubt some of the ideas in the initial list will prove to be entirely off the track, and some of the others will prove closer to the mark. As we philosophers like to say, humbly, that is an empirical question. But I hope the conceptual issues are becoming clearer.

4. This way of thinking about things allows one to make sense of an idea that is sometimes floated: that of a *consciousness module*. Sometimes this notion is disparaged; sometimes it is embraced. But of the methodology in the search for an NCC suggests that it is at least possible that there could turn out to be such a module. What would it take? It would require some

sort of functionally localizable, internally integrated area, through which all global availability runs. It need not be anatomically localizable, but to qualify as a module it would need to be localizable in some broader sense. For example, the parts of the module would have to have high-bandwidth communication among themselves, compared to the relatively low-bandwidth communication that they have with other areas. Such a thing *could* turn out to exist. It does not strike me as especially likely that things will turn out this way; it seems just as likely that we will find multiple independent mechanisms of global availability in the brain, scattered around without much mutual integration. If that is the result, we will probably say that there is no consciousness module after all. But that is another of those empirical questions.

If something like this module did turn out to exist in the brain, it would resemble Baars's conception of a global workspace: a functional area responsible for integrating information in the brain and disseminating it to multiple nonconscious specialized processes. In fact, many of the ideas I put forward here are compatible with things that Baars has been saying for years about the role of global availability in the study of consciousness. Indeed, this way of looking at things suggests that some of his ideas are almost forced on us by the methodology. The special epistemological role of global availability helps explain why the idea of a global workspace is a useful way of thinking about almost any empirical proposal about consciousness. If NCCs are identified as such precisely because of their role in global control, then at least on a first approximation we should expect the global-workspace idea to fit with any NCC.

5. We can also apply this picture to a question that has been discussed frequently at this conference: Are the neural correlates of *visual* consciousness to be found in V1, in the extrastriate visual cortex, or elsewhere? If our picture of the methodology is correct, then the answer presumably will depend on which visual area is most directly implicated in global availability.

Crick and Koch have suggested that the visual NCC is not to be found within V1, because V1 does not contain neurons that project to the prefrontal cortex. This reasoning has been criticized by Ned Block for conflating access consciousness and phenomenal consciousness (see Block, Chapter 29, this volume), but interestingly, the picture I have developed suggests that it may be good reasoning. The prefrontal cortex is known to be associated with control processes; so *if* a given area in the visual cortex projects to prefrontal areas, then it may well be a mechanism of direct availability. And if it does not project in this way, it is less likely to be such a mechanism; at best it might be *indirectly* associated with global availability. Of course we still have plenty of room to raise questions about the empirical details. But the broader point is that for the reasons discussed in (2) above, it is likely that the neural processes involved in *explaining* access consciousness will simultaneously be involved in a story about the *basis* for phenomenal consciousness. If something like this idea is implicit in their reasoning, Crick and Koch might escape the charge of conflation. Of course the reasoning depends on these somewhat shaky bridging principles, but then all work on the neural correlates of consciousness must appeal to such principles somewhere, and so this limitation cannot be held against Crick and Koch in particular.

6. Sometimes the neural correlate of consciousness is conceived of as the Holy Grail for a theory of consciousness. It will make everything fall into place. For example, once we discover the NCC, then we will have a definitive test for consciousness, enabling us to discover consciousness wherever it arises. That is, we might use the neural correlate itself as a sort of consciousness meter. If a system has 40-Hz oscillations (say), then it is conscious; if it has none, then it is not conscious. Or if a thalomocortical system turns out to be the NCC, then a system without such a system is unlikely to be conscious. This sort of reasoning is not usually put quite so baldly, but I think one finds some version of it quite frequently.

This reasoning can be tempting, but one should not succumb to the temptation. Given the very methodology that comes into play here, we have no way of definitely establishing a given NCC as an independent test for consciousness. The primary criterion for consciousness will always remain the functional property we started with: global availability, or verbal report, or whatever. That is how we discovered the correlations in the first place. The 40-Hz oscillations (or whatever) are relevant *only* because of their role in satisfying this criterion. True, in cases where we know that this association between the NCC and the functional property is present, the NCC might itself function as a sort of "signature" of consciousness, but once we dissociate the NCC from the functional property, all bets are off. To take an extreme example: If we have 40-Hz oscillations in a test tube, that condition almost certainly will not yield consciousness. But the point applies equally in less extreme cases. Because it was the bridging principles that gave us all the traction in the search for an NCC in the first place, it is not clear that anything follows in cases where the functional criterion is thrown away. So there is no free lunch here: one cannot get something for nothing.

Once we recognize the central role of preexperimental assumptions in the search for the NCC, we realize that there are limitations on just what we can expect this search to tell us. Still, whether or not the NCC is the Holy Grail, I hope I have said enough to make it clear that the quest for it is likely to enhance our understanding considerably. And I hope to have made a case that philosophy and neuroscience can come together to help clarify some of the deep problems involved in the study of consciousness.

NOTE

1. This chapter is an edited transcript of my talk at the second Tucson conference in April 1996 (omitting some diversions with a consciousness meter). A more detailed argument for some of the claims here can be found in Chapter 6 of *The Conscious Mind* (Chalmers 1996).

REFERENCES

Baars, B. J. 1988. *A Cognitive Theory of Consciousness*. Cambridge: Cambridge University Press.

Bogen, J. E. 1995. On the neurophysiology of consciousness, parts I and II. *Consciousness and Cognition* 4:52–62 and 4:137–158.

Cauller, L. J., and A. T. Kulics. 1991. The neural basis of the behaviorally relevant N1 component of the somatosensory evoked potential in awake monkeys: Evidence that backward cortical projections signal conscious touch sensation. *Experimental Brain Research* 84:607–619.

Chalmers, D. J. 1996. *The Conscious Mind: In Search of a Fundamental Theory*. Oxford: Oxford University Press.

Chalmers, D. J. 1997. Availability: The cognitive basis of experience? *Behavioral and Brain Sciences*. Also in N. Block, O. Flanagan, and G. Guzeldere, eds., *The Nature of Consciousness* Cambridge: MIT Press.

Cotterill, R. 1994. On the unity of conscious experience. *Journal of Consciousness Studies* 2:290–311.

Crick, F., and C. Koch. 1990. Towards a neurobiological theory of consciousness. *Seminars in the Neurosciences* 2:263–275.

Crick, F., and C. Koch. 1995. Are we aware of neural activity in primary visual cortex? *Nature* 375:121–123.

Edelman, G. M. 1989. *The Remembered Present: A Biological Theory of Consciousness*. New York: Basic Books.

Farah, M. J. 1994. Visual perception and visual awareness after brain damage: A tutorial overview. In C. Umilta and M. Moscovitch, eds., *Consciousness and Unconscious Information Processing: Attention and Performance*. Cambridge: MIT Press, p. 15.

Flohr, H. 1995. Sensations and brain processes. *Behavioral Brain Research* 71:157–161.

Gray, J. A. 1995. The contents of consciousness: A neuropsychological conjecture. *Behavioral and Brain Sciences* 18:659–722.

Greenfield, S. 1995. *Journey to the Centers of the Mind*. New York: W. H. Freeman.

Hameroff, S. R. 1994. Quantum coherence in microtubules: A neural basis for emergent consciousness? *Journal of Consciousness Studies* 1:91–118.

Leopold, D. A., and N. K. Logothetis. 1996. Activity changes in early visual cortex reflect monkeys' percepts during binocular rivalry. *Nature* 379:549–553.

Libet, B. 1993. The neural time factor in conscious and unconscious events. In *Experimental and Theoretical Studies of Consciousness* (Ciba Foundation Symposium 174). New York: Wiley.

Llinas, R. R., U. Ribary, M. Joliot, and X.-J. Wang. 1994. Content and context in temporal thalamocortical binding. In G. Buzsaki, R. R. Llinas, and W. Singer, eds., *Temporal Coding in the Brain*. Berlin: Springer-Verlag.

Logothetis, N., and J. Schall. 1989. Neuronal correlates of subjective visual perception. *Science* 245:761–763.

Milner, A. D., and Goodale, M. A. 1995. *The Visual Brain in Action*. Oxford University Press.

Shallice, T. 1988. Information-processing models of consciousness: Possibilities and problems. In A. Marcel and E. Bisiach, eds., *Consciousness in Contemporary Science*, Oxford: Oxford University Press.

Sheinberg, D. L. and Logothetis, N. K. 1997. The role of temporal cortical areas in perceptual organization. *Proceedings of the National Academy of Sciences USA* 94:3408–13.

Taylor, J. G., and F. N. Alavi. 1993. Mathematical analysis of a competitive network for attention. In J. G. Taylor, ed., *Mathematical Approaches to Neural Networks*. New York: Elsevier.

Tootell, R. B., J. B. Reppas, A. M. Dale, R. B. Look, M. I. Sereno, R. Malach, J. Brady, and B. R. Rosen. 1995. Visual motion aftereffect in human cortical area MT revealed by functional magnetic resonance imaging. *Nature* 375:139–141.

20 A Rosetta Stone for Mind and Brain?

Susan A. Greenfield

Tony Bland suffered serious head injuries when a football stadium collapsed at Hillsborough in the United Kingdom. Once it was established that he had no chance of ever regaining consciousness, all food was withheld. The brutal, if tacit message is that if you have no chance of regaining consciousness then you might as well be dead. Ultimately, all our endeavors are directed toward a payoff of deepened-heightened-blunted consciousness, be it achieved by downhill skiing, falling in love, or a good claret. Not only that: most people are in direct contact with children or pets with seemingly different types of consciousness, or they have been prescribed or have even abused drugs that dramatically modify "mood." Small wonder then that consciousness captures the imagination.

The direction to follow is far from obvious. No other topic has been so energetically appropriated by, on the one hand, the philosophers with their millennia of tradition, and on the other, the scientific Johnny-come-latelys with their privileged insight into brain operations, quantum mechanics, chaos theory, pharmacology, and so on. In this chapter I suggest one possible route through the current gridlock between the philosophers' agenda emphasizing subjectivity and the scientific strategy of monitoring objective brain features.

In my view, the answer lies in attempting to develop a theoretical Rosetta stone in which both the phenomenology of consciousness and the physiology of its physical infrastructure can be simultaneously described in terms of each other. We need a way of matching up parallel descriptions of subjective and physical phenomena. To achieve this goal we must step back from the physical brain, and indeed from the philosophers' usual deconstructionist labels, and try to identify just what we would be looking for in the physical brain that might accommodate subjective awareness. Clearly, we have to start with the state of consciousness itself and try to list phenomenological features that would need to be catered to.

The first property is inspired by a conundrum: When does a baby become conscious? Perhaps as the midwife dangles it by its ankles and slaps its behind, awareness slams into its brain like the bright lights suddenly going on in Oxford Street or at Rockefeller Center. Alternatively, consciousness might dawn sometime in infancy, but if so, when? Would any new mother affirm that her baby was merely in vegetable or robot status for the first month or so of life? The most plausible explanation is rather that consciousness has already been long under way in the womb. But if so, when did the baby become conscious, and what exactly is it conscious of?

We cannot expect a fetus to have the same consciousness as we because it has had no direct sensory experiences of the world. Moreover, we now know that although the human brain has an almost maximal number of neurons by the time the fetus reaches full term, a more telling feature in the adult brain are the connections between the neurons that infiltrate, penetrate, and iterate thousands and tens of thousands of times between one cell and the next like an incessant web spun by a demented, obsessive spider. Some of these connections are already present in the brains of fetuses, but it is during early life that their growth in density is conspicuous, during which time the environment crafts individual patterns of connectivity. Hence if the fetus is conscious, with its newly minted and modestly connected neurons, surely it cannot be expected to have the same type of consciousness as an adult or even a child.

The same riddle applies to animals. Again, it seems unlikely that human beings are conscious, but chimpanzees, who differ from us by only 1 percent in their DNA, are zombies. And moving still further from our own species in the animal kingdom, most pet owners would avow that their Fifi understood everything they said. If we carry on in this spirit, however, when do we stop? Some scientists, among them Gerald Edelman, have come clean and stated explicitly that "lower" animals are not conscious: he gives as an example the lobster. But where exactly *do* we draw the line? If it is by possessing a specific physical feature or region in the brain that one acquires consciousness, that structure must be the "seat of consciousness." The idea of a consciousness center, though seductive, is fallacious. No area in the brain can be shown to act as an autonomous minibrain with executive powers. Moreover, if animals with much simpler brains, lacking such a structure, exhibit periods of apparent sleep, or at least rest, then what is the state that dominates at other times?

To my mind a satisfactory way of accommodating all these problems about animal and neonatal consciousness is to turn one's back on the Oxford Street lights scenario. Instead, imagine a dimmer switch that, when on, can vary from almost imperceptible light—say consciousness in simpler animals and midterm fetuses; through moderate illumination—mammalian consciousness; to light from floodlit brilliance—adult human consciousness. Quite simply, consciousness could grow in degree as brain connectivity did. The first property that we could list, then, would be that consciousness is a continuum. Because the brain has no fixed consciousness center, we would have to imagine that consciousness arose from a growing assembly of neurons that were not preordained but just transiently large enough.

But what factor would determine this temporary recruitment? The answer to this question, in turn, prompts the idea about the second property of consciousness. It is a paradox in terms to be conscious of nothing. Hence, we must always be conscious of something. This is an idea currently being debated by philosophers, who refer to this type of consciousness as "representational." The issue for them is whether all forms of consciousness are representational. Obviously, if you look at a rose, that rose is the center of your consciousness for that moment; but what if you are having a fantasy, or a more abstract hope, or even more abstracted still, just feeling happy or anxious? Although philosophers have previously distinguished this more abstract "higher-order" consciousness from the brute sensual experience of smelling, holding, and starting at a rose, Michael Tye (for example), in his *Ten Problems of Consciousness*, now argues that really the two states are similar. The higher-order consciousness can be seen as a distillation or net product of the different individual sensory experiences flooding in. For our purposes we can still say, then, that whether it is sensory or more abstractly "cognitive," either way, consciousness entails some sort of focus or epicenter.

Again this "phenomenological" or subjective feature could easily have a physical counterpart: as mentioned earlier, it is through one's individual experience in life that the connections between sets of neurons become reinforced or "strengthened" according to idiosyncratic associations. A network of neurons assembled into this kind of hard-wired formation would be much smaller than that needed to generate appreciable consciousness, but on the other hand, could be the kind of epicenter around which a transient assembly is recruited. An alternative image might be that of a stone thrown into a puddle. The stone is relatively unchanging and fixed in size. When it hits the water, though, it sends out ripples that last only an instant but far exceed its own diameter.

Returning once more to the physiological level, we already have sufficient information to know that neurons can be transiently recruited in this way. Optical imaging in the frog's brain has revealed groups of neurons that grow slowly out over about half a second in response to flashes of light. Moreover, in human beings it is possible to record the sensation of a prick on the skin in the appropriate receiving area of the brain very quickly. Only after about half a second, however once the electrical signs of a response have spread over much wider areas, will subjects report that they are "conscious" of the tingle elicited by the prick.

Not only can science show that transient neuronal assemblies are a reality, but it can also provide us with clues about how they are formed. Certain chemicals, released according to different biorhythms and arousal levels, will "modulate" the ease with which neurons are corralled into joining a group activated by the pulling power of the epicenter. In this way the size of a transient assembly will depend on the strength of the stimulus epicenter, corresponding to how intense the stimulation, or indeed how many hard-wired connections it activated, namely its personal significance to you. But another equally important factor will be the availability of these modulation chemicals, depending in turn on time of day or arousal levels generally. It is from among this variety of chemicals that the selective targets of mood-modifying drugs such as Prozac or Ecstasy find their targets. At the phenomenological level, each drug alters consciousness in a different way, but physiologically this action is associated with an effect on a chemical system, hence on its modulating power to determine the sizes of transient neuronal assemblies.

If one goes along with this idea, then it is possible to circumvent another worry about consciousness when considering its physical basis, namely just what the magic extra ingredient might be. If we substitute the issue of quantity of neurons for any mysterious extra quality, then we will have a much better chance to accommodate the experience of consciousness in the physical brain. Because no brain region is magic or special, it is much more reasonable to envisage that appreciable consciousness appears as more and more neurons are connected, just as a photographic image slowly appears as more and more of the parts become clearer in the developing dish. Degree of consciousness can thus be seen as related to number of neurons recruited in a transient assembly, which in turn depends on several factors. Given such a scenario, what a relief it would be to abandon the quest for a magic bullet: how much more plausible to envisage instead that several factors, such as arousal levels, extent of epicenter associations, and stimulus strength are each necessary for consciousness, but sufficient only when present together in a specific way.

I discounted earlier the idea of a permanent and committed consciousness center, but on the other hand, if we take the physicalist stance—and it is hard for scientists to make much progress unless they do—then we must be able to pinpoint somewhere in the brain where it all happens. Where might these fluctuating assemblies occur in the brain? Again, the answer to this problem prompts the third possible property of consciousness. We saw with the neuronal correlate of the focus of consciousness that it could be a small network of neurons that were hard-wired but insufficient in size. Of course any one neuron could participate in many such networks simultaneously; it has, after all, thousands of connections with other neurons, any of which are there to be activated under the right conditions.

Imagine then that all over the brain are such connections with the potential to recruit sufficient additional neurons to generate consciousness. On the other hand, for most people most of the time we have only one consciousness at any one time. The third property of consciousness could then be that it is spatially (potentially) multiple but temporally unitary. Taking these three properties together, *conscious* could be described as:

Spatially multiple yet effectively single at any one time. An emergent property of nonspecialized and divergent groups of neurons that is continuously variable with respect to, and always entailing, a stimulus epicenter. The size of the assembly, hence the degree of prevailing consciousness, is a product of the interaction between degree of arousal and recruiting power of the epicenter. The recruiting power of the epicenter depends in turn on strength of stimulus signal and extent of associative neuronal connectivity.

Here then is an attempt at the type of Rosetta-stone description that could be applied to both phenomenological and physiological descriptions of consciousness. At the physical-brain level would be endless formation and reformation of large banks of neurons: we have seen that such a description would be valuable because we could then avoid problems posed by the conundrum about states of mind in neonates and animals, by the search for a special, magic ingredient, and by a specific location for consciousness in the brain. But what about the other side of the coin, the subjective world? How could the Rosetta stone be applied to different types of consciousness?

A good place to start is with an extreme. Could there be, for example, types of consciousness associated with neuronal assemblies that were particularly small? And if so, would those types of consciousness, even though they were in one sense very different in origin, nonetheless have something very fundamental in common? I think the answer is Yes.

If we were looking for a brain in which small assemblies were most likely, then a fetal brain would be highly appropriate. After all, we already know for certain that one factor governing neuronal size, namely neuronal connectivity to be forged in later life through experiential associations, is very modest at this stage. Thanks to the sensitivity of EEG recordings made from premature babies at 26 weeks old, we have a valuable clue to the type of consciousness they might be having. Fetuses at 26 weeks will exhibit in their brain for the first time consistent electrical activity indicative of a functioning "conscious" brain. Moreover, this pattern is similar to one seen in human adults. The big difference is that we display this state a few times a night, whereas the fetus generates it constantly. This electrical activity, indicative of a special type of sleep (rapid eye movement or REM sleep), is associated with dreaming.

An intriguing although speculative possibility then is that fetuses, with their potential for only small neuronal assemblies, have a dreamlike consciousness, and that, in turn, small neuronal assemblies will underlie our dreaming-consciousness. When we are asleep we are far less sensitive to the outside world: hence at this time we would have small assemblies, but for a different reason. Although our connectivity is intact, another important factor would be modified: the strength of the epicenter, not activated in the normal way by our sense organs, would be at best weakly stimulated. Most of us would acknowledge that dreams are a different experience from normal daytime awareness, with their ruptures in logic and sudden shifts in scene: it is tempting to imagine then that this type of consciousness did indeed correspond to a flimsy position far down the continuum.

The psychiatrist and sleep expert Alan Hobson has subjected reports of dreaming consciousness to a "mental-status" exam such as that used by psychiatrists, and found that dreaming has certain parallels to the state of mind of the schizophrenic; the only difference is that the schizophrenic is in a dream, or perhaps nightmare, much more of the time. In the schizophrenic brain, unlike that of a baby, the associative connectivity would be intact, but this time a problem might arise with another factor in determining size of neuronal assembly, namely arousal levels: we know that schizophrenia is alleviated by giving a drug that blocks availability of one "modulating" chemical that might be in functional excess in this condition. In this way then it is possible, at the phenomenological level, to link three very different conditions—dreaming, schizophrenia, and childhood—with a common type of consciousness. Such a consciousness would be disconnected and highly labile, as assembly after flimsy neuronal assembly formed and reformed almost as randomly and capriciously as clouds.

On a less extreme level, one could apply the model to oneself, envisaging that throughout the day, and indeed the night, the depth of our consciousness will be constantly changing, as we acknowledge when we speak of raising our consciousness, or blunting it. By keeping one toe in the subjective world of our own experiences, and seeking a physiological counterpart resulting from a confluence of factors that we can manipulate, we might more readily be able to describe individual types of consciousness with increasing specificity. Moreover, the great advances in noninvasive brain imaging, though their temporal or spatial resolution is currently too low to be appropriate, in a few years will presumably be sensitive enough that transient populations of neuronal assemblies will be monitored as they currently are with invasive optical methods in the frog brain.

Where might it all lead? Certainly we would have a common forum for scientists and philosophers, a descriptive framework of consciousness that tallies at both the physiological and phenomenological levels. It would be a significant, if nonglamorous and unspectacular step forward. But such a description is far from being an explanation: for the forseeable future; your private world is likely to remain inviolate from probings by scientists and philosophers alike.

REFERENCES

Hobson, A. 1994. *The Chemistry of Conscious States: How the Brain Changes Its Mind*. Boston: Little, Brown and Co.

Iye, M. 1995. *Ten Problems of Consciousness: A Representational Theory of the Phenomenal Mind*. Cambridge: The MIT Press.

21 Locating the Subjectivity Pump: The Thalamic Intralaminar Nuclei

Joseph E. Bogen

It is here proposed that subjectivity (hereafter, C) is engendered by neuronal activity in and immediately around the intralaminar nuclei (ILN) of each thalamus (Bogen 1993b). Falsification of this proposal is straightforward: find someone with essentially complete, bilateral destruction of ILN whom we would consider conscious. Absolute proof of this claim is unlikely, but I hope to make it plausible. One reason to consider it plausible is that many informed persons have long believed it, or something like it (including Rodolfo Llinas as well as Wilder Penfield and Herbert Jasper, of whom more later).

The physiologic evidence for this proposal has been presented often by Llinas and colleagues (e.g., Llinas and Ribary 1993, Pare and Llinas 1995). Hence, in this chapter I emphasize the anatomic and neurologic evidence.

BASIC DISTINCTION BETWEEN C AND THE CONTENT OF CONSCIOUSNESS

The crucial core of the many concepts of consciousness includes subjectivity, the ascription of self or "me-ness" to some percept or affect. Examples include: "It hurts me," "I see red," "I feel thirsty." This core of consciousness I call C. Consequently, *whatever else* consciousness involves, without C there is no consciousness.

Consciousness involves both a property C of varying intensity and a widely varying content. The content (commonly of cortical origin) is not our main interest here. This distinction between the core of consciousness and different *contents* of consciousness has been urged most recently by Baars (1993). The distinction has been made by others, such as Grossman (1980), who wrote: "We can also introspectively discriminate between the contents of consciousness ... and the quality of being conscious." Landesman (1967) quotes G. E. Moore:

The sensation of blue differs from that of green. But it is plain that if both are *sensations* they also have some point in common.... I will call this common element "consciousness." ... We have then in every sensation two distinct terms, (1) "consciousness," in respect of which all sensations are alike, and (2) something else [the object], in respect of which one sensation differs from another (*Philosophical Studies*, London 1922).

The entity call C is provided by some cerebral mechanism. In "cerebral" I mean to include cerebral cortex, underlying white matter, thalami, and basal ganglia. This view, though explicitly mechanistic, is not necessarily materialistic, fully deterministic, or solely reductionistic. I assume only that C requires neural activity whose nature is discoverable.

DISTINGUISHING C FROM THE MECHANISM THAT PRODUCES IT

It is the mechanism producing C that we hope to locate and ultimately analyze. Pointing to C may turn out to be like pointing to the wind. We do not actually see the wind. We can, however, point to the *effects* of the wind, and we can often give a good account of what *causes* the wind, the causes often being quite distant (in miles) from the effects.

We can ask: Which brain parts are essential for the "subjectivity pump," as Kinsbourne (1995) calls it? One important clue is that when a pattern of nerve-cell activity acquires subjectivity, it also acquires widespread access to other brain regions. This idea is basic to Baars's (1988) concept of a global workspace. Velmans (1991) called this procedure "information dissemination." And Van Gulick (1991) spoke of "broadcasting." Kinsbourne (1995) points out that identifying a neuronal system as a coordinator of either attention or action, or even both, does not suffice to identify it as a subjectivity pump. That a neuronal system, however, coordinates both attention and action is a necessary, though not sufficient, property, greatly narrowing our search.

LOCALIZING THE MECHANISM PRODUCING C

How some mechanism momentarily endows with C the percepts or affects represented by neuronal patterns situated elsewhere is more likely to be solved when the mechanism is located. Knowing the *where* will greatly facilitate finding out the *how*. That the mechanism is localizable can be argued variously.

The usual localizationist argument in neurology involves two findings: first, a large deficit in some function is produced by a small lesion in the "center" for that function [this statement does *not* imply that the representation is wholly contained within some sharp boundary—see Bogen 1976, Bogen and Bogen 1976]. Second, a large lesion elsewhere (the right hemisphere in the example of a right-hander's syntactic competence results in a small (or no) loss of the function. With respect to C, quite small bithalamic lesions involving both ILN typically impair C (see below), whereas large bicortical lesions (e.g., bioccipital, bifrontal, or bitemporal) typically do not (e.g., Damasio and Damasio 1989).

Another, less familiar argument analogizes neural circuits with single cells:

A primordial cell has the potential for a range of activities, including multiplication, detoxification, secretion, contraction, conduction, and so on. But cells come to specialize, so that skin cells multiply well, liver cells metabolize marvelously, pancreatic islet cells secrete superbly, muscle cells contract best, and the more familiar neurons conduct information better than they secrete, move, multiply, or metabolically adapt.

Analogously, neuronal aggregates form circuits that, starting early, have a wide spectrum of potential function. But some come to specialize in generating diurnal and other rhythms (e.g., suprachiasmatic nucleus), some in converting short-term memory to long (hippocampus), some in long-term storage (probably including neocortex), and so on.

Although any sufficiently sizable aggregate of neurons might from the start have a *potential* for producing C, only certain aggregates developmentally organize to do so (namely, "nonspecific" thalamus, especially ILN).

THE MECHANISM FOR C IS DOUBLE

In an intact cerebrum, the mechanism for C is double: *whatever* the anatomical basis, the anatomy exists in duplicate. That only one of the mechanisms suffices for C is clear from human hemispherectomy (Austin and Grant 1958; Smith 1966, Smith and Sugar 1975), as well as hemicerebrectomy in cats and monkeys (White et al. 1959, Bogen and Campbell 1960, Bogen 1974).

That with two hemispheres C can be doubled has been inferred from split-brain cats and monkeys (Sperry 1961) as well as human beings (Sperry et al. 1969). How such a structural duality could be handled by an intact cerebrum is a fascinating and important question (Bogen 1969, 1977, 1990, 1993a); but it is not the issue here. I consider here only how C is engendered in someone with just one cerebral hemisphere.

THE MECHANISM FOR C IS THALAMIC

That C is *not* produced by cerebral *cortex* was emphasized by Penfield and Jasper (1954). Their views were derived mainly from observations of epilepsy, including that consciousness could be absent during complex behavior (requiring neocortex). Conversely, severe disturbances of function either from cortical removals or cortical hyperactivity need not be accompanied by loss of consciousness. As early as 1937, Penfield wrote:

All parts of the brain may well be involved in normal conscious processes but the indispensable substratum of consciousness lies outside of the cerebral cortex, probably in the diencephalon (p. 241).

To their reasons for this auxiliary conclusion we can add these: some potential contents of consciousness are quite primitive; that is, unneedful of discrimination, association, or learning. Examples are nausea, fatigue, unelaborated pain (e.g., trigeminal neuralgia), thirst, and the like. Did C evolve to give these percepts greater potency, another layer of control over the starting and stopping of continuing action? Was C only recruited subsequently to serve so-called higher functions and more elaborate responses?

We understand that a mechanism might endow with C instances of complex cortical activity describable as "representations of representations" or "higher-order thoughts" (Rosenthal 1993). But these are special contents, not the crucial core of consciousness. Moreover, such special contents might very well influence other cerebral functions without reaching awareness (e.g., Kihlstrom 1987, Castiello, Paulignan, and Jeannerod 1991).

C DEPENDS ON THE INTRALAMINAR NUCLEI

Although large lesions elsewhere deprive the subject of conscious *content*, tiny bilateral lesions of the ILN can cause immediate unresponsiveness. Simultaneous bimedial thalamic infarction can occur because the medial parts of both thalami are occasionally supplied by one arterial trunk that branches, one branch to each thalamus. If the trunk is occluded before it branches, both thalami will be affected. When simultaneous, partial infarction of the two sets of ILN occurs, unresponsiveness typically ensues (see Table I in Guberman and Stuss 1980). Sudden onset of coma can occur even when the lesions are only a few cubic centimeters in volume, as in case 4 of Graff-Radford et al. (1990). This result contrasts with retention of responsiveness with very large lesions elsewhere. Even a quite large lesion involving one (and only one) thalamus rarely if ever causes coma (Plum and Posner 1988).

Emergence from unresponsiveness after bithalamic lesions (not causing death) is commonly accompanied by mental impairments variously described as contusion, dementia, and amnesia or hypersomnia or both. Which of these impairments dominates depends on precise lesion site as well as size (Castaigne et al. 1981, Gentilini, De Renzi, and Crisi 1987, Guberman and Stuss 1983, Meissner et al. 1987, Markowitsch, von Cramon, and Schuri 1993).

CONNECTIONS OF THE INTRALAMINAR NUCLEI

Ascending input to ILN can help explain C of primitive percepts. The input to ILN includes a large fraction of the ascending output of the brain-stem reticular formation, from a spinothalamic system conveying temperature and pain information, from the cerebellum, the superior colliculus, substantia nigra, and vestibular nuclei (Kaufman and Rosenquist 1985, Royce, Bromley, and Gracco 1991).

The existence of connections to ILN from globus pallidus suggests a monitoring of motor systems, as do the cortical projections a monitoring of motor systems, as do the cortical projections to ILN from sensorimotor and premotor cortex. A role in control of motor output is evident in the very substantial projections from ILN to striatum. Is this the pathway for the inhibition (or release from inhibition) supposed by Libet (1983, 1985) to stop (or release) developing motor plans? Is this the basis for a "volitional" decision?

If it is correct that subjectivity is generated within ILN (and environs), this connection bears immediately on the old question of epiphenomenality because ILN's principal output is to striatum. Hence, awareness of something (i.e., transient subjectivity of a particular content) will necessarily influence motor output.

It is now widely accepted that the reticular nucleus (nucleus reticular is thalami or nRt) of thalamus affords a physiologic basis for selective attention (Scheibel and Scheibel 1966, Yingling and Skinner 1977, Crick 1984, Mitrofanis and Guillery 1993). Associated with nRt is a plausible theory of C that I consider inadequate for several reasons. It assumes that the thalamocorticothalamic activity passing through nRt can, in one small locale, grow so large that it shuts down other activity by a sort of surround inhibition; this relationship would account for the focus of attention. Meanwhile, the level of activity in the small locale could rise above the "threshold for consciousness." Problems with this view include: (1) it does not account for C of primitive content; (2) there may well be focal attention without C (and possibly vice versa); and (3) it makes no provision for an immediate inhibition (or release) of a developing motor plan. That focal attention can be influenced by C could have its anatomical basis in collaterals of ILN efferents that terminate in nRt.

Interlaminal nuclei efferents, some of them collaterals of the ILN projection to striatum, are widely and sparsely distributed to most of neocortex. This distribution may provide continuous cortical computation with immediate notice of the aforementioned "volitional decision." In any case, one can see how ILN could directly influence ideation, insofar as ideation is a function of cortex.

Groenewegen and Berendse (1994) recently reviewed evidence that ILN *p. 244* are more specific than the traditional "nonspecific" label might suggest. They concluded that, "the major role of the midline–intralaminar nuclei presumably lies in the regulation of the activity and the ultimate functioning of individual basal-ganglia-thalamocortical circuits" (p. 56), and that, "the midline-intralaminar nuclei are positioned in the forebrain circuits like a spider in its web" (p. 57).

APPROPRIATE INTERACTION

I have implied that subjective experience of any content requires some as yet unspecified "appropriate interaction" between ILN and the neural representation of that content. It has been suggested (Crick and Koch 1990, Llinas and Ribary 1993) that the "appropriate interaction" involves synchronization of neuronal activity at 40 Hz.

As an example of "appropriate interaction" between ILN and cortex, we can consider awareness of the direction of motion of a stimulus. It is now widely understood that information on direction of motion is available in cortex of the superior temporal sulcus, especially area V_5, more commonly called MT (Allman and Kaas 1971, Boussaoud, Ungerleider, and Desimone

1990, Newsome et al. 1990, Rodman, Gross, and Albright 1990, Murasugi, Salzman, and Newsome 1993, Zeki 1993).

We expect that for direction of motion to have a subjective aspect (i.e., to acquire C) the "appropriate interaction" must occur between ILN and MT (or its targets). We keep in mind that activity in MT might well be available for adaptive behavior *whether or not* it acquires C.

In the neurally intact individual, the "appropriate interaction" can be on, or off, or in between, and is quickly adjustable. When V1 (striate cortex) has been ablated, however, the "appropriate interaction" for vision does not occur. That is, the information on direction of motion in MT is not available to verbal output (the individual denies seeing the stimulus). At the same time, that information may be available for some other behavior, and has come to be known as "blindsight" (Weiskrantz 1986, Stoerig and Cowey 1993). It appears (when we accept availability to verbal output as the index of awareness) that the "appropriate interaction" between MT and ILN does not occur in the absence of influences from ipsilateral striate cortex. (But cf. Barbur et al. 1993.)

UPDATING THE "CENTRENCEPHALON"

When Penfield and Jasper (1954) advocated the "centrencephalon" concept, they particularly stressed the role of ILN. Why was this idea eclipsed, to reappear some forty years later? At least three reasons can be readily seen:

1. The centrencephalon was supposed to be not only a mechanism for consciousness, but also a source of seizures that were "generalized from the start." The concept of "centrencephalic seizures" has mostly been abandoned by epileptologists. That Penfield and Jasper combined these two ideas, however, does not require that we do so; arguments for an ILN role in C can be made quite independently of theories about origin and spread of seizure.

2. Cerebral commissurotomy (the split brain) reinforced doubts about the existence of a centrencephalon (Doty 1975). The problem of localizing the mechanism for C can be approached, however, in terms of a single hemisphere (which we know can have C), postponing to the future the problem of integrating the two mechanisms, and how this integration bears on the "unity of consciousness."

3. Forty (even twenty) years ago, many doubted ILN projections to cortex, because unilateral decortication did not produce rapid degeneration in the ILN as it did in most of the ipsilateral thalamus. Another exception to rapid degeneration was nRt, which, indeed, we now believe does *not* project to cortex (Scheibel and Scheibel 1966, Jones 1985). More recent tracer techniques have shown, however, that ILN *do* project to cortex, and widely (Jones 1985).

The "centrencephalon" concept held a germ of truth that now needs to be nourished by considering ILN a major constituent of the mechanisms that provide us, and creatures like us, with consciousness.

SUMMARY

Understanding how some neural mechanism can momentarily endow neuronal activity patterns with subjectivity requires that we identify structures essential to that mechanism. A role for ILN in the awareness of primitive (i.e., not cortically computed) sensations is suggested by their connection from ascending pathways. A role for ILN in awareness of cortical activity is suggested by their widespread afference from cortex. A role for ILN in volition is suggested by their heavy projection to striatum. Unlike striatum, ILN also project widely to almost all neocortex, enabling an effect on ideation. And passage through nRt of ILN efferents to cortex could influence the attention-selective action of nRt. The loss of consciousness with bilateral thalamic lesions involving the intralaminar nuclei (ILN) contrasts with retention of C after large cortical ablations depriving consciousness of specific content. It is suggested here that the quickest route for better understanding consciousness involves more intensive study of ILN. No other structures seem, from current knowledge, to be more likely candidates for the neural mechanism responsible for subjective experience.

REFERENCES

Allman, J. M., and J. H. Kaas. 1971. A representation of the visual field in the caudal third of the middle temporal gyrus of the owl monkey (*Aotus frivirgatus*). *Brain Research* 31:85–105.

Austin, G. M., and F. C. Grant. 1958. Physiologic observations following total hemispherectomy in man. *Surgery* 38:239–258.

Baars, B. J. 1988. *A Cognitive Theory of Consciousness*. Cambridge: Cambridge University Press.

Baars, B. J. 1993. How does a serial, integrated and very limited stream of consciousness emerge from a nervous system that is mostly unconscious, distributed, parallel and of enormous capacity? In G. Broch and J. Marsh, eds., *Experimental and Theoretical Studies of Consciousness*. New York: John Wiley and Sons.

Barbur, J. L., J. D. G. Watson, R. S. J. Frackowiak, and S. Zeki. 1993. Conscious visual perception without V1. *Brain* 116:1293–1302.

Bogen, J. E. 1969. The other side of the brain. II: An appositional mind. *Bulletin of the Los Angeles Neurological Societies* 34:135–162.

Bogen, J. E. 1974. Hemispherectomy and the placing reaction in cats. In M. Kinsbourne and W. L. Smith, eds., *Hemispheric Disconnection and Cerebral Function*. Springfield, MA: C. C. Thomas.

Bogen, J. E. 1976. Hughlings Jackson's Heterogram. In D. O. Walter, L. Rogers, and J. M. Finzi-Fried, eds., *Cerebral Dominance BIS Conference Report* 42. Los Angeles: UCLA, *Brain Research Institute*.

Bogen, J. E. 1977. Further discussion on split-brains and hemispheric capabilities. *British Journal of the Philosophy of Science* 28:281–286.

Bogen, J. E. 1990. Partial hemispheric independence with the neocommissures intact. In C. Trevarthen, ed., *Brain Circuits and Functions of the Mind*. Cambridge: Cambridge University Press.

Bogen, J. E. 1993a. The callosal syndromes. In K. Heilman and E. Valenstein, eds., *Clinical Neuropsychology*, 3rd ed. New York: Oxford University Press, pp. 337–381.

Bogen, J. E. 1993b. Intralaminar nuclei and the where of awareness. *Proceedings of the Society for Neuroscience* 19:1446.

Bogen, J. E., and G. M. Bogen. 1976. Wernicke's region—where is it? *Annals of the New York Academy of Sciences* 280:834–843.

Bogen, J. E., and B. Campbell. 1960. Total hemispherectomy in the cat. *Surgical Forum* 11:381–383.

Boussaoud, D., L. G. Ungerleider, and R. Desimone. 1990. Pathways of motion analysis: Cortical connections of the medial superior temporal and fundus of the superior temporal visual areas in the macaque. *Journal of Comparative Neurology* 296:462–495.

Castaigne, P., F. Lhermitte, A. Buge, R. Escourolle, J. J. Hauw, and O. Lyon-Caen. 1981. Paramedian thalamic and midbrain infarcts: Clinical and neuropathological study. *Annals of Neurology* 10:127–148.

Castiello, U., Y. Paulignan, and M. Jeannerod. 1991. Temporal dissociation of motor responses and subjective awareness: A study in normal subjects. *Brain* 114:2639–2655.

Crick, F. 1984. Function of the thalamic reticular complex: The searchlight hypothesis. *Proceedings of the National Academy of Science U.S.A.* 81:4586–4590.

Crick, F., and C. Koch. 1990. Towards a neurobiological theory of consciousness. *Seminars in the Neurosciences.* 2:263–275.

Damasio, H., and A. R. Damasio. 1989. *Lesion Analysis in Neuropsychology.* New York: Oxford University Press.

Doty, R. W. 1975. Consciousness from neurons. *Acta Neurobiologiae Experimentalis* 35:791–804.

Gentilini, M., F. De Renzi, and G. Crisi. 1987. Bilateral paramedian thalamic artery infarcts: Report of eight cases. *Journal of Neurology, Neurosurgery and Psychiatry* 50:900–909.

Graff-Radford, N., D. Tranel, G. W. Van Hoesen, and J. P. Brandt. 1990. Diencephalic amnesia. *Brain* 113:1–25.

Groenewegen, J. J., and H. W. Berendse. 1994. The specificity of the "nonspecific" midline and intralaminar thalamic nuclei. *Trends in Neuroscience* 17:52–57.

Grossman, R. G. 1980. Are current concepts and methods in neuroscience adequate for studying the neural basis of consciousness and mental activity? In H. M. Pinsker and W. D. Willis, Jr., eds., *Information Processing in the Nervous System.* New York: Raven Press.

Guberman, A., and D. Stuss. 1983. The syndrome of bilateral paramedian thalamic infarction. *Neurology* 33:540–546.

Jones, E. G. 1988. *The Thalamus.* New York: Plenum Press.

Kaufman, E. F. S., and A. C. Rosenquist. 1985. Afferent connections of the thalamic intralaminar nuclei in the cat. *Brain Research* 335:281–296.

Kihlstrom, I. D. 1987. The cognitive unconscious. *Science* 237:1445–1452.

Kinsbourne, M. 1995. The intralaminar thalamic nuclei: Subjectivity pumps or attention-action coordinators? *Consciousness and Cognition* 4:167–171.

Kruper, D. C., R. A. Patton, and Y. D. Koskoff. 1961. Delayed object-quality discrimination in hemicerebrectomized monkeys. *Journal of Comparative Physiology and Psychology* 54:619–624.

Landesman, C. 1967. Consciousness. In P. Edwards, ed., *Encyclopedia of Philosophy*, vol. 2, pp. 191–195.

Libet, B. 1985. Unconscious cerebral initiative and the role of conscious will in voluntary action. *Behavioral and Brain Sciences* 8:529–566.

Libet, B., C. A. Gleason, E. W. Wright, and D. K. Pearl. 1983. Time of conscious intention to act in relation to onset of cerebral activities (readiness-potential): The unconscious initiation of a freely voluntary act. *Brain* 106:623–642.

Llinas, R., and U. Ribary. 1993. Coherent 40-Hz oscillation characterizes dream state in humans. *Proceedings of the National Academy of Science U.S.A.* 90:2078–2081.

Markowitsch, H. J., D. Y. von Cramon, and U. Schuri. 1993. Mnestic performance profile of a bilateral diencephalic infarct patient with preserved intelligence and severe amnesic disturbances. *Journal of Clinical and Experimental Neuropsychology* 15:627–652.

Meissner, I., S. Sapir, E. Kokmen, and S. D. Stein. 1987. The paramedian diencephalic syndrome: A dynamic phenomenon. *Stroke* 18:380–385.

Mitrofanis, J., and R. W. Guillery. 1993. New views of the thalamic reticular nucleus in the adult and the developing brain. *Trends in Neuroscience* 16:240–245.

Murasugi, C. M., C. D. Salzman, and W. T. Newsome. 1993. Microstimulation in visual area MT: Effects of varying pulse amplitude and frequency. *Journal of Neuroscience*. 13:1719–1729.

Newsome, W. T., K. H. Britten, C. D. Salzman, and J. A. Movshon. 1990. Neuronal mechanisms of motion perception. *Cold Spring Harbor Symposium on Quantitative Biology* 55:697–705.

Pare, D., and R. Llinas. 1995. Conscious and preconscious processes as seen from the standpoint of sleep–waking cycle neurophysiology. *Neuropsychologia* 33:1155–1168.

Penfield, W. 1937. The cerebral cortex and consciousness. *The Harvey Lectures*. Reprinted 1965 in R. H. Wilkins, ed., *Neurosurgical Classics*. New York: Johnson Reprint Corp.

Penfield, W., and H. H. Jasper. 1954. *Epilepsy and the Functional Anatomy of the Human Brain*. Boston: Little, Brown.

Plum, F., and J. B. Posner. 1985. *The Diagnosis of Stupor and Coma*. Philadelphia: F. A. Davis.

Rodman, H. R., C. G. Gross, and T. D. Albright. 1990. Afferent basis of visual response properties in area MT of the macaque. II. Effects of superior colliculus removal. *Journal of Neuroscience* 10:1154–1164.

Rosenthal, D. M. 1993. State consciousness and transitive consciousness. *Consciousness and Cognition* 8:355–363.

Royce, G. J., S. Bromley, and C. Gracco. 1991. Subcortical projections to the centromedian and parafascicular thalamic nuclei in the cat. *Journal of Comparative Neurology* 306:129–155.

Scheibel, M. E., and A. B. Scheibel. 1966. The organization of the nucleus reticularis thalami A Golgi study. *Brain Research* 1:43–62.

Smith, A. 1966. Speech and other functions after left (dominant) hemispherectomy. *Journal of Neurology, Neurosurgery and Psychiatry* 29:467–471.

Smith, A., and O. Sugar. 1975. Development of above-normal language and intelligence 21 years after left hemispherectomy. *Neurology* 25:813–818.

Sperry, R. W. 1961. Cerebral organization and behavior. *Science* 133:1749–1757.

Sperry, R. W., M. S. Gazzaniga, and J. E. Bogen. 1969. Interhemispheric relationships: The neocortical commissures: Syndromes of hemisphere disconnection. *Handbook of Clinical Neurology* 4:273–290.

Spiegel, D. In M. Velmans. 1991. Is human information processing conscious? *Behavioral and Brain Sciences* 14:651–725.

Stoerig, P., and A. Cowey. 1993. Blindsight and perceptual consciousness: Neuropsychological aspects of striate cortical function. In B. Gulyas, D. Ottoson, and P. E. Roland, eds., *Functional Organisation of the Human Visual Cortex*. Oxford: Pergamon Press.

Van Gulick, R. 1991. In M. Velmans. 1991. Is human information processing conscious? *Behavior and Brain Science* 14:651–725.

Velmans, M. 1991. Is human information processing conscious? *Behavioral and Brain Sciences* 14:651–725.

Weiskrantz, L. 1986. *Blindsight: A Case Study and Implications*. Oxford: Clarendon Press.

Wexler, Bruce E., S. Warrenburg, G. E. Schwartz, and L. D. Janer. 1992. EEG and EMG responses to emotion-evoking stimuli processed without conscious awareness. *Neuropsychologia* 30:1065–1079.

White, R. J., L. H. Schreiner, R. A. Hughes, C. S. MacCarty, and J. H. Grindlay. 1959. Physiologic consequences of total hemispherectomy in the monkey. *Neurology* 9:149–159.

Yingling, C. D., and J. E. Skinner. 1977. Gating of thalamic input to cerebral cortex by nucleus reticularis thalami. In J. E. Desmedt, ed., *Attention, Voluntary Contraction and Event-Related Cerebral Potentials* Basel: Karger, pp. 70–96.

Zeki, S. 1993. *A Vision of the Brain*. Oxford: Blackwell Scientific Publications.

22 Anterior Cingulate Cortex Participates in the Conscious Experience of Emotion

Richard D. Lane, Eric M. Reiman, Geoffrey L. Ahern, Gary E. Schwartz, Richard J. Davidson, Beatrice Axelrod, and Lang-Sheng Yun

Conscious awareness of emotion may be a double-edged sword. On the one hand, life without emotional experience would be joyless and barren. The ability to experience pleasure stems in part from the ability to experience and contrast it with its opposite (Dafter 1996). On the other hand, mental-health services, including psychotropic medications, are often sought to relieve excessive experiences of anxiety, depression, euphoria, or rage. Although coping strategies that draw attention away from emotional experience may relieve mental anguish (Lane et al. 1990a), a growing body of evidence in behavioral medicine suggests that nonexpression of emotion or deficits in the capacity to experience emotion are associated with physiological disregulation and disease (Taylor et al. 1997). Understanding the neural substrate of emotional experience is therefore relevant to fundamental aspects of normal mental life as well as certain classes of mental and physical disorders.

LEVELS OF EMOTIONAL AWARENESS

In an attempt to better understand the structure of conscious experience, Lane and Schwartz (1987) developed a conceptual framework and an associated measurement tool, the Levels of Emotional Awareness Scale (LEAS) (Lane et al. 1990b). The terms "awareness" and "experience" are used interchangeably, but the former is preferred to highlight the importance of conscious cognition in experience.

Lane and Schwartz (1987) propose that an individual's ability to recognize and describe emotion in oneself and others, called emotional awareness, is a cognitive skill that undergoes development similar to that which Piaget described for cognition in general. Lane and Schwartz's cognitive-developmental model posits five "levels of emotional awareness" that share the structural characteristics of Piaget's stages of cognitive development. The five levels of emotional awareness in ascending order are physical sensations, action tendencies, single emotions, blends of emotion, and blends of blends of emotional experience (the capacity to appreciate complexity in the experience of self and others).

"Structural characteristics" refers to the degree of differentiation and integration of the cognitive schemata used to process emotional information. The development of schemata, according to this model, is driven by the words used to describe emotion. Thus, the nature of conscious emotional experience and the ability to appreciate complexity in one's own experience and that of others are influenced by what one knows about emotion, which itself is based on the words with which one has described emotion in the past.

This position is consistent with that of successors to Piaget such as Karmiloff-Smith (1994), who holds that cognitive development in different domains of knowledge proceeds through "representational redescription." In essence, cognitive development from this theoretical perspective consists of transforming knowledge from implicit (procedural, sensorimotor) to explicit (conscious thought) through language (or other representation mode), which renders thought more flexible, adaptable, and creative. This viewpoint is consistent with a fundamental tenet in the LEAS model.

To measure their level of emotional awareness with the LEAS, subjects are presented with verbal descriptions of emotion-evoking situations involving two people and are asked to write down how self and other would feel in each situation. Scoring is based on specific structural criteria aimed at determining degree of differentiation in use of emotion words (degree of specificity in words used and range of emotions described) and differentiation of self from other. The LEAS has desirable psychometric properties, including high inter-rater reliability, high internal consistency, positive correlations with other cognitive–developmental measures (Lane et al. 1990b), positive correlation with the degree of right-hemispheric dominance in perception of facial affect (Lane et al. 1995), and a positive correlation with the ability to accurately recognize verbal and nonverbal emotion stimuli (Lane et al. 1996b).

LEVELS OF EMOTIONAL AWARENESS AND BLOOD FLOW IN THE ANTERIOR CINGULATE CORTEX

Because the biological basis of consciousness is unknown, any model addressing the neuroanatomical basis of the conscious awareness of emotion must be speculative. Clues to the underlying functional neuroanatomy of emotional awareness, however, come from a positron emission tomography (PET) study of emotion by Lane et al. (1996a, 1997a).

Subjects included twelve right-handed female volunteers who were free of medical, neurological, or psychiatric abnormalities. The LEAS and other psychometric instruments were completed prior to PET imaging. Happiness, sadness, disgust, and three neutral control conditions were induced by film and recall of personal experiences (12 conditions). Twelve PET images of blood flow (BF) were obtained in each subject, using the ECAT 951/31 scanner (Siemens, Knoxville, TN), 40 millicuries intravenous bolus injections of ^{15}O-water, a 15-sec uptake period, 60-sec scans, and an interscan interval of 10–15 min.

To examine BF attributable to emotion generally, rather than to specific emotions, one can subtract the three neutral conditions from the three emotion conditions in a given stimulus modality (film or recall). This difference, which can be calculated separately for the six film and six recall conditions, identifies regions in the brain where BF changes specifically attributable to emotion occur. These BF changes can then be correlated with LEAS scores to identify regions in the brain that are associated with the conscious experience of emotion.

These were our results. Correlations between LEAS and BF change due to emotion (3 emotions minus 3 neutrals) were each significant ($r \geq .63$, $p < .005$) in anterior cingulate cortex (ACC) for both the film-elicited and recall-elicited conditions. When correlating LEAS directly with the components of this difference however (i. e., the 3 emotions alone or the 3 neutrals alone), correlations between BF and LEAS were not significant in the ACC for either the film conditions or the recall conditions (four alternative correlations). Together these findings indicate that the LEAS correlates with activity in the ACC specifically during emotion.

ROLE OF ANTERIOR CINGULATE CORTEX IN CONSCIOUS EXPERIENCE OF EMOTION

These data are consistent with recent findings indicating that the ACC is important in attention to or conscious awareness of perceptual stimuli (Corbetta et al. 1990, 1991, Pardo et al. 1990, Bench et al. 1993, Petersen et al. 1988, Frith et al. 1991, Paus et al. 1993). For example, ACC activity increases as a function of the number of targets to be selected from competing inputs in a visual array, and decreases as task performance becomes automatic (Posner 1994). Activity in the ACC appears to be related to degree of mental effort involved in conscious attention (S. Petersen, personal communication June 1996). The anterior cingulate, together with the basal ganglia, have been described as serving an executive function consisting of attentional recruitment and control of brain areas involved in performing complex cognitive tasks (Posner and Dehaene 1994). Thus, the phrase "attention to action" has been used in describing this aspect of ACC function. Others, however (e.g., Cotterill [1995]), have drawn on these and other data and speculated that the ACC may have a broader role (the "master node") in mediating consciousness generally.

A role for the ACC in emotional experience has been hypothesized for some time (e.g., Papez 1937) and is well accepted in current neurosurgical practice. Surgical lesions are made in the ACC in treating intractable pain. Interestingly, patients report that they still feel the pain but "don't care" about it as much. Their relief appears related to removal of the emotional component of the pain. It has also been observed that approximately 50 percent of patients who undergo cingulotomy have blunted affect postoperatively (Devinsky, Morrell, and Vogt 1995). Surgical lesions in the ACC tend to be quite large and the precise locus of their effects on emotional experience is not known.

The link between these observations and the theory about levels of emotional awareness may be that language contributes to concept formation, which in turn affects allocation of attentional resources and discriminative performance. Thus, higher scores on the LEAS may reflect greater conscious attention to emotional experience and greater capacity to generate or perceive greater complexity (more "targets") in experience during emotional arousal. Thus, the degree to which emotion is consciously experienced (degree to which experience is differentiated and integrated) may in part be a function of the degree to which the ACC actively participates with other neural structures in the neural network mediating emotion.

It is notable that in the PET study described above, BF during both film- and recall-induced emotion was increased in Brodmann's area 9 (BA9) in medial prefrontal cortex. This finding of BF increase in BA9 during emotion was recently replicated in a PET study in which emotion was induced with pleasant and unpleasant pictures (Lane et al. 1997b). We (Reiman et al. 1996) have previously speculated that BA9 may be participating in some aspect of regulating conscious experience (Kihlstrom 1987). This is one of the brain areas that was destroyed in Phineas Gage, the railway worker who became childlike, irresponsible, and prone to emotional outbursts when a metal rod was propelled through his brain. This area could also be involved in emotion-related decision making (Damasio 1994) or inhibition in expressing emotion (Morgan, Romanski, and LeDoux 1993). These possibilities are not mutually exclusive. Interestingly, the LEAS did not correlate with BF in BA9.

One tentative hypothesis is that BA9 participates in the representation and voluntary regulation of emotional experience. If the ability to consciously experience emotion confers evolutionary advantage, it should operate automatically and not depend on learning or voluntary effort. Intelligent thought has been observed in the absence of language (Schaller 1992). Language, however, contributes to the creation of concepts and thus to the allocation of attentional resources and discriminative performance, in cognition generally as well as in emotion. The ACC may thus serve a different function than BA9 in the conscious experience of emotion consisting of the automatic influences of emotion and attention on each other. These two aspects of experience may be analogous to those involved in breathing, which proceeds automatically and involuntarily but may also be consciously controlled.

IMPLICATIONS FOR HEALTH

As mentioned in the introduction, deficits in the capacity to experience and express emotion appear to be associated with poorer health outcomes. *Alexithymia*, a name coined in 1972, meaning "the absence of words for emotion," is a phenomenon that is receiving more and more attention (Taylor et al. 1997). A fundamental assumption in alexithymia research is that a deficit in the capacity for symbolic representation of emotion is somehow associated with an alteration in the normal physiology of emotion. Findings with the LEAS (Lane et al. 1996a, 1996b), however, raise the possibility that alexithymia may fundamentally consist of a deficit in conscious awareness of emotion due to the tendency to fail to consciously attend to one's own emotional experience (Lane et al. in press). The lack of words for emotion and the relatively impoverished cognitive schemata for processing emotional information would be a result of this primary deficit.

To the extent that alexithymia is associated with physiological disregulation, this condition may arise from alteration in the functional neuroanatomy of emotion in these individuals. The leading neurological model of alexithymia is that of a functional commissurotomy (Hoppe and Bogen 1977). This model follows from the assumption that emotional information perceived in the right hemisphere is not transferred to the verbal left hemisphere in alexithymic individuals. The functional commissurotomy model, however, does not explain how a failure to transfer emotional information from the right to the left hemisphere could contribute to disease pathophysiology.

In contrast, the association between emotional awareness and the anterior cingulate cortex may provide a better explanation for the physiological basis of the association between deficits in experiencing and expressing emotion and physical disease, a problem that interested MacLean (1949) when he revised the Papez model of emotion. The ACC is a heterogeneous structure that helps orchestrate the motor, neuroendocrine, and autonomic responses to emotional stimuli (Vogt, Finch, and Olson 1992). For example, the ACC has direct monosynaptic connections to the vagal nuclei in the brain stem (Hurley et al. 1991). It is possible, for example, that transmission of information on interoceptive emotion to the ACC permits completion of a feedback loop to modulate sympathetic arousal, and that failure of such transmission could lead to exaggerated and persistent sympathetic discharge. To the extent that this interpretation is accurate, this alternative model provides a physiological basis for disregulation theory (Schwartz 1983), which states that conscious awareness of emotions promotes both psychological (promoting optimal adaptation by integrating all available information, including that derived from emotions) and physiological health.

REFERENCES

Bench, C. J., C. D. Frith, P. M. Grasby, K. J. Friston, E. Paulesu, R. S. J. Frackowiak, and R. J. Dolan. 1993. Investigations of the functional anatomy of attention using the Stroop test. *Neuropsychologia* 31(9):907–922.

Corbetta, M., F. M. Miezin, S. Dobmeyer, G. L. Shulman, and S. E. Petersen. 1990. Attentional modulation of neural processing of shape, color, and velocity in humans. *Science* 248:1556–1559.

Corbetta, M., F. M. Miezin, S. Dobmeyer, G. L. Shulman, and S. E. Petersen. 1991. Selective and divided attention during visual discriminations of shape, color, and speed: Functional anatomy by positron emission tomography. *Journal of Neuroscience* 11(8):2382–2402.

Cotterill, R. M. J. 1995. On the unity of conscious experience. *Journal of Consciousness Studies* 2(4):290–312.

Dafter, R. E. 1996. Why negative emotions can sometimes be positive: The spectrum model of emotions and their role in mind-body healing. *Advances* 12:6–19.

Damasio, A. R. 1994. *Descartes' Error*. New York: G. P. Putnam.

Devinsky, O., M. J. Morrell, and B. A. Vogt. 1995. Contributions of anterior cingulate cortex to behavior. *Brain* 118:279–306.

Frith, C. D., K. Friston, P. F. Liddle, and R. S. J. Frackowiak. 1991. Willed action and the prefrontal cortex in man: A study with PET. *Proceedings of the Royal Society of London B* 244:241–246.

Hoppe, K. D., and J. E. Bogen. 1977. Alexithymia in twelve commissurotomized patients. *Psychother Psychosom* 28:148–155.

Hurley, K. M., H. Herbert, M. M. Moga, and C. B. Saper. 1991. Efferent projections of the infra limbic cortex of the rat. *Journal of Comparative Neurology* 308:249–276.

Karmiloff-Smith, A. 1994. Précis of *Beyond Modularity*: A developmental perspective on cognitive science. *Behavioral and Brain Sciences* 17:693–745.

Lane, R. D. and G. E. Schwartz. 1987. Levels of emotional awareness: A cognitive-developmental theory and its application to psychopathology. *American Journal of Psychiatry* 144:133–143.

Lane, R., K. Merikangas, G. Schwartz, S. Huang, and B. Prusoff. 1990. Inverse relationship between defensiveness and lifetime prevalence of psychopathology. *American Journal of Psychiatry* 147:573–578.

Lane, R. D., D. Quinlan, G. Schwartz, P. Walker, and S. Zeitlin. 1990b. The levels of emotional awareness scale: A cognitive–developmental measure of emotion. *Journal of Personality Assessment* 55:124–134.

Lane, R. D., L. S. Kivley, M. A. DuBois, P. Shamasundara, and G. E. Schwartz. 1995. Levels of emotional awareness and the degree of right hemispheric dominance in the perception of facial emotion. *Neuropsychologia* 33:525–528.

Lane, R. D., E. Reiman, G. Ahern, G. Schwartz, R. Davidson, B. Axelrod, and L. Yun. 1996a. Anterior cingulate cortex participates in the conscious experience of emotion. *Neuroimage* 3:S229.

Lane, R. D., L. Sechrest, R. Riedel, V. Weldon, A. Kazniak, G. E. Schwartz, 1966b. Impaired verbal and nonverbal emotion recognition in alexithymia. *Psychosomatic Medicine* 58:203–210.

Lane, R. D., E. Reiman, G. Ahern, G. Schwartz, R. Davidson, B. Axelrod, L. Yun, N. Blocher, and K. Friston. 1997a. Neuroanatomical correlates of happiness, sadness and disgust. *American Journal of Psychiatry* 154:926–933.

Lane, R. D., E. M. Reiman, M. M. Bradley, P. J. Lang, G. L. Ahern, R. J. Davidson, and G. E. Schwartz. 1997b. Neuroanatomical correlates of pleasant and unpleasant emotion. *Neuropsychologia* 35:1437–1444.

Lane, R. D., G. L. Ahern, G. E. Schwartz, A. W. Kaszniak. (in press). Is alexithymia the emotional equivalent of blindsight? *Biological Psychiatry*.

MacLean, P. D. 1949. Psychosomatic disease and the visceral brain: Recent developments bearing on the Papez theory of emotion. *Psychosomatic Medicine* 11:338–353.

Morgan, M., L. Romanski, and J. LeDoux. 1993. Extinction of emotional learning: Contributions of medial prefrontal contex. *Neuroscience Letters* 163:109–113.

Papez, J. W. 1937. A proposed mechanism of emotion. *Archives of Neurology and Psychiatry* 38:725–734.

Pardo, J. V., P. J. Pardo, K. W. Janer, and M. E. Raichle. 1990. The anterior cingulate cortex mediates processing selection in the Stroop attentional conflict paradigm. *Proceedings of the National Academy of Sciences U.S.A.* 87:256–259.

Paus, T., M. Petrides, A. C. Evans, and E. Meyer. 1993. Role of the human anterior cingulate cortex in the control of oculomotor, manual, and speech responses: A positron emission tomography study. *Journal of Neurophysiology* 70(2):453–469.

Petersen, S. E., P. T. Fox, M. I. Posner, M. Mintun, and M. E. Raichle. 1988. Positron emission tomographic studies of the cortical anatomy of single-word processing. *Nature* 331:585–589.

Posner, M. I. 1994. Attention: The mechanisms of consciousness. *Proceedings of the National Academy of Sciences U.S.A.* 91:7398–7403.

Posner, M. I., and S. Dehaene. 1994. Attentional networks. Trends in Neurosciences 17:75–79.

Reiman, E. R., R. D. Lane, G. L. Ahern, G. E. Schwartz, and R. J. Davidson. 1996. Positron emission tomography, emotion and consciousness. In S. R. Hameroff, A. W. Kaszniak, and A. C. Scott, eds., *Toward a Science of Consciousness—The First Tucson Discussions and Debates.* Cambridge: MIT Press, pp. 311–320.

Schaller, S. 1992. *A Man Without Words.* New York: Summit Books.

Schwartz, G. E. 1983. Disregulation theory and disease: Applications to the repression/cerebral disconnection/cardiovascular disorder hypothesis. *International Review of Applied Psychology* 32:95–118.

Taylor, G. J., R. M. Bagby, and J. D. A. Parker. 1997. *Disorders of Affect Regulation—Alexithymia in Medical and Psychiatric Illness.* Cambridge: Cambridge University Press.

Vogt, B. A., D. M. Finch, and C. R. Olson. 1992. Functional heterogeneity in cingulate cortex: The anterior executive and posterior evaluative regions. *Cerebral Cortex* 2(6):435–443.

23 Toward the Neurobiology of Consciousness: Using Brain Imaging and Anesthesia to Investigate the Anatomy of Consciousness

Michael T. Alkire, Richard J. Haier,
James H. Fallon

Where does consciousness exist? Is it a cosmic phenomenon that pervades the universe? Or is it a limited entity, a property of biological neuronal systems that exists primarily within the human mind? Crick has offered an "Astonishing Hypothesis" (1994) suggesting that the latter idea might be more nearly correct. He proposes that those interested in scientifically studying consciousness might do well to begin investigating with the simplifying assumption offered by that astonishing hypothesis. In other words, it will probably be easier to gain a scientific understanding of human consciousness specific to the human brain than it will be to scientifically understand whatever "universal" consciousness may turn out to be.

Agreeing with Crick, we have decided to limit our investigation of consciousness to phenomena that can be measured within the human brain. Furthermore, we have decided to experimentally address only a small portion of the consciousness problem as we attempt to answer the specific question: where in the human brain does consciousness reside? Does consciousness arise within individual sensory systems, or does it require a more global integration of brain functioning? To address these questions, we have taken a novel approach to the problem: we are experimenting on "consciousness" itself. We are experimentally manipulating consciousness as a variable using anesthetic agents in volunteers and visualizing the resulting functional brain changes at various levels of consciousness with advanced brain imaging technology.

By reducing a person's level of consciousness stepwise, we can identify the specific cognitive and motor behaviors seen at specific levels of consciousness and correlate those behaviors with the underlying functional neuroanatomy responsible for them. Subtracting functional brain images obtained at one level of consciousness from images obtained at a slightly different level should also reveal the neuroanatomic regions that underlie behaviors evident during the more conscious condition, but lost during the less conscious condition. Thus, by combining experimental manipulation of consciousness with functional brain imaging we should be able to identify the fundamental links between the specific cognitive functions associated with consciousness and their underlying anatomic substrates.

A number of techniques are available for assessing the human brain's functioning *in vivo* (Neil 1993, Naatanen, Ilmoniemi, and Alho 1994, Perani et al. 1992, Wyper 1993, Mullani and Volkow 1992). These techniques are often referred to as functional brain imaging techniques to distinguish them from the commoner structural brain imaging techniques computed tomography (CT) and magnetic resonance imaging (MRI). We distinguish between structural and functional because structural imaging (with CT or MRI) demonstrates brain structure and shows the same "picture" of the brain, regardless of what the subject does while the brain "picture" is taken. With functional imaging, though, the brain can be viewed as it appears while performing a specific function. With structural imaging, a person's brain will appear the same whether the subject is awake or asleep. With functional imaging, however, the brain "picture" of a subject in non-REM sleep looks substantially different from that of a person awake (Buchsbaum et al. 1989).

Functional imaging works because the neurons that are responsible for processing a stimulus will do more work than their surrounding unstimulated companions. As the stimulus-specific neurons increase their rate of work, they will also increase their underlying rate of metabolism. This shift will then drive an increase in regional blood flow that supports the increased metabolism. Therefore, by assessing stimulus-specific changes in either regional blood flow or regional metabolism, we can identify the specific groups of neurons involved in processing a presented stimulus. A study in which researchers are looking for the group of neurons responsible for processing a stimulus is often referred to as an "activation" study. This terminology implies a cause-and-effect relationship between the stimulus used and the resulting regional increase in local neuronal activity. In other words, some regions in the brain will be "activated" by the test stimuli. Similarly, some regions may decrease activity with a stimulus and are often referred to as "deactivated" regions. These stimulus-specific activated (and deactivated) regions can be visualized with brain-imaging technology and their precise anatomic loci within the brain can then be determined. Thus, functional brain imaging offers the researcher a powerful tool for identifying specific structure and function relationships within the living human brain.

Most functional brain-imaging research uses positron emission tomography (PET), single photon emission computed tomography (SPECT), and functional magnetic resonance imaging (fMRI) (Neil 1993). Functional imaging techniques are used primarily to assess changes in regional blood flow, regional metabolic states, and regional receptor–ligand interactions (Saha, MacIntyre, and Go 1994). Each of these physiologic processes can be imaged with PET and SPECT, and fMRI may prove useful in estimating changes in regional blood flow.

Functional brain-imaging technology is exciting because these relatively noninvasive techniques can reveal patterns of brain functioning previously invisible to researchers. The inherent value of functional imaging increases as the cognitive process being studied becomes more complex, and more difficult to study by other means. One interesting finding is that visual neurons in the visual cortex are activated in response to a visual stimulation during a PET study (Phelps et al. 1981). If, however, the same visual neurons are seen to be activated when a subject simply imagines seeing a visual stimulus, then something quite intriguing has been learned about the functional neuroanatomy of imagination (Kosslyn et al. 1993).

Functional brain imaging has allowed researchers to gain significant insights into the structure and function of many higher-order cognitive processes that are intimately involved with consciousness, such as learning, memory, attention, and reasoning (Pardo, Fox, and Raichle 1991 , Haier et al. 1992, Squire et al. 1992, Schachter et al. 1996, and Haier et al. 1988). Only a handful of studies, though, have looked at brain functioning during altered levels of consciousness such as sleep or coma (Buchsbaum et al. 1989; Tommasino et al. 1995) and none have yet attempted to experimentally manipulate "consciousness" as a variable.

To begin our investigation, we studied the functional brain anatomy associated with the anesthetic state during different types and depths of anesthesia in human volunteer subjects. We also assessed the specific cognitive function of auditory verbal memory during normal waking consciousness and unconsciousness produced by the general anesthetic agent propofol. We used the correlational approach to relate each subject's performance on tests of auditory verbal memory back to the functional brain activity that was evident (assessed by PET) when subjects were exposed to the memory stimulus in both the conscious and unconscious states.

To study human regional utilization of cerebral glucose, a positron-labeled deoxyglucose tracer is used, such as ^{18}fluorodeoxyglucose (FDG) (Phelps et al. 1979). This tracer is taken up by active brain neurons as if it were glucose. Once inside a cell, however, ^{18}fluorodeoxyglucose is phosphorylated by hexokinase to ^{18}fluorodeoxyglucose-6-phosphate, which is not a substrate for glucose transport and cannot be metabolized by phosphohexoseisomerase, the next enzyme in the glucose metabolic pathway. Thus, labeled ^{18}fluorodeoxyglucose-6-phosphate becomes metabolically trapped within the intracellular compartment. The amount of radioactive label that occurs in each discrete part of the brain and body is related to the glucose uptake of that discrete region. The more metabolism occurring in a brain region, the more glucose, or tracer, will be taken up (Huang et al. 1980).

We use the FDG technique in our studies. Regional glucose utilization may more accurately assess regional metabolism than would a blood-flow based technique in the presence of an anesthetic, for anesthetics directly affect the regional cerebral blood flow and regional cerebral metabolism coupling relationship (Michenfelder 1988). The standard FDG technique used in humans utilizes a 30- to 45-minute uptake period. Uptake of FDG and metabolic trapping of FDG in the brain as FDG-6-phosphate is 80–90 percent complete at 32 min (Huang et al. 1980, Sokoloff et al. 1977). The actual scanning begins after the uptake period, once the remaining labeled nonphosphorylated FDG has been cleared from the plasma. The eventual images represent the accumulated regional FDG-6-phosphate distribution that occurred during the corresponding uptake period while the study subject was exposed to the experimental conditions.

We have been able to develop a substantial database on how anesthetic agents affect the human brain. We have now obtained enough data that we can begin to see some patterns that may be fundamentally important in eventually understanding consciousness. In our first study we examined global and regional brain metabolic responses to unconsciousness produced by propofol anesthesia (Alkire et al. 1995). These were data from the first systematic study to use functional brain-imaging technology to investigate changes in brain metabolism associated with the anesthetized state in the human brain. Six volunteers were studied twice in two states of consciousness. In one condition the subjects were fully awake and aware, and in the other they were rendered unconscious with the general anesthetic agent propofol. Figure 23.1 is a representative PET image of one subject studied when awake and again when anesthetized with propofol to the point of unconsciousness (defined as loss of responsiveness to verbal or tactile stimulation).

The figure shows regional brain glucose metabolism plotted on a color scale for both the awake and the anesthetized conditions. The absolute rate of glucose metabolism in an area can be determined by comparing the color in that region with the corresponding color on the color scale bar. For example, most of the activity in the awake brain is in the yellows and reds range and thus has regional metabolic rate values of around 30 to 40 micromol/100 gm/min. In the anesthetized brain, however, the colors are in the purples and blues range and thus have values around 5 to 20 micromol/100 gm/min of glucose utilization. These PET images are quantified and placed on the same color scale. Thus we can see at a glance that the amount of regional metabolic activity (an indicator of underlying regional neuronal activity) in an anesthetized brain is dramatically lower than that of an awake brain. In fact, with propofol, the average percentage of reduction in whole-brain glucose metabolism from the awake to the anesthetized condition was 55 ± 13 percent. This metabolic reduction was global and fairly uniform throughout the brain. It was not completely uniform, however, for some brain regions were affected more than others. Most important, the cerebral cortex was significantly more depressed metabolically than subcortical gray matter.

These data revealed that unconsciousness produced by propofol anesthesia was associated with both a global effect on the brain and specific regional effects. Which of these two functional brain changes is more important in producing the unconscious state cannot be determined from this one study alone. To investigate this issue further, we brought back a number of the original subjects and gave them an intermediate dose of propofol. In this second study, we titrated the anesthetic level so that each subject was heavily sedated but remained awake and aware. A graph of our pilot data for the intermediate effect is shown in Figure 23.2A (Alkire et al. 1996).

For the intermediate-dose study the awake whole-brain glucose metabolic rate (GMR) averaged 32 ± 7 μmol/100 /gm/min. Sedation (i.e., intermediate

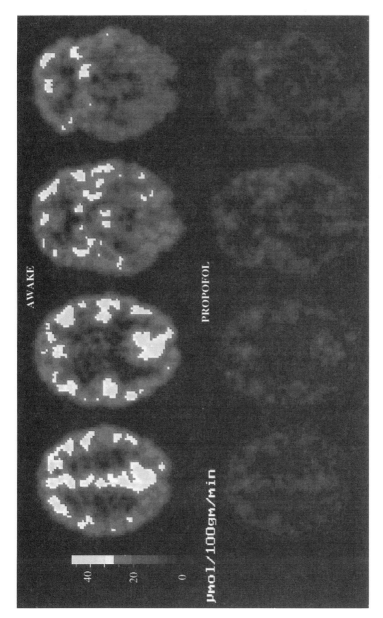

Figure 23.1 PET images of regional cerebral glucose metabolism (micromol/100 gm/min) during normal wakefulness (upper images) and during propofol anesthesia (lower images). The comparison is within one representative subject's brain. These are horizontal slices through the brain (as if the top of the head had been cut off above the ears and we are looking down on the remaining brain tissue). The slices proceed from higher (near the top of the head) to lower (with cerebellum) from left to right the front of the brain is toward the top of the picture and the left side of the image is the left side of the brain. All images are on the same color scale of absolute glucose metabolism. This quantified image demonstrates that propofol anesthesia is associated with a dramatic, fairly uniform reduction in whole-brain metabolism. In this subject, unconsciousness was associated with a whole-brain metabolic reduction (from baseline) of 62%.

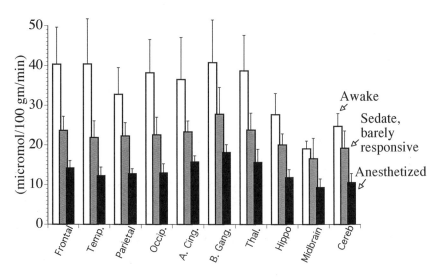

Figure 23.2A Regional cerebral glucose metabolism (micromol/100 gm/min) during awake (light bars) sedated (gray bars), and anesthetized (dark bars) conditions. The figure shows the regional metabolic variability that occurs in response to the anesthetic agent propofol. A dose-response relationship is clearly evident in which higher drug doses further decrease brain metabolism. Because subjects remained aware during the sedation scans, these data suggest that unconsciousness results only when global neuronal functioning is reduced below some critical threshold required to maintain consciousness.

dose) GMR and anesthetized GMR averaged 21 ± 4, and 12 ± 2 μmol/100 gm/min, respectively. Thus, loss of consciousness for this sample of subjects occurred at a mean 62 percent metabolic reduction during propofol anesthesia and sedation occurred at a mean 34 percent whole-brain metabolic reduction. The point that matters in Figure 23.2A is that the pattern of metabolic reduction caused by propofol appears nearly identical in the sedate and anesthetized conditions. Figure 23.2B is a redrawn version of Figure 23.2A in which the intermediate and anesthetized data are so displayed as to better represent the similarity in pattern of regional metabolic changes evident between the two states of awareness.

This similarity in the drug's regional effect suggests that the loss of consciousness associated with propofol was caused by no specific regional shift in metabolism (i.e., it was not caused by changes within a specific consciousness circuit), but rather by the further uniform global reduction in neuronal functioning produced by the increased dose of the drug. Moreover, these findings suggest that loss of consciousness occurs when global neuronal functioning is reduced below some critical threshold required for maintaining consciousness. Thus, these data suggest that whatever or wherever consciousness is, it appears to be a phenomenon well distributed in the human brain.

A few considerations prevent us, though, from fully accepting the well-distributed idea of consciousness. Perhaps the findings with propofol were specific to this anesthetic agent. Other agents, with potentially different

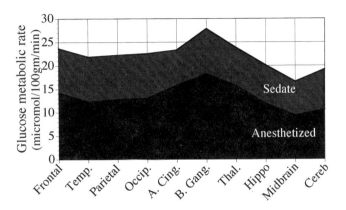

Figure 23.2B The intermediate (i.e., sedation) and anesthetized data from Figure 23.2A are replotted to emphasize the uniformity in the metabolic reduction associated with unconsciousness. This figure shows that a similar pattern in regional metabolism is evident during both sedation and anesthesia with propofol. The primary difference between conscious and unconscious conditions appears to be a global, fairly uniform, further reduction in brain metabolism from the sedated to the anesthetized condition.

mechanisms, might produce regional metabolic findings very different from those of propofol. Another consideration is that the PET spatial resolution may not be sufficient to image the consciousness control circuits within the human brain (though the recent high-resolution functional-imaging demonstration of human brain attention-arousal circuitry certainly suggests otherwise) (Kinomura et al. 1996).

In our next experiment we attempted to address these questions by studying a completely different class of anesthetic agent and using a new, higher-resolution PET scanner. Under a similar protocol to the propofol study, we have now studied the effects of the inhalational anesthetic agent isoflurane on human brain metabolism (Alkire et al. 1997). Figure 23.3 shows the regional cerebral glucose metabolic effects of isoflurane anesthesia titrated to the point of unconsciousness in the brain of one representative subject. The display is similar to that for the propofol data. This subject's whole-brain metabolic reduction during isoflurane anesthesia was 46 percent, which was at the group mean of 46 ± 11 percent.

The anesthetic state (i.e., unconsciousness) is again associated with a rather dramatic reduction in whole-brain metabolism. Moreover, the pattern of regional metabolism seen during isoflurane anesthesia did not significantly differ from the pattern evident when the subjects were awake. This similarity suggests that isoflurane produced the unconscious state by causing a global uniform reduction in brain functioning, rather than by specifically affecting one consciousness circuit. One cannot, however, rule out the possibility that isoflurane's effects simply were as potent on the brain's specific consciousness neurons as on all other neurons in the brain. Nonetheless, the uniformity in metabolic reduction during isoflurane anesthesia, coupled with the fairly uniform metabolic reduction during propofol anesthesia both seem to

Michael T. Alkire, R. J. Haier, J. H. Fallon: Toward the Neurobiology of Consciousness

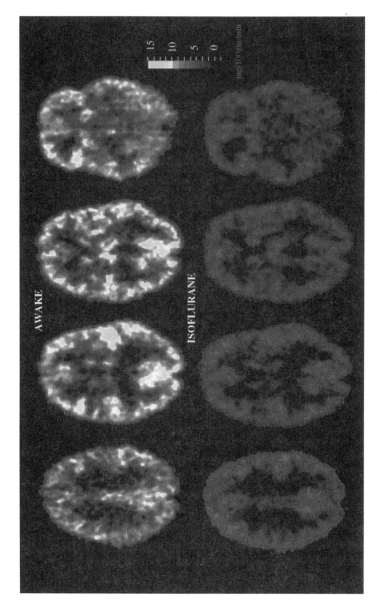

Figure 23.3 PET images of regional cerebral glucose metabolism (mg/100 gm/min) during normal wakefulness (upper images) and during isoflurane anesthesia (lower images). The comparison is within one representative subject's brain. The picture orientation is the same as in Figure 23.1. Notice the increased scanner resolution. The slice levels are selected to match those of Figure 23.1. The image shows that isoflurane anesthesia dramatically reduces whole-brain metabolism in a fairly uniform manner. For this representative subject, isoflurane anesthesia produced a whole-brain metabolic decrease (from baseline) of 46 percent. This subject participated in both the propofol and the isoflurane studies and is the one displayed in the propofol example above (see Figure 23.1). Having studied the same subject under two anesthetics, titrated to similar clinical endpoints, we could see that this person's brain appeared to require a minimum whole-brain metabolic reduction of at least 46 percent to render it unconscious.

suggest that consciousness may be a phenomenon widely distributed in the human brain.

Thus, after studying only two anesthetic agents in the human brain, we may be seeing a pattern in global versus regional metabolic changes produced by anesthesia. Two classes of anesthetic agents each produced unconsciousness by reducing global brain functioning below some specific level. In both the loss of consciousness appeared to be associated more with the global whole-brain metabolic reduction produced by each agent than with any specific regional metabolic change produced by each agent. Moreover, the dose-response effect of propofol on whole-brain glucose metabolism clearly suggests that sedation and anesthesia result from global rather than regional decreases in neuronal functioning.

Certainly, though, some parts of the brain must be more important than others for consciousness to occur. After all, it is well known that large parts of brain can be surgically removed without necessarily altering a person's consciousness. Our recent findings related to conscious versus unconscious verbal memory distinctions suggest that the thalamus may significantly influence the subjective quality of a person's conscious experience (Alkire et al. 1996).

In our memory study (Alkire et al. 1996) we examined how performance on verbal tests of free-recall and forced-choice recognition correlated with regional brain metabolism measured with PET during encoding of the verbal stimuli. In one encoding condition the subjects remained fully awake, whereas in the other the subjects were rendered unconscious with propofol general anesthesia. As one might expect, following the anesthesia condition none of the subjects had objective recall of any information that was presented to them when they were unconscious. Nonetheless, when these subjects were tested on a forced-choice recognition test they did better than expected by chance at selecting the words they had been exposed to a day earlier when unconscious under general anesthesia. Furthermore, following the forced-choice testing, each subject was specifically asked if the recognition test had triggered memories for the words previously presented. All subjects emphatically denied any memory for any of the test words. Thus our unconscious-memory data represent a real examination of implicit memory effects that is beyond possibility of contamination from conscious memory processing.

To find the anatomic loci of the conscious and unconscious memory effects we subsequently correlated, pixel by pixel, the memory-performance scores with the regional metabolic data obtained at the time of memory encoding. We can think of these correlational PET-memory images as regional anatomic maps of brain regions in which significant correlated activity occurred between relative glucose metabolism and memory performance. These correlational maps demonstrated that conscious recall and unconscious recognition share much regional anatomic overlap.

In fact, conscious and unconscious correlations showed much more regional anatomic overlap than regional differences. For both conscious and unconscious conditions the correlational PET images revealed significant correlations in brain regions known to be involved with auditory verbal memory (Mazziotta et al. 1982, Pawlik et al. 1987, Grasby et al. 1993), including the frontopolar cortices (Brodmann's area 9, 10), dorsolateral prefrontal cortex (BA 46), Broca's area (BA 44, 45), Wernicke's area (BA 22), angular gyrus (BA 39), the ideational speech area of the supramarginal gyrus in the inferior parietal lobule (BA 40), the ventral precuneus (BA 31), the dorsal parahippocampal/hippocampal region, as well as perirhinal cortex (BA 35) bordering the temporal parahippocampal region. Negative correlations were found to overlap between conscious and unconscious conditions in the regions of the visual association cortices and the white matter deep to areas 39/40. Negative correlations unique to the unconscious condition were found within the right caudate.

The most revealing difference between the two states of consciousness occurred in the mediodorsal thalamic nucleus. In the conscious condition, memory performance scores correlated highly with values of relative glucose metabolic rate measured in the region of the mediodorsal nucleus at time of encoding. In the unconscious condition, memory performance scores were almost perfectly, uncorrelated (i.e., $r = +0.01$) to values of relative glucose metabolic rate within the mediodorsal nucleus at time of encoding. This difference, between the level of correlated thalamic activity across conditions, was statistically significant ($p < 0.01$, two-tailed).

Data from patients with Korsakoff's syndrome and stroke damage suggests that the thalamus is highly influential in human memory (Cole et al. 1992). It is known too that bilateral damage to either the hippocampus (Winocur 1990, Winocur 1985, Markowitsch et al. 1985, Mishkin 1982). Or the diencephalon (Graff-Radford et al. 1990, Aggelton and Mishkin 1983, McKee and Squire 1992, Vogel et al. 1987, Malamut et al. 1992) can produce global anterograde amnesia. Such lesions usually produce deficits only of conscious explicit memory and not of unconscious implicit memory, suggesting that conscious and unconscious memory may reside in separate neural systems (Squire 1992). Animal lesion studies suggest that the diencephalon (i.e., the region of the thalamus) is more important for conscious memory processing than for unconscious memory phenomena (Winocur 1985, Cahill et al. 1996).

Our findings with the correlational memory data support and, in essence, were predicted by the animal literature, for we found correlated thalamic activity only in the conscious state. In other words, according to the animal data, conscious memory requires thalamic activity, whereas unconscious memory does not. This effect is exactly what our human PET data revealed. In our data, subjects with "better" explicit recall of the auditory information were the same ones who had relatively more metabolic activity within the thalamus at the time they were "memorizing" the auditory information. Thus, thalamic activity at time of encoding predicts subsequent ability in long-term free recall of verbal information. A similar relationship is reported for emotional memory and amygdala activity (Cahill et al. 1996).

A number of roles could be postulated for this thalamic conscious activity. Some suggest that the thalamus may affect memory processing by regulating or controlling attention (LaBerge and Buchsbaum 1990, Posner 1994). Alternatively, it has been suggested that thalamic activity may be required for proper memory encoding (Graff-Radford et al. 1990, Squire 1981, Huppert and Piercy 1979). The encoding hypothesis would be consistent with our finding that level of relative metabolic activity at time of encoding determined subsequent recall ability. One recent PET report, however, demonstrated thalamic activity during retrieval, but not encoding, of auditory verbal memory (Fletcher et al. 1995). Thus, it appears that the thalamus could influence both encoding and retrieval of information with a different "type" of activity required for each process.

This apparent role for thalamic activity during both encoding and retrieval of information, coupled with our finding that the thalamus is important in conscious versus unconscious memory distinctions, suggests the hypothesis that the thalamus, especially the MD nucleus, might serve an important gatekeeper function in partially regulating the information that gains access to the conscious mind. Essentially, the thalamus may be the site at which information is kept about where conscious memories are stored within the brain. This idea is analogous to a disk directory's way of "knowing" where all the information on a computer hard disk is stored. It is not itself the storage site for the data, but it "knows" how to get access to all the bits of data that make up a file. This analogy might explain why, following the unconscious condition, the subjects in our study had no free recall of the verbal stimuli even though the verbal memory data appeared to be within their brains on the PET images. In the anesthetized condition, the thalamus, which should have been on-line, monitoring where information was being stored in the brain, was inhibited from doing so by the anesthetic agent. Thus, when the subjects tried to recall the verbal memory data that were in their brains they had no way of consciously retrieving it because they did not know where each of the bits of data were stored.

SUMMARY

Our search for the specific site of consciousness in the human brain is only just beginning. Nonetheless, even at this early stage we have found interesting aspects about the neurobiology of consciousness. Our data indicate that the unconscious state produced by anesthesia appears to be associated with a fairly uniform whole-brain metabolic reduction. These early experiments have not yet found specific consciousness-control circuitry. The global whole-brain metabolic reduction seen with the two types of anesthetic agents studied so far suggests that consciousness may be evident in the human brain only when some critical threshold amount of global neuronal activity is present.

Many current theories about the neurobiology of consciousness have been proposed and many seem to involve the thalamus or cortical-thalamic interactions (Crick 1994, Baars 1988, Llinas and Ribary 1993). We have found that conscious and unconscious verbal memory processing share much regional anatomic overlap, but do not show functional overlap within the thalamus. Therefore, the thalamus (centering on the mediodorsal nucleus) appears to be particularly important in conscious versus unconscious verbal memory distinctions. Based on the neuroanatomy of this brain region and its involvement with memory functioning, we speculate that this region may be influential in the subjective sensation of consciousness because it facilitates continually comparing the present moment with the past. It may be that subjective awareness of this comparison procedure is a large part of what an organism an organism experiences as consciousness.

It is our hope that our empirical data and our experimental approach to the consciousness problem may ultimately help to answer at least some of the fundamental questions about the neurobiology of consciousness.

REFERENCES

Aggleton, J. P., and M. Mishkin. 1983. Visual recognition impairment following medial thalamic lesions in monkeys. *Neuropsychologia* 21:189–197

Alkire, M. T., R. J., Haier, S. J. Barker, and N. K. Shah. 1996. Positron emission tomography assessment of cerebral metabolism during three different states of human consciousness. *Anesthesia and Analgesia* 82:S7 (abstract).

Alkire, M. T., R. J. Haier, S. J. Barker, N. K. Shah, J. C. Wu, and Y. J. Kao. 1995. Cerebral metabolism during propofol anesthesia in humans studied with positron emission tomography. *Anesthesiology* 82:393–403, discussion 27A.

Alkire, M.T., R. J. Haier, J. H. Fallon, and S. J. Barker. 1996. PET imaging of conscious and unconscious verbal memory. *Journal of Consciousness Studies* 3:448–462.

Alkire, M. T., R. J. Hairer, N. K. Shah, and C. T. Anderson. 1996. Positron emission tomography study of regional cerebral metabolism in humans during isoflurane anesthesia. *Anesthesiology* 86:549–557.

Baars, B. 1988. *A Cognitive Theory of Consciousness.* Cambridge: Cambridge University Press.

Buchsbaum, M. S., J. C. Gillin, J. Wu, E. Hazlett, N. Sicotte, and W. E. Bunney, Jr. 1989. Regional cerebral glucose metabolic rate in human sleep assessed by positron emission tomography. *Life Sciences* 45:1349–1356.

Cole, M., M. D. Winkelman, J. C. Morris, J. E. Simon, and T. A. Boyd. 1992. Thalamic amnesia: Korsakoff syndrome due to left thalamic infarction. *Journal of the Neurological Sciences* 110:62–67.

Cahill, L., R. J., Haier, J. H. Fallon, M. T. Alkire, C. Tang, D. Keator, J. C. Wu, and J. McGaugh. 1996. Amygdala activity at encoding correlated with long-term, free recall of emotional information. *Proceedings of the National Academy of Sciences U.S.A.* 93:8016–8021

Crick, F. 1994. *The Astonishing Hypothesis.* New York: Charles Scribner's Sons, Macmillan Pub. Co.

Fletcher, P. C., C. D. Frith, P. M. Grasby, T. Shallice, R. S. Frackowiak, and R. J. Dolan. 1995. Brain systems for encoding and retrieval of auditory-verbal memory. An in vivo study in humans. *Brain* 118:401–416.

Graff-Radford, N. R., D. Tranel, G. W. Van Hoesen, and J. P. Brandt. (1990) Diencephalic ammnesia. *Brain* 113:1–25.

Grasby, P. M., C. D. Frith, K. J. Friston C. Bench, R. S. Frackowiak, and R. J. Dolan. 1993. Functional mapping of brain areas implicated in auditory-verbal memory function. *Brain* 116:1–20.

Haier, R. J., B. Siegel, and K. H. Nuechterlein. 1988. Cortical glucose metabolic rate correlates of reasoning and attention studied with positron emission tomography. *Intelligence* 12:199–217.

Haier, R. J., B. J. Siegel, A. MacLachlan, E. Soderling, S. Lottenberg, and M. S. Buchsbaum. 1992. Regional glucose metabolic changes after learning a complex visuospatial/motor task: A positron emission tomographic study. *Brain Research* 570:134–143.

Huang, S. C., M. E. Phelps, E. J. Hoffman, K. Sideris, G. J. Selin, and D. E. Kuhl. 1980. Noninvasive determination of local cerebral metabolic rate of glucose in man. *American Journal of Physiology* 238:E69–82.

Huppert, F. A., and M. Piercy. 1979. Normal and abnormal forgetting in organic amnesia: Effect of locus of lesion. *Cortex* 15:385–390.

Kinomura, S., J. Larsson, B. Gulyas, and P. E. Roland. 1996. Activation by attention of the human reticular formation and thalamic intralaminar nuclei. *Science* 271:512–515.

Kosslyn, S. M., N. M. Alpert, W. L. Thompson, and V. Maljkovic. 1993. Visual mental imagery activates topographically organized visual cortex: PET investigations. *Journal of Cognitive Neuroscience* 5:3:263–287.

LaBerge, D., and M.S. Buchsbaum. 1990. Positron emission tomographic measurements of pulvinar activity during an attention task. *Journal of Neuroscience.* 10:613–619.

Llinas, R., and U. Ribary. 1993. Coherent 40-Hz oscillation characterizes dream state in humans. *Proceedings of the National Academy of Sciences U.S.A.* 90:2078–2081.

Markowitsch, H. J., J. Kessler, and M. Streicher. 1985. Consequences of serial cortical, hippocampal, and thalamic lesions and of different lengths of overtraining on the acquisition and retention of learning tasks. *Behavioral Neuroscience* 99:233–256.

Mazziotta, J. C., M. E. Phelps, R. E. Carson, and D. E. Kuhl. 1982. Tomographic mapping of human cerebral metabolism: Auditory stimulation. *Neurology* 32:921–937.

McKee, R. D., and L. R. Squire. 1992. Equivalent forgetting rates in long-term memory for diencephalic and medial temporal lobe amnesia. *Journal of Neuroscience* 12:3765–3772.

Mishkin, M. 1982. A memory system in the monkey. *Philosophical Transactions of the Royal Society of London B Biological Sciences* 298:83–95.

Malamut, B. L., N. R. Graff-Radford, J. Chawluk, R. I. Grossman, and R. C. Gur. 1992. Memory in a case of bilateral thalamic infarction. *Neurology* 42:163–169.

Michenfelder, J. D. 1988 *Anesthesia and the Brain.* New York: Churchill Livingstone.

Mullani, N. A., and N. D. Volkow. 1992. Positron emission tomography instrumentation: A review and update. *American Journal of Physiologic Imaging* 7:121–135.

Naatanen, R., R. J. Ilmoniemi, and K. Alho. 1994. Magnetoencephalography in studies of human cognitive brain function. *Trends in Neurosciences* 17:389–395.

Neil, J. J. 1993. Functional imaging of the central nervous system using magnetic resonance imaging and positron emission tomography. *Current Opinions in Neurology* 6:927–933.

Pardo, J. V., P. T. Fox, and M. E. Raichle. 1991. Localization of a human system for sustained attention by positron emission tomography. *Nature* 349:61–4.

Pawlik, G., W. D., Heiss C. Beil G. Grunewald, K. Herholz, K. Wienhard, and R. Wagner. 1987. Three-dimensional patterns of speech-induced cerebral and cerebellar activation in healthy volunteers and in aphasic stroke patients studied by positron emission tomography of 2 (18F)-fluorodeoxyglucose. In J. S. Meyer, H. Lechner, M. Reivich, and E. O. Ott, eds., *Cerebral Vascular Disease*. Amsterdam: Excerpta Medica, pp. 207–210.

Peinado-Manzano, M. A., and R. Pozo-Garcia. 1991. The role of different nuclei of the thalamus in processing episodic information. *Behavioural and Brain Research* 45:17–27.

Perani, D., M. C. Gilardi, S. F. Cappa, and F. Fazio. 1992. PET studies of cognitive functions: A review. *Journal of Nuclear Biology and Medicine* 36:324–336.

Phelps, M. E., S. C. Huang, E. J. Hoffman, C. Selin, L. Sokoloff, and D. E. Kuhl. 1979. Tomographic measurement of local cerebral glucose metabolic rate in humans with (F-18) 2-fluoro-2-deoxy-D-glucose: Validation of method. *Annals of Neurology* 6:371–388.

Phelps. M. E., D. E. Kuhl, and J. C. Mazziota. 1981. Metabolic mapping of the brain's response to visual stimulation: Studies in humans. *Science* 211:1445–1448.

Posner, M. I. 1994. Attention: the mechanisms of consciousness. *Proceedings of the National Academy of Sciences U.S.A.* 91:7398–7403.

Saha, G. B., W. J. MacIntyre, and R. T. Go. 1994. Radiopharmaceuticals for brain imaging. *Seminars in Nuclear Medicine* 24:324–349.

Schacter, D. L., N. M. Alpert, C. R. Savage, S. L. Rauch, and M. S. Albert. 1996. Conscious recollection and the human hippocampal formation: Evidence from positron emission tomography. *Proceedings of the National Academy of Sciences U.S.A.* 93:321–325.

Sokoloff, L., M. Reivich, C. Kennedy, R. M. Des, C. S. Patlak, K. D. Pettigrew, O. Sakurada, and M. Shinohara. 1977. The [14C] deoxyglucose method for the measurement of local cerebral glucose utilization: Theory, procedure, and normal values in the conscious and anesthetized albino rat. *Journal of Neurochemistry* 28:897–916.

Squire, L. R., J. G. Ojemann, F. M. Miezin, S. E. Petersen, T. O. Videen, and M. E. Raichle. 1992. Activation of the hippocampus in normal humans: A functional anatomical study of memory. *Proceedings of the National Academy of Sciences U.S.A.* 89:1837–1841.

Squire, L. R. 1992. Memory and the hippocampus: A synthesis from findings with rats, monkeys, and humans. *Psychological Review* 99:195–231.

Squire, L. R. 1981. Two forms of human amnesia: An analysis of forgetting. *Journal of Neuroscience* 1:635–640.

Tommasino, C., C. Crana, G. Lucignani, G. Torri, and F. Fazio. 1995. Regional cerebral metabolism of glucose in comatose and vegetative state patients. *Journal of Neurosurgical Anesthesiology* 7:109–116.

Vogel, C. C., H. J. Markowitsch, U. Hempel, and P. Hackenberg. 1987. Verbal memory in brain damaged patients under different conditions of retrieval aids: A study of frontal, temporal, and diencephalic damaged subjects. *International Journal of Neuroscience* 33:237–256.

Winocur, G. 1990. Anterograde and retrograde amnesia in rats with dorsal hippocampal or dorsomedial thalamic lesions. *Behavioural and Brain Research* 38:145–154.

Winocur, G. 1985. The hippocampus and thalamus: Their roles in short- and long-term memory and the effects of interference. *Behavioural and Brain Research* 16:135–152.

Wyper, D. J. 1993. Functional neuroimaging with single photon emission computed tomography (SPECT). *Cerebrovascular and Brain Metabolism Review* 5:199–217.

24 Neuronal Mechanisms of Consciousness: A Relational Global-Workspace Framework

Bernard J. Baars, James Newman, and
John G. Taylor

In this chapter we explore a remarkable convergence of ideas and evidence, previously presented in separate places by its authors. That convergence has now become so persuasive that we believe we are working within substantially the same broad framework. Taylor's mathematical papers on neuronal systems involved in consciousness dovetail well with work by Newman and Baars on the thalamocortical system, suggesting a brain mechanism much like the global-workspace architecture developed by Baars (see references below). This architecture is relational, in the sense that it continuously mediates the interaction between input and memory. Although our approaches overlap in a number of ways, each of us tends to focus on different areas of detail. We believe the most striking and significant condition about our work is the extent of consensus, which we believe to be consistent with other contemporary approaches by Weiskrantz, Gray, Crick and Koch, Edelman, Gazzaniga, Newell and colleagues, Posner, Baddeley, and others. We suggest that cognitive neuroscience is moving toward a shared understanding of consciousness in the brain.

Here we outline some elements in this emerging framework.

1. Consciousness is an architectural aspect of the brain's organization. It has global influences and effects.

    "Global workspace theory," developed by Baars (1983, 1988, 1997, and in press) has three fundamental constructs, best illustrated by a theatrical metaphor. Consciousness corresponds to the bright spot on stage, and unconscious systems operate "in the dark" backstage and in the audience. Thus we have

    1.1 The active bright spot on the stage of working memory.
    1.2 Contextual systems that reside "backstage," shaping the content of consciousness without themselves entering consciousness.

    Last,

    1.3 The "audience," with specialized sources of knowledge that are unconscious, ranging from long-term memories to motor automatisms. This audience is sitting in the dark, receiving information from the bright spot on stage.

    Only the global workspace (GW) is conscious at any given moment; contextual elements backstage are unconscious, as are the specialized systems in the brain that can receive information from the bright spot in the darkened theater.

2. A number of brain mechanisms could serve such functions.

    2.1 The active bright spot may be closely associated with sensory projection areas that provide the detailed content of sensory consciousness, closely supported by subcortical systems in the thalamus, basal ganglia, hippocampus, and brain stem. An attentional system selects which of several potential inputs will become conscious at any one time. The reticular nucleus in the thalamus (nRt), with its ability to gate traffic from sensory surfaces to cortex, is one natural candidate for such a selective attention mechanism (Newman and Baars 1993, Baars 1993, 1997, in press). Posner (1994) has found evidence for several other brain loci for visual attention, notably the anterior cingulate, which may be associated with effortful attention.

    2.2 Contextual systems that are unconscious but still shape conscious content may be found in, among other places, the dorsal visual pathway, including right parietal cortex, which provides the object-centered "framework" for visual perception (Baars 1997, in press)

    2.3 The theater audience, which includes specialized sources of knowledge that receive conscious input, include frontal cortex, memory-related systems such as the hippocampus, brain mechanisms for automatic routines such as the basal ganglia, and mediating emotional processes such as the limbic system and amygdala.

    2.4 How could visual conscious content be distributed to its audience? The brain's gross anatomy shows massive fiber tracts leading from posterior to anterior cortex, from one hemisphere to the other, and from cortex to thalamus and back again. Each of these massive fiber tracts is known to map significant features of conscious information from one location to another. For example, the famous work on split-brain patients by Sperry, Gazzaniga, and Bogen shows that cutting the transverse fiber tracts between hemispheres blocks the normal flow of consciously available information between right and left hemispheres. Thus broadcasting of cortical sensory information may occur in several directions from sensory cortex: from back to front, from side to side, and from cortex to midbrain and back again.

        Baars (1988) hypothesized that the neural substrate of this GW was an "extended reticular thalamic activating system" (ERTAS). The acronym emphasizes that this system (though it includes the classic reticular activating system), is *centered on the thalamus* with its rich, reciprocal projections with the cortex. Newman and Baars (1993) also cite the significance of layer I of the cortex, often viewed as a "feltwork" of neurons that permit not just axonal transmission but horizontal spread of activation. Layer I may also provide a channel for global broadcasting; however, it seems better suited to connectionist propagation than to high-fidelity corticocortical transmission. In more recent developments, cortical sensory projection areas seem more plausible loci for a conscious GW, at least for sensory consciousness.

3. Conscious experience involves ceaseless interaction between input (from outside and within the brain) and memory.

In the vocabulary that Taylor suggests, it is relational: "The conscious content of a mental experience is determined by the evocation and intermingling of suitable past memories evoked by the input giving rise to that experience". Such a relational feature implies a ceaseless dialogue between conscious content and unconscious systems, notably the hippocampus, basal ganglia, and unconscious regions of cortex.

3.1 The "intermingling" of past and present requires both long-range intermodal and short-range intramodal competition. Taylor has explored the problem of intermodal (global) inhibition via the nucleus reticularis thalami (nRt) (1992). The nRt seems a beautiful device for achieving global input competition, being composed solely of inhibitory cells and also having remarkable lateral connectivity similar to that of the outer plexiform layer in the retina (Taylor 1990). Taylor suggests the phrase "Conscious I" for the nRt contribution to global competition (1993), with the notion that nRt may bind activities across modalities. He believes that nRt supports a far more complex form of spatial competition, however, than given by a simple winner-take-all (WTA) form, because it produces as winner a wave over the whole of the coupled thalamic–nRt–cortical system (Alavi and Taylor 1993, 1995). Such a winner will have many spatial regions over cortex that have nonzero activity.

3.2 In a target article for *Brain and Behavioral Science*, Jeffrey Gray (1995) reviews a wealth of data supporting a model for "the generation of the contents of consciousness … correspond[ing] to the outputs of a comparator that, on a moment-by-moment basis, compares the current state of the organism's perceptual world with a predicted state" (p. 659). The heart of this "comparator system" is the hippocampus; but its activities are also closely tied to those of the basal ganglia and cortex.

Newman (1995b) offers the alternative hypothesis that Gray's comparator provides feedback to the ERTAS, "flagging" present perceptions as "expected/familiar" or "unexpected/novel." A novel/ unexpected flag interrupts continuous behavior, causing an ERTAS-mediated orienting response. Conversely, an expected/familiar flag would produce habituation or, in goal-directed behavior, a shift in attention to the next step in the current program.

In his response to the BBS commentaries, Gray (1995) offers an extension to his original model "that links the outputs of the

Bernard J. Baars, James Newman, and J. G. Taylor: Neuronal Mechanisms of Consciousness comparator system to the reticulo-thalamic core which, as set out by Newman, seems likely to underlie the generation of consciousness-as-such (p. 716)." He describes findings by Lavin and Grace (1994) showing that the fornix also projects to areas in the basal ganglia, which project to the nRt. The nRt's possible role in selective attention and conscious processing is pointed out by Crick (1984), and Taylor (1992) incorporates it into a neural-network model. Notice that, because the output to these neurons is itself inhibitory, its activation disinhibits these sensory-relay pathways; that is, it increases entry to the cerebral cortex by stimuli that are currently engaging the thalamocortical loops (Gray 1995, p. 712).

4. Cortical foci of activity appear to provide the content of consciousness.

    Taylor suggests that the crucial aspect for consciousness arising from nonconscious neural activity is creation of relatively lasting "bubbles" of activity in cortex by local recurrence (Amari 1977). It is proposed (Taylor 1996b) that such activity singles out cortical regions with highest density of cells in layers 2 and 3, which appear to be identical to the sites with highest coding in cortex. This model then allows some crucial aspects of qualia (transparency, ineffability, intrinsicality) to be derived (Taylor 1996b), and also gives a neural underpinning to the "global-workspace" idea (Baars 1988) by means of the excellent intercortical connectivity of such regions in parietal, inferotemporal and frontal cortices. Thus detailed coding of the content of consciousness appears to be cortical. How much the thalamus is involved in this coding is still to be determined. This view seems in complete accord with extension of the ERTAS system (Newman and Baars 1993) and helps flesh it out further.

5. At any one time, different sensory inputs, including such "inner" inputs as visual imagery and inner speech, compete for access to consciousness. Other possible inputs include abstract conscious content such as beliefs and ideas.

    The material selected to be conscious involves both top-down influences and bottom-up inputs. Top-down influences include goal systems associated with frontal cortex, and emotional and motivational systems combining limbic and right frontal cortex. Thus conscious content reflects an endless interplay of competition and cooperation between possible inputs and top-down influences.

    Taylor points out a further totally inhibitory system that greatly contributes to global competition, the basal ganglia. These are expected to be able to support the comparison and buffering needed in developing sequence learning (schemata) and in forming rules and reasoning; all are involved in anterior cortex (C_a). This system's analysis and modeling are explored in Bapi et al. (1996), fully discussing a neural model of frontal-lobe executive function. The psychological aspects of such an architecture for temporal tasks (such as delayed-matching tasks) are explored by Monchi and Taylor (1996). The principles of such an architecture have also been explored as part of the ACTION network (Taylor 1995, Taylor and Alavi 1993).

6. The brainstem-thalamocortical axis supports the state, but not the detailed content of consciousness, which is produced by cortex.

Newman and Baars (1993) describe in detail the anatomy and putative functions of a "neural global workspace." Reviewing a half century of research, they describe an architecture extending from the midbrain reticular formation to prefrontal cortex. The midbrain core of this system is the classic ascending reticular activating system, including the intra-laminar complex (ILC). Integrated with this reticular core is a "global attentional matrix," centered nRt, which both "gates" information flow to and from the cortex and regulates electrical oscillatory patterns throughout the cortex.[1]

When Newman and Baars (1993) was published the authors were unaware of Taylor's model for "global guidance," mediated by nRt. Newman refers to this form of resource allocation as "global attention." Its core neural mechanism is an *array of gating circuits* in the nRt, which covers the lateral surfaces of the thalamus. Through it pass nearly all the pathways coursing between the thalamus and cerebral hemispheres. Via these reciprocal nRt circuits, the cerebral cortex and brainstem reticular formation *selectively modulate their own information-processing activities* in serving conscious perceptions, and intentions or plans or both.

7. A selective attention system, including the nRt, selects among multiple possible conscious contents.

Attentional selection of conscious content appears to operate by means of the nRt, influenced by several centers from brain stem to pre-frontal cortex. The nRt is believed to "gate" the sensory thalamic nuclei, which flow up to the primary projection areas in the cortex, and is therefore in the most strategic position for controlling sensory input. We know that almost ten times as many visual neurons go down from visual cortex to the thalamus as the other way, suggesting continuous and intimate looping between thalamus and cortex, controlled by nRt.

A voluntary component may also act via the anterior cingulate gyrus and the vigilance network of prefrontal cortex, indentified by Posner (1994). Attentional selection is also influenced by the content of con-sciousness, suggesting that reentrant loops from sensory cortex descend to the major sensory nuclei of the thalamus to create a self-sustaining feed-back loop, again under nRt control (Edelman 1989, Newman 1995a, b).

8. Posterior cortex provides sensory conscious content, and anterior cortex is involved in active, voluntary control; both seem to be necessary for normal conscious experience and control.

From Taylor's point of view, it is possible to discern at least two main components of consciousness, which we denote C_p and C_a. The former, C_p, is the part of consciousness containing phenomenal experience, the "raw feels." The subscript $_p$ denotes the passive condition of C_p, without active transformations by frontal motor cortical systems such as those involved in thinking and reasoning. The subscript can also be used to denote siting of this component in posterior cortical systems and their related thalamic structures. The memorial structures needed to give content to C_p are those of the primary sensory, postprimary, associative, and heteromodal cortices, all of which are posterior.

Further, we have the antithetical C_a, in which "$_a$" denotes *active*—that is, involved in thinking and planning as well as responding in a willful manner. Its major activity is involved with anterior cortical, related thalamic, and basal-ganglia neural sites, which are known to be crucially involved with actions of either direct (motor action) or higher-order (thought, planning) form. Baars would emphasize that such frontal activity was voluntary. A more thorough analysis is presented in Taylor, (in preparation).

Newman writes,

> The aspect of consciousness most extensively controlled by these parallel distributed circuits is immediate perception, mainly supported by posterior cortical modules, allowing them to be interpreted as a passive part of the complex that is the totality of conscious experience. It is nRt that allows arrays of modular processors to compete for access to the cortical GW. Because of the dendrodendritic connections among nRt neurons, which create coherent, nRt-wide activation/inhibition patterns, this competition is global. This nRt coherence mediates the global allocation of the processing resources in this posterior corticothalamic system.

9. Interaction between self-structures and consciousness.

Baars (1997, in press) proposes a framework in which one necessary condition for consciousness is providing information to a self-system, a stable contextual system that provides predictability in varied situations. The left-hemisphere "narrative interpreter" that Gazzaniga and colleagues have discovered may be one such self-system.

Taylor suggests further components, such as a self-structure of consciousness (C_s) and an emotional part (C_e). The former, undoubtedly present, is sited in the meso-orbital frontal region (as indicated by lesion studies of frontal patients, starting with the famed Phineas Gage case); it is not clear that the latter has any specific cortical site, but it is more diffusely distributed from limbic systems, especially by the dopaminergic and related aminergic neurotransmitter systems.

10. Layers of visual consciousness.

Blindsight is one empirical source for any approach to visual consciousness. It seems to show that the first visual projection area in the cortex, the first place where the visual tract reaches cortex, is a necessary condition for conscious vision, but not for unconscious visual knowledge. Blindsight patients, who lack parts of this area (V1) have unconscious (implicit) visual knowledge about objects, such as location, color, motion, and even object identity. But they passionately protest that they have no conscious visual experience in the damaged parts of the visual field.

Crick and Koch (1995) point out a significant paradox in blindsight: Area V1 is known to represent points (center-surround), and spatial intervals (spatial frequencies), but it does not represent color, motion, or visual form. And yet these higher-level visual features drop from visual consciousness when damage occurs to V1, as shown by blindsight patients. Crick and Koch say that V1 does not "explicitly" represent color and form because it has no cells that are sensitive to color, and so on. And yet conscious appreciation of color and form is destroyed by damage to V1, a contradiction that we call "the paradox of area V1." An adequate theory of visual consciousness must account for this paradox.

In contrast to the V1 puzzle, damage to higher visual areas of cortex creates only selective loss of conscious features. Thus damage to area MT destroys conscious perception of motion, but not of color, form, or retinal locus. From that point of view, V1 is especially important because its absence abolishes all visual conscious features, including those not explicitly represented in V1.

We must consider the remarkable interconnectivity among all parts of the brain. In the visual system we find top-down feedback from each "higher" visual area to lower areas, as well as a bottom-up flow going the other way. Indeed, in thalamocortical loops, the downflowing neurons outnumber the upgoing ones by a ratio of almost ten to one. This imbalance makes sense when we consider classical neural-net approaches, in that multiple layers, when their patterns of activation are consistent, enhance each other, but nonconsistent layers tend to compete and decrease activation patterns. This result has been called the rich-get-richer principle (McClelland and Rumelhart 1986).

How does visual consciousness relate to other kinds of sensory and non-sensory consciousness? Evidence has been found for blindsight analogues in auditory and somatosensory cortex. These may work much like the early visual areas. One can think therefore of the early sensory-projection areas as several theater stages, each with its own bright spot, alternating rapidly so that at any moment only one spotlight is on. As the most active, coherently paced sensory cortex becomes conscious, its content is broadcast widely throughout the brain, simultaneously suppressing the other sensory cortices for a cycle time of approximately 100 milliseconds (msec), the time needed for perceptual integration. The most highly amplified sensory-projection area in any 100 msec time cycle may send conscious information to spatial, self, and motor maps via massive fiber tracts, some going through thalamus, others via the corpus callosum, and yet others through massive cortico-cortical connections within each hemisphere. Thus rapid switching can take place between different sensory cortices, integrated by multimodal neurons in association cortex and elsewhere.

SUMMARY

Any theory of consciousness must satisfy extensive empirical constraints that are quite well established (Baars 1983, 1988, 1996). Together, these sources of evidence implicate a global-workspace system that is most easily understood via the theater-of-consciousness metaphor. Thus, consciousness corresponds to the bright spot on the stage of a theater, shaped by context systems that are invisible behind the scenes, and being broadcast to receiving processors in the unconscious audience. Taylor emphasizes the need to include a memory-matching component, which he calls "relational," leading to a relational global-workspace framework. We believe this framework captures our current understanding of the psychological and brain evidence.

NOTES

1. A more recent and broadened discussion of this architecture is available at the Association for the Scientific Study of Consciousness web site (<http://www.phil.vt. edu/ASSC/esem.html). It is part of an electronic seminar led by Newman (1996).

REFERENCES

Alavi, F., and J. G. Taylor. 1993. A global competitive network for attention. *Neural Network World* 5:477–502.

Alavi, F., and J. G. Taylor. 1995. A global competitive neural network. *Biological Cybernetics* 72:233–248.

Amari, S.-I. 1977. Dynamics of pattern formation in lateral-inhibition type neural fields. *Biological Cybernetics* 27:77–87.

Baars B. J. 1983. Conscious contents provide the nervous system with coherent, global information. In R. Davidson, G. Schwartz, and D. Shapiro, eds., *Consciousness and Self-Regulation.* New York: Plenum Press, pp. 45–76.

Baars, B. J. 1988. *A Cognitive Theory of Consciousness.* New York: Cambridge University Press.

Baars, B. J. 1993. How does a serial, integrated and very limited stream of consciousness emerge from a nervous system that is mostly unconscious, distributed, and of enormous capacity? In G. Bock and J. Marsh, eds., *CIBA Symposium on Experimental and Theoretical Studies of Consciousness.* London: Wiley, pp. 282–290.

Baars, B. J. 1997. *In the Theater of Consciousness: The Workspace of the Mind.* Oxford: Oxford University Press.

Baars, B. J. (in press) Metaphors of Consciousness and Attention in the Brain. *Trends in Neurosciences.*

Bapi, R., G. Bugmann, D. Levin, and J. G. Taylor. 1996. *Analyzing the Executive Function of the Prefrontal System: Towards a Computational System.* KCL preprint.

Bogen, J. E. 1995. On the neurophysiology of consciousness. *Consciousness and Cognition* 4:52–62.

Crick, F. 1984. Function of the thalamic reticular complex: The searchlight hypothesis. *Proceedings of the National Academy of Sciences U.S.A.* 81:4586–4590.

Crick, F. H. C. 1994. *The Astonishing Hypothesis*. Cambridge: Cambridge University Press.

Crick, F. and C. Koch. 1990. Towards a neurobiological theory of consciousness. *Seminars in Neuroscience* 2:263–275.

Crick, F., and C. Koch. 1995. The location of visual consciousness. *Nature* 375:121–123.

Edelman, G. M. 1989. *The Remembered Present: A Biological Theory of Consciousness*. New York: Basic Books.

Gray, J. A. 1995. The contents of consciousness: A neuropsychological conjecture. *Behavioral and Brain Sciences* 18:659–722.

McClelland, J. L. 1986. The programmable blackboard model of reading. In J. L. McClelland and D. E. Rummelhart, eds., *Parallel Distributed Processing*. Cambridge: MIT Press, ch. 16.

McClelland, J. L., and D. E. Rumelhart. 1986. The lexical superiority effect. *Psychological Review*.

Newman, J. 1995a. Review: Thalamic contributions to attention and consciousness. *Consciousness and Cognition* 4:172–193.

Newman, J. 1995b. Commentary: Reticular–thalamic activation of the cortex generates conscious contents. *Behavioral and Brain Sciences* 18:691–692.

Newman, J. 1996. Thalamocortical foundations of conscious experience. Association for the Scientific Study of Consciousness: <http://www.phil.vt.edu/ASSC/esem.html>.

Newman, J. (in preparation). Putting the puzzle together: Toward a general theory of the neural correlates of consciousness.

Newman, J., and B. J. Baars. 1993. A neural attentional model for access to consciousness: A Global Workspace perspective. *Concepts in Neuroscience* 4 (2):255–290.

Parent, A., and L.-N. Hazrati. 1995. Functional anatomy of the basal ganglia. I. The cortico-basal ganglia-thalamo-cortical loop. *Brain Research Reviews* 20:91–127.

Posner, M. I. 1994. A visual attention network of the brain. *Proceedings of the National Academy of Sciences U.S.A.*

Scheibel, A. B. 1980. Anatomical and physiological substrates of arousal: A view from the bridge. In J. A. Hobson and M. A. B. Brazier, eds., *The Reticular Formation Revisited*. New York: Raven Press, pp. 55–66.

Taylor, J. G. 1990. Analysis of a silicon model of the retina. *Neural Networks* 3:171–178.

Taylor, J. G. 1992. Towards a neural network model of the mind. *Neural Network World* 2:797–812.

Taylor J. G. 1993. *When the Clock Struck Zero*. London: Picador Press.

Taylor, J. G. 1995. Modules for the mind of psyche. *Proceedings of the WCNN'95* 2:967–972, INNS Press.

Taylor J. G. 1996a. A competition for consciousness? *Neurocomputing* 11:271–296.

Taylor, J. G. 1996b. How and where does consciousness arise in cortex? KCL preprint.

Taylor, J. G., and F. N. Alavi. 1993. Mathematical analysis of a competitive network for attention. In J. G. Taylor, ed., *Mathematical Approaches to Neural Networks*. New York: Elsevier Science Publishers B.V., pp. 341–387.

Taylor, J. G. 1997. *The Emergent Mind*. Cambridge: MIT Press (forthcoming).

25 Creeping up on the Hard Question of Consciousness

Jeffrey A. Gray

That there is a "hard question" of consciousness has been passionately pro-claimed by some and denied by others for many years. But the debate now attracts much wider attention than it once did. It would be comforting to think that this change has occurred because the problem has entered the realm of solubility, and thus is coming of age for serious scientific treatment (Medawar 1967). Certainly, many scientists who once would have banned any talk of consciousness as dealing with the devil now suppose that their routine study of electrophysiology or psychology *ipso facto* takes them ever closer to a detailed understanding of how consciousness works. This think-ing may be self-deception, however; we are perhaps witnessing no more than a change in intellectual fashion. The change, nonetheless, has been pro-found. A quarter century ago I published a paper setting out the hard ques-tion as I then saw it (Gray 1971). The paper attracted zero comment—in the next decade I had two requests for reprints. Now we find large and enthusi-astic audiences, as at the Tucson conferences on consciousness, for talks on these same topics. Is this change happening because we are now much closer to finding answers to the hard question (or at least reaching a consensus that the hard question does or does not exist) than we were in 1971? I think not: I can make essentially the same points now as then; they still have the same cogency (or lack thereof); and they still occasion the same fierce debates (Gray 1995a). The accumulation over the intervening years of clin-ical and experimental data, often in highly sophisticated psychological or physiological paradigms, has sharpened the issues, but done little to resolve them.

One thing that has become clearer, or at least more widely appreciated, is that consciousness becomes a problem only at the point at which subjective experience occurs. We have no problem understanding in principle (though, of course, vast amounts of detail remain to be worked out) how brains can carry out the processing of information that is required to link input from the environment through to subsequent behavior. The hard problem, however, is that we have no understanding about how, in this sequence of presumed events, the activities of brains give rise to conscious experience. Nor do we have any scientific reason to postulate the occurrence of such experiences in the explanatory chain that links input to brain function to behavioral output. If we do postulate them, we do so simply on the grounds that, from our own subjective experience, we know them in fact to occur; but this inductive leap provides them with no explanatory force (Gray 1971). This distinction between aspects of psychological processes that pose no problem in principle—Chalmers's (1995) "easy problems"—and those which constitute the "hard problem," has been extensively discussed in recent years in various terminological guises, such as Nagel's (1974) concept of "what-it-is-like-to-be" (hard), Jackendoff's (1987) distinction between primary (hard) and reflective (easy) awareness, Block's (1995) between phenomenal (hard) and access (easy) consciousness, and Chalmers's (1996) between the phenomenal (hard) and psychological (easy) aspects of mind. In each explanation, the hard category covers, roughly, the perceived world with all its qualities (visual, auditory, olfactory, etc.), but also bodily sensations, proprioception, emotional feelings, dreams, hallucinations, mental images, and internal speech. It seems likely that, if we could once see how to integrate into the rest of science the qualitative aspects of our perceptions of the external world (e.g., the color red, the smell of a rose, the feel of cold water on the tongue, the feel of velvet on the skin), the more internal aspects of conscious experience (mental images, internally spoken or imaged thoughts, dreams, etc.) would pose no additional problem (other than the detailed extension to this more ghostly realm of whatever explanation one had crafted).

This, then, is the hard problem: how to provide an account, integrated with the rest of our scientific understanding of the world, of the links between, on the one hard, brain plus behavior plus information processing by the brain and, on the other, conscious experience. Such an account would need to deal both with the sheer occurrence of conscious experience (why do we experience anything rather than nothing at all?) and with the nature of the contents of consciousness (why does red or the smell of vanilla or the sound of a cello have the qualitative feel that each severally has?). Any such theory, furthermore, would need to be tightly linked to the rest of biology and physiology.

Many distinguished scientists and philosophers, of course, do not accept a hard problem of consciousness, stated in this or any other way (e.g., Dennett 1991). But those who do would all agree that we are a long way from having answers to these questions. A further divide, then, separates those who believe that, hard though it may be, the problem of consciousness eventually will have a solution, which will form part of general scientific theory (though by that time scientific theory will perhaps have greatly changed, partly because of the very need to produce a solution to the problem of consciousness), and those who believe that no such solution can ever be found by the normal means of scientific inquiry, whether empirical or theoretical. I see no reason to adopt the latter, pessimistic stance; though, until a solution is in fact provided, whether it will ever be forthcoming can only be a matter of opinion.

CRITERIA FOR A SUCCESSFUL THEORY OF CONSCIOUSNESS

If we had a successful theory of consciousness, it would need to answer four key questions (Gray 1971). The first two have to do with the place of consciousness in evolution: (1) How did conscious experiences evolve? and (2) How do such experiences confer survival value upon organisms possessing them? In asking these questions, I take it as axiomatic that no characteristic of such evident importance as consciousness could have arisen other than by natural selection. Notice, however, that this way of putting the matter implies that consciousness must confer survival value beyond that conferred by whichever brain processes are associated with the occurrence of conscious experience. And yet this inference is strongly resisted by many scientists and philosophers, who fear that it opens the door to a now mostly discredited Cartesian dualism. Nonetheless, because of Darwinian theory's overwhelming success in biology generally, I believe the inference to be necessary.

The other two questions are mechanistic: (3) How do conscious experiences arise out of brain events? and (4) How do these experiences alter the behavior with which they are associated? The mechanistic questions are, of course, closely linked to the evolutionary ones: Darwinian selection can be exerted only toward specific behavioral consequences (which must aid survival or reproduction or both) of consciousness. Thus it would be particularly helpful if we knew how consciousness gives rise to such useful behavioral consequences. Now, this part of the problem of consciousness is the hardest to put across to the ordinary person, for the experimental evidence from which it derives flagrantly contradicts our everyday experience. It is obvious to everyone, is it not, that consciousness is full of useful behavioral consequences? What then is the problem? But recall that it is also obvious to everyone that the sun goes around the earth. And the one appears to be almost as much an illusion as the other.

The burned child (as illustrated in Descartes's famed drawing—see Figure 25.1) withdraws his hand from the flame, but he does it before he feels the pain. We now have a multitude of experimental demonstrations that this general kind of observation—that consciousness comes too late to affect the processes to which it is apparently linked—is valid for a range of other activities, including selection of sensory stimuli for attention and perceptual analysis, learning and memory, and producing sequences of movement requiring great planning and creativity, such as speaking English or playing tennis (Velmans 1991). In each activity, the conscious events follow the information processes to which they are related. As an example, listen to yourself thinking in your head: you will find that you are completely unaware of all the elaborate computations that have gone into composing the grammatically, semantically, and phonetically correct words you hear there. You do not become consciously aware even of what you are thinking until after you have thought it!

A more dramatic example comes from competition tennis. The speed of play in a Wimbledon final is so great, and the rate at which percepts enter

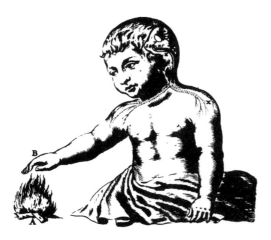

Figure 25.1 Descartes's drawing of the hand withdrawn from the flame. We feel the pain after withdrawing the hand.

consciousness so slow, that the response to a typical serve has to be completed before the player has consciously seen the ball come over the net (I owe this example to John McCrone). Although it is logically impossible that the whole of consciousness could be an illusion, it is certain that much about conscious experience is illusory. In the tennis example is an illusory experience that one consciously sees the ball and then hits it. What actually happens is that one hits the ball (based upon a great deal of extremely rapid unconscious processing of visual information), consciously sees it, and then consciously experiences the hitting, thus preserving in consciousness the temporal order of events that took place unconsciously. What then does conscious seeing add to the unconscious processing of visual information that is on its own sufficient to permit the extraordinarily high-precision performance seen in competition tennis? In spite of the many achievements in the experimental study of behavior, it is still remarkably difficult to answer this question. A recent experiment by Kolb and Braun (1995) starkly illustrates this difficulty. These workers were able to demonstrate "blindsight," originally observed by Weiskrantz and Warrington (see Weiskrantz 1986) in patients with scotomata caused by damage to the occipital cortex, in perfectly normal observers. The subjects had to detect a target that appeared in one quadrant in a display presented on a video monitor. Kolb and Braun manipulated the display's characteristics so that, in one set of conditions, subjects reported consciously seeing the target and, in another, they were unable to do so; confidence ratings confirmed that this manipulation was efficient. Yet the accuracy of target detection was identical in the two conditions.

Thus, at present, the experimental study of conscious experience gives no clear answer to the question: What does conscious experience add to behavior that the unconscious information processing carried out by the brain cannot do by itself? (This, by the way, is not the Freudian unconsciousness. Along with everything else that Freud got wrong, he also wrongly treated the unconscious as a mystery. It is not. As indicated above, we have no difficulty in understanding in principle, nor increasingly in detail, how neural events can carry out all the complex informational processes needed to mediate behavioral transactions between the organism and its environment. It is the fact that some of these processes become conscious that is the mystery.) Where then shall we begin the search for answers to the four key questions?

CONSCIOUSNESS AND THE BRAIN

The one thing we know for sure about consciousness is that it is in some way related to brain function. One place to start then is by asking how we should think about the brain. The trouble is that we have many ways in which to do so. Thus, the brain can be regarded as (1) a system which (2) processes information so as (3) to display behavior in (4) an environment, and which (5) is composed of physical matter or, more specifically, (6) biological tissue (cells, neurons, etc.). Thus if we consider the question, "What are the distinguishing features of those processes that we know to be accompanied by consciousness in the human brain?" at least these answers are possible:

1. All the conditions (1–6) are necessary for consciousness; that is, only biological nervous systems can produce it.

2. Only conditions 1–4 are essential. This statement implies that, if we put together the right kind of robot and allowed it to interact with the right kind of environment in the right way, it would have conscious experiences.

3. Only the nature of the information-processing system (1 and 2) matters. This statement implies that, if we mimicked the system correctly on a computer (e.g., so that it passed the famous Turing Test, by answering questions indistinguishably from the answers given by a human being), conscious experiences would occur in the computer.

4. It is all in the physics (5), a view recently advocated by Hameroff and Penrose (1996). This statement implies that consciousness might occur in nonbiological physical systems in which the critical physical parameters happened to be satisfied.

5. Only condition (4) matters; that is, conscious experience is somehow a property of biological cells, or perhaps of nerve cells only. If so, a small quantum of consciousness might reside even in a single cell or neuron.

This list of possibilities is not exhaustive, but surely it is long enough. It provides another way to demonstrate just how deep the problem of consciousness is. All these answers have been seriously—and usually dogmatically—proposed; worse still, we have no solid grounds for ruling out any of them! Against this wide-open background, then, I may have license to add a brief account of a hypothesis of my own. This hypothesis does not, however, address the main problem of consciousness—that is, how the brain comes to generate any kind of conscious experience—but

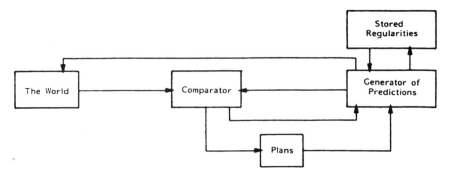

Figure 25.2 Information processing involved in the comparator system.

rather the somewhat more limited (but nonetheless still "hard") problem: Given that the brain is able to create conscious experiences, why do the contents of consciousness take the forms that they do?

THE COMPARATOR HYPOTHESIS

The hypothesis extends previous work in which my colleagues and I have developed a neuropsychological model with the aim of explaining, initially, the emotion of anxiety (Gray 1982) and, subsequently, the bizarre aberrations of conscious experience that characterize acute schizophrenia (Gray et al. 1991). A key feature of the model is a comparator system that has the general function of predicting, moment by moment, (where "a moment" is about a tenth of a second long), the next perceived state of the world, comparing this state to the next perceived state, and determining whether the predicted and actual states do or do not match (see Figure 25.2). In the model, this comparator system's functions are discharged by a complex set of brain mechanisms. The details about this machinery are not relevant here; let us call it the "subicular comparator" for short, after the subicular region of the hippocampal formation where the key comparisons are postulated to take place. The hypothesis about consciousness then takes this form: the contents of consciousness consist of activity in the subicular comparator, together with feedback from the comparator to the sets of neurons in perceptual systems that have just provided input to the comparator for the current comparison. This hypothesis can provide a plausible rationale for many known features of the contents of consciousness (see Table 25.1, based on Gray 1995a), including the finding that, as mentioned above, consciousness comes too late to affect on-line behavior (as in playing tennis or detecting visual targets).

This is not the place to defend the comparator hypothesis. Rather, I shall use it to demonstrate again the nature of the problem of consciousness.

Like most current accounts in cognitive neuroscience, the hypothesis provides statements that (1) certain neural circuits carry out (2) certain kinds of information processing and result in (3) certain kinds of behavior, all this accompanied—or not—by (4) certain kinds of conscious experience (Gray

Table 25.1 Features of the contents of consciousness for which the comparator hypothesis (Gray 1995a,b) offers an account.

Conscious experience is closely linked to current action plans
One is conscious of the outputs of motor programs, not of the program itself
Consciousness occurs too late to affect outcomes of the processes to which it is apparently linked
Conscious events occur on a time scale about two orders of magnitude slower than that of the neural events that underlie them
Conscious experience has a spatiotemporal unity quite unlike the patterns of neuronal events that underlie it
Conscious experience consists of a series of constructions based on a model of the world, not direct reflections of inputs from the world
Consciousness is highly selective
Neuronal events operate in parallel; consciousness operates serially
Conscious experience is closely linked to memory

1995a). In principle, and sometimes even in practice, it is known how to construct detailed accounts of the links between steps 1 to 3 in this type of chain; but, if one goes on to ask for details about how 1 to 3 are linked to 4 (the hard question about consciousness), no principled answer can as yet be given. In the example considered here, the comparator hypothesis can be seen as setting up a four-way set of equivalences: activity in a neural circuit (hippocampal formation, subicular area, etc.—see Gray et al. 1991) = information processing of a specific kind (the comparator function) = detection of degrees of match or mismatch between current and predicted inputs to perceptual systems = generation of the contents of consciousness.

The comparator hypothesis may appear to be satisfyingly comprehensive, cutting as it does across four levels of explanation, all obviously relevant to the problem of consciousness. But the price for this comprehensivity is that one is left straddling nearly all the fences so carefully laid out above (see part on Consciousness and the Brain). The hypothesis—and all like it—beg such questions as whether one should seek explanations for the occurrence of conscious experiences in neural events alone, information processing alone, these two jointly, or even at some deeper level in the physics of brain events (Penrose 1989). This hypothesis has nothing to say, for example, in answer to these more specific questions: (1) Suppose we changed the neural circuitry instantiating the comparator function while retaining the information processing—would the contents of consciousness remain the same? (2) Suppose we changed the information processes performed by the subicular circuitry: Would the same neuronal activity still generate the same conscious contents as before? A well-constructed scientific theory should be able to predict the outcome of such gedanken experiments, or at least show why, according to the theory, the questions are ill formed. (Notice, however, that even if the theory could deal with questions 1 and 2, we would still be left with the hardest of the hard questions. Suppose the answers to these questions are that one must preserve both the neural machinery and the information-processing functions to generate conscious experience: Why does this combination produce any kind of conscious experience rather than none?)

At present quite different types of answer to these questions are assumed to be correct in different types of general approach to the problem of consciousness: functionalists assume that conscious experience is tied to information processing, proponents of the mind–brain identity approach assume that it is tied to neural function, and still others assume that it is tied to both (for examples, see Blakemore and Greenfield 1987, Marsh 1993, and commentaries on Gray 1995a, as summarized in Gray 1995b). Each of these assumptions is equally lacking in empirical justification, nor, apparently, have attempts yet been made to gather relevant experimental evidence. It will perhaps be possible to do so, however, by studying brain function in synesthesia.

SYNESTHESIA

Synesthesia is a condition in which the individual experiences a sensation in one sensory modality triggered involuntarily and automatically by a sensation in a different sensory modality (Motluk 1994). The condition appears to be consistent all through the individual's lifetime, and is present from as early in childhood as the individual can recall. It can occur between any two sensory modalities, though in practice some combinations are more common. The commonest form appears to be seeing colors when hearing sounds. Typically, in "colored hearing," the person sees a different color when hearing a different sound, but consistently. For example, when hearing speech, each word heard triggers a different color, and the same word always triggers the same color.

One hundred years ago, synesthesia stirred much scientific interest (Binet 1893, Galton 1883, Myers 1911, 1914). By the 1940s, the topic had just about vanished from science, for two reasons: introspection had become a disrespectable method for collecting data in experimental psychology, and no objective way seemed available for validating that synesthesia was actually occurring, beyond self-report data from the subject. Skepticism about whether synesthesia was real or not is understandable, though many psychiatric phenomena (hallucinations, delusions, etc.) rely purely on data obtained via self-report.

Simon Baron-Cohen's group started studying the condition at the Institute of Psychiatry in the mid-1980s (Baron-Cohen et al. 1987), reporting one case (E. P.)—a woman with synesthesia. A first aim in this research was to overcome the problem posed by potentially unreliable self-report data. Baron-Cohen et al. showed that, when E. P. was given a long word list and was asked to describe the colors triggered by each word in the list, she gave very detailed descriptions (e.g., the word "Maria" triggered a dark purple with a shiny texture, and with speckled spinach-green at the edges). When retested on the same word list a year later, without warning, she was 100 percent

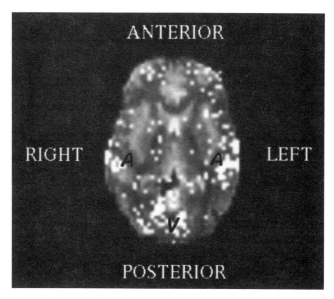

Figure 25.3 Functional MR image from one case with synesthesia (colored–speech perception). The data show a *t*-test map at 97.5 percent confidence (white pixels) of imaged pixels responding in synchrony with the external stimulus. These data are superimposed on one of the original echoplanar images acquired in the near-axial. This example shows clear activation of both auditory (A) and visual (V) cortices even though, during the condition, our subject was simply hearing words.

consistent in the colors she described for each word. In contrast, a normal control subject, matched for intelligence and memory, who was asked to associate colors with words in the same word list, and who had the advantage of being warned that she would be retested after two weeks (and so could attempt to use mnemonics), was only 17 percent consistent (Baron-Cohen et al. 1987). Because a memory strategy could not plausibly account for such performance, it was concluded that synesthesia is a genuine phenomenon. This finding was replicated with a larger group of synesthetes in a later study (Baron-Cohen et al. 1993).

Establishing that synesthesia is highly consistent in an individual is one way of testing its genuineness. A second way has been to apply functional neuroimaging to investigate if the condition the a neural basis. In a first study with positron emission tomography (PET), Paulesu et al. (1995) compared six synesthetic women with six matched controls. They found that, when hearing words, the group of synesthetes showed abnormal activation in some visual-cortex areas (e.g., the left lingual gyrus, a putative portion of human area V2) relative to controls. We have found support for this result in a pilot study of one synesthete using functional magnetic resonance imaging (fMRI). This study showed clear activation of the visual cortex when the subject listened to words, unlike a normal control (see Figure 25.3). This is clearly an abnormal finding, and suggests that visual imagery indeed occurs when synesthetes hear words.

These results suggest the possibility that there is abnormal neuronal connectivity between auditory and visual cortical areas, and so a neural basis for synesthesia. A further line of evidence that synesthesia has a biological basis is the suggestion that it may be genetic. First, following science programs (British Broadcasting Company, Radio 4) on synesthesia, Baron-Cohen (personal communication) heard from 600 individuals who claimed to have synesthesia, more than 95 percent of them female. Because listeners to the program were predominantly male, this result is unlikely to be due to a trivial sex bias in responding, and suggests that the condition may be sex-linked for genetic reasons. Baron-Cohen has also carried out a questionnaire survey of 565 of these individuals with synesthesia and asked about family relatives. In 132 of these responses, another family relative is reported to have the condition, and in all these the affected relatives are female. Cytowic's (1994) studies also suggest a predominance of females in samples of synesthetes.

IS SYNESTHESIA RELEVANT TO THE STUDY OF CONSCIOUSNESS?

The study of synesthesia may be relevant to consciousness in three ways:

1. Fodor's (1983) view that the sensory systems are modular has received much discussion in neuroscience. Synesthesia, as a mixing of the senses, may be a natural experiment demonstrating the consequences of "a breakdown in modularity" (Baron-Cohen et al. 1993). This view of synesthesia suggests that the normal individual must have a mechanism, possibly under genetic control, which leads to modularization of the senses, and which thus prevents most of us from having synesthesia. Studying this condition may therefore illuminate the organization of the normal brain, as well as that of the synesthetic brain.

2. One possibility is that synesthesia results from disruption in the normal selective neuronal cell death during infancy. In the normally developing brain in many species, many more neuronal connections are made than are finally retained (e.g., Dehay et al. 1984), redundant or maladaptive connections being "pruned" during infancy. In synesthesia, the suggestion is that these connections may persist. This interpretation has led some (e.g., Maurer 1993) to argue that perhaps synesthesia has its origins in infancy. The study of synesthesia may therefore elucidate mechanisms of neural development (see Baron-Cohen 1995).

3. Two hypotheses about how synesthesia occurs in the brain are most pertinent to the major line of argument pursued here. One is that permanent neural connections occur between modalities that are not normally present (e.g., Baron-Cohen et al. 1993), perhaps due to the processes indicated in (2). The other is that synesthesia simply results from learned associations between stimuli (reflecting vagaries in individual life events). The choice between these hypotheses is a specific instance of one general issue about consciousness outlined above: viz., the choice between neuronal events and

information processing as the critical level that determines conscious experience. Does a synesthete experience color upon hearing a word because of a special type of information processing (an association formed between word and color) or a specific type of neuronal event (activity in specific neurons in a specific part of the visual system)? If we could choose between the two types of hypothesis in synesthesia, this choice might have important implications for constructing a general theory of consciousness. It might, of course, be impossible to make this choice because the experiments are too coarse. A more interesting possibility is that the choice might be impossible because conscious experiences depend upon both appropriate information processing and appropriate neuronal events, the two being indissolubly linked in some as yet unknown way. Only by the attempt to dissociate information processing from neuronal events, however, is one likely to uncover such a tight linkage.

To differentiate between these two hypotheses we have commenced a study using fMRI, to measure regional cerebral blood flow (rCBF). We plan to measure rCBF (1) in synesthetes exposed to verbal stimuli that spontaneously evoke experiences of color; (2) in normal controls exposed to the same verbal stimuli during and after associative learning in which they are paired with visual stimuli comparable to those described as part of the synesthetes' experience; (3) in normal controls exposed to the same verbal stimuli but with no prior associative learning task; (4) in synesthetes given associative learning tasks involving stimuli to which they do not have a spontaneous associative response; and (5) in normal controls given the same tasks as for (4). If the special features of the synesthetic experience are due to hard wiring between normally separate, modality-specific regions, we would expect to see activation patterns (including, in particular, activation of visual color cortex by words) in condition (1) which differ from those seen in the remaining four conditions. In contrast, if the synesthetic experience reflects prior associative learning, the results in conditions 1, 2, 4, and 5 should all resemble each other, but differ from those in condition 3. Finally, if synesthetes differ from normals in their associative learning, their results in conditions 1 and 4 should differ from those seen in the controls in conditions 2, 3, and 5.

An outcome from these experiments consistent with the "hard-wiring" hypothesis (above) would have the furthest-reaching implications for a general theory of consciousness. If synesthetes have color experiences when they hear words because unusual patterns of neuronal connectivity lead to activity in brain circuits, with no need for a life history of associative learning, this would imply that the features characterizing specific conscious experiences depend upon neuronal events, not upon information processing. If correct, this inference would further imply that much current effort to explain consciousness by appealing simply to informational transactions that could go on in nonneuronal systems, such as computers (e.g., Johnson-Laird 1987), is fundamentally misdirected.

REFERENCES

Baron-Cohen, S. 1995. Is there a phase of synaesthesia in normal development? *Psyche* 2(27), URL: http://psyche.cs.monash.edu.au/volume2-1/psyche-96-2-27-syn_development-baron_cohen.html.

Baron-Cohen, S., M. Wyke, and C. Binnie. 1987. Hearing words and seeing colours: An experimental investigation of a case of synaesthesia. *Perception* 16:761–767.

Baron-Cohen, S., J. Harrison, L. Goldstein, and M. Wyke. 1993. Coloured speech perception: Is synaesthesia what happens when modularity breaks down? *Perception* 22:419–426.

Binet, A. 1893. L'Application de la psychométrie à l'étude de l'audition colorée. *Recherches Philosophiques* 36, 334–336.

Blakemore, C., and S. Greenfield, eds. 1987. *Mindwaves*. Oxford: Basil Blackwell.

Block, N. 1995. On a confusion about a function of consciousness. *Behavioral and Brain Sciences* 18:227–247.

Chalmers, D. J. 1995. Facing up to the problem of consciousness. *Journal of Consciousness Studies* 2:200–219.

Chalmers, D. J. 1996. *The Conscious Mind*. Oxford: Oxford University Press.

Cytowic, R. 1994. *The Man Who Tasted Shapes*. Archer/Putnam.

Dehay, C., J. Bullier, and H. Kennedy. 1984. Transient projections from the fronto-parietal and temporal cortex to areas 17, 18, and 19 in the kitten. *Experimental Brain Research* 57:208–212.

Dennett, D. C. 1991. *Consciousness Explained*. Boston: Little, Brown.

Fodor, J. 1983. *The Modularity of Mind*. Cambridge: MIT/Bradford Books.

Galton, F. 1883. *Enquiries into the Human Faculty*. London: Denton.

Gray, J. A. 1971. The mind–brain identity theory as a scientific hypothesis. *Philosophical Quarterly* 21, 247–252.

Gray, J. A. 1982. *The Neuropsychology of Anxiety*. Oxford: Oxford University Press.

Gray J. A. 1995a. The contents of consciousness: A neuropsychological conjecture. *Behavioral and Brain Sciences* 18:659–722.

Gray, J. A. 1995b. Consciousness and its (dis)contents. *Behavioral and Brain Sciences* 18:703–722.

Gray, J. A., J. Feldon, J. N. P. Rawlins, D. R. Hemsley, and A. D. Smith. 1991. The neuropsychology of schizophrenia. *Behavioral and Brain Sciences* 14:1–84.

Hameroff, S., and R. Penrose. 1996. Orchestrated reduction of quantum coherence in brain microtubules—A model for consciousness. In S. Hameroff, A. Kaszniak, and A. Scott, eds., *Toward a Science of Consciousness: Contributions from the 1994 Tucson Conference*. Cambridge: MIT Press.

Jackendoff, R. 1987. *Consciousness and the Computational Mind*. Cambridge: MIT Press.

Johnson-Laird, P. 1987. How could consciousness arise from the computations of the brain? In C. Blakemore and S. Greenfield, eds., *Mindwaves*. Oxford: Basil Blackwell, pp. 247–257.

Kolb, F. C., and J. Braun. 1995. Blindsight in normal observers. *Nature* 377:336–338.

Marsh, J., ed. 1993. Experimental and theoretical studies of consciousness. *Ciba Foundation Symposium* 174. New York: John Wiley & Sons.

McCrone, J. 1993. Good timing. *New Scientist Supplement* 9 October, pp. 10–12.

Maurer, D. 1993. Neonatal synaesthesia: Implications for the processing of speech and faces. In B. de Boysson-Bardies, S. de Schonen, P. Jusczyk, P. McNeilage, and J. Morton, eds., *Developmental Neurocognition: Speech and Face Processing in the First Year or Life*. Dordrecht: Kluwer Academic Publishers.

Medawar, P. B. 1967. *The Art of the Soluble*. London: Methuen.

Motluk, A. 1994. The sweet smell of purple. *New Scientist* 13 August, 33–37.

Myers, C. 1911. A case of synaesthesia. *British Journal of Psychology* 4:228–238.

Myers, C. 1914. Two cases of synaesthesia. *British Journal of Psychology* 7:112–117.

Nagel, T. 1974. What is it like to be a bat? *Philosophical Review* 4:435–450.

Paulesu, E., J. Harrison, S. Baron-Cohen, J. D. G. Watson, L. Goldstein, J. Heather, R. S. J. Frakowiac, and C. D. Frith. 1995. The physiology of coloured hearing: A PET activation study of colour-word synaesthesia. *Brain* 118:661–676.

Penrose, R. 1989. *The Emperor's New Mind*. Oxford: Oxford University Press.

Velmans, M. 1991. Is human information processing conscious? *Behavioral and Brain Sciences* 14:651–726.

V   Vision and Consciousness

OVERVIEW

Petra Stoerig

When are we conscious of visual events?

As we pursue our neuroscientific inquiry into consciousness and how it is mediated by the brain, we must distinguish two primary meanings of consciousness. For the first we consider being conscious in the sense of being in a conscious state, as opposed to being dreamlessly asleep or in a coma. The neuronal processes and anatomical structures involved in regulating the conscious state in its different degrees are addressed in work by J. Bogen, J. A. Hobson, and R. Llinas. Their results, as we would expect, point to an unspecific system comprising brain-stem and thalamic nuclei. Without this system's proper function, consciousness is disturbed, and without being conscious one cannot be conscious of something. Any conscious content—image, melody, mathematical theorem, or smell of sauerkraut—requires the organism to be in a conscious state. Once one is conscious, one is usually conscious of something; after all, we require long practice in meditation to achieve a state of consciousness devoid of sensory information, memories, and thoughts. The second meaning of consciousness requires conscious representation: How does information come to be represented in conscious form? We address this question in the next chapters. The senses are prime providers of conscious content, and the visual system is the best-studied sensory system. Therefore we focus here on the visual modality and investigate how visual information can be used and manipulated to reveal the underlying processes that distinguish the consciously represented information from the extensive part that can be processed without becoming conscious.

Stoerig distinguishes both between and within unconscious and conscious visual processes from extensive neuropsychological evidence. Unconscious vision includes neuroendocrine reactions, reflexes, and responses observed in patients with blindsight (see Chapters 32 and 33; see Stoerig and Cowey 1997 for review). These kinds of unconscious visual processing involve different neuronal pathways, as do the kinds of conscious processing that include phenomenal vision, object vision, and object recognition. Phenomenal vision appears to depend on crosstalk between striate and extrastriate visual cortical areas: destroying striate cortex causes a cortical blindness, and selectively destroying extrastriate cortical areas causes selective blindness for submodalities such as color and motion. Phenomenal vision also corresponds to the lowest level of conscious vision, which provides the biologically necessary basis for object vision and recognition, and consequently for the infinite number of conscious manipulations we can perform. This conjecture starkly contrasts to the numerous hypotheses advocating that qualia are mysteriously added to cognitive–computational visual processes than could easily (and much more conveniently for the researcher) take place without them. Much less controversial is Block's distinguishing between two kinds of visual consciousness, that between a phenomenal (p) representation and conscious access (a) to visual information. Referring to a report by Hartmann et al. (1991) on a neuropsychological patient who denied his visual capacities, Block argues that a- and p-consciousness are independent from each other. Consequently, they may well have different neural correlates, and primary visual cortex may be involved in the phenomenal representation.

Block's philosophical critique of Crick and Koch's (1995) assigning visual consciousness to frontal cortex (which denies an important function to primary visual cortex) receives experimental support from Ishai and Sagi. With intricate psychophysics, they demonstrate inhibitory influence by visual imagery on visual perception whose properties implicate primary visual cortex as mediator. Iwasaki and Klein give further examples of how psychophysics can be used to explore properties of conscious and unconscious perception. Iwasaki describes digit identification under backward-masking conditions, thus aiming at temporal constraints on conscious vision, and Klein focuses on signal-detection methodology and double-judgment psychophysics, required to disentangle visual performance from the conscious representation of stimulus. Although Klein restricts himself to a theoretical application to blindsight, Weiskrantz describes experimental work on the subject in Chapter 33. He exemplifies two "modes of blindsight," both in a patient with almost complete but relative cortical blindness, GY. Adjusting stimulus parameters such as contrast and speed, and using four response keys for the patient to indicate (1) direction of stimulus motion (two keys) and (2) whether or not he was aware of the stimulus (two keys), an unconscious but highly effective mode was distinguished from a similarly effective one that was accompanied by some kind of conscious event (Weiskrantz, Barbur, and Sahraie 1995). Having teased apart the parameters required for the two modes, Weiskrantz and colleagues proceeded to use fMRI on the patient's brain as he performed the motion-direction discrimination while alternating between the modes. The preliminary results reported here show that the superior colliculus, often thought to be responsible for mediating blindsight, was activated in the unaware mode only, as were parts of frontal cortex. In contrast, ipsilesional extrastriate cortical areas were visually responsive in both conditions, demonstrating that their activation alone cannot account for visual awareness.

Logothetis and Leopold again address how striate and extrastriate visual cortical areas influence visual perception, combining psychophysical with electrophysiological methods in their attempts to tackle the link between neuronal activity and conscious visual perception. Making use of unstable perceptual phenomena initiated through ambiguous figures or binocularly rivalrous stimulation, and recording the monkeys' perception-related responses throughout the recording, the authors found perception-related neuronal activity in area MT and also in V1, V4, and, when rivalry was initiated between faces or other complex figures, also in inferotemporal cortex. At the same time, they found neurons that did not correspond to the monkeys' perception, demonstrating both that the visual cortical areas contain the full equipment necessary for reciprocal inhibition, attentional modulation, and task requirements, and that no one visual cortical area is likely to turn out to be *the* site for conscious perception. Crick and Koch suggested one site for conscious vision, hypothetically assigning it to frontal cortex. In these chapters, with unfortunately do not include these authors, this hypothesis receives no support: Not only does destruction of the frontal lobes not cause loss of conscious vision but, more in line with traditional neurologists from Brodmann to Holmes, all authors who address the question about the neuronal substrate of conscious vision suggest that visual cortex is involved. Concerted activity in striate and extrastriate visual cortical areas, together with parts of the frontal cortex, and, suggested and illustrated by Bachmann, together with the unspecific nuclei of the thalamus assumed to maintain the states and degrees of consciousness irrespective of its content, all appear to be part of a network whose integrated function underlies our visual experiences. To further study the properties of this network, from the anatomical links and single-cell mechanisms to the perceptual processes and the multiple uses to which they can be put, remains a challenging task.

REFERENCES

Crick, F., and C. Koch. 1995. Are we aware of neural activity in primary visual cortex? *Nature* 375:121–123.

Hartmann, J. A., W. A. Wolz, D. P. Roeltgen, and F. L. Loverso, 1991. Denial of visual perception. *Brain and Cognition* 16, 29–40.

Logothetis, N. K., and J. D. Schall. 1989. Neuronal correlates of subjective visual perception. *Science* 245:761–763.

Stoerig, P., and A. Cowey. 1997. Blindsight in man and monkey. *Brain* 120 (pt. 3):535–559.

Weiskrantz, L., J. L. Barbur, and A. Sahraie. 1995. Parameters affecting conscious versus unconscious visual discrimination with damage to the visual cortex (V1). *Proceedings of the National Academy of Sciences U.S.A.* 92:6122–6126.

26 Varieties of Vision: From Blind Responses to Conscious Recognition

Petra Stoerig

Most neuroscientists who study the neuronal correlate(s) of consciousness assume that a consciously represented neuronal process must differ in some measurable way from the simultaneous processes that are not, now or in principle, represented in this form. As the best-studied sensory system, the visual has been the focus of such empirical approaches. If organizational principles are discovered in one sensory system, they may well apply to the others, no matter whether direct projections to prefrontal areas (Crick and Koch 1995) back-projections from higher cortical areas to primary sensory cortex (Cauller and Kulics 1991), synchronization of neuronal firing (Crick and Koch 1990), certain cortical (Goodale and Milner 1992) or subcortical areas in the brain (Bogen 1995), specific neurons (Crick and Koch 1995, Cauller 1995), or neurotransmitters (Flohr 1995) are needed for the sensory information to be consciously represented.

Neuropsychological evidence demonstrates that visual processes take conscious as well as unconscious form; both shape the patient's behavior. The evidence demonstrates too that different stages in blind as well as conscious vision must be distinguished, and that they require functional integrity in different parts of the system. Consequently, we need to clarify which of the dissociable conscious visual processes we mean when we suggest a neuronal correlate.

UNCONSCIOUS VISION

The legal definition of blindness specifies visual acuity reduced to an incapacitating fraction, but absolute blindness means total absence of visual information processing. A baby born prematurely without eyes is an example of this rare condition. An adult who has lost the function of his or her eyes is not covered by this definition, because once the visual system has worked normally it may remain capable of endogenous vision, as we learn from reports of visual hallucinations in blindness caused by ocular and retinal pathology (Lauber and Lewin 1958). The form of blindness closest to absence of all visual function we can observe in patients who have lost their vision because of damage that destroys the parallel retinofugal projections except for the pathway to the hypothalamus. Although neither a pupil reflex nor any dim perception of light can be evoked, these patients may still suppress melatonin secretion when exposed to bright light (Czeisler et al. 1995).

Reflexive responses such as the pupil light reflex, the photic blink reflex, and optokinetic nystagmus form the second level of visual functions. Although often subnormal, the reflexes can also be demonstrated in the absence of conscious light perception, in comatose patients (Keane 1979), and in patients who have suffered lesions that abolish the retinal input to the geniculo-striate cortical projection but spare the retinofugal pathways to the extrageniculate nuclei, which are known to mediate the visual reflexes.

Patients with lesions that destroy or deafferent the primary visual cortex also lack conscious vision in those parts of the visual field that correspond topographically to the damaged region. Nevertheless, various visual functions can be demonstrated in their homonymous visual-field defects. Beyond reflexive responses (Weiskrantz 1990), two methodologically distinct classes of functions persist. The first is implicit processing of a visual stimulus in the field defect, which affects the response to a second one presented in the normal visual field. An example is the effect that a light shown in the field defect (without telling the patient) exerts on reaction time to a consciously seen stimulus presented in the normal field (Marzi et al. 1986). Another example is the change in induced color caused by replacing with a different color the part of the inducing stimulus configuration that falls into the defect (Pöppel 1986).

The second class of visual responses that can be evoked from a cortically blind field represents the highest level of visual processing with no conscious perception. It is that of forced-choice responses to stimuli presented within the field defect. When the patients are made to guess whether a stimulus has been presented, or which one of a limited number it may have been, the results significantly differ from chance. The functions that have been demonstrated thus include localizing, by saccadic eye movements or hand pointing, stimuli presented at different eccentricities in the field defect; detecting stimuli presented briefly and in random alternation with no-stimulus (blank) trials; discriminating the velocity of a moving stimulus and its direction, and the orientation and wavelength of stationary stimuli (for reviews, see Weiskrantz 1990, Cowey and Stoerig 1991, Stoerig and Cowey 1996). Under optimal conditions—variables including contrast, speed, wavelength, size, adaptation level, and retinal position—the patients can respond correctly up to 100 percent of the time and show loss of sensitivity ranging from only 0.4 to 1.5 log units (Stoerig and Cowey 1997).

In an absolute field defect, the patients are cortically blind, meaning they have lost all conscious sensation of light or color (Wilbrand and Sänger 1904). Similarly, monkeys with unilateral striate cortical ablation who in forced-choice detection show sensitivity and levels of performance very much like the patients', classify stimuli in the affected half-field as nonstimuli or blanks (Cowey and Stoerig 1995).

Blind visual responses thus encompass four levels: neuroendocrine responses, reflexes, effects on conscious visual responses, and "informed"

Glossary

Kinds of blindness	
Absolute blindness	No visual information can be processed
Legal blindness	An incapacitating reduction in acuity (In Germany defined as 1/25–1/50 of normal)
Cortical blindness	Complete absence of conscious visual sensation
Hemianopia	Cortical blindness in one visual half-field
Blindsight	In cortical blindness, visual functions that remain
Apperceptive agnosia	Disturbance in object vision
Associative agnosia	Disturbance in object recognition
Prosopagnosia	Disturbance in face recognition
Kinds of conscious vision	
Phenomenal vision	Lowest level of conscious vision; provides an image consisting of qualia
Qualia	Phenomenal representation of physical properties, such as wavelength as color, and intensity as brightness and darkness
Object vision	Ability to see shape, to segment the image, and to bind the qualia into objects
Object recognition	(1) Ability to classify the visual object ("fork," "cat"); (2) ability to register the objects's individuality and meaning ("my cat," "your face")

guesses about presence and properties of stimuli that are not consciously perceived (see Table 26.1).

CONSCIOUS VISION

Conscious vision is first found in patients with lesions beyond the primary visual cortex that do not disconnect it from extrastriate cortical areas; deafferentation from both the geniculate fibers and the surrounding cortical areas cause cortical blindness (Bodis-Wollner et al. 1977, Horton and Hoyt 1991). If the lesions are confined to subsets of extrastriate visual cortical areas in the vicinity of V1/V2, they cause such selective visual deficits as cortical color, motion, stereo blindness, or a combination of these (see Cowey 1994 for review). The visual world that these patients consciously see lacks color or depth; it may look like a dirty black-and-white television screen or a slow-running movie, but it looks like *something*: the patients have phenomenal vision that lacks only specific qualia.

Patients with apperceptive visual agnosia, which also results from extrastriate cortical damage, may consciously see the full repertoire of qualia. But they lack object vision. They differ from patients with selective qualia-specific cortical blindness, who can construct objects from the reduced set of qualia available to them; and the apperceptive agnosic is unable to segment the visual image into background and foreground, to fuse the impressions into shapes and object (Grüsser and Landis 1991). A good example is Benson and

Table 26.1 Levels of blind vision: If the damage is in the eye but spares retino-hypothalamic fibers, neuroendocrine responses can be observed that influence the circadian rhythm. Reflexive responses like the pupil light reflex are the second level. Implicit blindsight responses, such as completion triggered when the blind field is stimulated in addition to the normal field, constitute the third level. Forced-choice responses, such as localization of stimuli in the cortically blind field, are the highest level of blind visual processing.

Damage	Pathways spared	Remaining response	Function
Ocular or optic nerve	Retino-hypothalamic pathway	Endocrine	Sleep–wake cycle
(Pre-)geniculate	Extra-geniculate pathways	Reflexive	Pupil
Post-geniculate	Extra-geniculo-striate pathways	Implicit	Reaction to seen stimulus
Post-geniculate	Extra-geniculo-striate pathways and extra-striate cortical areas	Forced-choice guessing	Detection of unseen stimulus

Greenberg's patient, who showed normal visual acuity, "keen ability to distinguish light intensity, object size, color, and direction, but could not differentiate simple forms" (Benson and Greenberg 1969, p. 89). The image segmentation and construction of visual objects can be disturbed in the absence of sensory deficits, and patients with more severe sensory deficits need not present with difficulties in object vision (Ettlinger 1956, De Haan et al. 1995).

In normal observers, object vision usually is achieved effortlessly from experience, but active seeing requires a noticeable amount of time when difficult-to-structure scenes such as those shown in Figure 26.1 need to be appropriately grouped.

Once the grouping is accomplished, the objects forming the visual scene need to be recognized. Again, object recognition is complex and inhomogeneous (Logothetis and Sheinberg 1996). The object's classification can be disturbed—a coin can be called a knife, even when the object's representation is well-enough defined to allow the patient to draw or copy it (Lissauer 1890). Classification can occur at different levels, and depends on individual experience and knowledge. Looking at Figure 26.1, only a few readers will be able to give more than the generic class of the entity depicted.

Once the classification is achieved, the object's individuality and meaning need to be recognized. This step can dissociate from object vision, as shown by patients with a form of associative agnosia that allows them to see and classify objects. They may recognize a car as a car and a face as a face, but nevertheless have a conscious percept that is "stripped of its meaning" (Teuber 1968). The percept does not evoke the associations that apply to its use, its proprietor, or its history. This "pure" loss has been reported in face agnosia (prosopagnosia), where the patient is rendered incapable of

---

*Two African butterflies (*Pontia helice*).

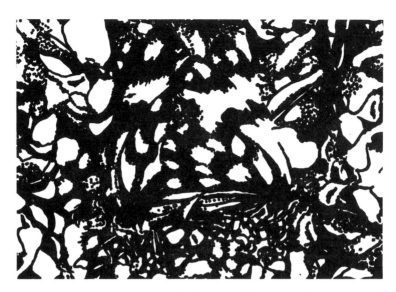

Figure 26.1 The image is perceived as phenomenal but ungrouped for as long as the viewer has not achieved the segmentation into visual objects. Once the objects are defined, they are seen quickly upon consecutive presentations. Conscious recognition follows; its extent and content (naming and associations) depend on the individual's background knowledge. (See footnote* for answer)

recognizing a face as her own, her husband's, or her daughter's (Damasio, Damasio, and van Hoesen 1982).

The labels "modality-specific cortical blindness," "apperceptive," and "associative agnosia" here supply points of reference even though no generally accepted clear-cut nomenclature appears. In clinical practice it is rare to find pure cases; more often, a patient with cerebral color blindness also has a partial defect in the visual field, and a patient with prosopagnosia also has achromatopsia or a sensory deficit. This continuum has provoked a debate about the distinctiveness of the disturbances, particularly apperceptive and associative agnosia (Grüsser and Landis 1991, Lissauer 1890, and Farah 1990). In this context, however, it is sufficient if we have at least one patient who can consciously see but not draw or copy objects (Benson and Greenberg 1969), one patient who can draw and copy but not classify (Lissauer 1890, Rubens and Benson 1971), and one who can classify but not recognize the meaning and individuality (Damasio, Damasio, and van Hoesen 1982, DeRenzi et al. 1991). These patients' symptoms demonstrate that object vision and recognition are dissociable. Consequently, conscious vision has (at least) three parts: phenomenal vision gives an image; grouping gives visual objects, and recognition gives their class and meaning in relation to one's history, experience, knowledge, and intentions (see Table 26.2).

FUNCTIONS OF VISION

All levels of vision are behaviorally relevant. The neuroendocrine response of melatonin suppression sets the circadian clock that regulates sleeping and

Petra Stoerig: Varieties of Vision: From Blind Responses to Conscious Recognition

Table 26.2 Levels of conscious vision: Phenomenal vision, the lowest form of conscious perception, is lost in cortical blindness. For object vision the appropriate qualia must be grouped in space and time. Recognition of objects, lost in patients with associative agnosia, gives their meaning in the individual context.

Level	Gives	Allows	Is lost in
Phenomenal vision	Image, qualia	Normal acuity, color, motion, and contrast	Cortical blindness
Object vision	Shapes, objects	To draw, copy, match	Apperceptive agnosia
Object recognition	Meaning, individuality	Appropriate use and description	Associative agnosia

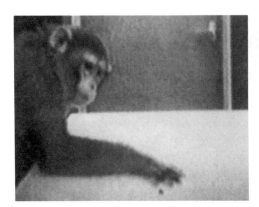 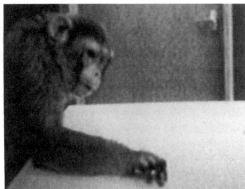

Figure 26.2 Despite her complete cortical blindness, monkey Helen could accurately grasp a raisin. (Reprinted with kind permission of N. K. Humphrey.)

waking patterns, saving the patients from the sleep disorders that often accompany total blindness (Czeisler et al. 1995). The visual reflexes protect the organism from harm. Blindsight shapes the visually guided behavior, although this function is not obvious in patients with partial-field defects who use the normal field—often more than a half-field—for all conscious visual purposes, such as exploration, navigation, and identification. Bilateral absolute cortical blindness, which could establish the extent of blindsight-guided behavior, is generally caused by lesions so extensive that they leave the patient incapacitated and unfit for in-depth testing and training. Therefore the remarkable extent of visual behavior that is possible with blindsight can at present best be demonstrated in monkeys with bilateral occipital lobectomy. Helen, the most extensively studied example, not only learned to orient toward visual stimuli, to reach for, discriminate, and avoid them, but to effectively navigate in her environment (Humphrey 1974).

The behavioral relevance of phenomenal vision is controversial; after all, qualia have long been declared mysterious addenda to perception (see Metzinger 1995 for current debate). Nevertheless, from neuropsychological evidence and contrary to views ascertaining that qualia are somehow added to a fully formed percept, I suggest that phenomenal vision is the prerequisite for object vision and recognition: it represents the lowest level of conscious vision. A reverse disorder—intact conscious vision-based recognition in the absence of phenomenal vision—has, to my knowledge, never been reported. If qualia are necessary for the grouping that is the basis for object vision and disturbed in apperceptive agnosia, blindsight patients should be unable to construct visual objects and discriminate objects embedded in a scene. Although this theory has not been extensively tested, the notion gains support from the lack of form discrimination that is independent of cues from orientation and length of contour in blindsight (Weiskrantz 1987). Some information about objects must, however, be available to allow the cortically blind monkey Helen to avoid obstacles, grasp raisins, and catch cockroaches (Humphrey 1974). Possibly the motor system can access this information, which would agree with the accurate grasping of objects differing in shape that has been demonstrated in an apperceptive agnosic patient (Goodale et al. 1994).

If objects cannot be consciously formed without qualia, conscious recognition will be equally impossible (although implicit recognition is possible (Bruyer et al. 1983)). Even after years of experience, cortically blind monkeys show no evidence of visually recognizing complex objects (Humphrey 1974). consequently, cortical blindness would necessarily include "psychic blindness" (agnosia). This dependence appeared sufficiently obvious to William James to be included in his definition: "Hemianopic disturbance comes from lesion of either [occipital lobe], and total blindness, sensorial as well as psychic, from destruction of both (James 1890, p. 47).

Even as they provide the basis for object vision and recognition, qualia may be required for all functions that act on a phenomenal representation of a physical-stimulus property and not on that property itself. For example, wavelength is phenomenally represented as color, and color constancy could conceivably be lost in patients who lack this quale, either because of cortical blindness or because of cortical color blindness. Recent evidence shows that color constancy is impaired along with color identification in a patients with incomplete achromatopsia (Kennard et al. 1995), indicating that constancy indeed depends on the quale. Last but not least, phenomenal vision may be a prerequisite for conscious access to visual information. Blindsight patients experience themselves as blind, as only guessing whether a stimulus has appeared in their blind field, and they seem unable to consciously remember anything they have "blind-seen" (Stoerig and Cowey 1996).

Conscious object vision, the next stage and preserved in associative agnosia, permits the patient to match, copy, and draw seen objects. Depending on which recognition process is disturbed, assigning the object to a class may or may not be possible. Patients who can classify objects can visually search for a set of keys in an array of other objects, an exceedingly difficult task for an apperceptive agnosic (Sparr et al. 1991).

Finally, full conscious recognition is the basis for the vast repertoire of the conscious vision-based behaviors: We explicitly recognize almost anything we see; we can grasp, manipulate, imagine, and rotate visual objects in our minds, we can draw them thirty years after having seen them, reinterpret them in a dream, and distort them in a novel. The possibilities are endless, at least as long as the covert or overt output is intact. If the muscles that close the lid in the photic-blink reflex are paralyzed, the visual information is processed to no effect, and a patient who has a severe aphasia will be unable to describe any object consciously recognized. The function of all levels of vision depends not just on the visual system's integrity but on that of the pathways and structures responsible for the many uses we can make of the visual information. Highly specific deficits such as color anomia (Oxbury, Oxbury, and Humphrey 1969) and optic aphasia (Lhermitte and Beauvois 1973) demonstrate the intricate connectivity between vision and behavior.

NEURONAL CORRELATES OF VISION

The lesion-induced dissociations demonstrate that (at least to some extent) different neuronal circuits and mechanisms underlie the distinct processing stages. A subset of retinal ganglion cells that project directly to the hypothalamus provides the information on light levels required for the circadian clock (Moore, Speh, and Card 1995). A subset of ganglion cells that project to extrageniculate nuclei mediate the visual reflexes (e.g., Hoffman 1989). Ganglion cells that project (via subcortical nuclei) to extrastriate visual cortical areas provide the information needed for the forced-choice visual responses demonstrated in blindsight patients (Stoerig and Cowey 1996). Lesions that destroy or disconnect the primary visual cortices cause cortical blindness (Wilbrand and Sänger 1904, James 1890); bilateral lesions around the fusiform and lingual gyri cause cortical color blindness (Zeki 1990); bilateral lesions around the middle temporal area cause cortical motion blindness (Zeki 1991); insufficiently specified lesions (often carbon-monoxide poisoning) of occipito-parieto-temporal cortex cause apperceptive agnosia (Grüsser and Landis 1991, Farah 1990, Goodale et al. 1994); bilateral lesions in inferior occipital and temporal visual cortical areas cause associative prosopagnosia (Damasio, Damasio, and van Hoesen 1982), and lesions destroying the connections between the extrastriate visual cortex and the memory structures in the temporal lobe cause associative object agnosia (Albert et al. 1979).

Phenomenal vision is lost in patients whose primary visual cortices are inactivated, destroyed, or disconnected. Specific qualia are selectively lost in patients with circumscribed extrastriate cortical lesions. Together, this loss indicates that both primary and secondary visual cortical areas are involved in phenomenal vision.

The exact function that primary visual cortex has in phenomenal vision has not been sufficiently studied. It appears that phenomenal images could be generated in its total absence only when massive excitation of temporal visual cortex is induced. Occipital-lobe destruction, assumedly through a release excitation, can be followed by a period of intense visual (pseudo-)

hallucinations, which disappear in a matter of weeks (Grüsser and Landis 1991, Kölmel 1985). No other form of phenomenal vision has yet been reported in patients with complete striate cortical destruction. The faint conscious experiences caused by certain types of visual stimulation (Weiskrantz, Barbur, and Sahraie 1995), and the perceptual completion of afterimages that extend into the cortically blind field when it is stimulated in conjunction with the normal field (Bender and Kahn 1946), have been demonstrated only in patients with incomplete striate cortical destruction. Consequently, they could result from topographically imprecise projections to and from residual striate cortex, a possibility strengthened by recent demonstrations of unsuspected plasticity in primary visual cortex in response to adaptive challenge (Sugita 1996). The "internal screen" onto which mental images are projected has also been shown to shrink in tandem with the visual field when the occipital cortex is ablated (Farah, Soso, and Dasheiff 1992). Whether means like magnetic or electrical stimulation could produce images in patients with complete destruction of primary cortex, whether such patients have visual dreams in the hemianopic field, and whether any conscious vision could be reinstated in such patients through rehabilitative measures all remain to be seen. The answers will further illuminate the role primary visual cortex plays in phenomenal vision.

Reciprocal projections between striate and extrastriate areas may also be involved in the grouping that requires binding the results from the areas specialized for different visual qualities into, say, the running figure of a person clad in red. Timing of neuronal events could be a unifying parameter, temporal synchronization of discharges of neurons in different cortical areas mediating the binding of what-belongs-to-what (Engel, Kreiter, König, and Singer 1991). Finally, recognition depends on the connections between visual cortex and memory systems. The behaviors consciously initiated using conscious recognition involve the complex links between vision and language, evaluation, emotion, planning, and action systems. Consequently they may be lost selectively when any of these systems is destroyed or disconnected from the visual information, even when conscious visual recognition remains fully intact.

It follows that different aspects of blind and conscious vision require different structures and algorithms that can be studied empirically. The recently proposed hypotheses on the neuronal basis of conscious vision are aimed at different parts of an inhomogeneous process. They need not therefore be mutually exclusive.

ACKNOWLEDGMENT

This chapter is dedicated to the late Norton Nelkin, who helped me understand what I knew. It is a pleasure to thank Nick Humphrey for allowing me to use a still from his film of Helen. The work was supported by the Deutsche Forschungsgemeinschaft.

NOTES

1. Reprinted with permission from Elsevier Science Publishers. Originally published in *Trends in Neurosciences* (1996), vol. 19. Varieties of vision: from blind responses to conscious recognition. *Trends in Neurosciences* 19(9):401–406.

REFERENCES

Albert, M. L., D. Soffer, R. Silverberg, and A. Reches. 1979. The anatomic basis of visual agnosia. *Neurology* 29:876–879.

Bender, M. B., and R. L. Kahn. 1949. After imagery in defective fields of vision. *J. Neurol Neurosurg Psychiatry* 12:196–204.

Benson, D. F., and J. P. Greenberg. 1969. Visual form agnosia: A specific defect in visual discrimination. *Archives of Neurology* 20:82–89.

Bodis-Wollner, I., A. Atkin, E. Raab, and M. Wolkstein. 1977. Visual association cortex and vision in man: Pattern-evoked occipital potentials in a blind boy. *Science* 198:629–631.

Bogen, J. E. 1995. On the neurophysiology of consciousness: I. An overview. *Consciousness and Cognition* 4:52–62.

Bruyer, R., C. Laterre, X. Seron, P. Feyereisen, E. Strypstein, E. Pierrard, and D. Rectem. A case of prosopagnosia with some preserved covert remembrance of familiar faces. *Brain and Cognition* 2:257–284.

Cauller, L. 1995. Layer I of primary sensor neocortex: Where top-down converges upon bottom-up. *Behavior and Brain Research* 71:157.

Cauller, L., and A. T. Kulics. 1991. The neural basis of the behaviorally relevant N1 component of the somatosensory-evoked potential in SI cortex of awake monkeys: Evidence that backward cortical projections signal conscious touch perception. *Experimental Brain Research* 84:607–619.

Cowey, A. 1994. Cortical visual areas and the neurobiology of higher visual processes. In M. J. Farah and G. Ratcliff, eds., *Object Representation and Recognition*. Hillsdale, NJ: Lawrence Erlbaum, pp. 1–31.

Cowey, A., and P. Stoerig. 1991. The neurobiology of blindsight. *Trends in Neuroscience* 14:140–145.

Cowey, A., and P. Stoerig. 1995. Blindsight in monkeys. 1995. *Nature* 373:247–249.

Crick, F., and C. Koch. 1995. Are we aware of visual activity in primary visual cortex? *Nature* 375:121–123.

Crick, F., and C. Koch. 1990. Towards a neurobiological theory of consciousness. *Seminars in the Neurosciences* 2:263–275.

Czeisler, C. A., T. L. Shanahan, E. B. Klerman, H. Martens, D. J. Brotman, J. S. Emens, T. Klein, and J. F. Rizzo 3rd. 1995. Suppression of melatonin secretion in some blind patients by exposure to bright light. *New England Journal of Medicine* 332:6–11.

Damasio, A. R., H. Damasio, and G. W. van Hoesen. 1982. Prosopagnosia: Anatomic basis and behavioral mechanisms. *Neurology* 32:331–341.

De Haan, E. H. F., C. A. Heywood, A. W. Young, N. Edelstyn, and F. Newcombe. 1995. Ettlinger revisited: The relation between agnosia and sensory impairment. *Journal of Neurology, Neurosurgery and Psychiatry* 58:350–356.

De Renzi, E., P. Faglioni, D. Grossi, and P. Nichelli. 1991. Apperceptive and associative forms of prosopagnosia. *Cortex* 27:213–221.

Engel, A. K., A. K. Kreiter, P. König, and W. Singer. 1991. Synchronization of oscillatory neuronal responses between striate and extrastriate visual cortical areas of the cat. *Proceedings of the National Academy of Sciences U.S.A.* 88:6048–6052.

Ettlinger, G. 1956. Sensory deficits in visual agnosia. *Journal of Neurology, Neurosurgery and Psychiatry* 19:297–308.

Farah, M. J. 1990. *Visual Agnosia.* Cambridge: MIT Press.

Farah, M., M. J. Soso, and R. M. Dasheiff. 1992. Visual angle of the mind's eye before and after unilateral occipital lobectomy. *Journal of Experimental Psychology, Human Perception and Performance* 18:241–246.

Flohr, H. 1995. An information-processing theory of anaesthesia. *Neuropsychologia* 33:1169–1180.

Goodale, M. A., J. P. Meenan, H. H. Bülthoff, D. A. Nicolle, K. J. Murphy, C. I. Racicot. 1994. Separate neural pathways for the visual analysis of object shape in perception and prehension. *Current Biology* 4:604–610.

Goodale, M. A., and A. D. Milner. 1992. Separate visual pathways for perception and action. *Trends in Neuroscience* 15:20–25.

Crüsser, O.-J., and T, Landis. 1991. Visual agnosias and other distubances of visual perception and cognition. *Vision and Visual Dysfunction,* vol. 12. New York: Macmillan.

Hoffmann, K.-P. 1989. Control of the optokinetic reflex by the nucleus of the optic tract in primates. *Progress in Brain Research* 80:173–182.

Horton, J. C., and W. F. Hoyt. 1991. Quadrantic visual-field defects: A hallmark of lesions in extrastriate (V2/V3) cortex. *Brain* 114:1703–1718.

Humphrey, N. K. 1974. Vision in a monkey without striate cortex: A case study. *Perception* 3:241–255.

James, W. 1890. *The Principles of Psychology.* New York: Macmillan.

Keane, J. R. 1979. Blinking to sudden illumination: A brain-stem reflex present in neocortical death. *Archives of Neurology* 36:52–53.

Kennard, C., M. Lawden, A. B. Morland, and K. H. Ruddock. 1995. Colour identification and colour constancy are impaired in a patient with incomplete achromatopsia associated with prestriate cortical lesions. *Proceedings of the Royal Society of London* B 260:169–175.

Kölmel, H. 1985. Complex visual hallucinations in the hemianopic field. *Journal of Neurology, Neurosurgery, and Psychiatry* 48:29–38.

Lauber, H. L., and B. Lewin. 1958. Über optische Halluzinationen bei Ausschaltung des Visus, klinisch und tiefenpsychologisch betrachtet. *Archiv für Psychiatrie und Zeitschrift für die Gesamte der Neurologie* 197:15–31.

Lhermitte, F., and M. F. Beauvois. 1973. A visual-speech disconnexion syndrome: Report of a case with optic aphasia, agnostic alexia and colour agnosia. *Brain* 96:695–714.

Lissauer, H. 1890. Ein Fall von Seelenblindheit nebst einem Beitrage zur Theorie derselben. *Archiv für Psychiatrie und Nervenkrankheiten* 21:222–270.

Logothetis, N. K., and S. Sheinberg. 1996. Visual object recognition. *Annual Review of Neuroscience* 19:577–621.

Marzi, C. M., G. Tassinari, S. Aglioti, and L. Lutzemberger. 1986. Spatial summation across the vertical meridian in hemianopics: A test of blindsight. *Neuropsychologia* 24:749–758.

Metzinger, T., ed. 1995. *Consciousness Experience.* Paderborn: Schöningh.

Moore, R. Y., J. C. Speh, and J. P. Card. 1995. The retinohypothalamic tract originates from a distinct subset of retinal ganglion cells. *Journal of Comparative Neurology* 352:351–366.

Oxbury, J. M., S. M. Oxbury, and N. K. Humphrey. 1969. Varieties of colour anomia. *Brain* 92:847–860.

Pöppel, E. 1986. Long-range colour-generating interactions across the retina. *Nature* 320:523–525.

Rubens, A. B., and D. F. Benson. 1971. Associative visual agnosia. *Archives of Neurology* 24:305–316.

Sparr, S. A., M. Jay, F. W. Drislane, and N. Venna. 1991. A historic case of visual agnosia revisited after 40 years. *Brain* 114:789–800.

Stoerig, P., and A. Cowey. 1997. Blindsight in man and monkey. *Brain* 120 (pt. 3)535–559.

Sugita, Y. 1996. Global plasticity in adult visual cortex following reversal of visual input. *Nature* 380:523–526.

Teuber, H.-L. 1968. Alteration of perception and memory in man. In L. Weiskranz, ed., *Analysis of Behavioral Change*. New York: Harper and Row, pp. 268–375.

Weiskrantz, L. 1987. Residual vision in a scotoma: A follow-up study of form discrimination. *Brain* 110:177–192.

Weiskranz, L. 1990. The Ferrier Lecture, 1989: Outlooks for blindsight: Explicit methodologies for implicit processes. *Proceedings of the Royal Society of London* B 239:247–278.

Weiskranz, L., J. L. Barbur, and A. Sahraie. 1995. Parameters affecting conscious versus unconscious visual discrimination with damage to the visual cortex (V1). *Proceedings of the National Academy of Science of the U.S.A.* 92:6122–6126.

Wilbrand, H., and A. Sänger. 1904. *Die Neurologie des Auges*, vol. III. Wiesbaden: J. F. Bergmann.

Zeki, S. 1990. A century of cerebral achromatopsia. *Brain* 113:1721–1777.

Zeki, S. 1991. Cerebral akinetopsia (visual motion blindness): A review. *Brain* 114:811–824.

27 Single-Neuron Activity and Visual Perception

Nikos K. Logothetis and David A. Leopold

SENSATION AND PERCEPTION

Numerous observations support the idea that part of what we perceive comes through our senses from the "things" around us, and another part—which is most likely to be the largest part—comes out of our own mind. Figure 27.1 brings out this point clearly. From top, left to right, bottom, the panels show nonsense lines (A), nonsense patterns (B), discontinuous parallel lines (C), a woman's face (D), a cube (E), and a vase (F). Are the lines and patterns in panel A meaningless? Or do they outline a washerwoman with a bucket at her right side? If we look at panel A again, we will probably see the lines turn into borders of a solid shape representing a well-known object—indeed, a woman with a bucket at her right side. Similarly, the figure in panel B turns into a face once we have been told that indeed it is a face. We can see panel D as an "old" woman or as a "young" girl (published in *Puck* in 1915 by the cartoonist W. E. Hill with the title, "My wife and my mother-in-law"). Panel E has two possible perspectives, and F has the celebrated faces-and-vase figure-ground reversal introduced by Danish psychologist Edgar Rubin in 1915. It can be perceived as either a goblet or a pair of faces. The perceptual changes occurring when we view ambiguous figures have been shown to occur even when these figures are stabilized in the retina and thus even under conditions in which the retinal stimulus remains entirely unchanged. Finally, in panel C the absence of visual stimulation appears to serve as input to our perception, as we see a white "filled" high-contrast circle in the middle and a concentric ring around it. Clearly our brain sees more than our eyes. The latter receive patterns of energy that are converted into patterns of neural excitation, but the former seldom sees such patterns. Instead our brain sees objects, which most often have meaning and history. Here is an important question: How does the brain derive descriptions of definite objects from the hodgepodge of visual elements provided through the sensory organs?

Pioneering research initiated by David Hubel and Torsten Wiesel shows that the visual cortex has all the machinery required to form neural descriptions of objects. Neurons have topographic organization, high selectivity for distinct stimulus attributes, and receptive field complexity that increases in

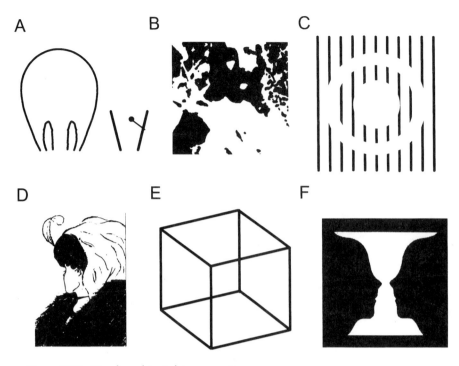

Figure 27.1 Stimuli used in studying perception.

successively higher visual cortical areas. Cells in the retina and the dorsal lateral geniculate nucleus (a small thalamic structure that receives direct input from the retina and relays it to the primary visual cortex) respond to light spots; neurons in primary visual cortex respond selectively to the orientation or direction of motion of line segments, and cells in the inferior temporal cortex (a large area in the temporal lobe) may respond selectively to very complex patterns, including animate objects such as faces or body parts.

Loosely speaking, retinal processing is optimized to detect intensity and wavelength contrast, early cortical areas extract fundamental stimulus descriptors, such as orientation and curvature, spatial frequencies and stimulus velocities, and high visual areas in the parietal and temporal lobe process information respectively about the spatial relationships and the identity of visual objects. And yet, despite the plethora of data on the properties of individual neurons, we know very little about how their responses contribute to unified percepts, and how these percepts lead to semantic knowledge about objects. Not only do we not know how inputs from a "face-selective" neuron in the inferior temporal cortex are organized, and thus how such a neuron comes to acquire such amazing configurational selectivity, but we do not even know how responses by such selective cells relate to any perceptual event. Do such cells mediate recognition of an object? Do they represent the stage at which information is routed to the motor planning or motor areas? We do know that many of these neurons respond vigorously when presented a specific stimulus, even when the animal is anesthetized. Do they then really relate to conscious perception? Which cells then code for this hodgepodge of visual primitives and which relate directly to our knowledge of familiar objects?

UNSTABLE PERCEPTS: THE MIND AT WORK

Visual stimuli such as the ambiguous figures in Figure 27.1 (panels D, E, and F) are excellent tools for addressing such questions. Normally, when we look steadily at the picture of a real object the information the retina receives mostly remains constant, as does perception of the object, presumably because the rich information derived by integrating a large number of visual cues establishes an unambiguous, unitary interpretation of a scene. In such cases neural responses that may underlie our perception of a stimulus are confounded with sensory responses to the stimulus or parts thereof. When the visual cues provided, however, do not suffice for one unitary interpretation, then rival possibilities can be entertained and perception becomes ambiguous, swiftly switching between two or more alternatives without concomitant change in the message received from the eye. Classic examples of figures eliciting different perceptions are the figure-ground and depth reversals shown in figures 27.1E and 27.1F. The question we must ask is: Would a cell that responds selectively to, say, the profile of a face, discharge action potentials only when the faces in panel F are perceived, though the pattern that can be interpreted as face is always available to the visual system? Addressing this question directly in invasive laboratory-animal experiments is extremely difficult for two reasons. First, an animal, presumably a monkey, must learn to report subtle configurational changes for one of the handful of known multistable stimuli. Second, individual neurons must be isolated that specifically respond to this stimulus, with the hope that alternate perceptual configurations will differentially activate the cell.

Fortunately, perceptual bistability can also be elicited by simply presenting a conflict to the two eyes, where the monocular images differ substantially in their spatial organization, color, or direction of motion. Rarely will non-matching stimuli be binocularly fused into a stable coherent stimulus; instead, each monocular pattern takes its turn at perceptual dominance, only to be overtaken by its competitor after a number of seconds. This phenomenon, known as *binocular rivalry*, was first noticed more than two centuries ago (DuTour 1760) and its phenomenology has been studied extensively for three decades in the context of binocular vision (for a review, see Blake 1989). Some psychophysical experiments have initially suggested a peripheral inhibitory mechanism for rivalry, specifically involving competition between the two monocular pathways. Rivalry therefore has generally been considered a form of interocular rather than perceptual competition. In other words, perceiving a stimulus was thought to amount to "dominance" by the eye viewing this stimulus. We have, however, recently shown that the eye-dominance notion fails to account for the long perceptual dominance by a stimulus presented alternately to one eye and then to the other (Logothetis, Leopold, and Sheinberg 1996), as described in the next section.

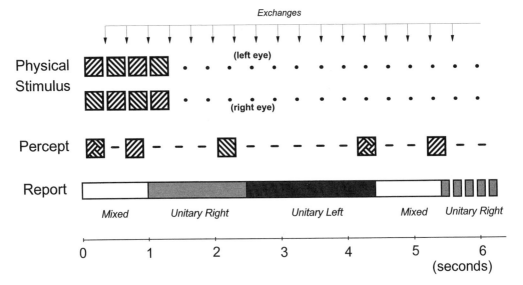

Figure 27.2 Psychophysical "switch" paradigm. The stimulus consisted of a pair of sinusoidal gratings of 20 percent contrast and 2.5 cycles per degree spatial frequency, which were orthogonally oriented in the two eyes. The stimuli were flickered on and off at 18 Hz, and exchanged between the eyes every 333 msec. Despite the constantly reversing stimulus, perception was dominated by prolonged periods of leftward and rightward unitary dominance, with intervening periods of mixed rivalry. Subjects viewed the stimulus for two-minute periods and held down buttons on a computer mouse to indicate leftward, rightward, or mixed perceptual dominance.

BINOCULAR RIVALRY: INTEROCULAR OR INTERSTIMULUS COMPETITION?

We presented to human observers incongruent stimuli via a mirror stereoscope, a device permitting independent stimulation of each eye under normal eye movement conditions, and asked them to report periods of sustained dominance of a left- or right-tilted grating pattern by pressing and holding the left and right computer-mouse buttons respectively. Our experimental paradigm is outlined in Figure 27.2. As in many other experiments on binocular rivalry, the visual stimuli were simple, consisting of square patches of sinusoidal gratings that were orthogonally oriented in the two eyes. Unlike all other experiments, however, the two monocular stimuli in our paradigm were exchanged between the eyes (three times each second), resulting in periodic orientation reversals of each monocular stimulus. The gratings were also flickered on and off 18 times a second to minimize perception of transients caused by the physical exchanges. What would one expect to see under these stimulation conditions? Traditional wisdom would predict that perception would be dominated by a grating regularly switching orientations, as it would if the subject closed one eye. If the perceptual rivalry were some form of competition between the central representations of the stimuli, though, one would expect slow alternations in perceived orientation that are uncorrelated to the physical exchange of the monocular stimuli. All observers indeed reported seeing prolonged periods of unitary dominance of each orientation, lasting up to several seconds.

The mean dominance duration exceeded two seconds, spanning seven physical exchanges of the gratings. Subjects reported that they rarely saw a grating rapidly changing its orientation at the exchange frequency, as "eye dominance" would predict; such changes could easily be observed by closing one eye. To compare rivalry during the "switch" paradigm with conventional rivalry, the statistics of the alternation phases were evaluated. First, we showed that successive dominance phases were independent both by auto-correlation analysis and the Lathrop test for sequential dependence (Lathrop 1996), in agreement with conventional rivalry (Fox and Herrmann 1967). Second, we found that the distribution of these durations (Figure 27.3c, pooled for 3 subjects) closely resembled those obtained during conventional rivalry for a human being (panel A) and a monkey (panel B), both of which match those previously reported in the literature (Walker 1975, Fox and Herrmann 1967, Leopold and Logothetis 1996).

Finally we examined how the strength of one stimulus affected the mean dominance and suppression of each. The contrast of one of the orientations was systematically varied while the other was held constant. Again, the pattern during "switch" rivalry (panel F, average of 3 subjects) resembles those from a human being (panel D) and a monkey (panel E) during conventional rivalry. In all cases the contrast of one orientation primarily affects the mean dominance time of the other orientation. Notice that in the "switch" condition each eye sequentially sees both the fixed- and variable-contrast stimuli, and it is therefore the strength of the competing *stimuli* rather than the strength in the two *eyes* that governs this effect. Our analysis shows that the rivalry experienced when monocular stimuli are continually swapped between the eyes is indistinguishable from conventional binocular rivalry.

Our finding clearly suggests that the perceptual alternations experienced during binocular rivalry involve perturbations in the same neural machinery involved in other multistable perceptual phenomena, such as monocular rivalry (Campbell and Howell 1972) and ambiguous figures, which incidentally show dynamics similar to those of binocular rivalry (Borsellino et al. 1972). Thus dichoptic stimulation, in which arbitrary combinations of conflicting stimuli can be brought into competition for dominance, can be an excellent tool for studying the physiology of perceptual organization and visual awareness in experimental animals. Next, we briefly describe one such physiological experiment.

CELL RESPONSES IN EARLY VISUAL CORTEX TO AMBIGUOUS STIMULI

To examine the neural responses in the primary visual cortex and the early extrastriate visual areas (of visual areas surrounding and receiving input from primary visual cortex) we trained monkeys to report the perceived orienta-

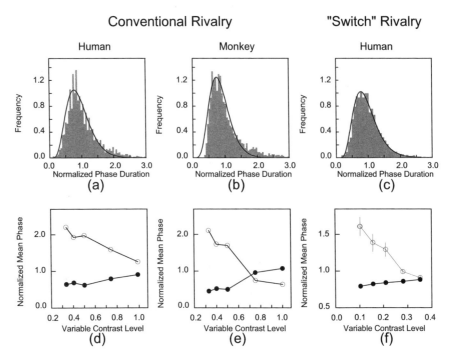

Conventional Rivalry   "Switch" Rivalry

Human   Monkey   Human

(a)   (b)   (c)

(d)   (e)   (f)

Figure 27.3 Statistics on perceptual-rivalry alternations. The temporal dynamics of rivalry during the switch paradigm were identical with those in conventional rivalry. (A–C) Distribution of dominance-phase durations expressed as a fraction of their mean. Data are shown for conventional rivalry from a human subject (A) and a monkey (B), and for switch rivalry pooled from three human subjects (C). The thin dark lines illustrate the approximation of the histogram data with a gamma function. (D–F) Effect of contrast from each rivaling stimulus. The abscissa shows the contrast of one stimulus, and the other was held fixed. Open circles represent the mean dominance for the fixed-contrast stimulus, and closed circles for the variable stimulus. This relation is shown for conventional rivalry form a human subject (D) and a monkey (E) and for switch rivalry averaged from three human subjects (F). The fixed-contrast values were held at 1.0 and 0.35 for the conventional switch rivalry, respecively.

tion of a stimulus under conditions of congruent and dichoptic stimulation (Leopold and Logothetis 1996). During the initial shaping and training phase each monkey was shown monocular grating patterns on a computer monitor and taught to press one of two levers according to whether the grating was tilted left or right of vertical. The animal eventually learned to respond to several successive changes in orientation, receiving a juice reward only at the end of each observation period (Figure 27.4). Once nearly perfect performance was achieved, training was continued with stimuli that mimicked the stochastic changes in stimulus appearance during binocular rivalry. Simulating perception during rivalry with composed, mixed, nonrivalrous stimuli allowed the monkey to grow accustomed to the "feel" of rivalry but still afforded us full control over the animal's behavior, because incorrect responses would abort the observation period. Gradually, periods of real binocular rivalry were introduced into the emulation, during which orientations in

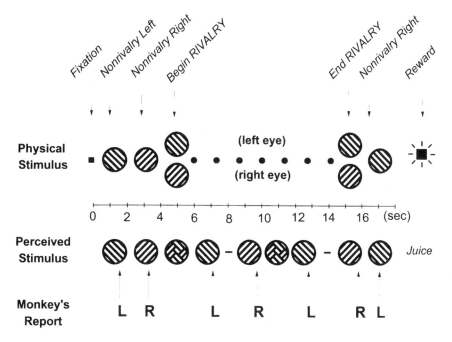

Figure 27.4 The monkey fixated a small spot and maintained fixation as nonrivalrous (monocular or binocular) and rivalorus grating patterns were presented. The animal signal-led perceptual transitions between the two orientations by pressing one of two levers (R or L) mounted on the primate chair. During the rivalry period the perceived transitions were not accompanied by changes in the physical stimulus. Incorrect responses for a nonrivalry trial, or failure to maintain accurate fixation (within a 0.8° window) resulted in aborting the 15 to 25-sec observation period, and the monkey would forfeit his juice reward.

right and left eyes were perpendicular. During these periods the monkeys continued to respond to orientation reversals, but now these changes were purely subjective because the physical stimuli remained unaltered, hence feedback for inappropriate responses was impossible. The accuracy of response during these periods was, however, indirectly probed by introducing *catch* trials, in which one of the gratings was smoothly reoriented after a lever response to yield a coherent binocular stimulus. The monkey was expected to respond either immediately or not at all, depending on whether the catch-trial orientation was perpendicular to or the same as that indicated by the previous response, a test in which each monkey consistently performed above 95 percent.

Two additional psychophysical controls were employed to show that the monkey was faithfully reporting his perception during rivalry. First, we compared distribution of dominance-phase durations to that for those obtained from human beings under identical stimulus conditions. The normalized distribution of monkeys' phases (panel B) resembled that obtained from a human observer (panel A), and both were representative of those described previously for both monkey and human subjects (Walker 1975, Myerson, Miezin, and Allman 1981). We got even stronger evidence on

Nikos K. Logothetis and David A. Leopold: Single-Neuron Activity and Visual Perception reliability of the monkeys' reports by studying how interocular contrast differences affected the mean phase duration. During rivalrous stimulation, increasing the stimulus strength in one eye increases the visibility of that stimulus, not by increasing its mean dominance phase, but by decreasing the mean period for which this stimulus remains suppressed (Levelt 1965, Fox and Rasche 1969). The data obtained from the monkey (panel E) show the same relation between stimulus strength and eye dominance as do the human data in this (panel D) and other studies. No random tapping of the levers could possibly yield this type of consistency, nor is it likely that animals or human beings systematically adjust their behavior for different interocular contrasts.

During the behavioral-testing sessions we isolated single neurons in the central representations of the fourth visual area (V4) as well as the border of striate cortex and V2 (V1/V2). As the monkey fixated a small point, each individual cell was evaluated for its orientation selectivity and binocularity by a computer-automated procedure. Specialized glasses worn by the animal produced complete isolation of the right and left monocular images. Rivalry stimuli were constructed based on the preferred attributes of the specific cell, where the preferred attributes of the specific cell, where the preferred orientation was placed in one eye and the orthogonal orientation in the other, whereas nonrivalry stimuli consisted of either the preferred or nonpreferred orientation presented either monocularly or binocularly. During testing, a typical observation period consisted of several nonrivalry periods, each lasting 1 to 5 sec, and one rivalry period, lasting up to 15 sec (Figure 27.4). The monkey responded to orientation changes during the nonrivalry periods and to *perceived* orientation changes during rivalry, and individual neurons in his brain were monitored by standard extracellular recording techniques (see Leopold and Logothetis 1996). Especially interesting were the rivalry periods, during which neurons exhibited diverse responses, and often modulated their activity according to the monkey's perceived stimulus.

Figure 27.5 illustrates four representative examples of the cell types encountered. For each cell, the left and right plots represent the activity averaged over numerous *perceptual* transitions to the preferred and null orientations, respectively. The activity is shown as a function of time, centered on the monkey's lever responses (vertical lines). Roughly one in three neurons that we tested modulated its activity in accord with the perceptual changes. These modulating cells were almost exclusively binocular, and had a higher preponderance in area V4 (38%) than in V1/V2 (18%). Most modulating cells increased their firing rate a fraction of a second before the monkey reported perceiving the cell's preferred orientation. Most often this elevation was temporary, declining to the base rate after several hundred msec (panel A), although for some cells it was sustained significantly longer (panel B). One class of neurons became most active when the nonpreferred stimulus was perceived, and the preferred stimulus was perceptually suppressed (panel C). Finally, many cells in all areas were generally uninfluenced by the animal's perceptual state (panel D).

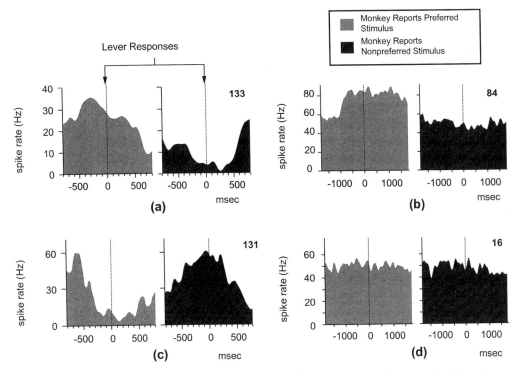

Figure 27.5 Four examples of the various cell types encountered during rivalry. For each pair of plots, the shaded regions correspond to the cell's activity during rivalry around the time of a perceptual transition. The lighter shading represents trials in which the monkey reported a transition to the cell's preferred orientation, and the darker shading to the nonpreferred. The plots are centered on the animal's lever responses (vertical lines) and the activity is shown before and after the response. (A) The commonest class of modulating cell, which increased its firing shortly before the monkey reported seeing a transition to the cell's preferred orientation and decreased before the nonpreferred orientation. (B) A cell whose elevation in activity was sustained as the monkey perceived the preferred orientation. (C) A cell that was representative of some cells in V4 that became more active when the monkey reported seeing the cell's nonpreferred orientation. (D) A nonmodulating cell, whose activity was not influenced by the monkey's perceptual state.

NEURONS AND PERCEPTION

The study described above makes a few new points about both binocular rivalry and perception in general. First, the physiological results—just like those described earlier—are incompatible with the hypothesis that phenomenal suppression during binocular rivalry results from a blockade of information emanating from either eye. Eye-specific inhibition would almost certainly be reflected by decreased activity of monocular neurons (Blake 1989), yet most monocular cells remained entirely unaffected during rivalry suppression. Instead, the highest fraction of perception-related neurons were binocular and encountered in the extrastriate area V4. Moreover, the inferior temporal cortex appears to contain and even higher fraction of modulating cells when rivalry is initiated between faces or other complex images (Sheinberg, Leopold, and Logothetis 1995).

Second, it is interesting, though not entirely unexpected (given the responses in the anesthetized preparation), that neural activity in visual cortex does not always predict awareness of a visual stimulus. Although some neurons appear to modulate their activity in perfect correlation with the animal's changing perception, many others continue firing whether or not the stimulus is perceived. It will be greatly interesting to determine whether the different response properties of the reponse-modulating neurons are in any way correlated with the anatomical location and connectivity patterns (Crick and Koch 1995). Unpublished observations (records of electrode position during recording, NKL) suggested that many of the modulating neurons in the middle visual area, MT, are in deep cortical layers. No histological data are currently available though, and localizing individual recording sites with high precision in the alert-monkey preparation will not be a trivial task.

Finally, the data presented here suggest (agreeing with a number of studies on the physiology of visual attention; for a review see Desimone and Duncan 1995) a prominent role for early extrastriate areas in image segmentation and grouping. These areas appear to have neurons that respond during perception but also during suppression of the stimulus, and therefore appear to have the entire neural substrate of a system of reciprocal inhibition, explaining the many characteristics of rivalry. They also have neurons, whose response depends on the task requirements, and whose activity is modulated by selective attention. Active inhibition, influences of attention, and selectivity of responses to complex two-dimensional patterns all strongly suggest an important part for early visual cortex in perceptual organization.

In the introduction we ask which cells code for the hodgepodge of visual elements and which relate directly to our knowledge of familiar objects. Obviously our experiments do not purport to answer this question, nor did we expect to understand perceptual organization in a few experiments or by studying only single cells and examining their average rate of firing. The study of dynamic interactions among neurons within and between areas (for review, see Singer and Gray 1995) will be greatly important for understanding image segmentation, as will be identifying different types of modulating neurons and their connectivity. Combining such techniques in experiments with alert, trained animals using stimuli that instigate perceptual multistability may help us gain insight into the neural processes that underlie the conscious perception of a visual stimulus.

REFERENCES

Blake, R. 1989. A neural theory of binocular rivalry. *Psychological Review* 96:145–167.

Borsellino, A., A. De Marco, A. Allazetta, S. Rinesi, and B. Bartolini. 1972. Reversal time distribution in the perception of visual ambiguous stimuli. *Kybernetik* 10:139–144.

Campbell, F., and E. Howell. 1972. Monocular alternation: A method for the investigation of pattern vision. *Journal of Physiology* (London) 225:19P–21P.

Crick, F., and C. Koch. 1995. Are we aware of neural activity in primary visual cortex? *Nature* 375:121–123.

Desimone, R., and J. Duncan. 1995. Neural mechanisms of selective visual attention. *Annual Review of Neuroscience* 18:193–222.

DuTour, M. 1760. Discussion d'une question d'optique (Discussion on a question of (optics)). Mémoires de Mathématique et de Physique Présentés par Divers Savants. Paris: Académie des Sciences.

Fox, R., and J. Herrmann. 1967. Stochastic properties of binocular rivalry alternations. *Perception & Psychophysics* 2:432–436.

Fox, R., and F. Rasche. 1969. Binocular rivalry and reciprocal inhibition. *Perception & Psychophysics* 5:215–217.

Lathrop, R. 1966. First-order response dependencies at a differential brightness threshold. *Journal of Experimental Psychology*. 72:120–124.

Leopold, D., and N. Logothetis. 1996. Activity changes in early visual cortex reflect monkeys' percepts during binocular rivalry. *Nature* 379:549–553.

Levelt, W. 1965. *On Binocular Rivalry*. Assen: Royal VanGorcum.

Logothetis, N., D. Leopold, and D. Sheinberg. 1996. What is rivalling during binocular rivalry? *Nature* 380:621–624.

Myerson, J., F. Miezin, and J. Allman. 1981. Binocular rivalry in Macaque monkeys and humans: A comparative study in perception. *Behav. Anal. Lett.* 1:149–159.

Sheinberg, D., D. Leopold, and N. Logothetis. 1995. Effects of binocular rivalry on face cells activity in monkey temporal cortex. *Society for Neuroscience Abstracts* 21:19.

Singer, W., and C. M. Gray. 1995. Visual feature integration and the temporal correlation hypothesis. *Annual Review of Neuroscience* 18:555–586.

Walker, P. 1975. Stochastic properties of binocular rivalry alternations. *Perception & Psychophysics* 18:467–473.

28 Visual Imagery and Visual Perception: The Role of Memory and Conscious Awareness

Alumit Ishai and Dov Sagi

In this chapter we review several aspects of visual imagery, as an example demonstrating interactions among perception, memory, and consciousness.[1] Visual imagery is the natural ability to invent or re-create an experience that resembles the experience of actually perceiving an object or an event, with no retinal input. Visual imagery and perception share several functional properties, and apparently underlying brain structures, too. That cortical structures common to visual imagery and perception are involved is supported by studies employing evoked potentials (Farah, Peronnet, and Gonon 1988), regional cerebral blood flow (Goldenberg et al. 1989), positron emission tomography (PET) (Kosslyn et al. 1993, Kosslyn et al. 1995, Roland et al. 1987, Roland and Gulyas 1995), and functional magnetic resonance imaging (fMRI) (LeBihan et al. 1993). Neuropsychological case studies support the hypothesis that visual imagery and perception have the same neural substrate (Bisiach and Luzzatti 1978, Mehta, Newcombe, and DeHaan 1992), and yet brain-damaged patients demonstrate double dissociation between imagery and perception, possibly because visual areas subserving visual imagery are a subset of those in visual perception (Behrmann, Winocur, and Moscovitch 1992, Jankowiak et al. 1992). Data indicating activity in early visual areas during visual imagery suggest that identical visual areas subserve both systems (LeBihan et al. 1993, Kosslyn et al. 1995). These areas are not activated during visual imagery in all subjects, however, and are activated mainly by tasks that require high-resolution images (Roland and Gulyas 1994, Sakai and Miyashita 1994).

That visual imagery influences visual perception is controversial, but many studies show that imagery interferes with perceptual processes. An early study by Perky (1910) demonstrated that when subjects were told to imagine looking at an object (such as a banana) on a supposedly blank screen while actually being shown a faint picture of the object, they did not see the object (Perky 1910). Segal and Fusella (1970) found that perceptual sensitivity was maximally reduced when the images modality matched that of the target—it was harder to detect a faint geometric form when imagining a visual scene than when imagining a familiar sound (Segal and Fusella 1970). Craver-Lemley and Reeves (1987) have explored the imagery-induced interference (the so called Perky effect) with a vernier acuity task. Imagery consisting of vertical or horizontal lines affected performance, but only when the image overlapped or was very close to the target (Craver-Lemley and Reeves 1987). Imagery reduces visual acuity by reducing sensitivity—that is, it reduces the target energy in the region of the visual field where the images are located (Craver-Lemley and Reeves 1992).

Can visual imagery facilitate visual perception? Neisser (1976) has proposed that images generally function as perceptual "anticipations"—imagining an object would speed up perception by initiating the appropriate perceptual processes in advance (Neisser 1976). Farah (1985) showed that subjects more accurately detected letters (H or T) when images of the letters matched the targets in both shape and location relative to the control condition, in which detection was performed without imagery (Farah 1985). The facilitation effect, however, was probably due to a spatially localized shift of criterion rather than to a change in sensitivity (Farah 1989). Thus, facilitation may reflect processes other than changes in visual sensitivity. McDermott and Roediger (1994) reported that imagery can promote priming on implicit memory tests. Imagery produced selective facilitation-imagining *pictures* primed picture-fragment identification but not word-fragment completion, whereas imagining *words* primed word-fragment completion but not picture-fragment identification (McDermott and Roediger 1994).

We have recently explored psychophysically the interactions between visual imagery and visual perception, using a lateral masking detection paradigm (Ishai and Sagi 1995, 1997a, 1997b). We review here results showing that imagery-induced facilitation and interference depend on memory: image generation from long-term memory (LTM) interferes with perception, but on short-term memory (STM) tasks, facilitation can be attained. We discuss here the implication for memory representation, and the function of conscious awareness.

SHORT-TERM MEMORY MEDIATES IMAGERY-INDUCED FACILITATION

The psychophysical paradigm was a detection task with a foveal Gabor target flanked by Gabor masks placed at different eccentricities (for a detailed description of the experimental procedure, see Ishai and Sagi 1995, 1997b). Observers were instructed to perform the detection task under three conditions: (1) perception, in which the target was flanked by the masks; (2) control, in which the masks were excluded; and (3) imagery, in which observers were instructed to imagine the previously presented Gabor masks while detecting the isolated target. Each experiment included alternating tasks, either with perception followed by control, or with perception followed by imagery (see Figure 28.1). The results were surprising. As previously reported, the presence of the flanking masks at an optimal distance enhanced detection of the target (Polat and Sagi 1993). As Figure 28.2 shows, in the perception condition a threshold reduction was seen. In the control condition, where no masks were presented, contrast thresholds were slightly higher than the base-

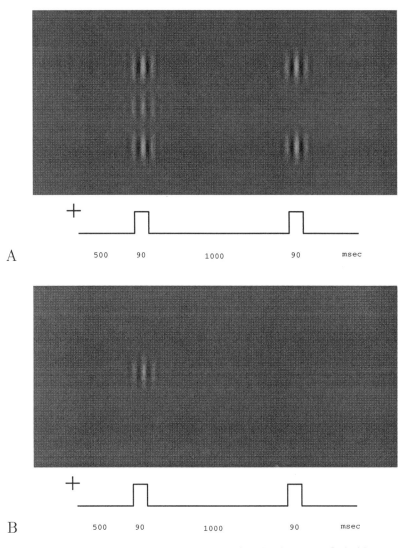

Figure 28.1 Temporal sequence of a trial. (A) A foveal Gabor target flanked by two high-contrast Gabor masks, at a distance of 3λ, used for the perception condition. Observers had to detect the target in the presence of the peripheral masks. (B) An isolated Gabor target used for the control and imagery conditions. In the imagery experiments, observers detected the isolated target while imagining the peripheral masks.

line threshold. In the imagery condition, where observers were imagining the masks, a threshold reduction was obtained (Ishai and Sagi 1995, 1997a). The only difference between control and imagery conditions was the instruction to imagine the previously presented masks (physically, in both conditions the same stimulus was presented—one Gabor target). The imagery instruction had a surprising effect—it reduced target threshold. When observers were aware of the flanking masks in the imagery experiment, they were able to detect the target better, yet when awareness was not required during the control experiments, the perceived masks had no effect on target threshold.

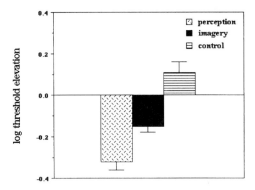

Figure 28.2 Enhancement area, averaged for six observers. The area from 2 to 12λ was computed for each session. The imagery-induced facilitation was 50 percent relative to the perceptual enhancement. In the control condition, contrast threshold was slightly higher than baseline threshold, because no cue appeared on the screen.

The imagery-induced facilitation has characteristics similar to those of the perceptual enhancement and is subserved by stimulus-specific short-term memory (Ishai and Sagi 1995, 1997a). The memory trace is specific to the orientation of the stimulus, as well as to the eye used in the task. When a vertical target is flanked by horizontal masks, no facilitation is obtained in either perception or imagery tasks. Moreover, when the perceptual task is performed with one eye covered[2] and the imagery task is done with the other eye covered, the imagery-induced facilitation disappears (Ishai and Sagi 1995, 1997a). The imagery-induced facilitation is based on recent memory, established a few minutes prior to the imagery task. Introducing a delay period longer than 5 min, between the perceptual and imagery tasks reduces the imagery-induced facilitation (Ishai and Sagi 1995). The need to perform the perceptual task before the imagery task and the stimulus specificity of the effect indicate that short-term memory is involved. Interestingly, this low-level memory system, which stores the images and enables reactivation of quasi-pictorial representations by top-down processes, is exposed only when conscious awareness is required.

LONG-TERM MEMORY MEDIATES IMAGERY-INDUCED INTERFERENCE

Using the lateral masking paradigm, we have found an imagery-induced facilitation, and yet we saw no interference (e.g. Perky effect), even when observers imagined Gabor stimuli on top of the Gabor target (Ishai and Sagi 1995, 1997a). Attempting to attain imagery-induced interference, we introduced a new experimental procedure. Observers had to detect a vertical Gabor target under three conditions: (1) control, (2) imagery of vertical lines, and (3) imagery of horizontal lines. Before the imagery experiments, observers were presented a picture with vertical and horizontal lines. Surprisingly, we saw an orientation-specific interference: imagery of vertical lines

Part V: Vision and Consciousness

elevated target threshold, and yet imagery of horizontal lines had no effect on target threshold (Ishai and Sagi 1997b). Notice again that the only difference between imagery and control conditions was the instruction to the observer. This Perky effect could have been due to the imaginary lines, as opposed to the imaginary Gabor stimuli, or it could have been caused by the experimental procedure—generating line images from LTM rather than STM. To test this hypothesis, we designed further experiments. Observers had to detect a Gabor target with *vertical lines* superimposed on it in the perception condition, to detect an isolated target in the control condition, and to imagine the absent lines in the imagery condition. Each experiment included alternating tasks of perception followed by control or perception followed by imagery. The results show that presence of the lines in the perceptual task increased target threshold, but imagery of the lines did not affect target threshold (Ishai and Sagi 1997b). Thus, when the imaginary lines were generated from STM, not LTM, no interference was seen. But when observer detected a vertical target in the presence of *horizontal* lines in the perception conditions, and were instructed to imagine *vertical* lines in the following imagery task, an elevated threshold was obtained (Ishai and Sagi 1997b). These results indicate interaction between STM and LTM.

It is possible that the lines create an excitatory trace in STM, balancing the inhibitory effect of generating images from LTM. Is this additivity specific for imaginary lines, or is it a general characteristic of visual memory systems? To test the additivity hypothesis, observers performed a detection task of a vertical Gabor target flanked by peripheral Gabor masks at a distance of 3λ. We have previously shown that the optimal target for mask distance created an excitatory trace that subserved the imagery-induced facilitation (Ishai and Sagi 1995, 1997a). In the following imagery task, observers imagined vertical lines. The results were surprising: although the standard enhancement was obtained in the perception condition, imaging vertical lines did not suppress target threshold, although the task required image generation from LTM (Ishai and Sagi 1997b).

It seems that indeed some mechanisms for comparing and subtracting present input and representation in LTM are involved—when an excitatory trace is created in STM, the suppressive effect of generating images from LTM is reduced. When the imagery task is based solely on LTM, maximal interference is seen. We summarize results from the imaginary-lines experiments in Figure 28.3. These findings imply interactions between actual inputs and stored representations, which may subserve object recognition. Moreover, the differences between image generation from LTM, as opposed to STM, and the differences between lines and Gabor stimuli, suggest that short-term visual memory maintains low-level descriptions, but long-term visual memory preserves structural descriptions.

SUMMARY

Using alternating tasks in perception followed by control, or perception followed by imagery, we have exposed a low-level memory system that

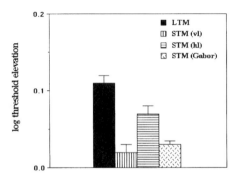

Figure 28.3 Effects of imaginary vertical lines on target threshold of a vertical Gabor signal. Imagery-induced interference was maximal when line images were generated from long-term memory. Excitatory trace in short-term memory (produced by either lines or Gabor stimuli) reduced the effect.

subserves imagery-induced facilitation (Ishai and Sagi 1995, 1997a). In our experiments the only difference between control and imagery conditions was the instruction given to observers. In the control task, detection of an isolated Gabor target was required, but in the imagery task awareness of the previously presented flanking masks was also necessary. To our surprise, we have discovered a stimulus-specific STM trace that enables target threshold to be reduced only in the imagery tasks. The memory trace was accumulated during the perceptual tasks (Ishai and Sagi 1995, 1997a), and yet only the imagery instruction enabled access to this trace. For visual imagery to facilitate visual perception, observers need conscious awareness of the perceptual input.

Imagery-induced interference was obtained when observers generated lines from LTM, but not STM (Ishai and Sagi 1996a). The differences between lines and Gabor stimuli, as well as between image generation from LTM and STM, support the idea of two types of representation in visual memory. In STM tasks the visual system utilizes low-level representations (Gabor), but in LTM tasks structural descriptions of common objects (lines) dominate. These two representations are interfaced at some visual-processing module, perhaps at the so-called visual sketch pad (Baddeley 1986).

We suggest that our data provide psychophysical evidence for involvement of early visual areas in visual imagery, due to low-level features of the effect: orientation specificity, monocularity, and locality (Ishai and Sagi 1995, 1997a). Crick and Koch (1995) hypothesized from macaque monkey neuroanatomy and human psychophysics that no conscious visual awareness lies in the primary visual area V1. They state, however, that these "ideas would not be disproved if it were shown convincingly that (for some people) V1 is activated during visual-imagery tasks. There is no obvious reason why such top-down effect should not reach V1. Such V1 activity would not by itself prove that people are directly aware of it" (Crick and Koch 1995, p. 123). We believe visual imagery can influence low-level perceptual processes when conscious awareness is involved. Further physiological and neuroimaging studies are needed to elucidate the neural correlates of visual awareness.

NOTES

1. In this chapter, consciousness implies the ordinary language sense of the relationship between an observer and a phenomenon—someone is aware of something.

2. The subject's eyes were covered with a blurring lens.

REFERENCES

Baddeley, A. 1986. *Working Memory*. Oxford: Oxford University Press.

Behrmann, M., G. Winocur, and M. Moscovitch. 1992. Dissociation between mental imagery and object recognition in a brain-damaged patient. *Nature* 359:636–637.

Bisiach, E., and C. Luzzatti. 1978. Unilateral neglect of representational space. *Cortex* 17:129–133.

Craver-Lemley, C., and A. Reeves. 1987. Visual imagery selectively reduces vernier acuity. *Perception* 16:599–614.

Craver-Lemley, C., and A. Reeves. 1992. How visual imagery interferes with vision. *Psychological Review* 99:633–649.

Crick, F., and C. Koch. 1995. Are we aware of neural activity in primary visual cortex? *Nature* 375:121–123.

Farah, M. 1985. Psychophysical evidence for a shared representational medium for mental images and percepts. *Journal of Experimental Psychology: General* 114:91–103.

Farah, M. 1989. Mechanisms of imagery-perception interaction. *Journal of Experimental Psychology: Human Perception and Performance* 15:203–211.

Farah, M., F. Peronnet, and M. Gonon. 1988. Electrophysiological evidence for a shared representational medium for visual images and visual percepts. *Journal of Experimental Psychology: General* 117:248–257.

Goldenberg, G., I. Podreka, M. Steiner, K. Willmes, E. Suess, and L. Deecke. 1989. Regional cerebral blood flow patterns in visual imagery. *Neuropsychologia* 27:641–664.

Ishai, A., and D. Sagi. 1995. Common mechanisms of visual imagery and perception. *Science* 268:1772–1774.

Ishai, A., and D. Sagi. 1997a. Visual imagery facilitates visual perception: psychophysical mevidence. *Journal of Cognitive Neuroscience* 9:476–489.

Ishai, A., and D. Sagi. 1997b. Visual imagery: Effects of short- and long-term memory. *Journal of Cognitive Neuroscience* 9:734–742.

Jankowiak, J., M. Kinsbourne, R. Shalev, and D. Bachman. 1992. Preserved visual imagery and categorization in a case of associative visual agnosia. *Journal of Cognitive Neuroscience* 4:119–131.

Kosslyn, S., N. Alpert, W. Thompso. V. Maljkovic, S. Weise, C. Chabris, S. Hamilton, S. Rauch, and F. Buonanno. 1993. Visual mental imagery activates topographically organized visual cortex: PET investigations. *Journal of Cognitive Neuroscience* 5:263–287.

Kosslyn, S., W. Thompson, I. Kim, and N. Alpert. 1995. Topographical representations of mental images in primary visual cortex. *Nature* 378:496–498.

LeBihan, D. L., R. Turner, T. Zeffiro, C. Cuendo, P. Jezzard, and V. Bonnerot. 1993. Activation of human primary visual cortex during visual recall: A magnetic resonance imaging study. *Proceedings of the National Academy of Sciences U.S.A* 90:11,802–11,805.

McDermott, K., and H. Roediger. 1994. Effects of imagery on perceptual implicit memory tests. *Journal of Experimental Psychology: Learning, Memory and Cognition* 20:1379–1390.

Mehta, Z., F. Newcombe, and E. DeHaan. 1992. Selective loss of imagery in a case of visual agnosia. *Neuropsychologia* 30:645–655.

Neisser, U. 1976. *Cognition and Reality*. San Francisco: W. H. Freeman.

Perky, C. 1910. An experimental study of imagination. *American Journal of Psychology* 21:422–452.

Polat, U., and D. Sagi. 1993. Lateral interaction between spatial channels: Suppression and facilitation revealed by lateral masking experiments. *Vision Research* 33:993–999.

Roland, P., L. Eriksson, S. Stone-Elander, and L. Widen. 1987. Does mental activity change the oxidative metabolism of the brain? *Journal of Neuroscience* 7:2373–2389.

Roland, P., and B. Gulyas. 1994. Visual imagery and visual representation. *Trends in Neuroscience* 17:281–287.

Roland, P., and B. Gulyas. 1995. Visual memory, visual imagery, and visual recognition of large field patterns by the human brain: Functional anatomy by positron emission tomography. *Cerebral Cortex* 5:79–93.

Sakai, K. and Y. Miyashita. 1994. Visual imagery: An interaction between memory retrieval and focal attention. *Trends in Neuroscience* 17:287–289.

Segal, S., and V. Fusella. 1970. Influence of imaged pictures and sounds on detection of visual and auditory signals. *Journal of Experimental Psychology* 83:458–464.

29 How Not to Find the Neural Correlate of Consciousness

Ned Block

Two concepts of consciousness that are easy to confuse are access-consciousness (a-consciousness) and phenomenal-consciousness (p-consciousness). Just as water and H_2O are different concepts of the same thing, however, so too the two consciousness concepts may come to the same thing in the brain. We focus in this chapter on the problems that arise when these two concepts are conflated. I argue that John Searle's reasoning about the function of consciousness goes wrong because he conflates the two senses. And Francis Crick and Christof Koch fall afoul of the ambiguity in arguing that visual area V1 is not part of the neural correlate of consciousness. Crick and Koch's work raises issues suggesting that these two concepts of consciousness may have different (though overlapping) neural correlates—despite Crick and Koch's implicit rejection of this idea.

I start with two quotations from Searle. You will see what appears to be a contradiction, and I claim that the appearance of contradiction can be explained if one realizes that he is using different concepts of consciousness. I will not yet explain the two concepts of consciousness; that will come later, after I have presented Searle's contradiction and Crick and Koch's surprising argument.

SEARLE'S APPARENT CONTRADICTION

Searle discusses my claim that there are two concepts of consciousness, arguing that I have confused modes of one kind with two kinds:

There are lots of different degrees of consciousness, but doorknobs, bits of chalk, and shingles are not conscious at all.... These points, it seems to me, are misunderstood by Block. He refers to what he calls an "access sense of consciousness." On my account there is no such sense. I believe that he ... [confuses] what I would call peripheral consciousness or inattentiveness with total unconsciousness. It is true, for example, that when I am driving my car "on automatic pilot" I am not paying much attention to the details of the road and the traffic. *But it is simply not true that I am totally unconscious of these phenomena. If I were, there would be a car crash.* We need therefore to make a distinction between the center of my attention, the focus of my consciousness on the one hand, and the periphery on the other (italics added) (Searle 1990).

Notice that Searle claims that if I became unconscious of the road, the car would crash. Now compare the next argument.

> ... *the epileptic seizure rendered the patient totally unconscious,* yet the patient continued to exhibit what would normally be called goal-directed behavior.... In all these cases, we have complex forms of apparently goal-directed behavior without any consciousness. Now why could all behavior not be like that? Notice that in the cases, the patients were performing types of actions that were habitual, routine and memorized ... normal, human, conscious behavior has a degree of flexibility and creativity that is absent from the Penfield cases of *the unconscious driver* and the unconscious pianist. Consciousness adds powers of discrimination and flexibility even to memorized routine activities ... one of the evolutionary advantages conferred on us by consciousness is the much greater flexibility, sensitivity, and creativity we derive from being conscious (Searle 1992).

Notice that according to the first quotation, if I were to become unconscious (and therefore unconscious of the road and traffic), my car would crash. But in the second quotation he accepts Penfield's description ("totally unconscious") as applying to the petit mal patient who drives home while having a seizure. Thus we have what looks like a contradiction.

CRICK AND KOCH'S PECULIAR ARGUMENT

I now shift to Crick and Koch's recent article in *Nature* (1995) arguing that V1 is not part of the neural correlate of consciousness (that which they call the NCC). Crick and Koch say that V1 is not part of the NCC because V1 does not directly project to frontal cortex. (They extrapolate (tentatively) from no direct connections being known in macaques to no connections in human beings.) Their reasoning makes use of the premise that part of the function of visual consciousness is to harness visual information to serve direct control of reasoning and decision making that controls behavior. On the hypothesis that the frontal areas are involved in these mental functions, they argue that a necessary condition of inclusion in the NCC is direct projection to frontal areas. Though something seems right about their argument, it has nonetheless puzzled many readers. The puzzle is this: Why could not there be conscious activity in V1 despite its lack of direct connection to frontal cortex? This is Pollen's (1995) worry: "I see no a priori necessity for neurons in perceptual space to communicate directly with those in decision space." The possibility of conscious activity in V1 is especially salient considering Crick and Koch's suggestion that visual consciousness is reverberatory activity in pyramidal cells of the lower layers in the visual cortex involving connections to the thalamus (Crick 1994). One wonders how they have ruled out the possibility that such activity *exists* in V1 despite the lack of direct connection between V1 and frontal cortex. They do not address this possibility at all. The overall air of paradox is deepened by their claim that, "Our hypothesis is thus rather subtle; if it [no direct connection] turns out to be true it [V1 is not part of the NCC] will eventually come to be regarded as completely obvious" (p. 123). But the reader wonders why this statement is true at all, much less obviously true. When such accomplished researchers say such puzzling things, one has to wonder if one is understanding them properly.

I argue that once the two concepts of consciousness are separated, the argument turns out to be trivial on one reading and not clearly compelling on the other reading. That is the critical part of my comment on Crick and Koch, but I have two positive points as well. I argue that nonetheless their conclusion about V1 should be accepted, but for a different reason, one which they implicitly suggest and which deserves to be opened up to public scrutiny. Further, I argue that the considerations they raise suggest that the two concepts of consciousness correspond to different neural correlates despite Crick and Koch's implicit rejection of this idea.

THE TWO CONCEPTS

Phenomenal-consciousness and *access*-consciousness are the two concepts of consciousness (Block 1995). Phenomenal-consciousness is just *experience*; a-consciousness is a kind of direct control. More exactly, a representation is a-conscious if it is poised for direct control of reasoning, reporting, and action.

One way to see the distinction between the two concepts is to consider the possibility of one without the other. Here is an illustration of access without p-consciousness. In Anton's Syndrome, blind patients do not realize that they are blind (though implicit knowledge of blindness can often be elicited). Hartmann, et al. (1991) report a case of "Reverse Anton's Syndrome" in which the patient does not realize that he is *not* really blind. The patient regards himself as blind, and he is at chance at telling whether a room is illuminated or dark. But he has a small preserved island of V1 that allows him to read individual words and recognize faces and facial expressions if they are presented to the upper-right part of the visual field. When asked how he knows the word or the face, he says "it clicks" and denies that he sees the stimuli. No obvious factor in his social situation would favor lying or self-deception. Besides the damage in V1, he has bilateral parietal damage, including damage to the left inferior parietal lobe. Milner and Goodale (1995) have proposed that p-consciousness requires ventral-stream activity plus attention, and that the requisite attention can be blocked by parietal lesions. Perhaps then this is a case of visual access without visual p-consciousness. (Notice that Milner and Goodale's account does not conflict with Crick and Koch's claim that V1 is not part of the NCC if activity in V1 is not the object of attentional processes.)

We see then that a-consciousness without p-consciousness makes sense and may even exist in a limited form. What about the converse, p-consciousness without access? For an illustration at the conceptual level, consider the familiar phenomenon in which we notice that the refrigerator has just gone off. Sometimes we have the feeling that we have been hearing the noise all along, but without noticing it until it went off. One of the many possible explanations illustrates p-consciousness without a-consciousness: Before the refrigerator went off, you had the experience (p-consciousness) of the noise (let us suppose) but insufficient attention was directed toward it to allow direct control of speech, reasoning, or action. There might have been *indirect* control (the volume of your voice increased to compensate for the noise) but not direct control of the sort that happens when a representation is poised for free use as a premise in reasoning and can be freely reported. (It is this free use that characterizes a-consciousness.) This hypothesis includes a period in which one has p-consciousness of the noise without a-consciousness of it. Of course, we have alternative hypotheses, including subtler ones that suggest degrees of access and degrees of phenomenality. One might have a moderate degree of both p-consciousness of and access to the noise at first, then filters might reset the threshold for access, putting the stimulus below the threshold for direct control, until the refrigerator goes off and one notices the change. The degree of p-consciousness and a-consciousness may always match. Although p-consciousness and a-consciousness differ conceptually (as do the concepts of water and H_2O), we do not yet know whether or not they really come to the same thing in the brain.

Once one sees the distinction, one sees many pure uses for both concepts. For example, the Freudian unconscious is *access*-unconscious. A repressed memory of torture in a red room could in principle be a phenomenally vivid image; it is unconscious in the Freudian sense because it comes out in dreams, slips, fleeing from red rooms, and the like rather than in directly controlling behavior. Thus in principle an image can be unconscious in one sense (not poised for access), yet experienced and therefore conscious in another sense (phenomenally).

SEARLE'S CONTRADICTION

Let us go back to Searle's contradiction. You will recall that he says if he were to become unconscious of the details about the road and traffic, the car would crash. "When I am driving my car 'on automatic pilot' I am not paying much attention to the details of the road and the traffic. But it is simply not true that I am totally unconscious of these phenomena. If I were, there would be a car crash." But he also says that Penfield's famous unconscious driver is "totally unconscious" and yet manages to drive home. Notice that no room remains for resolving the contradiction via appeal to the difference between "conscious" and "conscious of." If Penfield's driver is "totally unconscious," then he is not conscious *of* anything. And thus we have a conflict with the idea that if one were to become unconscious of the road and traffic, the car would crash. Can we resolve the contradiction by supposing that what Searle thinks is that *normally* if one were to become unconscious of the road the car would crash, but that the Penfield case is an abnormal exception? Not a likely choice, for Searle's explicit conclusion is that consciousness adds flexibility, creativity, and sensitivity to action—suggesting that he thinks consciousness is simply not necessary to routine activities like driving home.

I think appealing to the access/phenomenal distinction does resolve the contradiction. The resolution is that Searle presupposes that the Penfield petit mal seizure case loses p-consciousness but still has sufficient a-consciousness to drive. But when he says that if he were unconscious of the road the car would crash, he is thinking of losing both p- and a-consciousness—and it is loss of the latter that would make the car crash.

I find that audiences I have talked to about this issue divide roughly evenly. Some use "conscious" to mean p-consciousness—to the extent that they control their uses. Others use "conscious" to mean either a-consciousness or some kind of self-consciousness. But Searle's error shows how easy it is for people to mix the two concepts together, whatever their official stance.

HOW CRICK AND KOCH'S ARGUMENT DEPENDS ON A CONFLATION

Crick and Koch argue that V1 is not part of the neural correlate of consciousness because V1 does not project to frontal cortex. Visual consciousness is used in harnessing visual information for directly guiding reasoning and decision making, and direct projection to frontal cortex is required for such a use. But what concept of consciousness are Crick and Koch deploying? They face a dilemma. If they mean phenomenal-consciousness, then their argument is extremely interesting but unsound: their conclusion is *unjustified*. If they mean a-consciousness, their argument is *trivial*. Let us look at their argument more closely:

1. Neural machinery of visual consciousness harnesses visual information for direct control of reasoning and decision making.

2. Frontal areas subserve these functions.

3. V1 does not project directly to frontal cortex.

4. Therefore, V1 is not part of the neural correlate of consciousness.

Notice that the "direct" in premise 1 is necessary to generate the conclusion. But why should we suppose that there cannot be *some* neural machinery of visual consciousness—V1, for example—that is part of the machinery of control over reasoning and decision making, but only indirectly so? If by "consciousness" we mean *p-consciousness*, there is no such reason, and so premise 1 is unjustified. But suppose we take "consciousness" to mean *a-consciousness*. Then premise 1 is *trivially* true. *Of course* the neural machinery of a-consciousness harnesses visual information for *direct* control because a-consciousness just *is* direct control. But the trivial interpretation of premise 1 trivializes the argument. For to say that *if* V1 does not project directly to areas that control action, *then* V1 is not part of the neural correlate of a-consciousness is to say something that is very like the claim that *if* something is a sleeping pill, then it is dormitive. Once Crick and Koch tell us that V1 is not directly connected to centers of control, nothing is added by saying that V1 is not part of the neural correlate of consciousness in the *access* sense. For an a-conscious representation just *is* one that is poised for direct control of reasoning and decision making.

On this reading, we can understand Crick and Koch's remark about their thesis that "if it [V1 is not directly connected to centers of control] turns out to be true it [V1 is not part of the neural correlate of consciousness] will eventually come to be regarded as completely obvious." On the a-consciousness interpretation, this remark is like saying that if it turns out to be true that barbiturates cause sleep, their dormitivity will eventually come to be regarded as completely obvious.

To avoid misunderstanding, I emphasize that I am not saying that it is a triviality that neurons in V1 are not directly connected to frontal areas. That is an empirical claim, just as it is an empirical claim that barbiturates cause sleep. That which is trivial is that if neurons in V1 are not directly connected to frontal areas, then neurons in V1 are not part of the neural correlate of a-consciousness. Similarly, it is trivial that if barbiturates cause sleep, then they are dormitive.

That was the "a-consciousness" interpretation. Now let us turn to the phenomenal interpretation. On this interpretation, their claim is very significant, but not obviously true. How do we know whether activity in V1 is p-conscious without being a-conscious? As mentioned earlier, Crick and Koch's own hypothesis that p-consciousness is reverberatory activity in the lower cortical layers makes this a real possibility. They can hardly rule out this consequence of their own view by fiat. Crick and Koch (1995) say, "We know of no case in which a person has lost the whole prefrontal and pre-motor cortex, on both sides (including Broca's area), and can still see." But we have two concepts of seeing, just as we have two concepts of consciousness. If it is the phenomenal aspect of seeing that they are talking about, they are ignoring the real possibility that patients who have lost these frontal areas *can* see.

Crick and Koch attempt to justify the "directly" by appeal to representations on the retina. These representations control but not directly; and they are not conscious, either. Apparently, the idea is that if representations do not control directly, then they are not conscious. But this example cuts no ice. Retinal representations have *neither* p- *nor* a-consciousness. Thus they do not address the issue of whether V1 representations might have p- but not a-consciousness.

Crick and Koch therefore face a dilemma: their argument is either not substantive or not compelling.

IS THE POINT VERBAL?

Crick and Koch often seem to have p-consciousness in mind. For example, they orient themselves toward the problem of "a full accounting of the manner in which subjective experience arises from these cerebral processes.... Why do we experience anything at all? What leads to a conscious experience (such as the blueness of blue)? Why are some aspects of subjective experience impossible to convey to other people (in other words, why are they private)?" (1995).

Crick and Koch often use "aware" and "conscious" as synonyms, as Crick does in *The Astonishing Hypothesis*. For example, their thesis in the paper in *Nature* is that V1 is not part of the neural correlate of consciousness and also that V1 is not part of the neural correlate of visual awareness. But sometimes they appear to use "awareness" to *mean* a-consciousness. For example, "All we need to postulate is that, unless a visual area has a direct projection to at least one of [the frontal areas], the activities in that particular visual area will not enter visual *awareness* directly, because the activity of frontal areas is needed to allow a person to report *consciousness*" (p. 122, emphases added). What could "consciousness" mean here? "Consciousness" cannot mean *a*-consciousness, for reporting is a kind of accessing, and we have no issue of *accessing* a-consciousness. Consciousness in the sense in which they mean it here is something that might conceivably exist even if it cannot be reported or otherwise accessed. And consciousness in this sense might exist in V1. Thus when they implicitly acknowledge a distinction between a- and p-consciousness, the possibility of phenomenal without access consciousness looms.

My point is not a verbal one. Whether we use "consciousness" or "p-consciousness," "awareness" or "a-consciousness," the point is that there are two concepts of the phenomenon or phenomena that interest us. We have to acknowledge the possibility in principle that these two concepts pick out different phenomena. Two versus one: that is not a verbal issue.

ARE THE NEURAL CORRELATES OF THE TWO KINDS OF CONSCIOUSNESS DIFFERENT?

Perhaps there is evidence that the neural correlate of p-consciousness is exactly the same as the neural correlate of a-consciousness? The idea that this is a conceptual difference without a real difference would make sense both of much that Crick and Koch say and of much empirical work on consciousness. But paradoxically, the idea that the neural correlates of the two concepts of consciousness coincide is one that Crick and Koch themselves give us reason to *reject*. Their hypothesis about the neural correlate of visual *p*-consciousness is that it is localized in reverberatory circuits involving the thalamus and the lower layers of the visual cortex (Crick 1994). This is a daring and controversial hypothesis. But it entails a much less daring and controversial conclusion: that localization of visual p-consciousness *does not involve the frontal cortex*. Crick and Koch, however, think the neural correlate of *a*-consciousness *does* involve the frontal cortex. Even if they are wrong, it would not be surprising if the brain areas involved in visual control of reasoning and reporting are not exactly the same as those involved in visual phenomenality.

One way for Crick and Koch to respond would be to include the neural correlates of *both* a- and p-consciousness in the "NCC." To see what is wrong with this response, consider an analogy. The first sustained empirical investigation of heat phenomena was conducted by the Florentine Experimenters in the seventeenth century. They did not distinguish between temperature and heat, using one word, roughly translatable as "degree of heat," for both. This failure to make the distinction generated paradoxes. For example, when they measured degree of heat by the test "Will it melt paraffin?" heat source A came out hotter than B, but when they measured degree of heat by how much ice a heat source could melt in a given time, B came out hotter than A (Wiser and Carey 1983). The concept of degree of heat was a *mongrel* concept, one that lumps together things that are very different.

The suggestion that the neural correlate of visual consciousness includes both the frontal lobes *and* the circuits involving the thalamus and the lower layers in the visual cortex would be like an advocate of the Florentine Experimenters' concept of degree of heat saying that the molecular correlate of degree of heat includes both *mean* molecular kinetic energy (temperature) and *total* molecular kinetic energy (heat). The right way to react to the discovery that a concept is a *mongrel*, is to distinguish distinct tracks of scientific investigation corresponding to the distinct concepts, not to lump them together.

Another way for Crick and Koch to react would be to include both the frontal lobes and the circuits involving the thalamus and the lower layers in the visual cortex in the neural correlate of *p*-consciousness. (Koch seems inclined in this direction in correspondence.) But this would be like saying that the molecular correlate of *heat* includes both mean and total molecular kinetic energy. The criteria that Crick and Koch apply in localizing visual p-consciousness are very fine-grained, allowing them to emphasize cortical layers 4, 5, and 6 in the visual areas. For example, they appeal to a difference in those layers between cats that are awake and cats that are in slow-wave sleep, both exposed to the same visual stimuli. No doubt we would find many differences between the sleeping and the waking cats in areas outside the visual cortex. But we would need a very good reason to include any of those other differences in the neural correlate of visual phenomenology as opposed, say, to the nonphenomenal cognitive processing of visual information.

A BETTER REASON FOR NOT INCLUDING V1 IN THE NCC

Though I find fault with one strand in Crick and Koch's reasoning about V1, I think another strand in the chapter does justify the conclusion, but for a reason that it would be good to have out in the open and to distinguish from the reasoning just discussed. (Koch tells me that what I say in this paragraph is close to what they had in mind.) They comment that it is thought that representations in V1 do not exhibit the Land effect (color constancy). But our experience, our p-consciousness, does exhibit the Land effect, or so we would all judge. We should accept the methodological principle: *at this early stage of inquiry*, accept what people say about their own experience. Following this principle and assuming the claim that cells in V1 do not exhibit color constancy is confirmed, then we should accept for the moment that representations in V1 are not on the whole phenomenally conscious. This methodological principle is implicitly accepted throughout Crick's and Koch's work.

An alternative route to the same conclusion would be to assume that the neural correlate of p-consciousness is "part of" the neural correlate of a-consciousness (and so there can be no p- without a-consciousness). Phenomenal consciousness is automatically "broadcasted" in the brain, but perhaps there are other mechanisms for broadcasting. (Blindsight would be a weak example.) Even if the "reverse Anton's syndrome" case turns out to be a-without p-consciousness, then, Crick and Koch's conclusion might still stand. Notice that both reasons given here are *independent of whether or not there is a direct connection between V1 and frontal areas*. However, if a substantial direct link between V1 and frontal areas is found, we would have an interesting riddle—the question of why the color nonconstant information is not a-conscious. One possibility is that nonconstant information from V1 is broadcasted in the brain but "swamped" by color-constant information from higher visual areas. This could be a case of a-consciousness without p-consciousness, but one that would be hard to observe.

The assumption that p-consciousness is part of a-consciousness is very risky empirically. One empirical phenomenon that favors taking p- without a-conscious seriously is that p-consciousness has a finer grain than a-consciousness based on memory representations. For example, normal people can recognize no more than 80 distinct pitches, but it appears that the number of distinct pitch experiences is much greater. This excess is indicated (but not proven) because normal people can *discriminate* 1400 frequencies from one another. There are many more phenomenal experiences than there are concepts of them.

Despite these disagreements, I greatly admire Crick's and Koch's work on consciousness and have written a very positive review of Crick's book (Block 1996). Crick has written, "No longer need one spend time … [enduring] the tedium of philosophers perpetually disagreeing with each other. Consciousness is now mainly a scientific problem (1996)." I think this conceptual issue shows that even if mostly a scientific issue, it is not entirely that. Some value remains in a collaboration between philosophers and scientists on this topic.

ACKNOWLEDGMENTS

This chapter is a substantially revised version of a paper that appeared in *Trends in Neuroscience* 19,2(1996). I am grateful to audiences at the 1996 consciousness conference in Tucson, at the 1996 cognitive-science conference at the University of Sienna, at the University of Oxford, Department of

Experimental Psychology, at Union College Department of Philosophy, and at the Royal Institute of Philosophy. I am also grateful to Susan Carey, Francis Crick, Martin Davies, Christof Koch, David Milner, and to the editor of *Trends in Neuroscience* for comments on a previous draft.

NOTE

1. Reprinted with permission from Elsevier Science Publishers. Originally published in *Trends in Neurosciences* (1996) vol. 19.

REFERENCES

Block, N. 1995. On a confusion about a function of consciousness. *Behavioral and Brain Sciences* 18(2):227–247.

Block, N. 1996. Review of Francis Crick, *The Astonishing Hypothesis, Contemporary Psychology*, May.

Crick, F., and C. Koch. 1995. Are we aware of neural activity in primary visual cortex? *Nature* 375:121–123.

Crick, F. 1994. *The Astonishing Hypothesis*. New York: Scribner.

Crick, F., and C. Koch. 1995. Untitled response to Pollen. *Nature* 377:294–295.

Crick, F. 1996. Visual perception: Rivalry and consciousness. *Nature* 379:485–486.

Crick, F., and C. Koch. 1995. Why neuroscience may be able to explain consciousness. Sidebar in *Scientific American*, Dec. 1995, p. 92.

Hartmann, J. A., Wolz WA, Roeltgen DP, Loverso FL 1991. Denial of visual perception. *Brain and Cognition* 16:29–40.

Milner, A. D., and M. A. Goodale. 1995. *The Visual Brain in Action*. Oxford: Oxford University Press.

Pollen, D. 1995. Cortical areas in visual awareness. *Nature* 377:293–294.

Raffman, D. 1995. On the persistence of phenomenology. In T. Metzinger, ed., *Conscious Experience*. The German publisher is Schöningh, but the English publisher is Imprint Academic Exeter, U.K.

Searle, J. 1992. *The Rediscovery of the Mind*. Cambridge: MIT Press.

Searle, J. 1990. Who is computing with the brain? *Behavioral and Brain Sciences* 13(4):632–634.

Wiser, M., and S. Carey. 1983. When heat and temperature were one. In D. Gentner and A. Stevens, eds., *Mental Models*. Hillsdale, NJ: Lawrence Erlbaum.

30 Speeded Digit Identification under Impaired Perceptual Awareness

Syoichi Iwasaki

Consciousness is a subjective mental state that cannot be directly accessible to external observers. For us to know how another person feels or what kind of internal experience he or she possesses, we must rely on observing some kind of overt responses. Therefore, it is important to know exactly the relationship between overt responses and covert mental states and to distinguish responses more tightly linked to consciousness from those with a relatively weak association (Marcel 1993). In the current state of knowledge it seems unsafe simply to assume that ability to make any overt discriminatory response is direct evidence of conscious identification (see Holender 1986, p. 3).

One way to pursue this correspondence is to deteriorate internal representation and to see what happens to overt responses. For this purpose experimental psychologists have long relied on backward pattern masking. This is a procedure in which a target stimulus is closely followed by a second stimulus called *masker*. Performance is known to deteriorate when the interval between a target and a masker is gradually shortened (usually less than 100 msec). To explain the temporal paradox in this phenomenon, Breitmeyer and Ganz (1976) proposed a transient-sustained interaction theory, in which they explained the phenomenon by resorting to an interaction between two neural channels. According to the theory, the visual system has two functionally distinct channels. One is a slow-conducting, sustained channel that carries information about stimulus identity and the other is a faster transient channel that carries information about stimulus onset. The fast-conducting transient channel, which is triggered by a masker, catches up with the slow-conducting sustained channel, activated by a target, and thereby interrupts transmission of information on this channel.

In 1962, Fehrer and Raab demonstrated, with a metacontrast paradigm (one type of backward masking), that people can detect a masked target as fast as they do under normal viewing conditions. This and several similar findings (Neumann and Klotz 1994, Taylor and McCloskey 1990) are compatible with the Breitmeyer and Ganz theory, for detection of stimulus onset is considered to be based on information carried by the transient channel, which is not interrupted by subsequent masking stimuli. Unlike repeatedly shown normal performance on detection, little is known about the extent to which people can have immediate access to much deeper levels of information under the backward-masking condition. The traditional method for ascertaining unconscious semantic activation is to use indirect indices such as priming (e.g., Marcel 1983) and autonomic activation (Forster and Govier 1978, Von Wright, Anderson, and Stenman 1975). These indirect indices are claimed to be more sensitive to hidden semantic processing than overt discriminatory responses (Marcel 1983). This claim, however has been severely criticized (Cheesman and Merikle 1984, Holender 1986, and Purcell, Stewart, and Stanovich 1983).

In our study, subjects performed a manual-choice reaction-time (RT) task under backward-masking condition. Our everyday experience suggests that we can make an overt discriminatory response when conscious perception is not fully attained or gravely impaired. For example, when making a speedy response, as in a ball game, we often feel that response emission is unconsciously controlled. Likewise, laboratory subjects undergoing a choice reaction-time task often make a spontaneous corrective response after committing an error. These observations suggest that before fully attaining consciousness, processing that is initiated by a signal has already proceeded extensively, sometimes beyond voluntary interruption of overt responses.

METHOD

We performed two experiments with a backward-masking paradigm, in which a briefly presented target (digits 2 to 9) after randomly varying delay periods, was followed by a pair of masking stimuli (a row of three numbers), one for each visual field. A trial was initiated with a beep sound, followed by a fixation field (F) presented for 1.5 sec. Then a digit was flashed (df) for 5 msec randomly either in the left or right visual field. The distance between the fixation mark and the center of the target was 2.9° in visual angle. For both experiments the subject's task was to make an odd–even discrimination, using either left or right index finger, within 1.5 sec. Key assignment was counterbalanced among subjects. Both reaction time and accuracy were recorded. We used five stimulus-onset asynchrony conditions (SOAs, i.e., the interval between onset of a target and that of masking stimuli). In the first experiment, they were 20, 30, 40, 60, and 80 msec.

In the second experiment, the SOAs were −20, 20, 30, 40, and 70 msec. Here, the negative sign means that no target was supplied and the would-be SOA was 20 msec. The no-target condition, in which an empty frame was followed 20 msec later by the masker, was introduced as a baseline condition for measuring zero-level performance. In this experiment, along with manual key pressings the subjects were asked to rate clarity with which they perceived digits ("visibility score") on an analog scale of 0 to 10 immediately after having made a speeded-choice response.

For presenting the stimulus and registering responses we used Iwatsu-Aisel's AV-tachistoscope (IS-701B). This apparatus consisted of a 20-inch monochrome monitor and a controller device. It was designed to present

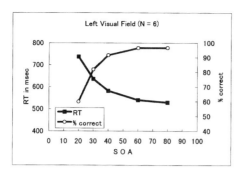

Figure 30.1 RT and accuracy as a function of SOA (left visual field). Performance gardually deteriorated as SOA shortened. Performance in the right visual field was virtually identical.

stimuli with maximum frame rate of 1000 Hz, which allowed us to control stimulus-presentation time with precision of up to 1 msec. Subjects faced the monitor at a distance of 1 m.

Six subjects (2 females and 4 males) including the author participated in experiment 1. Of these, 3 (all male) served again in experiment 2. In both experiments each subject underwent 3000 trials in all, over 10 sessions.

RESULTS

Experiment 1

As may be seen in Figure 30.1, our results differed from those in the detection task used by Fehrer and Raab: the subjects' responses became slower and accuracy declined as SOA was shortened. Two-way ANOVAs (SOA, Visual Field) separately performed on RTs and percentage of correct data confirmed the deterioration with the significant main effect on SOA (F = 45.3 for RT and F = 156.4 for accuracy, both df's = 4/20; both F's are highly significant). Performance in the right visual field tended to be better than that in the left (F = 4.2, $p < 0.1$ for RT and F = 3.2, $p > 0.1$ for accuracy, both df's =, 1/5). Although deterioration in performance was not unexpected, even in the shortest SOA of 20 msec, individual discrimination accuracy remained well above chance (the average scores were 59.8 percent correct for the left visual field and 64.7 percent correct for the right). Debriefing the subjects after the experiment revealed that in this shortest SOA they were barely aware of the digits. Indirect evidence for their claim was that they never showed spontaneous error-correction behavior or voluntarily commented on their errors under the two shortest SOAs (those of 20 and 30 msec), and they often made such confessions when they were tested under the longer SOAs (especially 60 and 80 msec). Maximum percentage of misses—that is, trials in which subjects failed to respond within the limit of 1.5 sec—was less than 5 percent even in the shortest SOA. Therefore it is unlikely that the result was due to the data obtained in the rare trials in which target stimulus happened to escape the effect of masking.

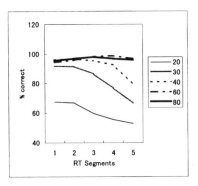

Figure 30.2 Average percentage of correct scores as a function of RT segment (left visual field). For the shortest three SOAs (20, 30, 40 msec) percentage of correct scores showed rapid decline at the slower RT segments.

To see how response latency was related to accuracy, all the successfully completed data including error trials were sorted by reaction time, from fastest to slowest, separately for each SOA and visual-field combination. These data sets were divided into 5 segments, the maximum number of which was 60 trials if no miss occurred, and percentage of correct scores was calculated for each segment. As shown in Figure 30.2, for the three shortest SOAs accuracy declined monotonically with increasing response latency. A three-way ANOVA (RT Segment, Visual Field, and SOA) confirmed this decline with a highly significant main effect of RT Segment (F = 46.3, df = 4/20, $p < 0.01$) and also significant interaction between SOA and RT Segment (F = 14.5, df = 16/80, $p < 0.01$). The finding suggests that reaction time can be used to sift out "good" trials (those in which response was driven by the stimulus) from "bad" ones (those in which response was endogenously driven). One objection to this idea is the possibility that different digits would not be equal in their discriminability. Therefore, the trials in which subjects reacted relatively faster were probably those in which easy-to-discriminate digits happened to be the target.

Experiment 2

The subjects could discriminate no-target trials from those in which a target was presented. This ability was shown by the finding that in each of the three measures (RT, percentage correct, and visibility score) performance of the three subjects was unanimously better even for the shortest SOA condition when a target was presented compared to no target.

Next, to ascertain exactly how they assigned each number to levels of visibility, at the experiment's end the subjects were asked for each number and exactly what they experienced when they used that number. The inquiry revealed that although some discrepancies appeared in the criteria with which they used some of the numbers, for 1 and 2 all the subjects reported that they felt something was presented but they could not discriminate

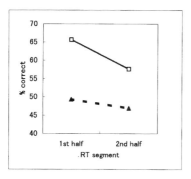

Figure 30.3 Average percentage of correct scores ($N = 3$) for low-visibility (thin solid line) and no-target (dotted line) conditions. Data were sorted by RT and divided into two segments to obtain percentage-correct score for each segment. Here, data from both visual fields were combined.

shapes of the digits. All they could see was a blob. When they felt nothing was presented they used zero. A level of awareness comparable to the present one was reported by some of the blindsight patients who, owing to lesions in occipital cortex had scotomas in the contralateral visual field. For example, the patient in the Weiskrantz et al. study (1974) reported that he sometimes felt something was in his scotoma when a stimulus was presented there, but could not tell what it was. Other patients (Blythe, Kennard, and Ruddock 1987) reported dark shadows in their "blind" fields. Thus even with limited visibility comparable to that of those experienced by the blindsight patients, all the subjects performed better when a target was actually presented than when they had none (Chi-squares were 14.02 for SI, 40.62 for SM, and 2.87 for OK; p's of the first two subjects were far below the conventional level of 0.01 and that of the third subject was 0.1 with df's of 1). Performance of the latter condition was, of course, no better than chance. Furthermore, when the data selected for the low-visibility scores were sorted by RT and then divided into two segments, here too the faster half segment was better in accuracy than the second half when a target was presented. But when they got no target the slope became much flatter (see Figure 30.3). In this respect the results of the three subjects were almost identical.

CONCLUSION

This study demonstrated that subjects can make speeded discriminatory responses to severely masked digits even with minimal awareness of them, suggesting that the manual response may be under direct control of stimulus parameters rather than mediated by consciousness (Marcel 1983, Neumann and Klotz 1994).

REFERENCES

Blythe, I. M., C. Kennard, and K. H. Ruddock. 1987. Residual vision in patients with retrogeniculate lesions of the visual pathways. *Brain* 110:887–905.

Breitmeyer, B. G., and L. Ganz. 1976. Implications of sustained and transient channels for theories of visual pattern masking, saccadic suppression, and information processing. *Psychological Review* 83:1–36.

Cheesman, J., and P.M. Merikle. 1984. Priming with and without awareness. *Perception and Psychophysics* 36:387–395.

Fehrer, E., and D. Raab. 1962. Reaction time to stimuli masked by metacontrast. *Journal of Experimental Psychology* 63:143–147.

Forster, P. M., and E. Govier. 1978. Discrimination without awareness. *Quarterly Journal of Experimental Psychology* 30:282–295.

Holender, D. 1986. Semantic activation without conscious identification in dichotic listening, parafoveal vision, and visual masking: A survey and appraisal. *Behavioral and Brain Sciences* 9:1–66.

Marcel, A. J. 1983. Conscious and unconscious perception: Experiments on visual masking and word recognition. *Cognitive Psychology* 15:197–237.

Marcel, A. J. 1993. Slippage in the unity of consciousness. In G. R. Bock and J. Marsh, eds., *Experimental and Theoretical Studies of Consciousness*. Chichester: John Wiley, pp. 168–186.

Neumann, O., and W. Klotz. 1994. Motor response to nonreportable, masked stimuli: Where is the limit of direct parameter specification? In C. Umilta and M. Moskovitch, eds., *Attention and Performance XV, Conscious and Nonconscious Information Processing*, Oxford: Academic, pp. 123–150.

Purcell, D. G., A. L. Stewart, and K. E. Stanovich. 1983. Another look at semantic priming without awareness. *Perception and Psychophysics* 34:65–71.

Taylor, J. L., and D. I. McCloskey. 1990. Triggering of preprogrammed movements as reactions to masked stimuli. *Journal of Neurophysiology* 63:439–446.

Von Wright, J. M., K. Anderson, and U. Stenman. 1975. Generalization of conditioned GSRs in dichotic listening. In P. C. Rabbit and S. Dornic, eds., *Attention and Performance V*. Oxford: Academic, pp. 194–204.

Weiskrantz, L., E. K. Warrington, M. D. Sanders, and J. Marshall. 1974. Visual capacity in the hemianopic field following a restricted occipital ablation. *Brain* 97:709–728.

31 Fast Dynamics of Visibility of Brief Visual Images: The Perceptual-Retouch Viewpoint

Talis Bachmann

Conscious perception of a visual object involves at least two cognitive events. The first is recognizing or identifying the object in the sense in which it is categorized with its defining characteristics. Categorization presupposes allocating respective specific representation for the object image in the cortical modules specialized for this purpose. (Let us denote the image A, and its specific, identifiable representation A'.) Categorizing is a choice among potentially available alternatives. The other event is the observer's becoming aware of A. Let us name this cognitive event B/A'. Based on conditions which we denote here B and which participate in perceiving the A in ensemble with the activity of A', the A' obtains the quality that allows us to deduce that conscious experience of A is a highly likely event.[1]

Some researchers assume a duality in neurophysiological processes that will enable us to find special mechanisms that could well stand for the equivalents of the activities that are responsible for B and A', respectively (cf. Koch and Crick 1991, Bogen 1995, Block 1995, Llinás 1996, Scheibel 1981, Bachmann 1984, 1994). The most popular choice is to relate B to the functions of the so-called nonspecific thalamus (e.g., Crick 1984, Bachmann 1984, LaBerge 1995). Others are more skeptical or simply more cautious and either reject the dual-process approach (e.g., Dennett this volume, Chapter 7) or assume that B/A' is rather a matter of some sort of widespread brain activity quantitatively accruing without "catastrophic" alternation between conscious and unconscious cognition as a function of the special physiological mechanisms for B (e.g., Greenfield 1994).

I favor the dual-process approach because it offers the possibility of building up a metatheory for perception of brief visual images that deals with quite widely varied psychophysical phenomena within a unitary theoretical framework, and at the same time provides means for falsifiability through psycho(physio)logical experiments (Bachmann 1985, 1994).

TWO TYPES OF BRAIN PROCESSES NECESSARY FOR CONSCIOUS PERCEPTION

Visual images are processed first by the ascending, afferent pathways that traverse the lateral geniculate body and project to primary (occipital) and further cortical centers that are organized in a modular manner. This specific system (SP) is set to encode many types of specific characteristics and features in the image; specialized subsystems are tuned to specific features in the image in parallel (they perform the function of analyzing the image into its elementary subcomponents and higher-order, integrated, complex characteristics). Selectively tuned neural systems for SP characteristics such as orientation, color, form, texture, and spatial frequency have been found (Zeki 1978, van Essen 1979, Livingstone and Hubel 1988, Kandel, Schwartz, and Jessell 1991, Churchland and Sejnowski 1992). This system for analyzing units in SP seems to be necessary and sufficient for exhaustively encoding any visual image A into its specific cortical representation A'. But relevant research has provided more and more converging evidence that SP processes are not sufficient to guarantee subjective awareness of A.

If sensory perceptual data have to become consciously experienced in the form of perceptual images, ascending activation from the so-called nonspecific thalamus and reticular formation (NSP) must participate in elaborating the afferent information that is processed in SP (Jasper et al. 1958, Magoun 1958, Lindsley 1960, Gellhorn 1961, Riklan and Levita 1969, Brazier 1977, Hassler 1978, Scheibel and Scheibel 1967, 1970, Scheibel 1981, Steriade 1981, Crick and Koch 1990, Llinás and Ribary 1993, Bogen 1995, Llinás 1996). According to Kimble (1977), SP provides the content of the conscious perceptual representation (the "what-it-is" of the image), whereas NSP provides necessary background activity or modulations for consciousness of the content of activated SP representations to appear. Thus SP is necessary but insufficient for conscious perception. Its interaction with NSP in a healthy, awake subject, however, seems to constitute the sufficient condition for any A to be represented in awareness as mediated by B/A' (Bachmann 1984, 1994, Baars 1995). At present it is unknown precisely how NSP helps to generate conscious quality of the perceptual information's representation in interaction with cortical SP modules, thus it would be more appropriate to speak about correlates of consciousness instead of causal relationships. (And no one can be sure if this "hard problem" can ever be solved from the natural-science point of view—see, e.g., Cogan 1995, Searle 1994.) We know quite a lot neurophysiologically, though, about interaction between NSP and SP.

Ascending afferents of both SP and NSP systems converge on the same set of cortical neurons. NSP provides primarily presynaptic excitatory influence that helps modulate the activity of the specific representational neurons activated by SP processes that signal the presence of the stimulus image's defining features. A stimulus that is presented to the observer not only causes specific processes of encoding in SP but also evokes NSP activity via the collaterals from ascending subcortical pathways of SP. Thus a bifunctional map of afference is built up (cf., e.g., Keidel 1971, Brazier 1977). Synaptic interaction of SP and NSP at the cortical level is neither rare nor very special: according to Akimoto and Creutzfeldt (cited in Brooks and Jung 1973), two thirds of the cortical neurons have converging afferents from both SP and

NSP. The latter provides mainly facilitatory effect (e.g., Livingstone and Hubel 1980, Scheibel and Scheibel 1967, 1970, Brazier 1977, Singer 1979, Purpura 1970, Steriade 1981).

The long list of the effects that NSP exerts on SP provides converging evidence favoring NSP modulation's decisive influence in creating awareness-related representations of the sensory–perceptual stimuli (consult studies by Bremer 1935, Magoun 1958, Jung 1958, Livingstone and Hubel 1980, Moruzzi and Magoun 1949, Riklan and Levita 1969, Doty 1970, Doty et al. 1973, Gouras and Padmos, cited according to Bridgeman 1980, Gusel'nikov 1976, Somjen 1972, Brooks and Jung 1973, Singer 1979, Worden et al. 1975, Libet 1978, Smirnov, Muchnik, and Shandurina 1978, Newman 1995). These effects and regularities are related to:

1. alternation of sleep and wakefulness.

2. EEG desynchronization.

3. detrimental effects of NSP-located injuries and tumors on patients' consciousness despite intact primary afferents via SP.

4. visual neglect.

5. high correlation between activities of cortical projections of the SP pathways and activity of the afferent neurons in the thalamic NSP.

6. strong NSP dependence of SP activity in total darkness.

7. dependence on NSP stimulation of the number of and size of the cortical area with active visual SP neurons.

8. artificial sensations or "phosphenes" that result from stimulation of the nuclei in NSP thalamus.

9. temporal stratification of the moments at which the sensations appear as dependent on NSP activation.

10. dependence on arousal responses of spatial organization and temporal stability of active visuocortical receptive fields.

11. stability of early cortical responses vis-à-vis variability of late-response components.

12. poorer spatial and temporal resolution of the receptive fields and conduction systems of NSP compared with those of SP.[2]

13. strong resistance to effects of anesthetics in SP neurons and high sensitivity to anesthetics in NSP.[3]

14. universality and nonspecificity of facilitatory effects of NSP modulation in the sense that resultant increase in firing frequency of cortical SP-neurons can spread to almost all classes of neural units—for example, to those responding to diffuse light, motion, combinations of hue and motion, and so on. Thus the NSP modulation is universal and nonspecific for formal characteristics of the stimulus image that are represented by the neural signals in SP, but it can be spatially selective (though with poorer spatial resolution than SP).

In earlier studies I proposed a special psychophysiological construct or operational concept to specify the process that seems to be necessary and decisive in creating conscious quality for perceptual representations of the stimuli (Bachmann 1984, 1985, 1994). I chose the label *perceptual retouch* (PR) for this purpose. By PR I denoted the allotting of conscious quality to perceptual representations that have been or are being formed or reactivated preconsciously in SP. The requirement for any representation A' to become "retouched" up to cognitively transparent, conscious status is modulation of its activity by NSP so that, as a result, the subject is aware of the respective stimulus A and able to report its presence or describe its qualities or both.

PERCEPTUAL-RETOUCH FRAMEWORK

Suppose for each stimulus image S a cortical SP unit D(S) is tuned to S and responds to it if S is exposed in its receptive field. Thus for S1 and S2 we have, respectively, D(S1) and D(S2). D(S) responds to S by a typical EPSP. We also have a thalamic NSP-modulator M that receives collaterals from the ascending SP pathways that feed D(S) upward. M shares receptive field with D(S). Because stimuli S1 and S2 fall within the receptive field of an invariant NSP modulator M(S), both of the respective specific encoding units, D(S1) and D(S2), can be modulated by the common M. The receptive field of M is considerably larger than that of D and nonspecific to formal characteristics of S.

The PR model has several outstanding features: (1) Slower latency of the main portion of the ascending NSP modulation by M to reach cortical SP units D compared to the latency with which EPSPs of D are evoked by the SP processes. This difference in effective time consists of at least 30 to 70 msec. (2) Coarse spatial resolution of the receptive fields of M compared to fine receptive fields of D. (3) Spatially selective mode of the direction of NSP modulation from M to D. These features of the model make it possible for an invariant system of modulation, M, to service alternative D(S1) and D(S2) that carry, respectively, the signals from the mutually different visual images S1 and S2. From the dual-process point of view and relying on features 1 to 3 of the theory, we can state that the slower subprocess within the domain of B (as effected by the NSP modulation) necessary for creating or mediating conscious quality for the specific representation A' (as embodied and exemplified in the primary activity of SP) and evoked by a first stimulus S1 may show its effects on another stimulus S2. In practice then, we must use very brief stimuli and short time intervals between the stimuli to "enter" into the time window where we find SP and NSP processes still temporally dissociated. By using this approach we will be able to analyze conscious perception in its emergence, in microdevelopment.

If two brief, consecutive stimulus images S1 and S2 are exposed to the observer within a common receptive field of M and with a time interval shorter than that which the standard SP plus NSP process normally takes (less than about 100 to 150 msec), then we expect that S2 will be a favored

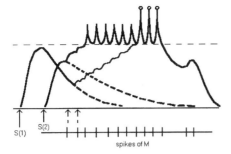

Figure 31.1 EPSPs of the specific cortical units D(S1) and D(S2) in response to successive exposure of stimulus images S1 and S2, respectively. Without the modulatory spikes from M, membrane potentials would have decayed (dashed part of the EPSPs). With modulatory spikes, EPSP levels are enhanced and neurons start firing, or increase their cumulative firing rate, or both. S2 gets advantage both in cumulative frequency of firing and in speed with which its neuron starts firing, because at the moment impulses arrive from M, the EPSP of D(S2) exceeds that of D(S1). The signal-to-noise ratio of the D(S2) activity is higher and, as a result, S2 should be represented in visual awareness more conspicuously or faster or both than S1.

stimulus compared with S1 in conscious perception. It should be favored because the main share of the temporally trailing, excitatory, presynaptic NSP modulation from M which is necessary for creating visible (conscious) qualities for the sensory information, and which was evoked by S1, will be effective only after some delay. At that moment, "fresh" SP signals of S2 arrive and the "older" signals of a very brief, preceding stimulus S1 have already been decayed. In Figure 31.1, this result is expressed by the larger cumulative frequency of the spikes produced by the neuron that encodes S2 compared with the S1 neuron. The other feature of this interaction is that the neuron for S2 starts firing relatively more quickly than the neuron for S1. This circumstance then predicts the speeding up of the subjective moment of S2's conscious perception, because it is exposed after the preceding, proactively employed S1. The basic predictions in the PR theory are thus related to the proactive facilitation effects with brief, rapidly alternated visual stimuli.

EXPERIMENTAL EVIDENCE FAVORING PREDICTIONS BY RETOUCH THEORY

In *mutual masking and metacontrast* we present an observer with two mutually different, but spatially overlapping (mutual masking), or closely or immediately adjacent (metacontrast) visual forms—S1 and S2, both for 10 msec. The SOA between exposures of these stimuli is systematically varied between 0 msec and about 150 msec. The PR theory predicts that with very short SOAs of fewer than 20 to 30 msec, SP representations for S1 and S2 are formed or allocated almost simultaneously and before the process B (from M in NSP) has had enough time to exert any substantial modulatory effect on respective EPSPs of D(S1) and D(S2). When this excitatory modulation arrives, respective EPSP levels are somewhat decayed, but at comparable

Talis Bachmann: Fast Dynamics of Visibility of Brief Visual Images

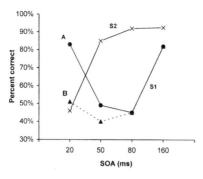

Figure 31.2 Typical functions for efficiency in perception for the brief stimuli that are exposed in rapid succession. In mutual masking, equal, though obscured visibility of S1 and S2 can be observed with shortest SOAs if stimulus intensities are compatible (cf. B). If the intensity of S1 much exceeds that of S2, then S1 will prevail in perception already with short SOAs (cf. A). With intermediate SOAs, S2 prevails in visibility anyway. In metacontrast the typical U-shaped function is obtained for S1 visibility (cf. A).

levels, because neither of them has much time shift compared to the other. As a result the observer will consciously experience the common, integrated visual image of both S1 and S2. In this compound image, neither of the stimuli dominates; their visibility is comparable. In mutual masking where alternative stimuli, S1 and S2, overlap in space, the result will be integrative masking, because it cannot be easy to discriminate one stimulus from the other in this compound image. In Figure 31.2, this relation is expressed in the variant "B," where with the shortest SOA value, recognition functions for S1 and S2 are compatible, but far from the very high level of recognition.

In metacontrast, where stimuli do not overlap in space and thus do not obscure each other when integrated, the target stimulus (S1) is easily visible at short SOAs (cf. variant "A" in Figure 31.2).

With intermediate SOAs (e.g., 40–90 msec), S2 will dominate in conscious perception over S1, although S2 has been exposed only after exposure of S1. We explain this somewhat paradoxical result thus: the B/A' type of modulatory process from M of NSP thalamus which is postulated to be necessary for creating conscious quality for the stimulus representations, and which was evoked by the signals from the preceding S1, begins to elaborate on EPSPs of D(S1) and D(S2) at the moment when the EPSP of D(S1) has been decayed much more than that of D(S2). As a consequence, the latter's firing will provide a higher signal-to-noise ratio for the neural processes that represent S2 (see Figure 31.1). In mutual masking, this result leads to strong predominance by S2 recognition and substantial deprivation of the S1 from the clear conscious representation with intermediate SOAs (see S1 and S2 recognition levels with SOAs of 50 msec and 80 msec in Figure 31.2). In metacontrast tasks in which subjects have to rate clarity of the test (S1) or identify it, intermediate intervals provide the lowest ratings or worst performance in identification (SOAs of 50 msec and 80 msec, variant "A" in Figure 31.2). The target is replaced by mask (S2) in consciousness. With SOAs

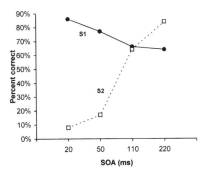

Figure 31.3 Unusual mutual masking functions obtained with parkinsonian patients whose nonspecific thalamus has been preliminarily activated via the chronically implanted electrodes (adapted from Bachmann 1994).

of more than 150 msec, two independent, noninteractive B/A′ processes (i.e., modulation of SP processes by NSP) are executed for two independent stimuli, and both stimuli are clearly visible at different moments in subjective time. The regularities in mutual masking and metacontrast described above have repeatedly been found (e.g., Werner 1935, Bachmann and Allik 1976, Michaels and Turvey 1979, Breitmeyer 1984, Bachmann 1994).

In Figure 31.3, we see results of the mutual-masking study employing patients suffering from Parkinson's disease whose NSP thalamus had been activated intracranially (Bachmann 1994). A qualitatively unusual picture has formed: S1 dominance in perception is strong and we do not find much of a typical pattern of relative S1 and S2 efficiencies where S2 should have clearly dominated. We interpret this result as reflecting either dopaminergic or cholinergic system deficiency or both, or as directly resulting from the NSP stimulation. The latter should support the PR theory because we should expect unusually efficient and fast perception of S1, given the preliminary and strong presynaptic activation from NSP. Recently we have completed a similar experiment with parkinsonian patients who did not belong to this unusual group of stereotactically treated subjects (Bachmann et al. 1996). We found typical mutual masking functions such as those in Figure 31.2. Thus it seems that indeed direct facilitatory activation of NSP is capable of qualitatively changing the psychophysical masking functions in the direction that goes hand in hand with the PR theory.

Proactive enhancement of contrast and speeding-up effect

I have also studied the effect of the preceding brief, spatially overlapping S1 on the contrast ratings of S2 as a function of SOA (Bachmann 1988). The average estimates in the single S2 exposure condition were taken as the baseline (zero-level contrast). The PR theory predicts that at intermediate SOAs, S2 contrast should be enhanced relative to its single-stimulus control condition level. Figure 31.4 displays basic results of that study. They are

Talis Bachmann: Fast Dynamics of Visibility of Brief Visual Images

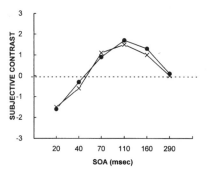

Figure 31.4 Subjective contrast ratings of a brief visual stimulus S2 as a function of SOA between the preceding S1 and succeeding S2. Intermediate SOAs lead to the proactive contrast enhancement. Zero-baseline level on the ordinate refers to the average of the S2 ratings in the conditions in which S2 is exposed alone. (Adapted from Bachmann 1988.)

consistent with the theoretical prediction: with intermediate SOAs, the non-specific modulatory impulses that were evoked by S1 reach presynaptic sites of D(S2) in SP when their EPSP level is maximized, and thus the cumulative frequency of firing of these S2-neurons will be much higher than it would have been in the conditions where modulatory impulses had to be evoked by the single S2 itself. In the latter condition the EPSP level should already have been considerably decayed when the presynaptic modulatory impulses arrive. In Figure 31.1, this condition was modeled by relative numbers of postsynaptic spikes. The more discharges we have in respective representational neurons in SP, the higher the subjective conspicuity of the respective stimulus in the conscious perceptual image.

Using the same theoretical rationale as in discussing masking and contrast enhancement helps to predict that if a stimulus S2 is exposed after the preceding stimulus S1 within optimal SOA, then the relative moment of S2's appearance in conscious awareness (the moment at which it establishes its visibility) will be shifted onto an earlier moment compared to the conditions in which S2 is exposed alone. This *speeding-up effect* is hypothesized because S1 should prepare the NSP modulation ahead of time so that D(S2) units that constitute S2 representation will start firing sooner than they would have without the prime. Now it takes fewer presynaptic inputs to modulate the EPSP up to the level of firing, thus saving some time. In Figure 31.1 we can easily see how much earlier on the time axis the neuron for S2 starts firing compared with the neuron for S1 that had no prime before it. Experimentally all this reasoning can be tested either by procedures in which subjects have to estimate the relative moments at which a visual test stimulus subjectively appears with regard to a sensory reference event—a temporal order judgment (TOJ), such as between visual form and an auditory click—or by the reaction time (RT) procedures. The TOJ method has successfully demonstrated proactive facilitation in studies by Neumann (1982), Bachmann (1989), and Neumann, Esselmann, and Klotz (1993). The facilitative effect of the preceding prime (S1) on the RT to the succeeding test stimulus (S2) was obtained by Bachmann (1994) and Klotz and Wolff (1995). In both of these studies S1 and S2 were either spatially overlapping or adjacent.

The Fröhlich Effect

If a laterally moving visual stimulus appears from behind the opaque screen, it will be visible first not at the objective spatial position where it first appeared (i.e., not at the edge of the occluding screen), but as somewhat shifted in space toward the direction of motion (Fröhlich 1923, Müsseler and Aschersleben 1996). The PR theory is consistent with this effect. The precise spatial position of a moving stimulus that abruptly appeared a moment ago changes during the time it takes for NSP impulses from M to reach respective SP units. The consciousness-related modulation mediates the first moment of visibility so as to represent the stimulus position as advanced in space, in the direction away from the edge.

The Tandem Effect and Visuo-Spatial Attention

The best account of the tandem effect appears in a thorough investigation by Müsseler and Neumann (1992). If a pair of small vertical bars—a "tandem" with interbar horizontal distance d—that is moving laterally behind the opaque screen appears in the aperture (the diameter of which measures D < d) and then disappears behind the other edge of the aperture, then in the newtonian-physics sense it is impossible for both bars to simultaneously occupy positions in the aperture. With optimal speed of motion and optimal interstimulus spatial distance, however, both stimuli will be seen in the window at once. This effect consists of compression in both subjective space and subjective time. The tandem effect can also be explained according to PR theory by the formally equivalent two-process account of SP encoding plus NSP modulation. The S1 that enters the window opens the modulatory process so that the following S2 benefits from it in a way analogous to that of the speeding-up effects, as described earlier. The conscious representation for the trailing S2 will be established relatively faster than respective representation for the leading S1. As a result, compression of subjective space-time occurs relativistically. In conscious representation, the element S2 of the tandem will be seen as shifted a bit more toward the S1 because the delay that is necessary for experiencing it will be shorter and the observer faster at noticing its advance position in space. Thus with S1 we live relatively more "in the past" with our subjective impression and with S2 relatively less.

In the innumerable experimental studies since the seminal work by Eriksen and Collins (1969) it has repeatedly been shown that a spatially selective peripheral pre-cue, if exposed before the target display within the optimal SOA, facilitates target processing (e.g., Eriksen and St. James 1986, Possamaï 1986, Warner, Juola, and Koshino 1990, Müller and Findlay 1988, Nakayama and Mackeben 1989, van der Heijden 1992, Cheal, Lyon, and Gottlob 1994). The facilitation effect in *selective spatial attention* manifests in speeded-up perception of the target or increased sensitivity. We explain the facilitation in a way equivalent to that proposed earlier. The optimal intervals for facilitating attention by physical pre-cues that have been found to take the actual values in the range of 60 to 150 msec satisfy our model.

Another interesting phenomenon is *binocular rivalry*. If two formally incompatible visual images are presented to the observer so that S1 stimulates one retina and S2 the retina in the other eye, then rivalry of the alternative subjective images will be experienced (Levelt 1968, Wolfe 1986). It has been argued that although conscious visibility of the images alternates, specific information about the currently suppressed image is still processed and represented (Dixon 1981, Varela and Singer 1987). We could speculate that if SP processes for the competing stimuli can proceed in parallel and specific input constantly arrives at cortical SP centers for S1 and S2, then NSP modulation from M that is necessary for rendering conscious quality to specific representations should alternate between two competing, specific excitatory constellations. In studies by Goldstein (1970), Anderson, Bechtoldt, and Dunlap (1978), and Wolfe (1983) it is shown that if two dichoptically competing stimuli are brief enough (shorter than, say, 100 msec), the so-called abnormal-fusion phenomenon appears. Two stimuli amalgamate into the composite as in monoptic or binocular conditions in mutual masking where with very short SOAs, NSP modulation is deprived of time for alternative retouch of alternative perceptual objects.

In dealing with the *stroboscopic-motion* phenomenon it is tempting to put forward this hypothesis: The impression of motion between S1 and S2 that we experience in our perceptual awareness (although just two stationary stimuli are successively flashed) is mediated by nonspecific modulation of the SP representations of actually absent but perceptually suggested stimuli that should occupy intermediate positions in space between S1 and S2. Similarity of time-course functions of apparent motion and metacontrast and similar space-time phenomena point toward this possibility. The studies that show close interdependence between motion-analyzing specific systems and the attentional system support this idea (e.g., Sekuler 1995, Stelmach, Herdman, and McNeil 1994, Yantis and Gibson 1994). Attention can considerably modulate the way of perceiving the otherwise invariant motion-inducing displays.

CONCLUSION

Because I have bypassed the "hard problem" and concentrated primarily on the pre-requisites for brief visual signals to achieve conscious visibility, I may risk disappointing those who seek to solve the mystery that is surrounding the very essence of perceptual awareness, and to solve it quickly and for good. On the other hand, for those educated in traditional psychology my approach may seem too physiological, and those educated and practicing in neurophysiology and neurology may find it too speculative and psychophysical. I believe interdisciplinary approaches encompassing subjective and objective in a unitary empirical framework are the strategy that sooner or later will bring us, if not to ultimately resolve the hard problem, then at least to more precisely understand where the explanatory gap opens up.

NOTES

1. Here I have ventured close to two intriguing, very complex philosophical problems—qualiae and intentionality. In this chapter, I avoid deeper involvement with such complexities, seldom straying from psychophysics and neuroscience.

2. This statement also means that two alternative visual stimulus images, say S1 and S2, with nonidentical specific receptive fields, can in principle be serviced by the common modulating unit located in NSP.

3. This picture is consistent with data from Doty et al. (1973), who found that in anesthetized monkeys diencephalic stimulation of NSP did not cause the effect of facilitating SP-responses, whereas in alert monkeys this effect was achieved (with peak latency equal to about 70 to 120 msec).

REFERENCES

Anderson, J. D., H. P. Bechtoldt, and G. L. Dunlap. 1978. Binocular integration in line rivalry, *Bulletin of the Psychonomic Society* 11:399–402.

Averbach, E., and A. S. Coriell. 1961. Short-term memory in vision. *Bell System Technical Journal* 40:309–328.

Baars, B. 1995. Tutorial commentary: Surprisingly small subcortical structures are needed for the *state* of waking consciousness, while cortical projection areas seem to provide perceptual *contents* of consciousness. *Consciousness and Cognition* 4:159–162.

Bachmann, T. 1984. The process of perceptual retouch: Nonspecific afferent activation dynamics in explaining visual masking. *Perception and Psychophysics* 35:69–84.

Bachmann, T. 1985. The process of perceptual retouch (in Russian). *Acta et Commentationes Universitatis Tartuensis* 722:23–60.

Bachmann, T. 1988. Time course of the subjective contrast enhancement for a second stimulus in successively paired above-threshold transient forms: Perceptual retouch instead of forward masking. *Vision Research* 28:1255–1261.

Bachmann, T. 1989. Microgenesis as traced by the transient paired-forms paradigm. *Acta Psychologica* 70:3–17.

Bachmann, T. 1994. *Psychophysiology of Visual Masking: The Fine Structure of Conscious Experience.* Commack, NY: Nova Science Publishers.

Bachmann, T., and J. Allik. 1976. Integration and interruption in the masking of form by form. *Perception* 5:79–97.

Bachmann, T., T. Asser, M. Sarv, P. Taba, E. Lausvee, E. Póder, N. Kahusk, and T. Reitsnik. 1996. The speed of elementary visual recognition operations in Parkinson's disease as measured by the mutual masking method. *Journal of Experimental and Clinical Neuropsychology* (paper submitted).

Block, N. 1995. On a confusion about a function of consciousness. *Behavioral and Brain Sciences* 18:227–287.

Bogen, J. E. 1995. On the neurophysiology of consciousness: I. An overview. *Consciousness and Cognition* 4:52–62.

Bogen, J. E. 1995. On the neurophysiology of consciousness: Part II. Constraining the semantic problem. *Consciousness and Cognition* 4:137–158.

Brazier, M. A. B. 1977. *Electrical Activity of the Nervous System*. London: Pitman.

Breitmeyer, B. G. 1984. *Visual Masking: An Integrative Approach*. Oxford: Clarendon.

Bremer, F. 1935. Cerveau "isolé" et physiologie du sommeil. *Comptes Rendus dela Société. Biologique* 118:1235–1241.

Bridgeman, B. 1980. Temporal response characteristics of cells in monkey striate cortex measured with metacontrast masking and brightness discrimination. *Brain Research* 196:347–364.

Brooks, B., and R. Jung. 1973. Neuronal physiology of the visual cortex. In R. Jung, ed., *Handbook of Sensory Physiology*, vol. VII/3: *Central Processing of Visual Information*. Part B. New York: Springer-Verlag, pp. 325–440.

Cheal, M. L., D. R. Lyon, and L. R. Gottlob. 1994. A framework for understanding the allocation of attention in location-precued discrimination. *Quarterly Journal of Experimental Psychology* 47A:699–739.

Churchland, P. S., and T. J. Sejnowski. 1992. *The Computational Brain*. Cambridge: MIT Press.

Cogan, A. I. 1995. Vision comes to mind. *Perception* 24:811–826.

Crick, F. 1984. Function of the thalamic reticular complex: The searchlight hypothesis. *Proceedings of the National Academy of Sciences* U.S.A. 81:4586–4590.

Crick, F., and C. Koch. 1990. Towards a neurobiological theory of consciousness. *Seminars in Neurosciences* 2:263–275.

Dixon, N. F. 1981. *Preconscious Processing*. Chichester: Wiley.

Doty, R. W. 1970. Modulation of visual input by brain-stem system. In F. A. Young and D. B. Lindsley, eds., *Early Experience and Visual Information Processing in Perceptual and Reading Disorders*. Washington, DC: National Academy of Sciences, pp. 143–150.

Doty, R. W., P. D. Wilson, J. R. Bartlett, and J. Pecci-Saavedra. 1973. Mesencephalic control of lateral geniculate nucleus in primates. I. Electrophysiology. *Experimental Brain Research* 18:189–203.

Eriksen, C. W., and J. D. St. James. 1986. Visual attention within and around the field of focal attention: A zoom lens model. *Perception and Psychophysics* 40:225–240.

Eriksen, C. W., and J. F. Collins. 1969. Temporal course of selective attention. *Journal of Experimental Psychology* 80:254–261.

Fröhlich, F. W. 1923. Über die Messung der Empfindungszeit. *Zeitschrift für Sinnesphysiologie* 54:58–78.

Gellhorn, E. 1961. Cerebral interactions: Simultaneous activation of specific and unspecific systems. In D. E. Scheer, ed., *Electrical Stimulation of the Brain*. Austin: University of Texas, pp. 321–328.

Goldstein, A. G. 1970. Binocular fusion and contour suppression. *Perception and Psychophysics* 7:28–32.

Greenfield, S. A. 1994. *Journey to the Centers of the Mind*. New York: Freeman.

Gusel'nikov, V. I. 1976. *Electrophysiology of the Brain* (in Russian). Moscow: Vysshaya Shkola.

Hassler, R. 1978. Interaction of reticular activating system for vigilance and the truncothalamic and pallidal systems for directing awareness and attention under striatal control. In P. A. Buser and A. Rougeul-Buser, eds., *Cerebral Correlates of Conscious Experience*. Amsterdam: North-Holland, pp. 111–129.

Jasper, H. H., L. D. Proctor, R. S. Knighton, W. C. Noshay, and R. T. Costello, eds. 1958. *Reticular Formation of the Brain*. Boston: Little, Brown.

Jung, R. 1958. Coordination of specific and nonspecific afferent impulses at single neurons of the visual cortex. In H. H. Jasper et al., eds., *Reticular Formation of the Brain*. Boston: Little, Brown, pp. 423–434.

Kandel, E. R., J. H. Schwartz, and T. M. Jessell, eds. 1991. *Principles of Neural Science*. Amsterdam: Elsevier.

Keidel, W. D. 1971. Sinnesphysiologie. Teil I. Allgemeine Sinnes-physiologie. *Visuelles System*. Berlin: Springer-Verlag.

Kimble, D. A. 1977. *Psychology as a Biological Science*. Santa Monica: Goodyear.

Klotz, W., and P. Wolff. 1995. The effect of a masked stimulus on the response to the masking stimulus. *Psychological Research/Psychologische Forschung* 58:92–101.

Koch, C., and F. Crick. 1991. Understanding awareness at the neuronal level. *Behavioral and Brain Sciences* 14:683–685.

LaBerge, D. 1995. *Attentional Processing*. Cambridge: Harvard University Press.

Levelt, W. J. M. 1968. *On Binocular Rivalry*. The Hague: Mouton.

Libet, B. 1978. Neuronal vs. subjective timing for a conscious experience. In P. A. Buser and A. Rougeul-Buser, eds., *Cerebral Correlates of Conscious Experience*. Amsterdam: North-Holland, pp. 69–82.

Lindsley, D. B. 1960. Attention, consciousness, sleep and wakefulness. In H. W. Magoun and V. E. Hall, eds., *Handbook of Physiology. Section I.: Neurophysiology* vol. 3. Washington, DC: American Physiological Society, pp. 1553–1593.

Livingstone, M., and D. Hubel. 1988. Segregation of form, color, movement, and depth: Anatomy, physiology and perception. *Science* 240:740–749.

Livingstone, M. S., and D. H. Hubel. 1980. Evoked responses and spontaneous activity of cells in the visual cortex during waking and slow-wave sleep. *ARVO 1980. Supplement to Investigative Ophthalmology and Visual Science* 223.

Llinás, R. 1996. Content and context in the thalamocortical system: The basis for cognition. Paper presented at Toward a Science of Consciousness 1996. Tucson II, International Conference, April 8–13, Tucson, AZ.

Llinás, R. R., and U. Ribary. 1993. Coherent 40-Hz oscillation characterizes dream state in humans. *Proceedings of the National Academy of Sciences* U.S.A. 90:2078–2081.

Magoun, H. W. 1958. *The Waking Brain*. Springfield: C. C. Thomas.

Michaels, C. F., and M. T. Turvey. 1979. Central sources of visual masking: Indexing structures supporting seeing at a single, brief glance. *Psychological Research* 41:1–61.

Moruzzi, G., and H. W. Magoun. 1949. Brain stem reticular formation and activation of the electroencephalogram. *EEG and Clinical Neurophysiology* 1:455–473.

Müller, H. J., and J. M. Findlay. 1988. The effect of visual attention on peripheral discrimination thresholds in single and multiple element displays. *Acta Psychologica* 69:129–155.

Müsseler, J., and G. Aschersleben. 1996. Localizing the first position of a moving stimulus: The Fröhlich Effect and an attention-shifting explanation. Max Planck Institute for Psychological Research, München, *Report 2*.

Müsseler, J., and O. Neumann. 1992. Apparent distance reduction with moving stimuli (Tandem Effect): Evidence for an attention-shifting model. *Psychological Research/Psychologische Forschung* 54:246–266.

Nakayama, K., and M. Mackeben. 1989. Sustained and transient components of focal visual attention. *Vision Research* 29:1631–1647.

Neumann, O. 1982. *Experimente zum Fehrer-Raab-Effekt und das Wetterwart-Modell der visuellen Maskierung*. Ber. Nr. 24/1982, Psychologische Institut der Ruhr-Universität Bochum, Arbeitseinheit Kognitionspsychologie.

Neumann, O., U. Esselmann, and W. Klotz. 1993. Different effects of visual-spatial attention on response latency and temporal-order judgment. *Psychological Research/Psychologische Forschung* 56:26–34.

Newman, J. 1995. Thalamic contributions to attention and consciousness. *Consciousness and Cognition* 4:172–193.

Paré, D., and R. Llinás. 1995. Conscious and preconscious processes as seen from the standpoint of sleep-waking cycle neurophysiology. *Neuropsychologia* 33:1155–1168.

Possamaï, C. A. 1986. Relationship between inhibition and facilitation following a visual cue. *Acta Psychologica* 61:243–258.

Purpura, D. P. 1970. Operations and processes in thalamic and synaptically related neural subsystems. In F. O. Schmitt, ed., *The Neurosciences. Second Study Program*. New York: Rockefeller University Press, pp. 458–470.

Riklan, M., and E. Levita. 1969. *Subcortical Correlates of Human Behavior: A Psychological Study of Thalamic and Basal Ganglia Surgery*. Baltimore: Williams & Wilkins.

Scheibel, A. B. 1981. The problem of selective attention: A possible structural substrate. In O. Pompeiano and C. Ajmone Marsan, eds., *Brain Mechanisms and Perceptual Awareness*. New York: Raven, pp. 319–326.

Scheibel, M. E., and A. B. Scheibel. 1967. Anatomical basis of attention mechanisms in vertebrate brains. In G. C. Quarton, T. Melnechuk, and F. O. P. Schmitt, eds., *The Neurosciences: A Study Program*. New York: Rockefeller University Press, pp. 577–602.

Scheibel, M. E., and A. B. Scheibel. 1970. Elementary processes in selected thalamic and cortical subsystems—the structural substrates. In F. O. Schmitt, ed., *The Neurosciences: Second Study Program*. New York: Rockefeller University Press, pp. 443–457.

Searle, J. R. 1994. The problem of consciousness. In A. Revonsuo and M. Kamppinen, eds., *Consciousness in Philosophy and Cognitive Neuroscience*. Hove: Erlbaum, pp. 93–104.

Sekuler, R. 1995. Motion perception as a partnership: Exogenous and endogenous contributions. *Current Directions in Psychological Science* 4:43–47.

Singer, W. 1979. Central core control of visual cortex functions. In F. O. Schmitt and F. G. Worden, eds., *The Neurosciences. Fourth Study Program*. Cambridge: MIT Press, pp. 1093–1110.

Singer, W. 1996. Putative functions of temporal correlations in neocortical processing. In C. Koch and J. Davis, eds., *Large Scale Neuronal Theories of the Brain*. Cambridge: MIT Press (in press).

Smirnov, V. M., and T. N. Resnikova. 1985. Artificial stable functional links as a method of research and treatment in the conditions of pathological state (in Russian). *Vestnik Akademii Meditsinskikh Nauk SSSR* 9:18–23.

Smirnov, V. M., L. S. Muchnik, and A. N. Shandurina. 1978. The outline and the functions of the deep structures of the brain (in Russian). In A. A. Smirnov, A. R. Luria, and V. D. Nebylitsyn, eds., *Estestvennonauchnye Osnovy Psikhologii*. Moscow: Pedagogika, pp. 76–108.

Somjen, G. 1972. *Sensory Coding in the Mammalian Nervous System*. New York: Appleton-Century-Crofts.

Stelmach, L. B., C. M. Herdman, and K. R. McNeil. 1994. Attentional modulation of visual processes in motion perception. *Journal of Experimental Psychology: Human Perception and Performance* 20:108–121.

Steriade, M. 1981. Mechanisms underlying cortical activation: Neuronal organization and properties of the midbrain reticular core and intralaminar thalamic nuclei. In O. Pompeiano and C. Ajmone Marsan, eds., *Brain Mechanisms and Perceptual Awareness*. New York: Raven, pp. 327–377.

van der Heijden, A. H. C. 1992. *Selective Attention in Vision*. London: Routledge.

van Essen, D. C. 1979. Visual areas of the mammalian cerebral cortex. *Annual Review of Neuroscience* 2:227–263.

Varela, F. J., and W. Singer. 1987. Neuronal dynamics in the visual corticothalamic pathway revealed through binocular rivalry. *Experimental Brain Research* 66:10–20.

Warner, C. B., J. F. Juola, and H. Koshino. 1990. Voluntary allocation versus automatic capture of visual attention. *Perception and Psychophysics* 48:243–251.

Werner, H. 1935. Studies on contour: I. Qualitative analyses. *American Journal of Psychology* 47:40–64.

Wolfe, J. M. 1983. Influence of spatial frequency, luminance, and duration on binocular rivalry and abnormal fusion of briefly presented dichoptic stimuli. *Perception* 12:447–456.

Wolfe, J. M. 1986. Stereopsis and binocular rivalry. *Psychological Review* 93:269–282.

Worden, F. G., J. P. Swazey, and G. Edelman, eds. 1975. *The Neurosciences: Paths of Discovery*. Cambridge: MIT Press.

Yantis, S., and B. S. Gibson. 1994. Object continuity in apparent motion and attention. *Canadian Journal of Experimental Psychology* 48:182–204.

Zeki, S. M. 1978. Uniformity and diversity of structure and function in rhesus monkey prestriate visual cortex. *Journal of Physiology* 277:273–290.

32 Double-Judgment Psychophysics for Research on Consciousness: Application to Blindsight

Stanley A. Klein

Can subjectivity be studied objectively? Over the past 100 years a field called psychophysics has developed with objective study of subjectivity as its goal. In this chapter, I develop a double-judgment psychophysical methodology that can help clarify experiments on blindsight. Blindsight is interesting for studying consciousness because it provides a tool for separating conscious from unconscious aspects of vision. A person with idealized blindsight acts as a "visual zombie" for certain stimuli, for he or she makes visual discriminations without visual awareness. A number of philosophers and artificial-intelligence researchers believe that if a person acts as if he sees then he does see. They believe performance alone is sufficient to ensure subjective awareness. The existence of individuals with blindsight makes one doubt this belief.

By comparing the neural circuitry of a blindsight observer to that of a sighted observer, one might learn about the circuitry that is specific to visual awareness. The question always remains, however, whether the blindsight findings are an artifact of methodology (Campion, Latto, and Smith 1983). For that reason it is my goal here to discuss psychophysical methodology in detail.

PURE DETECTION (SINGLE-JUDGMENT)

Let us start by considering the task of detecting a dim flash of light. Until about 1960, detection experiments were done by repeatedly presenting a range of stimulus levels and having the observer make a yes–no judgment on detection. The hit rate is the percentage of times the observer says yes to the stimulus. For example, if the observer saw the stimulus on 40 of the 100 times it was presented, then the hit rate would be 40 percent. The hit rate, p_h, at each stimulus strength was measured. Threshold was often defined as the light level for which the observer's hit rate was 50 percent. We will call this threshold the subjective threshold, $Th_{subjective}$.

After 1960, researchers became increasingly worried about "the criterion problem." It was found that different observers used different criteria for saying yes or no. A strict-criterion observer would reserve a yes judgment for stimuli seen with high confidence. An observer with a loose criterion would say yes at the slightest suspicion of signal. Or sometimes a person would just hallucinate or guess that a stimulus was present. A person with a loose criterion could have thresholds below those of someone with a strict criterion and could erroneously be thought of as having greater sensitivity, whereas in reality only the criterion had shifted.

Human performance is typically assessed by measuring the *psychometric function* that specifies percentage correct on some perceptual task as a function of stimulus strength. We focus on the example of detecting a spot of light whose contrast varies from 0 to 4 percent. Suppose the performance is given in Table 32.1.

Table 32.1

Stimulus contrast	0%	1%	2%	3%	4%
Probability correct (p_h)	2.5%	2.5%	16%	50%	84%
z-score	−2	−2	−1	0	1

The z-score (bottom row) is a function of probability correct and is often used in its place. The z-score is closely related to standard deviation and to cumulative normal distributions. The probabilities shown in the middle row were chosen to give simple z-score values.

To get a handle on the criterion (otherwise called the guessing or response-bias problem), one needs to measure the guessing rate (false-alarm rate), p_f, the percentage of times the observer said yes to a blank stimulus. In the example in Table 32.1, $p_f = 2.5$ percent because in the blank-field example the stimulus has 0 contrast. Two types of correction for guessing are commonly used:

1. the high-threshold correction

$$P = (p_h - p_f)/(1 - p_f) \qquad (32.1)$$

This formula is obtained by requiring P to equal zero when the blank stimulus is presented ($p_h = p_f$) and to equal unity when the hit rate is 100 percent correct ($p_h = 1$).

2. the signal-detection correction.

$$d' = z_h - z_f \qquad (32.2)$$

where z_f and z_h are the z-scores for the false alarms and hits. The left side of equation (32.2), called d', is a measure of detectability that is relatively insensitive to response bias. It is common to call the contrast producing $d' = 1$, the objective threshold, $Th_{objective}$. Given equation (32.2), this threshold occurs at the point where $z_h = z_f + 1$. The beauty in this definition of threshold is its relative independence of the subject's criterion (false-alarm rate).

In a typical pre-1960 experiment, the experimenters tried to keep the false-alarm rate very low. Suppose the hit rate was 50 percent and the false-alarm

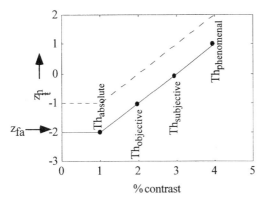

Figure 32.1 A possible psychometric function (transducer function) for a typical detection experiment.

rate was 0 percent. Then the d' would have a tremendous uncertainty because the false-alarm z-score would be poorly estimated. To establish a reliable false-alarm rate, modern psychophysicists attempt to get false-alarm rates greater than 10 percent. Unfortunately, in most clinical studies, including those on blindsight, it is rare to find the false-alarm rate measured accurately.

SUBJECTIVE AND OBJECTIVE THRESHOLDS

Figure 32.1 shows a possible psychometric function (also often called the transducer function) for a typical detection experiment. Figure 32.1 shows the hit rate (shown here as the z-score of the hit rate in Table 32.1) versus the stimulus strength. We chose a psychometric function with the shape shown both for simplicity in discussion and also because it is fairly realistic. Between 0 and 1 percent contrast we assume a dead zone in which the stimulus strength has no effect on the hit rate. Above 1 percent contrast we assume the psychometric function is linear, whereby for every 1 percent increase in contrast the z-score increases by 1 unit. The solid line shows the case in which the observer adopts a false-alarm rate of 2.5 percent (a z-score of $z_f = -2$). We indicate four possible definitions for *threshold*:

$Th_\text{absolute} = 1$ percent is the contrast that marks the transition from the "dead zone" (flat region) to the linear zone. Recent experiments in my laboratory in collaboration with Christopher Tyler and Tina Beard indicate that the psychometric-function shape shown in Figure 32.1 is quite close to the actual shape except that the transition is not as sharp as depicted. This definition of threshold is rarely adopted because the sharpness of the kink at 1 percent contrast depends on experimental conditions.

$Th_\text{objective} = 2$ percent is the contrast where $z_h = z_f + 1$. This is the signal-detection definition of threshold corresponding to $d' = 1$ (see discussion with equation 32.2). For the present example this hit rate would be $z_h = -1$

Stanley A. Klein: Double-Judgment Psychophysics for Research on Consciousness (corresponding to 16 percent correct) because the false-alarm z-score is $z_f = -2$.

$Th_{\text{subjective}} = 3$ percent is the contrast that marks the point where the hit rate is $p_h = 50$ percent corresponding to $z_h = 0$. This is the point that had been called threshold in pre–signal-detection days. It seemed natural to call threshold the point at which one sees the stimulus 50 percent of the time. For the psychometric function shown in Figure 32.1, the objective threshold is $2/3$ the subjective threshold.

$Th_{\text{phenomenal}} = 4$ percent. Here we are inventing a concept that may be relevant to blindsight. This would be the contrast at which the observer begins to have distinct visual subjective awareness of the stimulus. In normal observers it is expected that the phenomenal threshold will equal the subjective threshold. As we will discuss, blindsight observers might use nonvisual cues to set a subjective threshold that is below the phenomenal visual threshold.

The dashed curve in Figure 32.1 is similar to the solid curve except that it is displaced upward by one unit. This displacement is produced by having the observer adopt a looser criterion so that the false-alarm rate is increased from $z_{fa} = -2$ to -1 (probabilities of 2.5 percent and 16 percent). Here the subjective threshold has moved down from 3 percent to 2 percent, to equal the objective threshold. If the observer had instead chosen a stricter criterion, then the psychometric function would have been shifted downward, increasing the subjective threshold and widening the gap between the subjective and objective thresholds. Notice that as the criterion changes the subjective threshold changes, but the objective threshold stays the same because we are assuming the psychometric function keeps the same shape and just moves vertically. This is called the equal-variance assumption.

DETECTION AND IDENTIFICATION (DOUBLE-JUDGMENT)

We now turn to blindsight. An observer with blindsight claims to be blind but is still able to make forced-choice identification judgments. Typically these individuals have lost part of their visual cortex, but as we will discuss, blindsight effects can also be found in normal individuals.

Consider this task—not only detecting a spot of light but also discriminating its position. On one third of the trials we present a spot in position $P1$, on one third of them in position $P2$, and on the remaining third neither spot is presented. We ask the observer to make a yes–no detection decision and also a $P1$–$P2$ location judgment, even when the observer claimed not to see the spot. Let us examine how five types of observers might respond:

The numbers in each row are the four categories of possible responses, where we have presented 200 trials of each condition for 600 total. When doing this type of detection-identification experiment, many trials are needed to have sufficient responses in all the response categories. To clarify

Table 32.2

	"No" responses		"Yes" responses			d' values		
	$N - P1$	$N - P2$	$Y - P1$	$Y - P2$	Total	d_D	d_{In}	d_{Iy}
1. Blind observer								
P1 stimulus	84	84	16	16	200			
P2 stimulus	84	84	16	16	200	0	0	0
Blank stimulus	84	84	16	16	200			
2. High-threshold observer (guesses if no detection)								
P1 stimulus	50	50	84	16	200			
P2 stimulus	50	50	16	84	200	1	0	2
Blank stimulus	84	84	16	16	200			
3. Signal-detection (equal-variance) observer								
P1 stimulus	84	16	84	16	200			
P2 stimulus	16	84	16	84	200	1	2	2
Blank stimulus	84	84	16	16	200			
4. Idealized blindsight observer (not using detection information)								
P1 stimulus	141	27	27	5	200			
P2 stimulus	27	141	5	27	200	0	2	2
Blank stimulus	84	84	16	16	200			
5. Observer 3 again, with a different criterion								
P1 stimulus	141	27	27	5	200			
P2 stimulus	27	141	5	27	200	1	2	2
Blank stimulus	97	98	2	3	200			

the meaning of the table, consider observer 5. He was shown the stimulus in the P1 location 200 times. This observer correctly identified the position on 141 of the 168 times that he claimed not to see the stimulus. That could be considered a striking case of blindsight. Here is how we calculate the last three columns. The detection d', d_D is based on equation 32.2, where the hit rate is based on the responses to either the P1 or P2 stimulus (they are symmetric in each of the five observers in the table) and the false-alarm rate is based on responses to the blank stimulus. One ignores the P1–P2 identification judgment when calculating d_D. The identification d', d_I is shown in the rightmost two columns. It is calculated separately for the yes responses and no responses. Consider, for example, d_{Iy} for observer 2. On the yes responses, he had 84 percent correct ($z = +1$) on the P1 judgment and 84 percent correct ($z = +1$) on the P2 judgment. The identification d', is the sum of the two, giving $d_{Iy} = 2$. For the "no" responses he had only 50 percent correct leading to $d_{In} = 0$, as shown in the next-to-last column. Further details can be found in Klein (1985).

Stanley A. Klein: Double-Judgment Psychophysics for Research on Consciousness

The first observer is truly blind because the response to either light flash is the same as to the blank stimulus. The next two observers say yes in 100 of 200 trials for either the $P1$ or $P2$ stimulus corresponding to a 50 percent hit rate ($z_h = 0$) and say yes in 32 of 200 blank trials, corresponding to a 16 percent false-alarm rate ($z_f = -1$), giving $d_D = z_h - z_f = 1$ (third-to-last column) and so the stimulus is just at the objective detection threshold ($d_D = 1$ is the commonest definition of threshold in signal-detection theory). The 16 percent false-alarm rate corresponds to the dashed curve in Figure 32.1. The second observer does not have blindsight, for he has no position-identification information on the trials with a no response (the trials in which he misses the stimulus and must guess the position). That is, $d_{In} = 0$ in the second-to-last column. This observer follows the predictions of high-threshold theory. The third observer, following the predictions of signal-detection theory, has position information even if the detection signal is below his criterion and he says he doesn't see it. As we will discuss, this observer could be said to have blindsight. The fourth observer is of the type commonly considered an ideal blindsight observer, having no stimulus detection ($d_D = 0$), though making good position-identification judgments, $d_{In} = d_{Iy} = 2$. The last observer is the same as the third except with a different criterion, to make him look more like a typical blindsight observer. We have chosen the criterion and stimulus strength so that observer 5's responses to the stimuli are identical to those of observer 4. On the detection judgment, observer 5 has a false-alarm rate of 2.5 percent, the same as depicted by the solid line. Observer 4 is interesting. He is able to make the $P1$–$P2$ discrimination as well as the normal observer (5), but he did not detect the spot ($d_D = 0$). Two interpretations of observer 4's data are possible:

1. The observer had no awareness of the stimulus—he thought he was pressing the buttons on the response box at random and was surprised by the correct identifications. It turns out that this type of surprising behavior is not too unusual. It is quite common for new normal observers to have blindsight results on experiments. They are often surprised at how well they are doing even when they have no phenomenal awareness of the stimulus. With practice they typically become consciously aware of the proper cue (a cue they have previously been using unconsciously).

2. The observer had no *visual* awareness, but did have awareness either amodally (a feeling) or through a nonvisual modality, such as sensing that his eyes moved to $P1$ or $P2$. The observer could use this nonvisual information for the position judgments, but he decided not to use it for the detection judgment, possibly because he misinterpreted the instructions. Incidentally, eye-care clinicians report that patients are sometimes misdiagnosed as blind in peripheral vision because they misunderstand the clinician's instructions when their peripheral vision is measured. The instructions (fixate on a central dot while paying attention to their periphery) may be confusing.

The measurements leading to Tables 32.1 and 32.2 are usually thought of as objective measurements for which the person is using all available cues.

Thus the results of all observers other than the truly blind observer 1 might be examples of blindsight. Consider observer 2, whom we previously claimed to be devoid of blindsight. When the observer is says "yes, I see it," he may be using nonvisual cues, for although the stimulus is at the objective threshold ($d_D = 1$), he may be below the phenomenal threshold. Thus, even observer 2 might still be lacking visual awareness, the trait of blindsightedness.

For me, the most surprising aspect of actual research on blindsight (as opposed to the idealized gedanken experiment in Table 32.2) is that the methodology is sloppy. The tendency has been that because the subjects are patients one need not use careful psychophysical methods. More research is needed using double-judgment signal-detection methods such as those shown in Tables 32.1 and 32.2. The main signal-detection study on blindsight is that of Stoerig, Hobner, and Poppel (1985). She measured the hit rates for a range of false-alarm rates and found d' values between .1 and .9. These values are above the absolute threshold but below the objective threshold of $d_D = 1$. At these low d' levels we would expect the observer to be phenomenally blind. One does not begin to *see* stimuli until d_D values are 2 and above. It would have been interesting to know if Stoerig's subject could discriminate an X from an O with an identification d_I greater than 1 when the detection d', d_D, was less than 1.

It would be useful to have a blindsight study in which the observer's objective, subjective, and phenomenal detection thresholds were documented (defined above). It is claimed that some observers' phenomenal thresholds are so high that they cannot be measured. It would be nice to do careful experiments on these observers, measuring their identification threshold, d_I above and below their objective and subjective thresholds. To my knowledge this experiment has not yet been done. By sharpening our definitions of the multiple thresholds, we can bring greater clarity to blindsight studies.

BLINDSIGHT IN NORMAL OBSERVERS

One can find blindsight in normal individuals if eye movements are used as the motor response. One robust experiment was carried out by Scott Stevenson at the University of California Berkeley School of Optometry. He presented the same dynamic random dot noise to the observer's two eyes. A relative shift in the patterns to each eye was introduced. The amount of the shift is called the *disparity*. The observer's task was to keep the patterns fused. Stevenson found that the eyes were able to make the proper vertical or horizontal vergence eye movements (the vertical disparity range was limited to about 1°) to keep the two patterns in register. Practiced observers had absolutely no awareness of motion by the pattern or of their eyes for vertical motion, and yet the eyes "knew" how to move appropriately. For vertical greetings and horizontal motions, again the eyes automatically kept the gratings in register, but this time the observers had strong phenomenal awareness of depth corresponding to the disparity. The first case with the vertical disparity is blindsight because the eye-movement system responded correctly without subjective awareness. I like this example because simply rotating the stimulus by 90° turns subjective awareness on and off. The physiologists may be able to trace the circuitry of the vertical and horizontal disparity systems and discover what is special about horizontal disparities that produces phenomenal visual awareness. One possibility is that it is a learned response, whereby the horizontal separation of the eyes causes horizontal disparities to be correlated with depth. If an animal were raised from infancy with periscopes so that the eyes had a vertical optical separation, then the phenomenal awareness might switch, and vertical disparities might lead to phenomenal awareness.

One might not be surprised by Stevenson's result because it is well known that the neural pathway controlling eye movements goes through the superior colliculus subcortical pathway rather than through the V1 cortical pathway (which seems to be the consciousness pathway). It is commonly believed, however, that fusion of dynamic random dot patterns requires V1 processing. That requirement implies that both the consious horizontal disparity and the unconscious vertical disparities are to be found in V1 activity. By studying the differences in the two types of activity one might learn a good deal about the awareness pathways. Rafal et al. (1990) showed that a stimulus in the blind temporal visual field (the right field for the right eye) influences eye movements. These eye movements could be used as a cue to stimulus attributes, even though phenomenal awareness was missing. It is claimed that blindsight individuals can not only move their eyes to targets but also point and give oral reports about target location. This ability might be expected because all output systems are motor systems that might be linked. Reports that have really surprised me say that blindsight individuals can perform visual discriminations such as "X" from "O". Further controlled experiments such as those discussed earlier (with "X" and "O" replacing positions P1 and P2) should be carried out.

DISCUSSION

A number of controversial issues are associated with blindsight. Further discussion is needed among researchers working with blindsight patients and among philosophers who desire to clean up our choice of words for describing the blindsight phenomenon. The recent research of Stoerig and Cowey (1997) and Cowey and Stoerig (1997) does increase one's confidence that blindsight for detection is real and is associated with V1 lesions. That direction of research needs to be extended beyond detection to object discrimination, as discussed in the preceding paragraph.

ACKNOWLEDGMENTS

I thank Scott Slotnick and students in my freshman–sophomore seminar, "Will Robots See?" for their thoughtful comments on this manuscript. This research was partly supported by grant R01 04776 from the National Eye Institute.

REFERENCES

Campion, J., R. Latto, and Y. M. Smith. 1983. Is blindsight due to scattered light, spared cortex and near threshold effects? *Behavioral and Brain Science* 6:423–486.

Cowey, A. and P. Stoerig. 1997. Visual detection in monkeys with blindsight. *Neuropsychologia* 35:929–939.

Klein, S. 1985. Double-judgment psychophysics: Problems and solutions. *Journal of the Ophthalmological Society of America A* 2:1560–1585.

Rafal, R., J. Smith, J. Krantz, A. Cohen, and C. Brennan. 1990. Extrageniculate vision in hemianopic humans: Saccade inhibition by signals in the blind field. *Science* 250:118–121.

Stoerig, P. and A. Cowey. 1997. Blindsight in man and monkey. *Brain*, 120:535–559.

Stoerig, P., M. Hubner, and E. Poppel. 1985. Signal detection analysis of residual vision in a field defect due to a post-geniculate lesion. *Neuropsychologia* 23:289–599.

33 Consciousness and Commentaries

Lawrence Weiskrantz

Some neuropsychological states have a special bearing on the question of consciousness, because with appropriate experimental methods capacities can be revealed that may remain after brain damage, without the patient's awareness. In fact, in every realm of disorders in cognitive achievement, in impairments of perception, recognition memory and recall, language, problem solving, meaning, and motor-skill learning, robust hidden processes can be found. Striking dissociations separate that which can be processed and which aspect of that process is available to awareness (Weiskrantz 1991, 1997). These are sometimes called "implicit processes." Perhaps the most striking and counterintuitive of these is the blindsight phenomenon. It may also be the most promising example for analyzing the brain mechanisms involved, because much background neuroscience is known about of the intact visual system.

RESIDUAL VISUAL CAPACITY VIA EXTRASTRIATE PATHWAYS

The problem started with primate animal research. It is not always appreciated that the eye sends a projection via the optic nerve not only along the well-studied geniculostriate pathway, but over parallel pathways to nine other targets in the brain (Cowey and Stoerig 1991), such as the superior colliculus and the pretectum in the midbrain. The geniculostriate pathway is certainly the largest, but the nongeniculate components are not trivial—they comprise about 150,000 fibers from each eye in the primate. Therefore, when the striate cortical target is removed in monkeys, good visual capacity can still be demonstrated, although of course it is altered both quantitatively and qualitatively in ways that are not our topic here (cf. Weiskrantz 1986 for review).

If cortical input is absent or blockaded, the other nine pathways remain intact. Visual information has various routes by which it can reach not only the midbrain and diencephalon but also, via relays, the remaining visual "association" cortices, V2, V3, . . . , Vx, as well as nonvisual cortex, such as the frontal lobes. Moreover, the lateral geniculate itself does not degenerate absolutely as classically thought, but retains some intralaminar cells that project to the visual association cortex.

The paradox is then that human subjects—whose visual system is highly similar to that of the monkey—report that they are blind after visual-cortex damage in the part of the visual field affected by the damage (typically, after unilateral damage, in the larger part or all of the contralateral half visual field). Why do they not use the remaining nonstriate cortical pathways? The answer gradually came with research starting about 25 years ago. The strategy requires one to abandon the typical approach to visual testing with human beings, which stems from the typical oral instruction (even if not explicitly stated): "Tell me what [or whether] you *see*" (e.g., the smallest letter on the chart, or the color, or the pattern). Rather, a forced-choice discrimination, or a reaching action with a limb, or an eye movement to an event is required even if the event is not seen. The positive correlation of eye movements and the position of stimuli was the method used in the first study by Pöppel, Held, and Frost in 1973. In other words, the testing had to have a basis similar to that actually used in animal visual testing, where we cannot ask the animal to report what it *sees*, but we do ask that it make a discriminative choice and we reward choices selectively. Of course, we normally assume that the animal "sees"—has visual experience—but that is only an assumption.

BLINDSIGHT

The results were a surprise. Some patients could perform quite well on various visual discriminations even though they reported not actually "seeing" the stimuli projected to their "blind" fields. They were "guessing." My colleagues and I (Weiskrantz et al. 1974) dubbed this phenomenon "blindsight." We confirmed the findings by Pöppel et al. (1973), but also studied a number of other approaches and situations. Subjects could reach for stimuli with reasonable accuracy, discriminate their orientation, their rough shape, and even discriminate between colors. Not all patients could do all these tasks, and some could do none. The incidence and variations in blindsight are complex and far from settled; we discuss the subject elsewhere (Weiskrantz 1995, 1996). As in other areas of neuropsychology, much of the research has been focused on intensively studying a few patients who have a relatively pure defect, a reasonably restricted lesion (brain damage does not always conform to the analytical limits that would suit the experimenter), and are also willing to submit to the tens of thousands of testing trials that are entailed. One of these, subject G.Y., has figured in much of the work reported here. He has been studied by several groups in the United Kingdom and the United States and in continental Europe. He was brain-damaged in a road accident more than 30 years ago, when he was 8 years old. The MRI brain scans reveals a lesion including, but also extending somewhat beyond, striate cortex in the left hemisphere. A small remnant of striate cortex also lies at the occipital pole, which could explain why he has an area of intact, normal "macular sparing" of vision in his otherwise blind right field, consisting of a patch of vision 3° to 5° in radius from the fixation point. Needless to say, all testing has been carried on outside the macular-spared region so that the stimuli fall within his "blind" field, and both PET scans (Barbur et al. 1993) and functional MRI imaging (Sahraie et al., 1997) recorded while discriminating visual stimuli in the blind field show *no* excitation in the region corresponding to the macular sparing.

Although the subject never "sees" or experiences in any way stimuli in the affected field, color can be discriminated (e.g., red vs. green) even though the subjects never report any experience of color over thousands of trials (Stoerig and Cowey 1992, Brent, Kennard, and Ruddock 1994), an interesting situation arises with rapidly moving stimuli or stimuli that have sudden onset. With such stimuli, G.Y. (and also D.B., who was the subject of a ten-year study reported in book form—Weiskrantz 1986), report a kind of "feeling" or "awareness" that something has moved, and G.Y. (and D.B., although less reliably) reports being "aware" of the direction of movement if the stimulus moves rapidly enough and over a large enough excursion. This is still not normal "seeing"—G.Y. still says he does not "see" it but "knows" that something has happened. Nevertheless, the subject readily acknowledges conscious awareness of the event.

BLINDSIGHT TYPE 2 VERSUS TYPE 1

The special status afforded in the blind field to rapidly transient events, which may well reflect their importance as danger signals in an evolutionary context, I call blindsight type 2. It has been PET scanned in G.Y. (Barbur et al. 1993) and its spatiotemporal tuning curve has been described for the same subject (Barbur et al. 1994, Weiskrantz et al. 1997). I distinguish it from blindsight type 1, where the subject reports no experience. This mode includes discrimination (typically by "guessing") of color, orientation, reaching, and discrimination of slow movement or gradual onset of stimuli.

These two modes of blindsight have rarely been distinguished and compared by direct study. Indeed, type 2, if veridical, is so much easier to study, both for experimenters and subjects, that it has received most experimental inquiries on G.Y. Pure "guessing" for tens of thousands of trials is no one's favorite flavor, which is why indirect methods of testing for residual function are interesting (Weiskrantz 1990). With our original blindsight subject, D.B., it was the other way around: we had more evidence on type 1 than type 2 because he was confused in the type 2 mode—it gave rise to odd kinds of disturbing "waves," and so we especially arranged conditions typically to be of the type 1 variety (see Weiskrantz 1986).

THE COMMENTARY PARADIGM

A philosophical question tempted us to directly compare type 1 and type 2. The subject emanated from a report by Daniel Dennett based on a misunderstanding. Barbur and I some years ago made a videotape of G.Y. mimicking the various paths of rapid movement by an image projected onto a white screen by a handheld red-laser pointer. With his arm movement, G.Y. can minic these paths, while maintaining good and unchanging visual fixation on a fixation point, with remarkable skill (a schematic summary of his mimicry appears in Weiskrantz 1995). When performing this feat, he also reports "knowing," being "aware" of the movement (but not of actually "seeing" it). Daniel Dennett saw this film at a symposium and reported it in his book (1991). But he also reported that "if a light is *slowly* moved across his scotoma horizontally or vertically and he is prompted to guess "vertical or horizontal," he does extremely well, though denying all consciousness of the motion" (1991, p. 332, italics added). In other words, G.Y. has type 1 blindsight.

Now the problem is that we never actually did that type 1 experiment with G.Y. reported by Dennett. We could not, because it is almost impossible to move a laser pointer slowly and smoothly by hand, and we know that transients are important to control. It may be that we speculated about the outcome in informal discussion, or I may have referred to a rather different but similar published observation on another subject, but somehow this interesting experiment was considered in Dennett's book to have been done even though it had not. The project did seem well worth doing, for two reasons, but it entailed constructing appropriate apparatus (my colleagues John Barbur and Arash Sahraie did the work) that would move a laser image smoothly over many excursions, directions, and speeds.

The first reason we wanted to do the project was that it actually prompted us, indeed forced us—to apply the kind of "commentary-key" paradigm that we suggested some years ago, but never formally effected. If one is trying to decide how well a subject is doing, and also whether he is "aware" or "unaware" of an event, he must be interrogated about that distinction and his performance must be assessed. We must, that is, measure the discrimination and also give him a way of recording whether or not he is aware on each trial. And so we provided G.Y. with *four* response keys. With two of them he was to indicate whether (by guessing if necessary) the laser spot was moving in one direction or another. On the other two keys he was to indicate whether he had any experience of the event. It was repeatedly stressed that he was to press the "no" key only if he had absolutely no experience of any kind of the event, and the "yes" key even if he experienced just a tickle or a feeling. Using this paradigm, therefore, it should be possible to compare performance in the two types of blindsight, and indeed to see whether Dennett was actually prescient.

The answer is that with slow movement, and even more impressively with low contrast, G.Y. could perform very well by guessing the direction in which a laser-pointer image was moving even when he reported *no* awareness (Weiskrantz et al. 1995). The performance can reach 90 percent or better. Dennett was correct, even if only indirectly. The results were published in 1995, but since then we have replicated the findings in two extensive studies, as yet unpublished. (We consider it probably fortunate that the research emanated from using the handheld red laser pointer. Sufficient contrast is not generated on PC monitors, and moreover we have reason to think light at the red end of the spectrum is especially differentially important with G.Y. But these two factors need study in their own right.)

IMAGING

We come to the second reason we were interested in performing this experiment, and indeed it explains why we had to replicate the original findings in a different environment. Brain imaging might allow us to compare type 1 and type 2, and if discriminative performance were matched in the two modes, we might be able to determine whether different patterns of brain activity occur when the subject reports awareness and when he does not, meanwhile performing just as well in the two modes. We wished to do this task with functional MRI, especially because G.Y. recently had PET (and, since then, SPECT) radioactive injections. The visual environment of the brain imager made it necessary to design a battery-operated laser-beam projector and a portable viewing screen, which John Barbur and Arash Sahraie succeeded in doing.

The experiment has been done. Functional MRI has been carried out on G.Y. for stimuli associated with the type 1 and the type 2 blindsight modes—that is, when he is unaware versus when he is aware of the moving spot and its direction in the "blind" field, but is able to perform well each way. The results also allow comparison with his performance when the stimuli are projected into his *intact* half field of vision. The results have recently been published (Sahraie et al., 1997); they indicate that a rather different pattern of brain activity is seen in the two modes. They both share activity ipsilateral to the damage in Brodmann areas 18 and 19 (I prefer this way of describing the areas at this stage, for human V2, V3, and so on are still mainly defined circularly, unlike their definition in primates). Both modes have areas of frontal cortex that are active, but spatially they are quite distinct, and the type 2 mode also overlaps with the frontal area that is active with normal sighted viewing. The most intriguing difference, however, is that in the type 1 (unaware) mode—but only in that mode—the superior colliculus shows elevated activity, combined with activity in contralateral areas 18 and 19. These results must be treated with caution because further analysis is called for. That a different pattern can be found with the two modes, however, is to be expected from the behavioral evidence about a strong hint of a qualitatively different psychophysical function for movement in the two modes (Weiskrantz 1986, ch. 6), and also that double dissociation can be found between the blindsight field and the intact, sighted half field. That areas 18 and 19 remain active in the two modes also demonstrates that such activity, by itself, is not sufficient to differentiate between conscious awareness and the absence of awareness; some other structures are necessary. It may be that areas 18 and 19 are *necessary* for visual functioning, whether or not accompanied by awareness, but earlier important animal experiments (Nakamura and Mishkin 1980) removing all *nonvisual* cortex in the monkey, but leaving visual cortex intact, strongly suggest that visual cortex, including areas 17, 18, 19, and beyond, is not *sufficient* to sustain visual behavior. Just which pattern of activity occurring in association with visual awareness, if any, will turn out to be critical is, of course, greatly interesting.

The vital phrase is "pattern of activity," rather than "awareness center." That frontal lobes light up hardly distinguishes this paradigm from practically all other cognitive and emotional states, including happiness. The frontal lobes are democratic and keen participants in practically any cognitive function the imager pursues. Nor do frontal lesions usually lead to loss of conscious awareness. The superior colliculus may well be critical in sustaining function after visual cortex damage (Mohler and Wurtz 1977), but again it is not a candidate for an awareness center because on their own, lesions there produce only subtle and minor observable changes, and we found superior colliculus activity only in the "unaware" mode—that is, blindsight 1. Areas 18 and 19 may be necessary for awareness, but they are not sufficient for it.

COMMENTARIES AND COMPLETING THE ECLIPSE

Attributing awareness *requires* ability to respond potentially on a commentary key or its equivalent, including of course its verbal equivalent. The commentary is an essential component in the very meaning of awareness. We have no way of determining whether or not a subject is aware, or conversely is in a type 1 blindsight mode, short of asking the subject in a manner that is off-line to the discrimination itself. The commentary must, as a rule, be off-line in any neuropsychological syndromes in which covert processing is contrasted with overt processing. The commentary stage of the processing could involve various patterns of activity well removed from the visual-processing cortices, rather than any one "center." A link connects this approach and that of "higher-order thoughts" as necessary for rendering a thought conscious (as advanced by David Rosenthal 1992). Imaging conscious versus nonconscious states makes it possible to investigate the patterns of activity in such a process.

Finally, because the research started with animals, we may ask whether animals can also be asked an off-line question of the commentary type about their retained capacities. Do monkeys with V1 lesions have blindsight? Cowey and Stoerig (1995) have recently asked monkeys with unilateral V1 lesions whether the visual stimuli they clearly can discriminate in their affected hemifields are treated as *visual* stimuli by the animals. That is, do they classify a visual target as a nonlight, even though they can respond to it? The remarkable answer is that the animals, like a human blindsight subject, treat the visual target as a nonlight. And so, elliptically perhaps, the path is returning to its starting point.

REFERENCES

Barbur, J. L., J. D. G. Watson, R. S. J. Frackowiak, and S. Zeki. 1993. Conscious visual perception without V1. *Brain* 116:1293–1302.

Barbur, J. L., J. A. Harlow, and L. Weiskrantz. 1994. Spatial and temporal response properties of residual vision in a case of hemianopia. *Philosophical Transactions of the Royal Society* B 343:157–166.

Brent, P. J., C. Kennard, and K. H. Ruddock. 1994. Residual color vision in a human hemianope: Spectral responses and colour discrimination. *Proceedings of the Royal Society* B 256:219–225.

Cowey, A., and P. Stoerig. 1991. The neurobiology of blindsight. *Trends in Neuroscience* 29:65–80.

Cowey, A., and P. Stoerig. 1995. Blindsight in monkeys. *Nature* 373:247–249.

Dennett, D. 1991. Consciousness explained. London: Penguin Press.

Mohler, C. W., and R. H. Wurtz. 1977. Role of striate cortex and superior colliculus in visual guidance of saccadic eye movements in monkeys. *Journal of Neurophysiology* 43:74–94.

Nakamura, R. K., and M. Mishkin. 1980. Blindness in monkeys following non-visual cortical lesions. *Brain Research* 188:572–577.

Pöppel, E. R. Held, and D. Frost. 1973. Residual visual function after brain wounds involving the central visual pathways in man. *Nature* 243:295–296.

Rosenthal, D. 1992. Thinking that one thinks. In M. Davies and G. W. Humphreys, eds., *Consciousness, Psychology and Philosophical Essays.* edited by Oxford: Blackwell, pp. 198–223.

Sahraie, A., Weiskrantz, L., Barbur, J. L., Simmons, A., Williams, S. C. R., and Brammer, M. J. 1997. Pattern of neuronal activity associated with conscious and unconscious processing of visual signs. *Proceedings of the National Academy of Science, U.S.A.* 94:9406–9411.

Stoerig, P., and A. Cowey. 1992. Wavelength sensitivity in blindsight. *Brain* 115:425–444.

Weiskrantz, L. 1986. *Blindsight: A Case Study and Implications.* Oxford: Oxford University Press.

Weiskrantz, L. 1990. Outlooks for blindsight: Explicit methodologies for implicit processes. The Ferrier Lecture. *Proceedings of the Royal Society* B 239:247–278.

Weiskrantz, L. 1991. Disconnected awareness for detecting, processing, and remembering in neurological patients. *Journal of the Royal Society of Medicine* 84:466–6470.

Weiskrantz, L. 1995. Blindsight: Not an island unto itself. *Current directions in psychological science* 4:146–151.

Weiskrantz, L. 1996. Blindsight revisited. *Current opinion in neurobiology* 6:215–220.

Weiskrantz, L. 1997. *Consciousness lost and found. A neuropsychological exploration.* Oxford, England: Oxford University Press.

Weiskrantz, L., J. L. Barbur, and A. Sahraie. 1995. Parameters affecting conscious versus unconscious visual discrimination without V1. *Proceedings of the National Academy of Sciences, U.S.A.* 92:6122–6126.

Weiskrantz, L., E. K. Warrington, M. D. Sanders, and J. Marshall. 1974. Visual capacity in the hemianopic field following a restricted occipital ablation. *Brain* 97:709–728.

VI Biology, Evolution, and Consciousness

OVERVIEW

As far as we now know, consciousness exists only in living systems; thus, it is possible that consciousness is a particular life process. To come to grips with consciousness, we may have to understand life.

WHAT *IS* LIFE?

Beginning with the discovery of DNA structure and the cracking of its code, we have witnessed a series of revelations in biology. Once-mysterious genes are now tools of the trade and offer new hope for treatment of old and terrible diseases. Cell biomolecules are isolated and analyzed, enzyme cascades manipulated, and membrane components monitored. Drugs are tailored to specific receptors for particular clinical effects, and increasingly invasive techniques reduce cells and living systems to their basic elements. But what life actually *is* remains unknown.

Erwin Schrödinger saw the molecular basis for life as a "strange, aperiodic crystal," repeating and changing its structure as the organism evolves. Allen Watts described life as "a flowing event ... like a flame, or a whirlpool," Thomas Mann as a "rainbow on a waterfall," Ilya Prigogine as a type of dissipative system, Humberto Maturana and Francisco Varela as an "autopoietic," self-sustaining metabolism (Margulis and Sagan 1995). Some suggest nonlinear, self-organizing solitons and coherent phonons in proteins and DNA as examples of basic life; others see in life a quantum process.

If life is a process, is the material in which life operates critical? In the field of artificial life (AL), self-organization is simulated in computers. In the same way that some artificial intelligence (AI) proponents predict that conscious machines will soon be among us, certain AL afficionados foresee life that is based on silicon.

In biology, this mechanistic view stems from Darwinism, which quelled the tide of nineteenth century animism—the view that some vital force (or *elan vital*) permeates living systems. Biologists before Darwin imbued simple unicellular organisms not only with a vital essence, but also attributes of consciousness. Samuel Butler, for example, proposed that innumerable tiny decisions directed the course of evolution, an idea that may be worthy of re-examination. However animism was drowned by Darwinism and DNA as heredity, genetics and nucleotide structure fell prey to scientific method. In a significant revisionist perspective, Lynn Margulis and Dorion Sagan (1995) suggest that an alternative or middle ground may lie between the mechanization of life and the vitalization of matter. They see life operating on a grand, planetary scale, "surfing and sifting" through the universe.

In Chapter 34, primatologists James E. King, Duane Rumbaugh, and E. Sue Savage-Rumbaugh draw parallels between the evolutionary emergence of consciousness and that of learning and language. They cite the work of George Romanes (1888) whose "Comparative Psychology" espoused a mental continuity between animals and humans. Romanes suggested that consciousness first emerged when animals became able to adapt their behavior based on past experiences—that is, when learning was able to overcome reflex responses. Although these criteria place early consciousness at the level of simple coelenterates, the authors focus their attention on mammals, and in particular nonhuman primates. Evidence from brain size, emergent learning, and language suggest a fairly linear progression of mind from apes to humans.

Microbiologist Victor Norris suggests that rudimentary aspects of consciousness exist in simple bacterial cells, which lack the sophisticated cytoskeletons of eukaryotic cells. He argues that self-organizing processes, such as cell division, differentiation, and the origin of life, employ a primitive form of consciousness. Norris considers various possible biomolecular correlates of consciousness at the level of bacteria, such as an emergent property of cell–cell interaction in bacterial colonies, elementary forms of consciousness arising from information, and communication or coherent oscillations at the subcellular level.

In eukaryotic organisms, the cytoskeleton provides movement, sensory perception, separation of chromososmes, and cellular differentiation. Ezio Insinna describes a particular eukaryotic single cell organism, *Euglena gracilis*, with a specialized cytoskeletal (flagellar) photoreceptor. He examines the mechanism for directional photodetection and the capacity for rapid behavioral response. Insinna concludes that classical nonlinear dynamics is capable of explaining cytoskeletal function in these adaptive responses, and that such function was critical in the evolution of consciousness.

In Chapter 37 Stuart Hameroff looks for the emergence of consciousness during the course of evolution and concludes that it coincided with the striking acceleration in the rate of evolution—the Cambrian explosion—that occurred about 540 million years ago. At this time, small urchins, worms, and shellfish had developed nervous systems and specialized cytoskeletal appendages for intelligent adaptive behaviors favoring survival. The emergence of awareness would have been even more advantageous, Hameroff suggests, and it may have caused the explosion because the cytoskeletal complexity consistent with early Cambrian creatures (e.g., hundreds of neurons and 10^9 tubulins in microtubules) matches the requirements for the Penrose-Hameroff Orch OR model.

Whether consciousness emerged early or more recently in the course of evolution, it remains an exclusive feature of living systems. Until proponents of AI show us a conscious computer, the understanding of life looms as the next great problem for consciousness studies.

REFERENCES

Margulis L., and D. Sagan. 1995. *What Is Life?* New York: Simon & Schuster.

Romanes, G. J. 1888. *Animal Intelligence.* New York: D. Appleton.

34 Evolution of Intelligence, Language, and Other Emergent Processes for Consciousness: A Comparative Perspective

James E. King, Duane M. Rumbaugh, and E. Sue Savage-Rumbaugh

Psychologists have held a long fascination with the elusive concept of consciousness. Consciousness is expressed in several ways, such as an ability to recognize and reflect upon oneself, experience intentional states, and possibly recognize those states in others (Dennett 1995, 1996). Another expression of consciousness is an ability to control behavior independently of the constraints and nudges imposed by past experiences and by the immediate stimulus environment. This facet of consciousness, involving independent control of behavior, has unquestionably developed during a long evolutionary time, particularly in mammals.

This chapter proposes the hypothesis that the evolution of consciousness in mammals paralleled the development of independent control of behavior. In other words, as the sophistication of independent control has increased, we assume a corresponding increase in consciousness has occurred. Fortunately, the animal-learning literature during the past 70 years has provided abundant examples of independent control present in diverse phenomena ranging from simple instrumental conditioning in rats to language learning in apes.

ROMANES'S CRITERION OF MIND

George J. Romanes was highly interested in the evolution of intelligence and was a strong proponent of the mental continuity between animals and humans. In fact, Romanes coined the term *comparative psychology*. He stated that adaptive behavior, even if highly complex, was not indicative of mind or consciousness if it was controlled by "particular stimulations" (Romanes 1888). In other words, kineses, taxes, reflexes, and fixed-action patterns, all under direct control of stimuli impinging upon an organism, may occur independently of any manifestation of mind.

Consciousness and mind began to emerge during evolutionary development only when animals became capable of making adaptive adjustments consistent with their own past experiences, what is usually called "learning." Strict application of Romanes's learning criterion therefore imputes a trace of mind and consciousness to animals with as rudimentary a nervous system as that found in coelenterates (Ross 1965).

Persons who are philosophically inclined may strongly disagree with Romanes's liberal, possibly even cavalier, attribution of consciousness to primitive organisms. The utility of Romanes's criterion of consciousness is that it provides a solid, well-defined starting point from which increases in consciousness can be indexed in animals that exceed coelenterates in neurological sophistication.

LEARNING AND THE CAPACITOR MODEL

The simplest form of learning that shows independence from Romanes's particular stimulations is instrumental conditioning, a phenomenon occurring when a behavior is followed by a consequence that either increases or decreases the future likelihood of the behavior. If the consequence increases the probability of the behavior, it is a positive reinforcer; if it decreases the probability, it is a punisher. This statement is Thorndike's (1911) law of effect. The accumulation of reinforcement-based behavior can be likened to the experience-based associations inscribed on John Locke's (1690) *tabula rasa*, or, to use a modern metaphor, the accumulations of electrical charges on a capacitor. The appeal of the law of effect is that it seems to describe human everyday experience. In addition, the law of effect has an obvious evolutionary validity because animals that did not respond appropriately to positive reinforcers and punishers suffered fatally diminished fitness.

The Thorndike-based assumption that response strength increases monotonically with the number of reinforced responses was incorporated into early animal learning theory (e.g., Hull 1943; Guthrie 1952); to many researchers, that theory embodies the heart of behaviorism. Because most of the interesting new phenomena that animal learning research has recently discovered (e.g., Roitblat 1987) entail clear violations of the capacitor model, the theory has been a convenient "straw man" for advocates of the cognitive-like aptitudes of animals. However, the capacitor model provides a baseline against which to assess animals' abilities to adapt in ways independent of strict adherence to the law of effect, an independence that is particularly evident in primates.

EMANCIPATION FROM THE CAPACITOR MODEL OF LEARNING

Evidence of mammalian emancipation from strict control from the law of effect was emerging during the 1930s. For example, Tolman and Honzik (1930) ran a group of rats through a complex maze for ten trials without any food reward at the end. When food was placed in the goal box at the end of the eleventh trial, the rats showed dramatically increased performance on the twelfth trial and committed no more errors than another group of rats that had previously been rewarded after each trial.

This phenomenon is called latent learning and has been interpreted in a variety of ways including rats' presumed talent for purposive behavior (Tolman 1932), and a disposition to remember foraging experiences (Olton,

Collison, and Werz 1977). However, the broader implication of latent learning is that early evidence shows that, even in the rat, learning is best interpreted as acquiring knowledge about related events and that behavior attributed to learning is simply an expression of that knowledge. These related events may include rewards and punishers, but the events do not directly drive learning in the Thorndikian sense.

Conventional reinforcers do not even have to be present for learning to occur. Harlow, Harlow, and Meyer (1950) showed that rhesus monkeys learned an extended sequence of responses to disassemble mechanical puzzles constructed from hasps, hooks, and pins although no food or other external reward was presented after successful solutions. Furthermore, after the monkeys had learned the puzzles, introduction of food impaired performance instead of improving it (Harlow and McLearn 1954). Food-related response impairment was also described by Schiller (1952, 1957), who described how chimpanzees given two sticks joined them together more readily in the absence of food than when food available outside their cages could be retrieved by the joined sticks.

We now know that learning can occur in the absence of behavior later shown to be a manifestation of the learning. This type of learning is called "silent" learning (Flaherty 1985). Rumbaugh, Savage-Rumbaugh, and Washburn (1996) described an interesting example of silent learning. A rhesus monkey was initially trained to use its foot to manipulate a joystick in a visual-motor pursuit task presented on a video screen. The joystick controlled a cursor that the subject moved to intercept an erratically moving target. After the monkey became skillful at the pursuit task, it was allowed to control the joystick with its hand. The result was an immediate, high level of response, markedly higher than the monkey's best proficiency with the foot. The proficiency of hand-directed pursuit could not be explained by previous reinforcement of hand responses because there had been none. Any explanation of this behavior as having involved response generalization is unconvincing because completely different muscle groups controlled the monkey's foot and hand responses.

Two other somewhat paradoxical effects illustrate the way in which reinforcers may fail to control behavior in the rigid way implied by the capacitor model of learning. The first is the well-known partial reinforcement effect (PRE), in which the number of trials to extinction is increased as the proportion of reinforced responses during the preceding acquisition phase is decreased (Barker 1997). The PRE is a robust and pervasive effect that has been repeatedly demonstrated across many mammalian and avian taxa. In most experimental designs demonstrating the PRE, partially reinforced and continuously reinforced groups receive equal numbers of trials during the acquisition phase to ensure that the partially reinforced group receives fewer reinforcements than the continuously reinforced group. Because the number of trials to extinction has been a common measure of response strength, the paradox is that response strength increases as the number of reinforced responses decreases.

The second paradoxical effect is the phenomenon of maximizing during probability learning. Subjects in probability learning tasks are presented with two response alternatives in each trial. The probability that one alternative (e.g., the red stimulus) is rewarded is different from that of the other alternative (e.g., the green stimulus). A frequently used payoff ratio between the two alternatives is for the favored alternative (S+) to be rewarded on a randomly determined 70 percent of the trials and for the less favored alternative (S−) to be rewarded on the remaining 30 percent of the trials. Although there are some exceptions, mammals, including rats, usually learn to choose S+ on a proportion of trials approaching 1.0, a result known as *maximizing* because it achieves the highest possible reward payoff (Macphail 1982; Warren 1973).

Meyer (1960) reported a remarkable example of rhesus monkeys' ability to discriminate between reward probabilities of different responses. Meyer's monkeys were able to maximize when the payoff probabilities for the two alternatives were as similar as 55 percent and 45 percent. The paradoxical nature of probability learning occurs because the maximizing subject learns to avoid making a response despite that response having been reinforced in the past, a clear violation of the capacitor model of learning.

These examples represent a large body of research on learning, and they support the following conclusions:

1. External reinforcement of a response is not a necessary condition for learning; it may even impair learning.

2. A learned response does not have to occur during the time in which the learning takes place.

3. A decrease in the number of reinforcements can increase the strength of a learned response.

4. The effects of rewarding a response can be suppressed and thereby reduce the probability of the response to near zero.

We maintain that these manifestations of animals' abilities to emancipate their simple, learned adaptations from strict control by the law of effect occurred during an early stage of an evolutionary progression and led to far greater cognitive sophistication in primates. If we assume that consciousness is linked to independent control of behavior, it is not unreasonable to assume that consciousness also had its most primitive origins during the period in which our mammalian predecessors first became capable of expressing aptitudes for latent learning, curiosity-driven learning, partial reinforcement effects, and maximizing. Nevertheless, all the examples involve very simple, artificial examples of single-problem learning in a highly structured format.

EMERGENT LEARNING IN NONHUMAN PRIMATES

In the 1940s, Harry Harlow described the consequences of presenting a large number of object discrimination problems to rhesus monkeys (Harlow 1944,

1949). Each discrimination problem was defined by two objects. Responses to one object were always rewarded, and responses to the other object were never rewarded. In what became the most common paradigm for this procedure, each discrimination problem was presented for six trials. After exposure to about 300 of the six-trial problems, Harlow's monkeys were achieving nearly perfect performances on trial 2. Harlow referred to their one-trial learning as a discrimination learning set.

The term *learning set* refers to the learning of any general rule that can be applied to an unlimited number of specific problems (Fobes and King 1982). In a discrimination-learning set, the rule has been succinctly stated as "win-stay; lose-shift" (Levine 1959).

When nonhuman primates acquire learning sets, a wide variety of phenomena that are not seen in simple, single-problem learning emerge, which suggests that learning sets are an example of a type of learning qualitatively different from conventional discrimination learning. This type of learning has been characterized as "emergent" learning (Rumbaugh, Savage-Rumbaugh, and Washburn 1996; Rumbaugh, Washburn, and Hillix 1996). In emergent learning, a new adaptive capability, competency, or pattern of responding is acquired. Emergents generalize between contexts or problems based on general rules or relationships, but not on the basis of conventional stimulus or response generalization.

For example, simple primary stimulus generalization is a classic phenomenon accompanying single-problem learning. Continued reinforcement of one stimulus (S+) results in an increased tendency for an animal to respond to stimuli resembling S+. The height of the resultant stimulus generalization gradient typically increases with the degree to which the S+ has been learned.

However, the situation changes markedly when monkeys learn multiple-discrimination problems and acquire a discrimination learning set. Although the individual problems are learned to ever higher levels of proficiency, the level of stimulus generalization decreases, an effect called transfer suppression (Riopelle 1953). King (1966) showed that transfer suppression acquired by rhesus monkeys during a series of discrimination problems later interfered with their learning of a stimulus-based concept (red in the center of objects) that was the S+ across different problems. Transfer suppression is clearly adaptive in the context of a discrimination learning set because there is no stimulus-based rule to define the correct object between problems. Therefore, stimulus generalization can only diminish learning-set performance.

One of the old truisms about animal learning is that memory for simple problems can be remarkably long. For example, rhesus monkeys tested by Strong (1959) showed almost perfect retention of 72 discrimination problems as long as seven months after learning. However, a different emergent mechanism for learning and memory seems to arise in rhesus monkeys that have a long history of training in discrimination learning sets. Bessemer and Stollnitz (1971) showed that experienced monkeys, as expected, displayed nearly perfect trial 2 performance on new object discrimination problems.

However, when the problems were presented again on a test of retention 24 hours later, preexisting object preferences first expressed on trial 1 of the original learning reasserted themselves and thus lowered the trial 1 retention scores. Later tests showed that the reemergence of the object preferences occurred at full strength within a period as short as one hour after learning.

Bessemer and Stollnitz' rhesus monkeys thus displayed both rapid learning and rapid forgetting of discrimination problems in contrast to less experienced monkeys that displayed slower learning and slower forgetting of similar problems. The monkeys showing the rapid learning and forgetting were described as having become "hypothesis learners." Instead of gradually acquiring preferences for particular objects, they had acquired a general strategy, namely win-stay; lose shift, that led them to choose the object correctly on the previous trial but to forget the preference for that object when the problem was concluded. The hypothesis-learner monkeys are a clear example of emergent learning.

Because a discrimination learning set elicits emergent learning, one might expect that interspecies differences in performance would be reliably reflected in intelligence and relative brain size of those species. In fact, a large body of research data on both primate and nonprimate species has failed to confirm this assumption. Most interspecies variation in performance with discrimination learning sets can be accounted for by differences in sensory capability (Warren 1973).

However, a learning set-related measure, the transfer index (TI), has been remarkably successful in discriminating among primate species in a manner consistent with their relative brain size. The TI (Rumbaugh 1969, 1971; Rumbaugh and Pate 1984; Rumbaugh, Savage-Rumbaugh, and Washburn 1996) is based on a sequence of discrimination reversal problems. Each problem has an acquisition (learning) phase followed by a constant number of reversal trials in which the reward value of the stimuli are reversed. A new pair of stimuli are then introduced for the next problem and so on. Training on the acquisition phase of each problem continues until the overall percentage of correct responses is 67 percent or 84 percent. The mean proportion of correct responses on all reversals is then divided by either 0.67 or 0.84 to yield two types of TI.

Both classic transfer theory and the capacitor model of learning would predict that the 84 percent TI should be lower than the 67 percent TI. A more thoroughly learned acquisition phase should lead to more errors on reversal and consequent negative transfer because there is more to unlearn during reversal after 84 percent correct acquisitions.

Rumbaugh (1971) showed that TI values for a wide variety of species— cats, prosimians, New and Old World monkeys, lesser apes, and great apes— were meaningfully related to relative brain complexity and evolutionary status. The relationship between the 67 percent and the 84 percent TIs was particularly revealing. The prosimians, consistent with classic transfer theory, did display increased negative transfer as the acquisition learning was increased from 67 percent to 84 percent correct. However, the species most closely related to humans, namely, the great apes, displayed positive transfer from acquisition to reversal; their 84 percent TI values were actually higher than their 67 percent TI values.

To understand the relationship between these two types of transfer and brain complexity one must understand the determinants of brain size. As a general rule, big animals have bigger brains than do small animals. Most variation in brain weight among species can be accounted for by their different body weights. Plots of logarithmically scaled brain and body weights among closely related species (e.g., primates) typically show the different species aligned along a straight line with slope of about 0.75. (Aboitz 1996; Jerison 1988). However, the line is higher for primates than for other orders of mammals; for a given body weight, a primate has a heavier brain than a nonprimate. Neonatal nonprimate mammals have brains weighing about 6 percent of their total body weight. In primates, the proportion is about 12 percent (Sacher 1982).

Even after accounting for the effect of body weight on brain weight by the logarithmic function, some variation around the best-fitting straight line remains. Aboitz (1996) refers to two modes of brain growth during evolutionary development. Passive growth occurs predominately during early ontogenetic development, affects all parts of the brain about equally, and is determined solely by body weight, according to the logarithmic function. Active growth accounts for the deviation of brain weight from that expected by brain weight alone, does not necessarily affect all parts of the brain equally, and probably results from species' evolutionary adaptation to ecological, social, psychological, and other intellectual demands of its environment.

Finlay and Darlington (1995) showed that the primate isocortex grows faster than the remaining parts of the brain and that its neurons are generated relatively late in ontogenetic development. The primate isocortex would therefore reflect large amounts of active growth and variation in its size and would account for a large part of the variation around the body weight-determined regression line among different primate species.

Data on Rumbaugh's (1971) 67 percent and 84 percent TI values provide evidence that the ability to display positive transfer between acquisition and reversal, contrary to classic transfer theory, is closely related to the amount of extra or active brain growth. Specifically, Rumbaugh (1997) showed that transfer between acquisition and reversal had a correlation of 0.82 with Jerison's (personal communication) estimate of extra brain volume across different primate species and a correlation of 0.79 with his estimate of extra neurons across those species. The correlations constitute impressive evidence that comparative measures of emergent learning in laboratory conditions are measuring species' learning capabilities that are relating to brain sophistication and the evolutionary processes that led to the sophistication.

A final example of emergent process in primates involves numerical cognition by rhesus monkeys (Washburn and Rumbaugh 1991). Two monkeys were trained to choose one of two numerals that had the highest value. The rule was that selection of a numeral would result in the monkey receiving a corresponding number of food pellets. Thus, if a five were paired with a three, selection of the five would result in the delivery of five pellets and selection of the three would result in the delivery of three pellets. The monkeys were trained on all but 7 of the 45 possible combinations of the numerals 0 through 9. The seven unrepresented combinations were presented on later test trials for one trial each. On the first presentation of these previously nonpresented pairs, one monkey made no errors, and the other monkey made only two errors.

The results clearly indicate that the two rhesus monkeys had learned more than a specific set of associations. They had learned a complete set of relative values that could be applied to any pair of items within the set. Indeed, a common element in all emergent learning is that it involves some principle that transcends learning inherent in any particular problem.

LANGUAGE: THE ULTIMATE EXPRESSION OF EMERGENT LEARNING

The phenomena described in the preceding sections show examples of animals' ability to learn general rules from experience with particular instances independently of constraints from strict adherence to the law of effect. However, this type of learning is vastly different from humans' spontaneous use and understanding of word sequences with constantly changing syntax in an unlimited number of different contexts. If human language competence gradually evolved during human evolution, we might expect that the nonhuman primates in which this competence would be most closely approximated would be the two species comprising the genus *Pan*, namely, chimpanzees and bonobos. These apes shared a common ancestor with humans as recently as 4 to 6 million years ago (Sibley and Ahlquist 1987).

Measurement of brain endocasts from human predecessors indicates that the left temporal gyrus began expanding relative to the comparable area in the right hemisphere about 2 to 3 million years ago (Falk 1983). Mediation of human speech is concentrated in the left temporal lobe. In chimpanzees, the left hemisphere is dominant for processing meaningful lexigrams used for communication, but no cerebral lateralization is evident for lexigrams not used for language-related functions (Hopkins and Morris 1989). Therefore, if we assume that the evolution of consciousness, capability for emergent learning, and language aptitude were linked, we would expect to find abundant language-related abilities in chimpanzees and bonobos.

Early research on ape language emphasized training chimpanzees to make manual signs (Gardner and Gardner 1969) or to use noniconic and arbitrary symbols (Premack 1971; Rumbaugh 1977; Terrace 1979) to name or to request some external object or material, usually to obtain some contingent reward. The chimpanzees in these studies achieved impressive vocabularies and remarkable facility in using the signs in a variety of situations. The chimpanzees displayed far more sophisticated learning than that reported in any previous laboratory studies of complex learning that required the subjects to move objects and symbols around in a highly constant and structured setting for hidden food rewards.

The inevitable question was whether the signing any symbol-using chimpanzees were displaying language and, if not, what were they lacking? One important property of human language that was probably lacking in these early chimpanzee subjects was an association between the symbols and an internal representation of the symbols' referents. In other words, did the symbols have meaning or semanticity? A pigeon could be trained to peck at a red disk to obtain food when it is food deprived and to peck at a green disk to obtain water when it is water deprived. Yet we cannot conclude that red means water to the pigeon in any semantic sense; the pigeon's performance is best regarded as a learned association between a stimulus (red), a response (peck), and an outcome (food) in the presence of a particular motivational state (hunger).

Children learn to comprehend the meaning of single words long before they become capable of producing those words (Snyder, Bates, and Bratherton 1981; Benedict 1979; Goldin-Meadow, Seligman, and Gelman 1976). It is now well established that syntactic capabilities in apes is dependent upon symbols having a semantic or representational content (Savage-Rumbaugh, 1986, 1988).

Research at the Georgia State University Language Research Center has shown that chimpanzees are capable of learning to use symbols in a representational manner (Savage-Rumbaugh 1981). For example, two chimpanzees, Sherman and Austin, learned to associate arbitrary geometrical symbols (lexigrams) with three particular foods and three particular tools (Savage-Rumbaugh 1986). They also learned to classify the three foods in one lexigram-designated category and the three tools in another lexigram-designated category. The semantic content of the two new general lexigrams was tested by having Sherman and Austin use them to label 17 other previously learned lexigrams that stood for a variety of other foods, drinks, and tools. They accomplished the labeling with almost perfect accuracy.

Sherman and Austin were also able to look at a lexigram, reach into a box, and select a particular object from several others solely on the basis of tactual cues (Savage-Rumbaugh, Sevcik, and Hopkins 1988). Sherman and Austin's ability to perform the cross-modal identification without prior training is direct evidence of their semantic understanding of the lexigrams.

More recent studies at the Georgia Language Research Center have shown that the bonobo Kanzi (*Pan paniscus*) was able to acquire an impressive comprehension of spoken English without any formal training, thus duplicating the conditions in which human children acquire language (Savage-Rumbaugh, Murphy, Sevcik, Brakke, Williams, and Rumbaugh 1993). Kanzi was exposed to language between the ages of 6 and 30 months as a result of being present at her adoptive mother Matata's training sessions in which spoken English and lexigram training occurred. Matata's training was not successful, probably because of her relatively mature age, but Kanzi, by observing the unsuccessful attempts to tutor Matata, became proficient at comprehension of spoken English and at production of responses by pointing at lexigrams on a portable keyboard.

Kanzi's understanding of spoken English sentences was later demonstrated in an experiment in which he was presented with over 600 new sentences requesting some specific action. Correct responses to the requests often required an understanding of the syntax of the sentence, not just an understanding of particular words. For example, the two sentences "Take the potato outdoors" and "Go outdoors and get the potato" had similar word content, but the correct response required comprehension of their syntactic structure. Both Kanzi and a $2\frac{1}{2}$-year-old child who was similarly tested displayed about 70 percent accuracy in responding to the requests. Additional studies with Kanzi have shown that his ability to produce language by combining lexigrams with manual gestures is approximately equal to that of a $1\frac{1}{2}$-year-old child (Greenfield and Savage-Rumbaugh 1991, 1993).

The most significant aspect to Kanzi's success in responding correctly to sentence requests is that the sentences were ones that he had not heard before. Therefore, any explanation of his performance in terms of learned associations, even complex ones, is insufficient. The ability to comprehend and to produce novel sequences of known words that obey rules of syntax is called generativity. Generativity has long been regarded as the sine qua non of human language (Corballis 1992). Kanzi's accomplishments show that he is indeed at the brink of the human mind (Savage-Rumbaugh and Lewin 1994).

CONCLUSION

We believe that there is not a large, glaring discontinuity between the learning and cognitive abilities of humans (and apes) at one end of the cognitive continuum and the learning abilities of other animals at the other end of the continuum. One often sees animal learning described in a disparaging, almost comedic style: rats scurrying around in a maze, slowly learning which way to turn to get a 45 mg food pellet or Pavlovian dogs salivating in response to bells. These examples are sometimes taken to exemplify the limits of the animal mind.

In this chapter, the samples of animal learning capability, ranging from latent learning in rats to emergent learning in multiple-problem learning of monkeys to the language proficiency of Kanzi, are part of a much larger experimental literature showing a continuous gradation in learning complexity and sophistication. The gradation is clearly consistent with the assumption that the evolution of cognitive abilities was slow, gradual, and conservative.

We also believe that Romanes was fundamentally correct when he stated that the first traces of consciousness emerged when nervous systems became capable of learned actions independent of reflexlike simplicity. If consciousness is to become a scientific entity, not just a philosophical concept, it must be tied to multiple behavioral indices, including the abilities for complex emergent learning and, ultimately, language. If continuity in the evolutionary development of the behavioral manifestations of learning and language exists, obviously consciousness also evolved along similar paths.

ACKNOWLEDGMENTS

Preparation of this chapter was supported by a grant from the National Institute of Child Health and Development (HD-06016) and by the College of Arts and Sciences, Georgia State University.

REFERENCES

Aboitz, F. 1996. Does bigger mean better? Evolutionary determinants of brain size and structure. *Brain Behavior and Evolution* 47:225–245.

Barker, L. M. 1997. *Learning and Behavior: Biological, Psychological, and Sociocultural Perspectives,* 2nd ed. Upper Saddle River, NJ: Prentice Hall.

Benedict, H. 1979. Early lexical development: Comprehension and production. *Journal of Child Language* 6:183–200.

Bessemer, D. W., and F. Stollnitz. 1971. Retention of discriminations and an analysis of learning set. In A. M. Schrier and F. Stollnitz, eds., *Behavior of Nonhuman Primates,* vol. 4. New York: Academic Press.

Corballis, M. C. 1992. On the evolution of language and generativity. *Cognition* 44:197–226.

Dennett, D. C. 1995. *Darwin's Dangerous Idea: Evolution and the Meanings of Life.* New York: Simon & Schuster.

Dennett, D. C. 1996. *Kinds of Minds.* New York: Basic Books.

Falk, D. 1983. Cerebral cortices of East African early hominids. *Science* 221:1072–1074.

Finlay, B. L., and R. B. Darlington. 1995. Linked regularities in the development and evolution of mammalian brains. *Science* 268:1578–1584.

Flaherty, C. F. 1985. *Animal Learning and Cognition.* New York: Knopf.

Fobes, J. L., and J. E. King. 1982. Measuring primate learning abilities. In J. L. Fobes and J. E. King, eds., *Primate Behavior.* New York: Academic Press.

Gardner, R. A., and B. T. Gardner. 1969. Teaching sign language to a chimpanzee. *Science* 165:664–672.

Goldin-Meadow, S., M. E. P. Seligman, and R. Gelman. 1976. Language in the two-year-old. *Cognition* 4:189–202.

Greenfield, P., and E. S. Savage-Rumbaugh. 1991. Imitation, grammatical development, and the invention of protogrammar by an ape. In N. A. Krasnegor, D. M. Rumbaugh, R. L. Schiefelbusch, and M. Studdert-Kennedy, eds., *Biological and Behavioral Determinants of Language Development.* Hillsdale, NJ: Erlbaum.

Greenfield, P., and E. S. Savage-Rumbaugh. 1993. Comparing communicative competence in child and chimp: The pragmatics of repetition. *Journal of Child Language* 20:1–26.

Guthrie, E. R. 1952. *The Psychology of Learning.* New York: Harper.

Harlow, H. F. 1944. Studies in discrimination learning by monkeys: I. The learning of discrimination series and the reversal of discrimination series. *Journal of General Psychology* 30:3–12.

Harlow, H. F. 1949. The formation of learning sets. *Psychological Review* 56:51–65.

Harlow, H. F., M. K., Harlow, and D. R. Meyer. 1950. Learning motivated by a manipulation drive. *Journal of Experimental Psychology* 40:228–234.

Harlow, H. F., and G. E. McClearn. 1954. Object manipulation learned by monkeys on the basis of manipulation motives. *Journal of Comparative and Physiological Psychology* 47:73–76.

Hopkins, W. D., and R. D. Morris. 1989. Laterality for visual-spatial processing in two language trained chimpanzees (*Pan troglodytes*). *Behavioral Neuroscience* 193:227–234.

Hull, C. L. 1943. *Principles of Behavior*. New York: Appleton.

Jerison, H. J. 1973. Evolutionary biology of intelligence: The nature of the problem. In H. J. Jerison and I. Jerison, eds., *Intelligence and Evolutionary Biology*. NATO ASI Series. New York: Springer-Verlag.

King, J. E. 1966. Transfer relationships between learning set and concept formation in rhesus monkeys. *Journal of Comparative and Physiological Psychology* 61:416–420.

Levine, M. 1959. A model of hypothesis behavior in discrimination learning set. *Psychological Review* 66:353–366.

Locke, J. 1690. An essay concerning human understanding. Reprinted in E. Sprague and P. W. Taylor, eds., *Knowledge and Value*. New York: Harcourt Brace.

Macphail, E. M. 1982. *Brain and Intelligence in Vertebrates*. Oxford: Clarendon Press.

Meyer, D. R. 1960. The effects of differential probabilities of reinforcement on discrimination learning by monkeys. *Journal of Comparative and Physiological Psychology* 53:173–175.

Olton, D. S., C. Collison. and M. A. Werz. 1977. Spatial memory and radial arm maze performance of rats. *Learning and Motivation* 8:289–314.

Premack, D. 1971. On the assessment of language competence in the chimpanzee. In A. M. Schrier and F. Stollnitz, eds., *Behavior of Nonhuman Primates*, vol. 4. New York: Academic Press.

Riopelle, A. J. 1953. Transfer suppression and learning sets. *Journal of Comparative and Physiological Psychology* 46:28–32.

Romanes, G. J. 1888. *Animal Intelligence*. New York: D. Appleton.

Ross, D. M. 1965. Complex and modifiable patterns in *Calliactis* and *Stomphia*. *American Zoologist* 5:573–580.

Roitblat, H. L. 1987. *Introduction to Comparative Cognition*. New York: W. H. Freeman.

Rumbaugh, D. M. 1969. The transfer index: An alternative measure of learning set. In *Proceedings of the Second International Congress of Primatology*, Atlanta, Georgia 1968, vol. 1. Basel: Karger.

Rumbaugh, D. M. 1971. Evidence of qualitative differences in learning among primates. *Journal of Comparative and Physiological Psychology* 76:250–255.

Rumbaugh, D. M., Ed. 1977. *Language Learning by a Chimpanzee: The Lana Project*. New York: Academic Press.

Rumbaugh D. M. 1997. Competence, cortex, and animal models: A comparative primate perspective. In N. Krasnegor, R. Lyon, and P. Goldman-Rakic, eds., *Development of the Prefrontal Cortex: Evolution, Neurobiology, and Behavior*. Baltimore: Paul H. Brooks.

Rumbaugh, D. M., and J. L. Pate. 1984. The evolution of cognition in primates: A comparative perspective. In H. L. Roitblat, T. G. Bever, and H. S. Terrace, eds., *Animal Cognition*. Hillsdale, NJ: Erlbaum.

Rumbaugh, D. M., E. S. Savage-Rumbaugh, and D. A. Washburn. 1996. Toward a new outlook on primate learning and behavior: Complex learning and emergent processes in comparative perspective. *Japanese Psychological Research* 38:113–125.

Rumbaugh, D. M., D. A. Washburn, and W. A. Hillix. 1997. Respondents, operants, and emergents: Toward an integrated perspective on behavior. In K. Pribram, ed., *Learning as a Self-Organizing Process*. Hillsdale, NJ: Erlbaum.

Sacher, G. A. 1982. The role of brain maturation in the evolution of primates. In E. Armstrong and D. Falk, eds., *Primate Brain Evolution: Methods and Concepts*. New York: Plenum.

Savage-Rumbaugh, E. S. 1981. Can apes use symbols to represent their worlds? In T. A. Sebeok and R. Rosenthal, eds., The Clever Hans phenomenon: Communication with horses, whales, apes, and people. *Annals of the New York Academy of Sciences* 364:35–59.

Savage-Rumbaugh, E. S. 1986. *Ape Language: From Conditioned Response to Symbol*. New York: Columbia University Press.

Savage-Rumbaugh, E. S. 1988. A new look at ape language: Comprehension of vocal speech and syntax. In D. Leger, Ed., *Comparative Perspectives in Modern Psychology*. Lincoln: University of Nebraska Press.

Savage-Rumbaugh, E. S., and R. Lewin. 1994. *Kanzi: At the Brink of the Human Mind*. New York: Wiley.

Savage-Rumbaugh, E. S., R. A. Sevcik, and W. D. Hopkins. 1988. Symbolic cross-modal transfer in two species of chimpanzees. *Child Development* 59:617–625.

Savage-Rumbaugh, E. S., J. Murphy, R. A. Sevcik, K. E. Brakke, S. L. Williams, and D. M. Rumbaugh. 1993. Language comprehension in ape and child. *Monographs of the Society for Research in Child Development* 58(3 and 4):1–221.

Schiller, P. H. 1952. Innate constituents of complex responses in primates. *Psychological Review* 59:177–191.

Schiller, P. H. 1957. Innate motor action as a basis for learning. In C. H. Schiller, ed., *Instinctive Behavior*. New York: International Universities Press.

Sibley, C. G., and J. E. Ahlquist. 1987. DNA hybridization evidence of hominoid phylogeny: Results from an expanded data set. *Journal of Molecular Evolution* 26:99–121.

Snyder, L. S., E. Bates, and I. Bretherton. 1981. Content and context in early lexical development. *Journal of Child Language* 8:565–682.

Strong, P. N., Jr. 1959. Memory for object discriminations in the rhesus monkey. *Journal of Comparative and Physiological Psychology* 52:333–335.

Terrace, H. S. 1979. *Nim*. New York: Knopf.

Thorndike, E. L. 1911. *Animal Intelligence: Experimental Studies*. New York: Macmillan.

Tolman, E. C. 1932. *Purposive Behavior in Animals and Men*. New York: Appleton-Century Crofts.

Tolman, E. C., and C. H. Honzik. 1930. Degrees of hunger, reward and non-reward, and maze learning in rats. *University of California Publications in Psychology* 4:215–256.

Warren, J. M. 1973. Learning in vertebrates. In D. Dewsbury and D. Rethlingshafer, eds., *Comparative Psychology: A Modern Survey*. New York: McGraw-Hill.

Washburn, D. A., and D. M. Rumbaugh. 1991. Ordinal judgments of numerical symbols by macaques (*Macaca mulatta*). *Psychological Science* 2:190–193.

35 Bacteria as Tools for Studies of Consciousness

Victor Norris

The possible value of bacteria as theoretical and experimental tools for consciousness studies can be considered for a variety of hypotheses. These hypotheses are not mutually exclusive. Consciousness may act as an organizing force emerging from a critical mass or density of organization and helping generate, in the case of brains, coherent oscillations of neuronal membranes. Understanding such oscillations may require applying underused concepts in biology, such as piezoelectricity. A function for consciousness at the level of the single cell can be proposed for coherent oscillations because the oscillations may have their origins in regulating the cell cycle—the beautiful, mysterious sequence of organizations and reorganizations on which all cells depend.

Bacteria have many advantages as model systems for investigations in biology. *Escherichia coli*, for example, is more easily manipulated and better understood than most, if not all, other organisms. The *E. coli* genome is nearly sequenced, and most of its proteins can be readily identified by their electrophoretic properties. Bacteria are also simple in comparison with organisms (although they are complex in comparison with computers). *E. coli* contains a chromosome of 4.7 million base pairs of DNA that has to be packed into a cell 1,000 times shorter; this packing is such that it can be duplicated in 40 minutes while being transcribed simultaneously into mRNA. The mRNA is translated into the thousands of different sorts of proteins that are present, in some cases, in tens of thousands of examples.

Syntheses of these and other types of molecules have to be coordinated in response to internal and external signals to permit the bacterium to grow in different environments and to survive exposure to a wide variety of different stresses. The net result of growth through autosynthesis and autoassembly is that one bacterium generates two; this miraculous process, the cell cycle, can be accomplished in 17 minutes.

In this chapter, I discuss the similarities between bacteria and "higher" cells and use the definition that equates consciousness with the phenomenon of subjective experience to examine a number of hypotheses to illustrate the ways in which bacteria may make a contribution to studies of consciousness.

SIMILARITIES BETWEEN BACTERIA AND HIGHER CELLS

The similarities between prokaryotic cells (bacteria) and eukaryotic cells (plants and animals) extend from molecular and macromolecular constituents and intracellular structures to signaling mechanisms. Like eukaryotic cells, bacteria contain DNA, RNA, proteins, polyamines, and so forth surrounded by membranes composed of phospholipids and proteins. In addition, in many cases a cell wall in bacteria and plants resists the turgor pressure that develops inside. The cytoskeleton in eukaryotes can also resist turgor. The supposed absence of the cytoskeleton and of other intracellular structures in bacteria is often used to emphasize the differences between the phyla.

It is, however, becoming clear that bacterial cells are just as structured as eukaryotic ones. Like eukaryotic membranes, bacterial membranes reveal a considerable lateral heterogeneity (Glaser 1993; Tocanne et al. 1989; Vaz and Almeida 1993). Recent examples of heterogeneity in the cytoplasmic membrane of *E. coli* include the localization of chemotactic proteins to the poles (Maddock, Alley, and Shapiro 1993) and the Ras-like protein, Era, to small domains (Gollop and March 1991). Like eukaryotes, bacteria possess an enzoskeleton (Norris, Turnock, and Sigee 1996); this dynamic, labile structure is an interlinked and interlaced assembly of enzyme complexes that channels metabolites (Agutter 1994; Srere 1987) and that connects membranes and nucleic acids (DNA and RNA). The enzoskeleton helps to organize both the cytoplasmic membrane and the DNA and includes eukaryotic-like cytoskeletal structures and elements such as the FtsZ protein.

Tubulin has been proposed to be important in consciousness (Insinna 1992; Penrose and Hameroff 1995) (see below). In *E. coli*, FtsZ is a tubulin-like protein that is essential for a normal cell cycle. Purified FtsZ is a GTPase, possesses a tubulin signature sequence of seven amino acids involved in GTP-binding, and exhibits a GTP-dependent polymerization that produces structures compatible with tubules 17 nm in diameter containing 12 or 13 protofilaments of 3.5 nm (see Bramhill and Thompson 1994; Mukherjee and Lutkenhaus 1994 and references therein). Like eukaryotic tubulin, FtsZ is involved in the cell cycle and, at the start of cell division, FtsZ relocalizes from the cytoplasm to a contractile ring at the inner membrane at the midpoint of the cell.

Similar signaling mechanisms in bacteria and eukaryotic cells are responsible for transducing extracellular information into appropriate forms for intracellular responses. One signaling system is based on calcium. Bacterial proteins concerned with calcium regulation include primary and secondary transporters responsible for efflux, voltage-operated calcium channels responsible for influx, and calmodulin-like proteins (Norris et al. 1991). These proteins help to implicate calcium in the control of chemotaxis, differentiation, the cell cycle, and several other processes common to both bacteria and higher cells. A second signaling system is based on the phosphorylation of proteins by kinases (Saier 1993). A variety of such kinases, including those once believed specific to eukaryotes, are present in bacteria (Freestone, Grant, Toth, and Norris 1995; Freestone, Nyström, Trinei, and Norris 1997).

HYPOTHESIS 1: CONSCIOUSNESS IS AN EMERGENT PROPERTY

Consciousness is sometimes considered to emerge from interactions within a population of cells. In the soil bacterium, *Myxococcus xanthus*, four sequential intercellular signals control the differentiation of vegetative cells into spores and the formation of a mound-shaped structure (Kaiser and Losick 1993). This process involves about 10^5 cells. Does this approach a critical threshold for the emergence of consciousness? Two signals have been chemically identified and a large number of mutants are available. Many other bacteria also make use of chemical signals to detect cell density and respond accordingly (Kell, Kaprelyants, and Grafen 1995). Because mutants are readily available and some of these systems are well understood, if we had and idea of how to measure consciousness, such bacterial systems might be worth exploring.

HYPOTHESIS 2: CONSCIOUSNESS ARISES IN INFORMATION-PROCESSING SYSTEMS

There are several related ideas concerning the relationships between consciousness and information processing. One is that consciousness arises from relatively straightforward stimulus–response (input–output) informational relationships between environment and system as exemplified by a thermostat. Bacteria possess information-processing systems (similar to those found in eukaryotic cells) that allow them to grow in a wide variety of environments and to adapt to a correspondingly wide variety of environmental challenges. Extensive networks of genes are transcribed in response to heat shock, cold shock, osmotic changes, ultraviolet irradiation, starvation, entry into stationary phase, ethanol stress, exposure to antibiotics, dessication, encounters with host cells, altered levels of oxygen, carbon, nitrogen, phosphorus, and the like. Controls over these networks include transcriptional regulators; *E. coli*, for example, possesses 55 known transcriptional activators and 58 repressors (Ouzounis, Casari, Valencia, and Sander 1996).

A second idea is that consciousness arises from internal representations of the external environment; during chemotaxis, bacteria, for example, represent the nutritional gradient along their trajectory by the number of methyl groups on certain proteins. This process is quite well understood. Bacterial chemotaxis and motility involve about 50 genes in *E. coli* (Manson 1992). Hameroff and others have raised the possibility that the chemotactic responses of single-celled eukaryotes involve the cytoskeleton acting as a nervous system (Hameroff 1994). Bacterial chemotaxis appears to involve elements found in eukaryotic chemotaxis, such as calcium and voltage-operated calcium channels (Tisa, Olivera, and Adler 1993). If chemotaxis is intimately associated with consciousness and microtubules, it should be predictable that chemotaxis will not occur when the function of the tubulin-like

FtsZ protein is disrupted by either mutation or expression of inhibitory proteins.

A third idea is that consciousness is associated with the cycling of information. In the case of a brain, cycling could involve sequences of neuronal activity without input or output. In the case of a single cell, cycling of information could involve cascades of signal-transducing molecules (proteins, modifications to proteins, chemical alarmones, calcium, lipids and their breakdown products, etc.) transferring information that would remain internal to the system. A prime example of such cycling may be in the cell cycle itself (see below).

Thus, if information processing per se engenders conscious experience, a prokaryotic cell is as likely as a eukaryotic cell to have conscious experiences. Because a bacterial population can be maintained in a relatively homogeneous and constant environment within a chemostat or turbidostat, the exposure of such a population to a single stimulus such as heat shock might induce a single quale in its purest form.

HYPOTHESIS 3: CONSCIOUSNESS HAS A FUNCTION IN INDIVIDUAL CELLS

Assuming that bacteria do have conscious experiences, in which bacterial processes would consciousness be involved? One candidate process is the cell cycle that constitutes a series of major alterations in the organization of the cell. Radical changes in intracellular structure occur when chromosomes are replicated, folded, separated, and segregated; the cell itself is invaginated during septation by the cytoplasmic membrane, the peptidoglycan layer, and the outer membrane. Key players in the execution of the *E. coli* cell cycle include the tubulin-like protein, FtsZ, which relocalizes from the cytoplasm to a contractile ring at the inner membrane at the midpoint of the cell to accomplish cell division. Because mere possession of microtubules may not be sufficient to confer consciousness and microtubules may need to form parallel arrays as in neurones (Penrose and Hameroff 1995), could it be that bacteria are conscious only when their tubulin-like protein forms a ring? Are bacteria conscious only during birth?

Numerous types of control mechanisms for regulating the bacterial cell cycle have been proposed (for references, see Norris 1995). Most are prosaic and readily testable, but despite intense efforts, there is no consensus as to the fundamental nature of this mechanism. One very speculative possibility is that coherent oscillations are involved in organizing the cell cycle (see below and Hypothesis 8). Another possibility is that consciousness itself is involved—in which case, we must ask how consciousness generates the organization of microtubules (FtsZ, etc.) rather than how the organization of microtubules generates consciousness.

A second candidate process in which consciousness might be involved is that of differentiation. As with cell division, this process involves major changes in the organization of chromosomes and membranes. Differentiation in both prokaryotes and eukaryotes also entails the recruitment and dismissal of teams of transcription factors, proteases, kinases, and other proteins (Norris et al. 1996; Norris, Turnock, and Sigee 1996). As with cell division, there is no clear, unifying hypothesis that brings it all together. As with cell division, consciousness could play a role as organizer. For example, consciousness might orchestrate the multitude of actions necessary when bacteria sporulate in response to impending nutrient starvation. If so, the important question is: How?

A third candidate process is that of the origin of life itself. One approach to the origin of life is to consider that the constituents, the processes, and the principles important to modern cells were actually important to the first cells. The advantage of this approach is that it allows the formulation of a unifying hypothesis to explain the regulation of cell cycle, differentiation, and the origin of life. In such a hypothesis, the regulation of the processes whereby cells once originated and now grow, multiply, and differentiate is by consciousness itself.

HYPOTHESIS 4: CONSCIOUSNESS HAS A FUNCTION AT A COSMIC LEVEL

There are hypotheses in which the Earth itself is considered a superorganism and in which geophysiological regulation involves complex feedback between the biota and the physical world (climate, rock formation, etc.) (Kump 1996; Lovelock 1989). An obvious extension of these types of hypotheses is that the Earth itself is conscious. If consciousness were to have a function in some global entity, is there any way in which bacteria might be relevant? Bacteria constitute a substantial proportion of the Earth's biomass—could the Earth possess a bacterial id? If the global ecosystem really is conscious (as distinct from the entire Earth, rocks and all), did this consciousness precede the first life-forms, accompany them, or appear at some later stage?

HYPOTHESIS 5: CONSCIOUSNESS IS AN ORGANIZING FORCE

In this hypothesis, consciousness is involved in the process of transmitting, receiving, and condensing organization to a common pattern (Norris 1996). Consciousness is proposed as a force that acts on patterns so that they condense irrespective of their physical or physiological correlates. The force would be created by information and would act to create information. It would be proportional to the density of information, similar to the way gravity is proportional to the density of mass. Hence, when the density of patterns is high, the consciousness generated is a large force able to create more patterns. This would be the situation within a human brain—consciousness would be responsible for the convergence of numerous different patterns of neuronal activity on one common pattern.

Although the volume of an individual human brain is 15 to 16 orders of magnitude greater than that of an individual *E. coli* bacterium, equivalent (and much larger) volumes of bacteria can easily be grown. Moreover, the density of information or, put differently, the degree of organization, is arguably as high in a prokaryotic cell as it is in a eukaryotic cell. Can one devise an experiment with bacteria in which the creation of organization might be ascribed to the force of consciousness—an experiment, for example, in which reorganization would avoid death (the ultimate loss of organization for the individual)? Requiring bacteria to mutate to survive might constitute such an experiment. Adaptive mutations occur in some cells of *E. coli* when populations of this bacterium that have, for example, lost the ability to use lactose to grow are confronted with the need to require this ability (Cairns, Ovebaugh, and Miller 1988). However, it appears that known molecular mechanisms involving an alarmone, ppGpp, and single-stranded DNA are responsible (Wright 1996). There is no need to invoke a force of consciousness. The lesson is that when we do invoke such a force, its explanatory power may often be inferior to one invoking a mundane reductionist mechanism.

HYPOTHESIS 6: CONSCIOUSNESS IS A METAFORCE THAT RECRUITS OTHER ORGANIZING FORCES

Consciousness is a metaforce that recruits or creates other forces to produce organizations. In this case, consciousness has a quasidivine status responsible for altering physical laws or their chemical and biological interpretations so that organizations occur. This status circumvents the problem that is often encountered in looking for evidence to support Hypothesis 5—with Hypothesis 6, the existence of a molecular mechanism that explains adaptive mutations does not matter. Consciousness has recruited the mechanism. If consciousness had not recruited the ppGpp single-stranded DNA mechanism, it would have recruited another. At the level of a bacterium, this hypothesis is almost a reformulation of "Life will find a way." At the level of a brain, consciousness as a metaforce might be accepted, providing that the metaforce is proportional to the degree of organization in the entity that generates it, as in Hypothesis 5.

HYPOTHESIS 7: CONSCIOUSNESS INVOLVES A NOVEL FORM OF COMMUNICATION

A novel and potentially very exciting form of communication has been reported between bacteria; bacteria growing on one plate are allegedly able to stimulate the germination of spores on another plate by a nonchemical form of signaling (Matsuhashi et al. 1995). It is believed that this signal involves the bacterial walls (and has apparently been duplicated, or mimicked, by a sonic device). Discovering the exact nature of this mechanism in bacteria is of relevance to studies of consciousness (and certain psychic phenomena) because it is conceivable that similar signals are used by neurons (see Hypothesis 8). For example, one might subject a culture of bacteria to a heat shock and then look for induction of heat shock proteins in a neighboring unshocked culture.

HYPOTHESIS 8: THE NEURAL CORRELATES OF CONSCIOUSNESS ARE COHERENT OSCILLATIONS

Different authors have argued that coherence is important in intracellular organization (Ho 1993), in the behavior of membranes (Fröhlich 1968), and in consciousness (Insinna 1992; Penrose and Hameroff 1995), but see Grush and Churchland (1995). Recently, I proposed that consciousness may be generated by—and may even help generate—coherent oscillations of neuronal membranes (Norris 1996). The reasoning is as follows:

1. Each neuron has a particular spatial distribution of membrane domains because the membranes that surround cells are not homogeneous and proteolipid domains are present in almost all cells (Tocanne et al. 1994; Welti and Glaser 1994).

2. When a neuron fires, the plasma membrane vibrates to emit signals at a specific set of frequencies that reflect its domain distribution. The vibration may involve the piezoelectric effect because the swelling and shrinkage of nerves accompany the action potential and because mechanical stimuli act like cathodal electric shocks (for references, see Leuchtag 1987).

3. Other neurons firing simultaneously elsewhere converge à la Fröhlich on the same set of frequencies, which couples neurons that fire together (to form a thought) and couples sets of neurons that fire successively (to form a stream of thoughts).

4. Neurons that have a similar pattern of vibration then become physically connected, for example, by synapsing with one another.

To explore this hypothesis using bacteria, one might speculate that bacteria make use of coherent oscillations in some process that is ancestral to the neural correlates of consciousness (e.g., the regulation of the cell cycle or protein folding). Coherent oscillations in bacteria would be consistent with the triggering of biological processes by electromagnetic radiation at specific microwave frequencies. It has been reported that the growth of *E. coli* and other organisms may be decreased by irradiation at 39 to 42 and 70 to 75 GHz (Webb 1979) and that the lytic cycle of bacteriophage lambda may be induced at 70.5 GHz (Berteaud, Dardalhon, Rebeyrotte, and Averbeck 1975; Grundler 1981). Such reports should be confirmed or discounted by further experimentation.

REFERENCES

Agutter, P. S. 1994. Intracellular solute movements: A problem-orientated lecture for final year undergraduates. *Biochem Education* 22:32–35.

Berteaud, A.-J., M. Dardalhon, N. Rebeyrotte, and M. D. Averbeck. 1975. Action d'un rayonnement electromagnetique a longueur d'onde millimetrique sur la croissance bacterienne. *Comptes Rendu Hebdomadaires des Seances de l'Academie des Sciences*, Serie D. 281:843–846.

Bramhill, D., and C. M. Thompson. 1994. GTP-dependent polymerization of *Escherichia coli* FtsZ protein to form tubules. *Proceedings of the National Academy of Sciences USA* 91:5813–5817.

Cairns, J., J. Ovebaugh, S. Miller. 1988. The nature of mutants. *Nature* 335:142–145.

Freestone, P., S. Grant, I. Toth, and V. Norris. 1995. Identification of phosphoproteins in *Escherichia coli*. *Molecular Microbiology* 15:573–580.

Freestone, P., T. Nyström, M. Trinei, and V. Norris. 1997. The Universal Stress Protein UspA, of *Escherichia coli* is phosphorylated in response to stasis. *Journal of Molecular Biology* (in press).

Fröhlich, H. 1968. Long range coherence and energy storage in biological systems. *International Journal of Quantum Chemistry* 42:641–649.

Glaser, M. 1993. Lipid domains in biological membranes. *Current Opinion in Structural Biology* 3:475–481.

Gollop, N., and P. March. 1991. Localization of the membrane binding sites of Era in *Escherichia coli*. *Research in Microbiology* 142:301–307.

Grundler, W. 1981. Recent results of experiments on nonthermal effects of millimeter microwaves on yeast growth. *Collective Phenomena* 3:181–186.

Grush, R., and P. S. Churchland, 1995. Gaps in Penrose's toiling. *Journal of Consciousness Studies* 2:10–29.

Hameroff, S. R. 1994. Quantum coherence in microtubules: A neural basis for emergent consciousness? *Journal of Consciousness Studies* 1:91–118.

Ho, M.-W. 1993. *The Rainbow and the Worm: The Physics of Organisms*. Singapore: World Scientific Publishing.

Insinna, E. M. 1992. Synchronicity and coherent excitations in microtubules. *Nanobiology* 1:191–208.

Kaiser, D., and R. Losick. 1993. How and why bacteria talk to each other. *Cell* 73:873–885.

Kell, D. B., A. S. Kaprelyants, and A. Grafen. 1995. Pheromones, social behaviour and the functions of secondary metabolism in bacteria. *TREE* 10:126–129.

Kump, L. R. 1996. The physiology of the planet. *Nature* 381:111–112.

Leuchtag, H. R. 1987. Indications of the existence of ferroelectric units in excitable-membrane channels. *Journal of Theoretical Biology* 127:321–340.

Lovelock, J. 1989. *The Ages of Gaia*. Oxford: Oxford University Press.

Maddock, J. R., M. R. K. Alley, and L. Shapiro. 1993. Polarized cells, polar actions. *Journal of Bacteriology* 175:7125–7129.

Manson, M. D. 1992. Bacterial motility and chemotaxis. *Advances in Microbial Physiology* 33:277–346.

Matsuhashi, M., A. N. Pankrushina, K. Endoh, H. Watanabe, Y. Mano, M. Hyodo, T. Fujita, K. Kunugita, T. Kaneko, and S. Otani. 1995. Studies on carbon material requirements for bacterial proliferation and spore germination under stress conditions: A new mechanism involving transmission of physical signals. *Journal of Bacteriology* 177:688–693.

Mukherjee, A., and J. Lutkenhaus. 1994. Guanine nucleotide-dependent assembly of FtsZ into filaments. *Journal of Bacteriology* 176:2754–2758.

Norris, V. 1995. Hypotheses and the regulation of the bacterial cell cycle. *Molecular Micro-biology* 15:785–787.

Norris, V. 1997. Are bacteria 'conscious'? *Journal of Consciousness Studies*, submitted.

Norris, V., M. Chen, M. Goldberg, J. Voskuil, M. McGurk, and I. B. Holland. 1991. Calcium in bacteria: A solution to which problem? *Molecular Microbiology* 5:775–778.

Norris, V., S. Grant, P. Freestone, I. Toth, K. Modha, J. Canvin, N. Sheikh, and R. I. Norman. 1996. Calcium signalling in bacteria. *Journal of Bacteriology* 178:3677–3682.

Norris, V., G. Turnock, and D. Sigee. 1996. The *Escherichia coli* enzoskeleton. *Molecular Micro-biology* 19:197–204.

Ouzounis, C., G. Casari, A. Valencia, and C. Sander. 1996. Novelties from the complete genome of *Mycoplasma genitalium*. *Molecular Microbiology* 20:895–900.

Penrose, R., and S. Hameroff. 1995. What gaps? Reply to Grush and Churchland. *Journal of Consciousness Studies* 2:99–112.

Saier, M. H. 1993. Introduction: Protein phosphorylation and signal transduction in bacteria. *Journal of Cellular Biochemistry* 51:1–6.

Srere, P. A. 1987. Complexes of sequential metabolic enzymes 1, 2. *Annual Review of Biochemistry* 56:89–124.

Tisa, L. S., B. M. Olivera, and J. Adler. 1993. Inhibition of *Escherichia coli* chemotaxis by ω-conotoxin, a calcium ion channel blocker. *Journal of Bacteriology* 175:1235–1238.

Tocanne, J.-F., L. Cezanne, A. Lopez, B. Piknova, V. Schram, J.-F. Tournier, and M. Welby. 1994. Lipid domains and lipid/protein interactions in biological membranes. *Chemistry and Physics of Lipids* 73:139–158.

Tocanne, J.-F., L. Dupou-Cezanne, A. Lopez, and J.-F. Tournier. 1989. Lipid lateral diffusion and membrane organization. *FEBS Letters* 257:10–16.

Vaz, W. L. C., and P. F. F. Almeida. 1993. Phase topology and percolation in multi-phase lipid bilayers: Is the biological membrane a domain mosaic? *Current Opinion in Structural Biology* 3:482–488.

Webb, S. J. 1979. *Physics Letters A* 73:145.

Welti, R., and M. Glaser. 1994. Lipid domains in model and biological membranes. *Chemistry and Physics of Lipids* 73:121–137.

Wright, B. E. 1996. The effect of the stringent response on mutation rates in *Escherichia coli* K-12. *Molecular Microbiology* 19:213–210.

36 Nonlinear Dynamics in the Photoreceptor of the Unicellular Alga *Euglena gracilis*: An Application to the Evolutionary Aspects of Consciousness

Ezio M. Insinna

On the basis of recent hypotheses concerning the possibility of information processing in the cytoskeleton (Hameroff and Watt 1982; Hameroff, Smith, and Watt 1984; Hameroff 1987), there have been several attempts to hatch new theories combining microtubules (MT), quantum physics, and consciousness. Some theories directly involve MT as the major elements necessary for the emergence of consciousness (Penrose 1994; Hameroff 1994; Jibu et al. 1994; Penrose and Hameroff 1996a, b).

It is not my intention to question the correctness of some existing hypotheses—they might all be absolutely right. However, all the suggestions based on a quantum mechanical description of brain phenomena contain a major flaw—they are not falsifiable in the Popperian sense; that is, they can be neither proven nor disproved. Their contribution to a pragmatic scientific approach of the question is therefore ruined in advance by lack of falsifiability.

In addition, the theories have a second major (and probably more important) drawback—they represent a huge epistemological jump. They are a gap inside the continuity of science because they do not coherently merge with the field of present scientific knowledge.

In contemporary biology, not a single model is capable of accounting for the most basic phenomena involving MT, such as intracellular transport and ciliary beating, or more complex phenomena such as the dynamics of the spindle pole during mitosis or the function of centrioles in eukaryotic cells. Therefore, it is indispensable to first build the scaffold of a theory capable of accounting for "standard" applications of MT before turning to theories as the major components of consciousness.

Advances in the field of science are achieved through small steps that fit into the prevailing paradigm until they cause its downfall. Typically, a new, more coherent, vision of reality (or at least of what we believe to be physical reality) emerges from the ruins. Large steps often fail to establish the link with the existing consensus and thus contribute little or nothing to collapsing the old paradigm. On the contrary, far-fetched hypotheses may sometimes have the opposite effect by reinforcing reactionary scientific forces trying to keep the old paradigm alive.

The need for epistemological continuity has forced me to wander on pathways inside a coherent evolutionary context and to look for a model of MT dynamics fitting into a historically and epistemologically acceptable view of biological processes. I have, therefore, attempted to understand how MT have been utilized by evolution in connection with primitive forms of behavior such as those displayed by Protozoans.

Some primitive organisms such as *Euglena gracilis* display simple perceptive functions (phototaxis) that can be extrapolated to instinctive intelligent behavior. This unicellular organism offers the unique possibility to study the function of MT in primitive forms of behavioral responses, rather than the complex instinctive behavior of more intelligent life-forms involving sophisticated neural systems.

Several suggestions have been made to establish a connection between *Euglena*'s various phototactic strategies, the photoreceptor mechanism, and the beating flagellum. However, the various attempts have failed mainly because the molecular dynamics of the flagellum has not yet been elucidated.

On the basis of my first work on MT (Insinna 1989), I have developed a new model of MT dynamics with Zaborski and Tuszynski. The present model is capable of accounting for most phenomena associated with cell motility (Insinna et al. 1996). In addition, its heuristic capabilities have contributed new light on *Euglena*'s phototactic behavior and on some evolutionary steps leading from primitive sensory organs to more complex ones, such as the photoreceptors of vertebrates.

The model is based on classic nonlinear physics. No quantum-coherence phenomena need to be postulated in MT to explain lower (and perhaps even higher) degrees of perceptive and cognitive mechanisms.

MICROTUBULES, CLASSIC NONLINEAR DYNAMICS, AND CHARGE TRANSFER

Microtubules are ubiquitous components of the cytoskeleton in eukaryotic cells. They are associated with many dynamic phenomena ranging from the beating of cilia and flagella to chromosome movement during mitosis (Dustin 1984; Hyams and Lloyd 1994).

Dynamic cell processes connected with motility-related proteins such as dyneins, kinesins, or actins and myosins, presently lack a plausible model capable of accounting for synchronization of the contraction–motility process (Gibbons 1988; Vale 1987, 1993).

Insinna et al. (1996), suggested that the sequential activation of motor proteins (ATPases) is the result of charge transfer occurring inside the microtubular lattice (Figure 36.1). The basic premise views the entire MT as an array of dipole moment triangles that arise because of the presence of mobile electrons in hydrophobic pockets of the tubulin dimer. The electrons can switch their location from the alpha to the beta monomer and thereby reverse the orientation of the associated dipole moment of the tubulin dimer. The reversal mechanism is most likely triggered by GTP-GDP hydrolysis

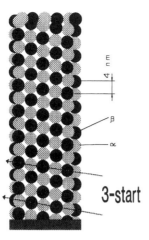

3-start

Figure 36.1 Structure of a microtubule (MT). The α and β globular tubulins are assembled in the form of a hollow cylinder about 240 Å (24 nm) in diameter. The model shows a microtubule constituted of thirteen protofilaments. A three-start helical family means that the microtubule is constituted of three helices stacked together. The pitch of a single helix is in this case 120 Å (12 nm). Charge transfer is suggested to occur along the lattice from bottom to top. (Modified from Insinna et al. 1996.)

(two energy-charged molecules). More specifically, the alpha state of the tubulin unit has its mobile electron in the top dimer (dipole moment up), and the beta state has its mobile electron in the bottom dimer (dipole moment down); the alpha state corresponds to the GTP-bound tubulin, and the beta state to the GDP-bound tubulin.

Therefore, a single hydrolysis event results in electron motion, which is also coupled to dipole reversal and an associated conformational change. It is conceivable that, under the influence of strong electric fields (which may arise in the cell's interior) or as a result of thermal effects, the mobile electrons can become completely delocalized and form a conduction band, which would directly lead to current flows along MT protofilaments or along specific helical paths of the microtubular lattice.

For example, Figure 36.2 shows the entire cycle of charge-activated, conformational changes of retrograde protein transport. The flow of an electron inside the helical MT lattice induces conformational changes within the ATP binding domain (motor domain) of the force-generating enzyme (site 2 on panel a), which allows an ATP (energy-charged) molecule to bind to the enzyme. Hydrolysis of the ATP molecule subsequently disconnects one of the protein heads from the MT. This head then binds very rapidly to the next site (site 3 on panel b) before the electron activates the ATP binding site of the second head (site 1 on panel b). The protein then waits for the next activation to continue its retrograde gliding walk along the track (panel c). A recovery time inherent in the mechanism prevents the head from reattaching to the same site immediately after ATP hydrolysis.

I have tentatively postulated that charge transfer-dependent protein activation is at the base of all MT-driven motility processes and that MT are the

Ezio M. Insinna: Nonlinear Dynamics in the Photoreceptor of *Euglena gracilis*

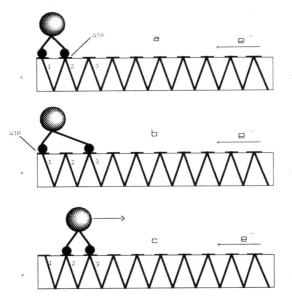

Figure 36.2 MT-based retrograde vesicle transport. (a) The charge transfer mechanism induces conformational changes both in the MT binding and in the dynein motor domain (site 1). (b) Subsequently, the ATP molecule binds to the enzyme and its hydrolysis allows the head to disconnect from the MT binding domain (site 2). The head then binds to site 3. (c) As soon as charge transfer reaches site 1, ATP hydrolysis allows the second head to disconnect and bind to site 2, which results in a retrograde transport along the MT lattice. (Modified from Insinna et al. 1996.)

clocking devices capable of coordinating the activity of all force-generating enzymes. Thus, MT deserve the name microtubular motors (MTM).

COORDINATION OF FLAGELLAR BEATING

Charge transfer inside the MTM is capable of accounting for ciliary and flagellar beating. In cilia and flagella, displacement of charges (electrons) occurs, in the normal state, distally (from the base to the tip) inside all MT fibers composing the axoneme (ciliary shaft).

In motile ciliary structures, a potential difference has to be maintained between the tip of the axoneme and the cell's interior for correct functioning of the beating mechanism (Insinna et al. 1996). In most cilia and flagella, such a potential difference (bias) is achieved through special membrane domains separating the ciliary membrane from the negative potential in the cell's interior and through sophisticated capping structures that terminate the distal ends of the axonemal MT (Dentler 1990).

The current model for ciliary and flagellar beating is based on the sliding MT hypothesis (Satir 1968; Sale and Satir 1977). Unfortunately, the model cannot account for the coordination of the axonemal components responsible for the generation of the bending wave. In ciliary and flagellar beating the smooth propagation of the bending wave along the axoneme presup-

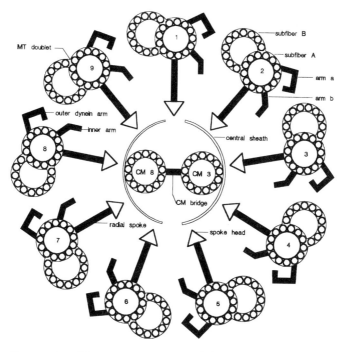

Figure 36.3 Schematic representation of the axonemal components. The cross section is viewed from base to tip. CM, central microtubule. (Modified from Warner and Satir 1974 and Insinna et al. 1996.)

poses not only the sequential activation of the dynein arms on each of the doublets, but also a sequential coordination of the entire force-generating mechanism.

The sequential activation of motility proteins is caused by the presence of electron transfer in the MTB subfibers to which the multiple heads of the dynein arms are attached (Figure 36.3). Activation of the ATPase in the motor domain of the dynein arms occurs through charge-transfer signaling at the site of attachment on the MTB subfiber. In addition to the activation of its motor domain (the head), a conformational change occurs at its distal part. This distal conformational change of the motor domain in motility proteins appears to be widely implemented by the cell to solve all synchronization problems inherent in ciliary and flagellar dynamics.

In the present model, the conformational-change mechanism plays a major role in connection with the radial spokes that connect the central pair MT to the peripheral doublets (see Figure 36.3). The radial spokehead ATPase is needed for signaling to, and control of, the MT doublet to which the radial spoke is attached distally. The conformational change occurring in the distal part of the radial spokes works as a gating mechanism as in semiconductor devices. When inactivated, the radial spokes block the current flow inside the corresponding MT B subfibers as long as the radial spokehead is not disconnected from the radial sheath of the central MT pair (CM 3 and CM 8) through ATP hydrolysis.

Ezio M. Insinna: Nonlinear Dynamics in the Photoreceptor of *Euglena gracilis*

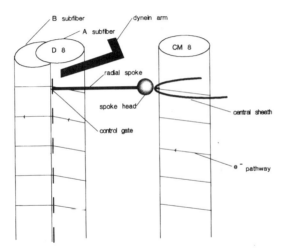

Figure 36.4 Suggested gating mechanism in cilia and flagella. Charge transfer inside the central MT (CM 8) induces conformational changes in the central sheath. The radial spoke head subsequently binds an ATP molecule and disconnects. A second conformational change occurs in the radial spoke and is transmitted to the MT doublet (D 8), which frees charge transfer and allows the activation of the binding domain of the dynein arm on the B subfiber. The arms of the preceding doublet (D 7) can then disconnect from D 8. The doublet numbers on the drawing are arbitrary and do not correspond to their true position. (Modified from Insinna et al. 1996.)

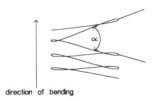

Figure 36.5 Spreading apart of the helically disposed axonemal components. The bending follows a helical path along the axoneme and tends to generate a purely helical beating. (Modified from Insinna et al. 1996.)

The gate mechanism also involves the participation of the radial or inner sheath, consisting of two rows of projections on each central MT (Witman, et al. 1976; Warner 1976). The role of these components is to distribute charge-transfer signaling from the central pair simultaneously to several radial spokes of the axoneme. A schematic representation of the gating mechanism is shown in Figure 36.4.

The dynein arms and the radial spokes are helically disposed along the axonemal structure. Combined with the charge-transfer activation of the motor proteins, the helical disposition results in a progressive spreading apart of a winding of the axonemal components under the action of CM 3 and MT 1 to MT 5 (Figure 36.5). Because of the mechanical constraints inherent in the axoneme (nexin bridges between the doublets), bending occurs in this particular zone of the flagellum. The progressive spreading apart of the imaginary winding continues along the entire structure through

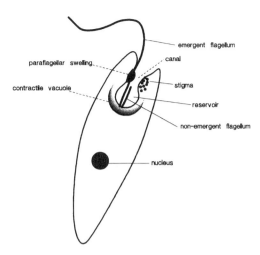

Figure 36.6 Major organelles of *Euglena gracilis*. The emergent flagellum is often accompanied by a nonemergent flagellum, which has no role in the phototactic response. The paraxial rod is parallel to the axoneme, as shown in the cross section of Figure 35.7. (Modified from Insinna et al. 1996.)

CM 8 and MT 6 to MT 9. A helical bending wave thus propagates progressively along the flagellum. According to this model, only a slight local sliding between MT is needed to produce the bending wave.

The heuristic capabilities of the model can be applied to the phototactic behavior of the Protozoan alga, *Euglena gracilis*. In *Euglena gracilis*, the locomotory flagellum (emergent flagellum, EF) is of the 9 + 2 type and is made up of nine doublet MT and a central MT pair as the majority of motile MT structures. The proximal part of the flagellum is located inside a membrane invagination (the reservoir), and its distal part emerges from it through a so-called canal. Another flagellum originating from a second basal body is much shorter and remains confined inside the reservoir (nonemergent flagellum, NEF) (Figure 36.6). Sometimes the axoneme of the NEF lacks the central pair, as is the rule in immobile flagella (Moestrup 1982). Longitudinally and circularly disposed MT surround the canal zone, probably associated to a matrix of longitudinal fibrils, the fibrillar sheath (Piccinni and Mammi 1978). A contractile vacuole has been observed at the base of the flagella, close to the reservoir. The vacuole pulsates in a rhythmic fashion and discharges every 20 to 30 seconds.

The motile flagellum carries along the entire length of its axoneme a hollow, rod-like structure with a diameter of 90 nm, the paraxial rod (PAR). The PAR is composed of seven 22-nm filaments coiled into a 7-start, left-handed helix (Hyams 1982). The pitch of the helix has been reported to be 45 degrees and the lattice periodicity 54 nm (Moestrup 1982). ATPase activity has also been detected in the rod of *Euglena* (Piccinni et al. 1975). Goblet-like projections have been observed to link the PAR with one of the MT doublets in the flagellar axoneme (Bouck et al. 1990), probably MT N.1.

Ezio M. Insinna: Nonlinear Dynamics in the Photoreceptor of *Euglena gracilis*

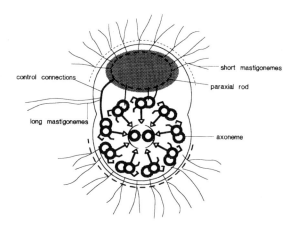

Figure 36.7 Cross section of emergent flagellum of *Euglena gracilis*. Control connections link the paraxial rod (PAR) to some of the A subfibers of the axoneme. The mastigonemes or flagellar hairs coating the flagellar membrane are also motile. The fact that the mastigonemes are attached to both the PAR and the axoneme suggests that their activation is also charge-transfer dependent and gives additional support to the present model. (Modified from Buck et al. 1990 and Insinna et al. 1996.)

However, other links seem to exist between the PAR and MT doublets N.2 and N.3 (Figure 36.7).

Located in the anterior part of the cell, between the reservoir and the canal, the paraflagellar body or paraflagellar swelling (PFS) is a visible, ovoidal protuberance on the motile emergent flagellum. At the level of the PFS, the paraxial rod seems to uncoil and completely surround the swelling (Gualtieri, 1990). Nowadays there is no doubt that in *Euglena* the PFS is the long-searched-for photoreceptive organelle (see Figure 36.6). Recently, Gualtieri et al. (1992) demonstrated the presence of rhodopsin in the PFS in *Euglena gracilis* and thereby confirmed that the PFS is the active location for photo-reception. The PFS contains as many as 1.5×10^7 rhodopsin molecules forming a crystalline-like lamellar structure (Leedale 1967; Wolken 1977; Piccinni and Mammi 1978).

The stigma, an orange-red organelle made of spheroidal granules located at the canal level and optically in line with the PFS, apparently plays the role of a shading device (Gualtieri et al. 1989). Long ago, Jennings (1906) and Mast (1911, 1914) proposed that positive phototaxis occurs through a series of corrective responses generated by the cell every time the stigma casts a shadow on the photoreceptor. These suggestions have now been widely accepted (Feinleib and Curry 1971; Feinleib 1985).

Euglena's phototactic behavior can be summarized as follows: The protist moves by the propulsive force of the 50-μm-long beating flagellum EF, in which roughly helical bending waves propagate along its structure. The 50 μm-long and 10 μm-wide cell moves in a helical path by spinning along its axis with a frequency of 1.2 to 1.8 Hz. In the phototactic strategy, the organism changes its direction in response to a light stimulus and swims

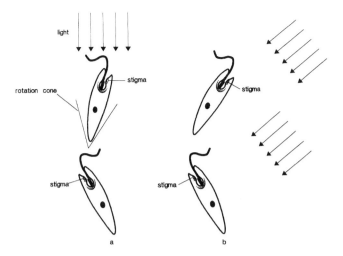

Figure 36.8 Phototactic behavior of *Euglena gracilis*. According to Mast (1917). The cell swims toward the light source as long as the incoming light is within the rotation cone. When the stigma casts a shadow on the photoreceptor, the flagellum is erected and the cell changes its direction accordingly. (Modified from Piccinni and Omodeo 1975 and Insinna et al. 1996.)

either toward (topotaxis) or away (negative phototaxis) from the light source. Positive phototaxis occurs through a series of corrective responses generated by the cell every time the stigma casts a shadow on the photoreceptor. The cell usually swims leaving its photoreceptor permanently illuminated (Figure 36.8). When the light beams are shaded by the stigma, the cell responds with an erection of the flagellum (shock or bending reaction), which results in a change of direction. Bancroft (1913) noted that the stiffening of the flagellum is proportional to the shading time.

Several suggestions have been made to connect *Euglena*'s various phototactic strategies with the photoreceptor mechanism (Insinna et al. 1996). None of these hypotheses have, however, resulted in a coherent and acceptable working model of *Euglena*'s "intelligent" phototactic response to light.

The basic principle of charge-transfer control previously postulated for the radial spokes of cilia and flagella is similarly implemented in *Euglena*'s photoreceptor architecture. Thus, the goblet-shaped projections connected to the doublets 1 to 3 of the axoneme (Figure 36.9) may be considered to work as gates for the control of the axonemal current. Activation of the gate projections happens through distally directed charge transfer occurring inside the helically disposed PAR filaments.

Euglena's phototactic capabilities can be outlined as follows: The incoming light bleaches the rhodopsin molecules contained in the paraflagellar swelling. An enzymatic cascade, following the isomerization of 11-*cis* retinal group to all-*trans*-retinal, induces changes in the charge transfer capability of PAR filaments.

As previously mentioned, ATPase activity has been detected in the rod of *Euglena* by Piccinni et al. (1975). Charge transfer activates the ATPase of the

Ezio M. Insinna: Nonlinear Dynamics in the Photoreceptor of *Euglena gracilis*

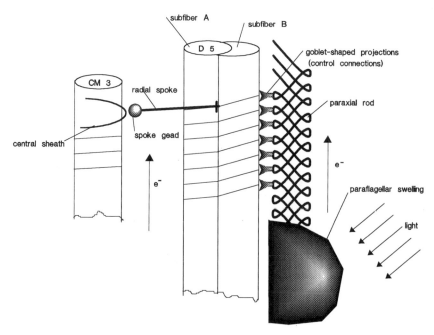

Figure 36.9 Phototactic response control mechanism in *Euglena gracilis*. The paraxial rod is shown with only three fibers instead of seven. Charge transfer inside the PAR is suggested to depend on the bleaching of rhodopsin molecules contained in the paraflagellar swelling, which in turn controls the activity of the axoneme via the goblet-shaped projections connected to the B subfiber. The cell can thus react to light changes. The phototactic response is based on a completely automatic mechanism. In the normal state (positive phototaxis), the more light that impinges on the paraflagellar swelling (PFS), the more the charge-transfer mechanism is activated inside the paraxial rod (PAR). As a result, the membrane (CM) conductance to cations decreases and the cell hyperpolarizes, which results in an increase in the beating frequency of the flagellum and in an acceleration of the cell in the medium (toward the light source). In negative phototaxis, proximity of the light source induces complete bleaching of the rhodopsin molecules. Charge transfer inside the PAR is stopped and the MTM is stalled. The membrane conductance to Ca increases and Ca^{++} enters the cell. The flagellum is first in a state of rigor, then, as soon as the Ca^{++} concentration is high enough, it starts beating in reverse until a regulating process (probably calmodulin) sets in and eliminates the surplus in Ca^{++}. (Modified from Insinna et al., 1996.)

gate projection on the paraxial rod. ATP hydrolysis induces a conformational change in the distal part of the gate projection attached to the axonemal MT doublet, and the conduction path is made free. The current flow on axonemal doublet MT 1 may thus occur as long as electron flow in the PAR continuously activates ATP hydrolysis. Both the charge transfer inside the PAR filaments and the subsequent ATP hydrolysis in the rod are light dependent.

To achieve more efficient response, the control pathway probably involves more than one MT doublet, as is shown in Figure 36.7. Every time light impinges on the detector, the current flow in the axonemal MT doublets is proportionally increased and determines the beat frequency of the flagellum. Casting a shadow on the stigma produces, instead, a decrease in ATP hydrolysis and current flow in the MT doublets, with a subsequent progressive stiffening of the corresponding axonemal components. The beating pattern of the flagellum and, thus, the cell's swimming path are modified accordingly. The stiffened fibers actually result in transforming the beat form of the flagellum so that it can work like a rudder. Therefore, shadowing of the PFS by the stigma helps *Euglena* find the direction of the light beam. The right trajectory is followed by means of successive corrections involving the flagellum beat direction.

Euglena's phototactic response to a sharp increase in light intensity consists of a shock reaction (phobotaxis) with a subsequent negative phototaxis. The flagellum is first completely straightened out and the cell subsequently moves backward during a short period (Bancroft 1913).

The model can easily explain how this occurs. On intense illumination, the sudden bleaching of the rhodopsin pigments completely stops charge transfer in the PAR. Consequently, all the gates connected to the relative MT doublets are closed (i.e., all electronic circuits along the entire length of the concerned MT axonemal doublets are switched off). This process results in complete stiffening of the flagellum. Subsequently, the Protozoan swims away from the light source via a depolarization of the cell membrane which induces a reversal of the MTM (Insinna et al. 1996).

MICROTUBULES, EVOLUTION, AND CONSCIOUSNESS

The Protozoan *Euglena gracilis* has been intentionally chosen because it is an ideal model to show how MT have been utilized by evolution to generate fast adaptive responses to environmental stimuli in primitive forms of life.

Eakin (1968) advanced that vertebrate photoreceptors and, by extension, all sophisticated sensory neurons implementing ciliary structures, are the result of an evolutionary pathway that has its origins in *Euglena*. Only the study of such primitive organisms will allow us to reach the vantage point from which we will be capable of understanding how perception has evolved into more sophisticated forms. Application of the new MT model to *Euglena* has allowed several questions to be clarified.

First, classic nonlinear dynamics is fully qualified to produce a consistent and heuristic model accounting for MT functioning and related protein activation. No global macroscopic quantum-coherent states are needed inside the MT lattice, although quantum phenomena such as electron tunneling should not be excluded and are most probably involved. It is even possible that macroscopic quantum states would represent an hindrance to local interactions, such as those needed for sequential protein activation.

Here, Occam's razor strikes again: Why should we appeal to quantum physics when it is known that quantum theory is burdened with problems such as linearity of Schrödinger's equation, energy conservation, and the like and thus is profoundly incompatible with the stable nonlinear (highly dissipative) processes of biological phenomena?

Second, it has been possible to give a plausible explanation for the functioning of *Euglena*'s protoeye. We are confronted here with a primitive form of a sensory neuron and related perception and sensory-motor reaction. The analysis of *Euglena*'s phototactic mechanism seems to lead to the following evolutionary steps: MT → centrioles → ciliated cells → sensory neurons → neuronal networks → brain.

Euglena further shows that the evolutionary process has led to the utilization of more complex processing of external stimuli through sensory cells and neurons. The conduction state of the MTM is used there to influence the membrane conductivity characteristics and subsequently cell polarization (Insinna et al. 1996). In sensory cells, the firing of the connected afferent neurons directly depends on MTM activity. Subsequently, the use of neurons for data storage and processing of sensory stimuli has been the most decisive step toward higher forms of behavior. However, MT and, as suggested, nonlinear dynamics seem to be fully involved in this process and represent a scientifically tenable alternative to quantum mechanics. This is why I believe that nonlinear dynamics has not even begun to show all its heuristical possibilities in the study of perceptive and cognitive processes and consciousness.

Third, it is epistemologically important to establish how consciousness and correlated functions such as awareness have evolved. In my opinion, speaking about consciousness outside its evolutionary context is impossible. Consciousness has evolved parallel to the development of sensory (perceptive) functions. Although consciousness cannot ultimately be reduced to sensory functions, the role of perceptive functions in its development is undeniable. We humans are what we are today because of our phylogenetic pathway. Consciousness and morphogenetical development cannot be separated into distinct processes. Jung's analytical psychology demonstrated that some unconscious psychic processes (dreams, etc.) display a symbolism that is intimately related to our phylogenetic evolution (Jung 1981). Edelmann (1992) stressed that "there must be ways to put the mind back into nature that are concordant with how it got there in the first place." The historical approach to consciousness will perhaps allow us to slowly build a bridge between mind and matter, between the biological and the psychic functions.

Euglena's instinctive behavior resulting from its automated sensory-motor capabilities (i.e., its responsiveness) might be assimilated to a primitive form of awareness. The question of how these proprioceptive capabilities are related to what we call consciousness is another story and cannot possibly be answered at this stage of preliminary investigations.

It might be plausible to think that instincts as innate, collective forms of behavior have emerged progressively in a feedback-loop phenomenon. Instincts are in the service of movement, and movement creates behavioral expression (in the service of instinct) in a mutual creative process. The process might perhaps be defined as a living phenomenon of collective nature whose evolutionary dynamics is the source of all forms of individual life. The creative feedback-loop process involving animate matter and an unknown memory substrate most probably resulted, after millions of years of interactions, in a differentiated collective psychic realm containing all evolutionary steps leading to higher forms of behavior and consciousness (i.e., Jung's collective unconscious). What *Euglena* teaches us, however, is that instincts are intimately linked with the perceptive (and proprioceptive) capabilities of the animate creature.

REFERENCES

Bancroft, F. W. 1913. Heliotropism, differential sensibility, and galvanotropism in *Euglena*. *Journal of Experimental Zoology* 15:383–428.

Bouck, G. B., Rosiere, T. K., Levasseur, P. J. 1990. *Euglena gracilis*: A model for flagellar surface assembly, with reference to other cells that bear flagellar mastigonemes scales. In R. A. Bloodgood, ed., *Ciliary and Flagellar Membranes*. New York: Plenum Press.

Dentler, W. L. 1990. Microtubule-membrane interactions. In R. A. Bloodgood, ed., *Ciliary and Flagellar Membranes*. New York: Plenum Press.

Dustin, P. 1984. *Microtubules*. Berlin: Springer.

Eakin, R. M. 1968. Evolution of photoreceptors. In T. Dobzhanski, M. K. Hecht, W. C. Steere, eds., *Evolutionary Biology*, vol. II. New York: Appleton-Century-Crofts.

Edelmann, G. 1992. *Bright Air, Brilliant Fire*. New York: Basic Books.

Feinleib, M. E. and G. M. Curry. 1971. The nature of the photoreceptor in phototaxis. In *Handbook of Sensory Physiology*, vol. I. Berlin: Springer-Verlag.

Feinleib, M. E. 1985. Behavioral studies of free-swimming photoresponsive organisms. In: Colombetti, G., ed., *Sensory Perception and Transduction in Aneural Organisms*. New York: Plenum Press.

Gibbons, I. R. 1988. Dynein ATPases as microtubule motors. *Journal of Biological Chemistry* 263:15837–15840.

Gualtieri, P., Barsanti, L., Passarelli, V. 1989. Absorption spectrum of a single isolated paraflagellar swelling of *Euglena gracilis*. *Biochimica et Biophysica Acta* 993:293–296.

Gualtieri, P., Barsanti, L., Passarelli, V., Verai, F., Rosati, G. 1990. A look into the reservoir of *Euglena gracilis*: SEM investigations of the flagellar apparatus. *Micron and Microscopica Acta* 21:131–138.

Gualtieri, P., Pelosi P. Passarelli V. Barsanti L. 1992. Identification of a rhodopsin photoreceptor in *Euglena gracilis*. *Biochimica et Biophysica Acta* 1117:55–59.

Hameroff, S. R. 1987. Ultimate computing: Biomolecular consciousness and nanotechnology. Amsterdam: Elsevier.

Hameroff, S. R. 1994. Quantum coherence in microtubules: A neural basis for emergent consciousness. *Journal of Consciousness Studies* 1:91–118.

Hameroff, S. R., and R. C. Watt. 1982. Information processing in microtubules. *Journal of Theoretical Biology* 98:549–561.

Hameroff, S. R., S. Smith, and R. C. Watt. 1984. Nonlinear electrodynamics in cytoskeletal protein lattices. In F. A. Lawrence and W. R. Adey, eds., *Nonlinear Electrodynamics in Biology and Medicine*. New York: Plenum Press.

Hameroff, S. R., and R. Penrose. 1996. Conscious events as orchestrated space-time selections. *Journal of Consciousness Studies* 3:36–53.

Hyams, J. S. 1982. The *Euglena* paraflagellar rod: structure, relationship to the other flagellar components and preliminary biochemical characterization. *Journal of Cell Science* 55:199–210.

Hyams, J. S., and C. W. Lloyd. 1994. *Microtubules*. New York: Wiley-Liss.

Insinna, E. M. 1989. Jungian synchronicity and biological morphogenesis. An application to the study of microtubules. Ph.D. thesis, Université Paris X, Nanterre.

Insinna, E. M., Zaborski, P., Tuszynski, J. 1996. Electrodynamics of microtubular motors: The building blocks of a new model. *BioSystems* 39 3:187–226.

Jennings. H. S. 1906. *Behavior of the Lower Organisms*. New York: Columbia University Press.

Jibu, M., S. Hagan, S. R. Hameroff, K. H. Pribram, and K. Yasue. 1994. Quantum optical coherence in cytoskeletal microtubules: Implications for brain function. *BioSystems* 32:95–209.

Jung, C. G 1981. *Collected Works*. London: Routledge and Kegan Paul.

Leedale, G. F. 1967. *The Euglenoid Flagellates*. Englewood Cliffs, NJ: Prentice-Hall.

Mast. S. O. 1911. *Light and the Behavior of Organisms*. New York: John Wiley and Sons.

Mast, S. O. 1914. Orientation in *Euglena* with some remarks on tropism. *Biologisches Zentralblatt* 34:641–664.

Moestrup, O. 1982. Flagellar structure in algae: A review, with new observations particularly on the *Crysophyceae, Phaenophyceae (Fucophyceae), Euglenophyceae* and *Reckertia. Phycologica* 21:427–528.

Penrose, R. 1994. *Shadows of the mind. A Search for the Missing Science of Consciousness*. New York: Oxford University Press.

Piccinni, E., Albergoni, V., Coppellotti, O. 1975. ATPase activity in flagella from *Euglena gracilis*. Localization of the enzyme and effects of detergents. *Journal of Protozoology* 22:331–335.

Piccinni, E., and M. Mammi. 1978. Motor apparatus of *Euglena gracilis*: Ultrastructure of the basal portion of the flagellum and the para-flagellar body. *Bollettino di Zoologia* 45:405–414.

Sale, W. S., and P. Satir. 1977. Direction of active sliding of microtubules in *Tetrahymena* cilia. *Proceedings of the National Academy of Sciences USA* 74:2045–2049.

Satir, P. 1968. Studies on cilia III. Further studies on the cilium tip and a "sliding filament" model of ciliary motility. *Journal of Cell Biology* 39:77.

Vale, R. D. 1987. Intracellular transport using MT-based motors. *Annual Review of Cell Biology* 3:347–378.

Vale, R. D. 1993. K. Thomas, and R. Vale, eds., *Guidebook to the Cytoskeletal and Motor Proteins*. New York: Oxford University Press, pp. 175–212.

Warner, F. D. 1976. Cross-bridge mechanism in ciliary motility: The sliding-bending conversion. In R. Goldman, T. Pollard, and J. Rosenbaum, eds. *Cell Motility*. Cold Spring Harbor, NY: Cold Spring Harbor Laboratory, pp. 891–914.

Witman, G. B., Fay, R., Plummer, J. 1976. *Chlamydomonas* mutants: Evidence for the roles of specific axonemal components in flagellar movement. In R. Goldman, T. Pollard, and J. Rosenbaum, eds., *Cell Motility*. Cold Spring Harbor, NY: Cold Spring Harbor Laboratory, pp. 969–986.

Wolken, J. J. 1977. *Euglena*: The photoreceptor system for photoxasis. *Journal of Protozoology* 24:518–522.

37 Did Consciousness Cause the Cambrian Evolutionary Explosion?

Stuart R. Hameroff

When and where did consciousness emerge in the course of evolution? Did it happen as recently as the past million years—for example, concomitant with language or tool making in humans or primates? Or did consciousness arrive somewhat earlier with the advent of mammalian neocortex 200 million years ago (Eccles 1992)? At the other extreme, is primitive consciousness a property of even simple unicellular organisms of several billion years ago, for example, as suggested by Margulis and Sagan (1995)? Or did consciousness appear at some intermediate points? If so, where and why? Whenever consciousness first occurred, did it alter the course of evolution?

CONSCIOUSNESS AND EVOLUTION

According to fossil records, life on Earth originated about 4 billion years ago (Figure 37.1). For about its first 3.5 billion years (pre-Cambrian period), life seems to have evolved slowly, producing only single cells and a few simple multicellular organisms. The most significant life-forms for the first 2 billion years of this period were algae and bacteria-like prokaryotes. Then, about 1.5 billion years ago, eukaryotic cells appeared—apparently as symbiotic mergers of previously independent organelles (mitochondria, plastids) with prokaryotic cells. According to biologist Lynn Margulis (Margulis 1975; Margulis and Sagan 1995), microtubules (MT) and the dynamically functional cytoskeleton were also outside additions and originated as independent motile spirochetes which invaded prokaryotes and formed a mutually favorable symbiosis. Prokaryotic cells provided a stable, nourishing environment and biochemical energy to the spirochetes, who reciprocated by cytoskeletal-based locomotion, sensation, mitosis, and differentiation.

Pre-Cambrian eukaryotic cells created by symbiosis continued to slowly evolve for another billion or more years, resulting only in simple multicellular organisms. Then, in a rather brief 10 million years, beginning about 540 million years ago (the beginning of the Cambrian period), a worldwide, dramatic acceleration in the rate of evolution apparently occurred: the Cambrian explosion. A vast array of diversified life abruptly emerged—all the phyla from which today's animals are descended (Gould 1989).

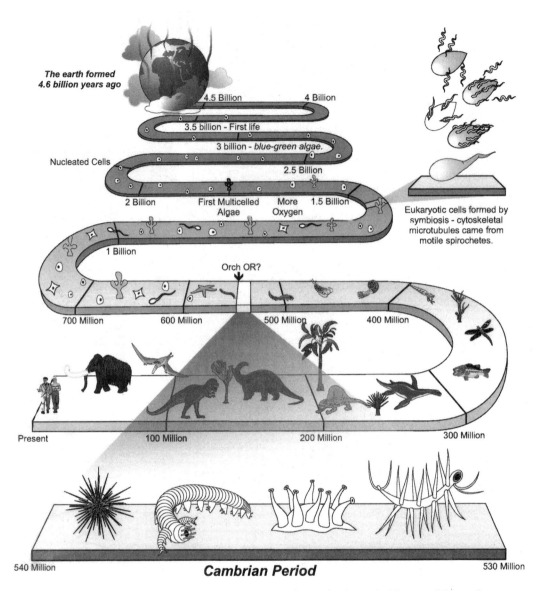

The earth formed 4.6 billion years ago

4.5 Billion

4 Billion

3.5 billion - First life

3 billion - *blue-green algae.*

Nucleated Cells

2.5 Billion

2 Billion   First Multicelled Algae   More Oxygen   1.5 Billion

Eukaryotic cells formed by symbiosis - cytoskeletal microtubules came from motile spirochetes.

1 Billion

Orch OR?

700 Million   600 Million   500 Million   400 Million

Present   100 Million   200 Million   300 Million

540 Million   ***Cambrian Period***   530 Million

Figure 37.1 The Cambrian explosion. According to fossil records, life on Earth began about 4 billion years ago but evolved slowly for the first 3.5 billion years (pre-Cambrian period). Beginning about 540 million years ago (the Cambrian period), a vast array of diversified life abruptly emerged: the "Cambrian explosion." Exemplary Cambrian organisms depicted are an urchin similar to modern *Actinosphaerium*, spiny worms, and a tentacled suctorian. (Artwork by Dave Cantrell and Cindi Laukes based on organisms in Gould 1989 and adapted from diagram by Joe Lertola, *Time*, December 4, 1995.)

The Cambrian explosion theory has been questioned. For example, using fossil nucleotide substitution analysis, Wray, Levinton, and Shapiro (1996) suggested a more linear process, with animals appearing about 1 billion years ago. But the more gradual, linear case assumes a constant rate of nucleotide substitution. It seems more likely that nucleotide substitution also increases during increased rates of evolution; thus, the abrupt Cambrian explosion theory still holds (Vermeij 1996).

What could have precipitated the Cambrian explosion? Were climate, atmosphere, environment, or external factors important or did a threshold of biological genetic complexity occur (Kauffman 1995; Dawkins 1989)? Can a particular biological functionality that critically enhanced adaptation, survivability, and mutation be identified? Did purposeful, intelligent behavior accelerate evolution?

The idea that behavior can directly alter genetic codes formed the basis of an eighteenth-century evolutionary theory by Jean-Baptiste Lamarck. No supportive evidence was found to show that behavior directly modified genetics, and "Lamarckism" was discredited. The question of whether behavior can alter the course of evolution *indirectly* was discussed by Schrödinger (1958), who offered several examples (Scott 1996). For instance, species facing predators and a harsh environment might best survive by producing a large number of offspring for cooperative support. Such a rapidly reproducing species is ripe for accelerated evolutionary development (Margulis and Sagan 1995). Another example is a species that finds a new habitat (moving onto land, climbing trees, etc.) to which adaptation is facilitated by supporting mutations. Changes in behavior can also favor chance mutations, which reinforce original changes and result in closed causal loops or positive feedback in evolutionary development (Scott 1996). Generally, intelligent behavior can enhance a species's survivability and enhance the opportunity for mutation to avoid extinction.

How did intelligent behavior come to be? Dennett (1995) described the "birth of agency"—the ability to perform purposeful actions—in complex macromolecules very early in the course of evolution. Dennett emphasized that agency and behavior at the macromolecular level are nonconscious and clearly preceded Cambrian multicellular organisms. For example, purposeful behavior surely occurred in unicellular eukaryotic ancestors of modern organisms such as *Paramecia* and *Euglena*, which perform rather complex adaptive movements. *Paramecia* swim in a graceful, gliding fashion via coordinated actions of hundreds of MT-based cilia on their outer surface. In this way they seek and find food, avoid obstacles and predators, and identify and couple with mates to exchange genetic material. Some studies suggest *Paramecia* can learn (e.g., they escape more quickly from capillary tubes with each subsequent attempt, Gelber 1958). Having no synapses or neural networks, *Paramecia* and similar organisms rely on their cytoskeleton for sensation, locomotion, and information processing. The cytoskeleton organizes intelligent behavior in eukaryotic cells.

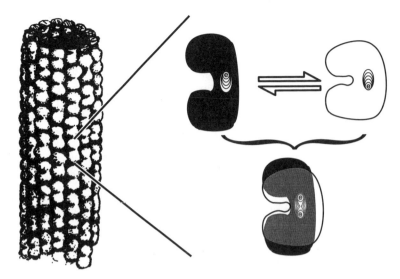

Figure 37.2 Left: Microtubule (MT) structure: a hollow tube of 25 nanometers diameter, consisting of 13 columns of tubulin dimers arranged in hexagonal lattice (Penrose 1994). Right (top): Each tubulin molecule can switch between two (or more) conformations, coupled to a quantum event such as electron location in tubulin hydrophobic pocket. Right (bottom): each tubulin can also exist in quantum superposition of both conformational states (From Hameroff and Penrose 1996).

THE CYTOSKELETON, INTELLIGENT BEHAVIOR, AND DIFFERENTIATION

Comprising internal scaffolding and external appendages of each eukaryotic cell, the cytoskeleton includes MT, actin filaments, intermediate filaments, and complex arrays of connected MT, such as centrioles, cilia, flagella, and axonemes.

MT are hollow cylinders 25 nanometers ("nm": 10^{-9} meter) in diameter (Figure 37.2). Their lengths vary and may be quite long within some nerve processes. MT cylinder walls are hexagonal lattices of tubulin subunit proteins—polar, 8-nm, peanut-shaped dimers that consist of two slightly different 4-nm monomers (alpha and beta tubulin). MT are interlinked by a variety of MT-associated proteins to form dynamic networks that define cell shape and functions. Numerous types of studies link the cytoskeleton to cognitive processes (Dayhoff, Hameroff, Lahoz-Beltra, and Swenberg 1994; Hameroff and Penrose 1996a). Theoretical models and simulations suggest that conformational states of tubulins within MT lattices are influenced by quantum events and can interact with neighboring tubulins to represent, propagate, and process information in classic cellular automata, or ferroelectric spin-glass-type computing systems (Hameroff and Watt 1982; Rasmussen et al. 1990; Tuszyński et al. 1995). Some authors suggest that quantum coherence may be involved in MT computation (Jibu, Hagan, Hameroff, Pribram, and Yasue 1994).

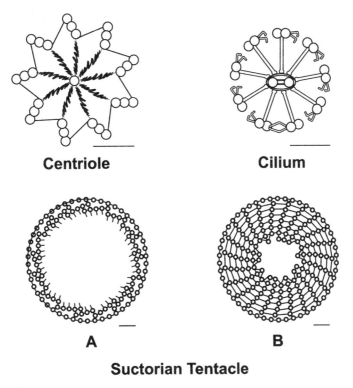

Centriole   **Cilium**

A   **B**

Suctorian Tentacle

Figure 37.3 Primitive appendages comprised of microtubules (MT, shown as circles. Top left: Cross section of a centriole. Nine microtubule triplets link to a single central MT. Top right: Cilium in cross section. Nine MT doublets link to a central MT pair. (See also Insinna, Chapter 36, Figures 36.3 and 36.7). Bottom left (A): cross section of a suctorian tentacle in an open, dilated phase. Bottom right (B): suctorian tentacle in a constricted phase. Scale bars: 100 nm. (Tentacle structure adapted from Hauser and Van Eys, 1976, by Dave Cantrell.)

MT are often assembled in nine MT doublets or triplets in a megacylinder found in centrioles, cilia, and flagella (Figure 37.3). Centrioles are two MT megacylinders in perpendicular array that control cell cycles and mitosis, form the focal point of the rest of the cell cytoskeleton, and provide cell navigation and orientation. Embedded in dense, electronegative material adjacent to the cell nucleus, the structural beauty, unfathomable geometry, and intricate behavior of centrioles have created an air of mystery: "biologists have long been haunted by the possibility that the primary significance of centrioles has escaped them" (Wheatley 1982; Lange and Gull 1996).

Cilia are membrane-covered megacylinders of nine MT doublets with an additional central MT pair that is both sensory and motor. Cilia can receive information and move in a coordinated fashion for locomotion, feeding, or movement of material. Flagella have the same 9 + 2 MT arrangement as cilia but are longer and more specialized for rapid cell movement. The basic microtubule doublet 9 + 2 (cilia, flagella, basal bodies, etc.) and 9 + 0 (centriole) arrangements apparently originated in spirochetes prior to eukaryotes. Their cytoskeletal descendants provided agency to eukaryotes by performing a variety of purposeful behaviors.

Cytoskeletal structures also provided internal organization, variation in cell shape, separation of chromosomes, and differentiation. An essential factor in evolution, differentiation involves emergence of specialized tissues and organs from groups of cells that started out alike but began to differ and develop specific and complementary form and functions (Rasmussen 1996, personal communication). Each eukaryotic cell contains all the genes of the organism but only a subset are selected; thus, for example, liver cells are distinct from lymphocytes. Puck (Puck and Krystosek 1992) showed appealing evidence to suggest that a cell's genes are activated and regulated by its cytoskeleton, and described how differentiation requires cooperative cytoskeletal function. Tissue specialization also required factors such as actingelation phases in cytoplasm, MT-based extensions (cilia, axonemes, etc.), and communication among cells. The most basic and primitive form of intercellular communication involves direct cell–cell channels such as gap junctions or electrotonic synapses (Lo 1985; Llinas 1985). Cytoskeletal cooperativity among neighboring cells enabled differentiation and allowed different types of tissues to emerge. Through benefit of the resultant division of labor, higher-order structures (e.g., axonemes, tentacles, eye cups, nervous systems, etc.) with novel functions appeared (Rasmussen 1996, personal communication), which in turn led to more intelligent behavior in small multicellular animals.

THE DAWN OF CONSCIOUSNESS

According to this scenario tissue differentiation, agency, and intelligent behavior were slowly occurring for a billion years from the symbiotic origin of eukaryotes until the Cambrian explosion (see Figure 37.1). What happened then? Was a critical level of intelligent behavior suddenly reached? Did consciousness appear? Could primitive consciousness have significantly improved fitness and survivability beyond previous benefit provided by non-conscious agency and intelligent behavior?

One possible advantage of consciousness for natural selection is the ability to make choices. As Margulis and Sagan observed (Scott 1996) (echoing similar, earlier thoughts by Erwin Schrödinger):

If we grant our ancestors even a tiny fraction of the free will, consciousness, and culture we humans experience, the increase in [life's] complexity on Earth over the last several thousand million years becomes easier to explain: life is the product not only of blind physical forces but also of selection in the sense that organisms choose.

By itself, the ability to make choices is insufficient evidence for consciousness (e.g., computers can choose intelligently). However, noncomputable, seemingly random, conscious choices with an element of unpredictability may have been particularly advantageous for survival in predator–prey dynamics (Barinaga 1996).

Another feature of consciousness favoring natural selection could be the nature of conscious experience—qualia, our "inner life"—in the sense of Chalmers' "hard problem" (Chalmers 1996a,b). Organisms that are not conscious but that have intelligent behavior are (in the philosophical sense) "zombies." If a zombie organism is threatened but has no experience of fear or pain, it may not react decisively. A conscious organism having an experience of fear or pain would be motivated to avoid threatening situations; one having experience of taste would be more motivated to find food. The experience of pleasure could well have promoted reproductive efforts.

Who were the early Cambrian organisms? Fossil records have identified a myriad of small worms, strange urchins, tiny shellfish, and many other creatures (Gould 1989, e.g. depicted at the bottom of Figure 37.1). Nervous systems in small Cambrian worms (by comparison with apparent modern cousins such as the nematode worm, *Caenorhabditis elegans*) may be estimated to contain roughly hundreds of neurons. Primitive eye cups and vision were also prevalent, as were tubelike alimentary systems with a mouth at one end and an anus at the other. Cambrian urchins and other creatures also featured prominent, spinelike extensions, which seem comparable to axoneme spines in modern echinoderms such as *Actinosphaerium*. The versatile axonemes (with MT arrays more complex than those of cilia and centrioles) are utilized for sensation, locomotion, and manipulation and provide perception, agency, and purposeful, intelligent behavior.

Because consciousness cannot be measured or observed in the best of circumstances, it seems impossible to know whether consciousness emerged in early Cambrian organisms (or at any other point in evolution). The simple (hundreds of neurons) neural networks, primitive vision, purposeful spinelike appendages, and other adaptive structures that characterize early Cambrian creatures depend heavily on cytoskeletal function, and they suggest the capability for agency, intelligent behavior, and the *possibility* of primitive consciousness. Perhaps coincidentally, a specific model (Orch OR, see below) predicts the occurrence of consciousness at precisely this level of cytoskeletal size and complexity.

CONSCIOUSNESS AND ORCHESTRATED OBJECTIVE REDUCTION

What is conscious experience? Believing that contemporary understanding of brain function is inadequate to explain qualia, or experience, a line of panpsychist—panexperiential philosophers (e.g., Leibniz, Whitehead, Wheeler, Chalmers) concluded that consciousness derives from an experiential medium that exists as a fundamental feature of reality. If so, conscious experience may be in the realm of space-time physics, and raw "protoconscious" information may be encoded in space-time geometry at the fundamental Planck scale (e.g., quantum spin networks, Penrose 1971; Rovelli and Smolin 1995a,b). A self-organizing, Planck-scale quantum process could select "fundamental" experience resulting in consciousness. Is there such a process?

A self-organizing quantum process operating at the interface between quantum and macroscopic states, objective reduction, is Penrose's (1989, 1994, 1996) quantum-gravity solution to the problem of wave function collapse in quantum mechanics. According to quantum theory (and repeatedly

Stuart R. Hameroff: Did Consciousness Cause the Cambrian Evolutionary Explosion?

verified experimentally), small-scale quantum systems described by a wave function may be "superposed" in different states or places simultaneously. Large-scale macroscopic systems, however, always appear in definite, classic states or places. The problem is that there is no apparent reason for the collapse of the wave function, no obvious border between microscopic quantum and macroscopic classic conditions. The conventional explanation—the Copenhagen interpretation—is that measurement or observation by a conscious observer collapses the wave function. To illustrate the apparent absurdity of this notion, Schrödinger (1935) described a now-famous thought experiment in which a cat was placed in a box into which poison is released when triggered by a particular quantum event. Schrödinger pointed out that, according to the Copenhagen interpretation, the cat would be both dead *and* alive until the box was opened and the cat observed by a conscious human.

To explain this conundrum, many physicists now believe that, intermediate between tiny, quantum-scale systems and large, cat-size systems, an *objective* factor disturbs the superposition and causes collapse or reduction to classic, definite states and locations. This putative process is called *objective reduction* (OR). One increasingly popular OR viewpoint, initiated by Károlyházy in 1966 (Károlyházy, Frenkel, and Lukacs 1986), suggests the "largeness" should be gauged in terms of gravitational effects—in Einstein's general relativity, gravity *is* space-time curvature. According to Penrose (1989, 1994, 1996), quantum superposition—actual separation (displacement) of mass from itself—causes underlying space-time to also separate at the Planck scale because of simultaneous curvatures in opposite directions. Such separations are unstable, and a critical degree of separation (related to quantum gravity) results in spontaneous self-collapse to particular states chosen noncomputably.

In Penrose's OR, the size of an isolated, superposed system (gravitational self-energy E of a separated mass) is inversely related to the coherence time T according to the uncertainty principle

$E = \hbar/T$

where $\hbar$ is Planck's constant over 2π and T is the duration of time for which the mass must be superposed to reach the quantum gravity threshold for self-collapse.

Large systems (e.g., Schrödinger's cat, roughly 1 kg) would self-collapse very quickly, in only 10^{-37} seconds. An isolated, superposed, single atom would not self-collapse for 10^6 years. Somewhere between those extremes are brain events in the range of tens to hundreds of milliseconds. A 25-msec brain event (i.e., one occurring in coherent 40-Hz oscillations) would require nanograms (10^{-9} gm) amounts of superposed neural mass.

In the Penrose–Hameroff Orchestrated Objection Reduction (Orch OR) model (Penrose and Hameroff 1995; Hameroff and Penrose 1996a,b), quantum coherent superposition develops in MT subunit proteins (tubulins) within brain neurons and glia. The quantum state is isolated from environmental decoherence by cycles of actin gelation and connected among neural and glial cells by quantum tunneling across gap junctions (Hameroff 1996). When the quantum-gravity threshold is reached according to $E = \hbar/T$, OR abruptly occurs. The prereduction, coherent superposition (quantum computing) phase is equated with preconscious processes, and each instantaneous OR corresponds with a discrete conscious event.

Sequences of events give rise to a "stream" of consciousness. MT-associated proteins "tune" the quantum oscillations and the OR is thus "orchestrated" (Orch OR). Each Orch OR event selects noncomputably the MT subunit states that classically regulate synaptic–neural functions. Because the superposed protein mass separation is also a separation in underlying space-time geometry, each Orch OR event selects a particular funda-mental experience.

For example, consider a low-intensity, conscious sensory perception such as activity in sensory cortex after lightly touching a finger. Such an event was shown by Libet, Wright, Feinstein, and Pearl (1979) to have a preconscious time of 500 msec until conscious awareness. For $T = 500$ msec of quantum coherent superposition, $E = $ self-collapse of approximately 10^9 tubulins. As typical neurons contain about 10^7 tubulins, Orch OR predicts involvement of roughly 10^2 to 10^3 neurons (interconnected by gap junctions) for rudimentary conscious events. For more intense conscious events, for example, events consistent with 25-msec "cognitive quanta" defined by coherent 40-Hz activity (Crick and Koch 1990; Llinas 1985; Joliot, Ribary, and Llinas 1994), superposition and self-collapse of 2×10^{10} tubulins (and 10^3–10^4 neurons) would be required.

How might Orch OR have happened? One possibility is that quantum coherence emerged in eukaryotic MT assemblies via the Fröhlich mechanism as a by-product of coordinated dynamics and biochemical energy (Fröhlich, 1968, 1970, 1975).

Quantum coherence could also be an intrinsic property of the structure and geometry of MT and centrioles—introduced to eukaryotes by spirochetes. Development of actin gels provided isolation for MT quantum states, and intercellular gap junction connections (suitable for quantum tunneling) enabled larger and larger quantum states among MT in many connected cells. At some point in the course of evolution, sufficient quantum coherence to elicit Orch OR by $E = \hbar/T$ was reached. Rudimentary "conscious" events then occurred. Organisms began to have experience and to make conscious, noncomputable choices.

THREE CANDIDATES FOR CAMBRIAN CONSCIOUSNESS

Three biological scenarios consistent with the Orch OR model for early Cambrian emergence of consciousness can be considered. Each case involves MT containing a minimum of 10^9 tubulins, sufficient for a 500-msec conscious event.

1. Sufficiently complex, gap-junction-connected neural networks (hundreds of neurons, e.g., small worms).

Many early Cambrian fossils are small worms with simple nervous systems. Hameroff and Penrose (1996b) speculated that, among current organisms, the threshold for rudimentary Orch OR conscious events (500-msec preconscious time) may be very roughly at the level of 300 neuron (3×10^9 neural tubulin) nematode worms, such as the well-studied *C. elegans*. This should be roughly the same neural network complexity as early Cambrian worms which could apparently burrow, swim, or walk the ocean floor with tentacles and spines (see Figure 1 in Gould 1989).

2. Primitive vision (ciliated ectoderm eye cup, e.g., small worms).

Another candidate for the Cambrian emergence of Orch OR consciousness involves the evolution of visual photoreceptors. Amoeba respond to light by diffuse sol-gel alteration of their actin cytoskeleton (Cronly-Dillon and Gregory 1991). *Euglena* and other single cell organisms have localized "eye spots," that is, regions at the root of the microtubule-based flagellum. Cytoplasm may focus incident light toward the eye spots and pigment material shields certain angles to provide directional light detection (Insinna, Chapter 36). *Euglena* swim either toward or away from light by flagellar motion. Having no neurons or synapses, the single-cell *Euglena*'s photic response (sensory, perceptive, and motor components) depends on MT-cytoskeletal structures.

Mammalian cells, including those of humans, can respond to light. Albrecht-Buehler (1994) showed that single fibroblast cells move toward red or infrared light by utilizing their MT-based centrioles for directional detection and guidance ("cellular vision"); he also pointed out that centrioles are ideally designed photodetectors (Figure 37.4). Jibu et al. (1994, Jibu, Pribam, and Yasue 1996) predicted that cellular vision depends on a quantum state of ordered water in MT inner cores (Figure 37.5). They postulated a nonlinear quantum-optical effect, "superradiance," that conveys evanescent photons by a process of "self-induced transparency" (the optical analogue of superconductivity). Hagan (1995, personal communication) observed that cellular vision may have provided an evolutionary advantage for single-cell organisms, with cilia, centrioles, or flagella capable of quantum coherence.

In simple multicellular organisms, eyes and visual systems began with groups of differentiated, light-sensitive ciliated cells that formed primitive eye cups (with as many as 100 photoreceptor cells) in many phyla including flatworms, annelid worms, molluscs, crustacea, echinoderms, and chordates—our original evolutionary branch, according to Cronly-Dillon and Gregory (1991).

The retinas in human eyes include over 10^8 rod and cone photoreceptors, each comprised of an inner and outer segment connected by a ciliated stalk. Because each cilium comprises about 300,000 tubulins, human retinas contain about 3×10^{13} tubulins per eye. Retinal rods, cones, and glia are interconnected by gap junctions (Leibovic 1990). Conventional vision science

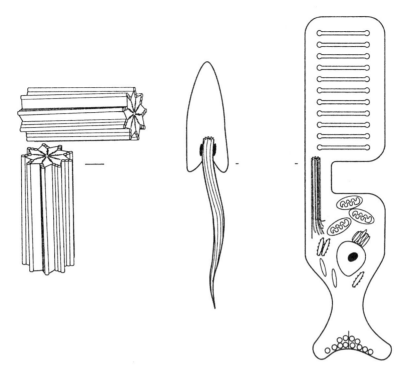

Figure 37.4 Photoreception/phototransduction mechanisms at all stages of evolution involve the nine MT doublet or triplet structures found in centrioles, cilia, flagella, and axonemes. Left: The centriole is a pair of MT-based megacylinders arrayed in perpendicular (Lange and Gull 1996). Albrecht-Buehler (1994) identified centrioles as the photoreceptor/phototransducer in photosensitive eukaryotic cells. Middle: Flagellar axonemes are the photosensitive structures in protozoa such as *Euglena gracilis* (see Insinna, Chapter 36). Right: Cilia in rod and cone retinal cells in vertebrate eyes (including humans) bridge two parts of the cells. Photosensitive pigment (rhodopsin) is contained in the outer segment (top); cell nucleus, mitochondria and synaptic connection are contained in the cell body (bottom). Light enters the eye (from the bottom in this illustration) and traverses the cell body and cilium to reach the rhodopsin-containing outer segment. Scale bars: 100 nm. (Adapted from Lange and Gull 1996 and Insinna, Chapter 36, by Dave Cantrell.)

assumes the cilium is purely structural, but the centriole–cilium–flagella MT structure, which Albrecht-Buehler analyzed as an ideal directional photoreceptor, may detect or guide photons in eye spots of single cells, primitive eye cups in early multicellular organisms, and rods and cones in human retinas. Quantum coherence leading to consciousness could have emerged in sheets of gap-junction-connected ciliated cells in eye cups of early Cambrian worms.

3. Geometrical microtubule arrays (e.g., axoneme spines in small urchins such as *Actinosphaerium*, tentacles in suctorians).

Perhaps consciousness occurred in even simpler organisms? Many Cambrian fossils are similar or related to current species that have particularly interesting MT geometrical arrangements. For example, *Actinosphaerium*

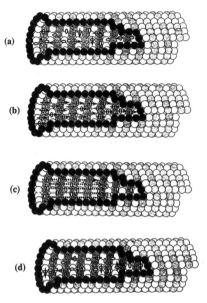

Figure 37.5 A schematic representation of the process of superradiance in a microtubule proposed by Mari Jibu et al. (1994). Each oval without an arrow stands for a water molecule in the lowest rotational energy state. Each oval with an arrow stands for a water molecule in the first excited rotational energy state. The process is cyclic ($a \rightarrow b \rightarrow c \rightarrow d \rightarrow a \rightarrow b$), and so forth. (a) Initial state of the system of water molecules in a microtubule. Energy gain caused by the thermal fluctuations of tubulins increases the number of water molecules in the first excited rotational energy state. (b) A collective mode of the system of water molecules in rotationally excited states. Long-range coherence is achieved inside a microtubule by means of spontaneous symmetry breaking. (c) A collective mode of the system of water molecules in rotationally excited states loses its energy collectively and creates coherent photons in the quantized electromagnetic field inside a microtubule. (d) Water molecules, having lost their first excited rotational energies by superradiance, start again to gain energy from the thermal fluctuation of tubulins, and the system of water molecules recovers the initial state (a). (From Jibu et al. 1994, with permission.)

(*Echinosphaerium*) *nucleofilum* is a modern echinoderm, a tiny sea-urchin heliozoan with about 100 rigid, protruding axonemes about 300 μm in length (see Figure 37.4). Appearing similar to spines of Cambrian echinoderms, *Actinosphaerium* axonemes sense and interact with environment, provide locomotion, and each comprise several hundred MT interlinked in a double spiral (Figure 37.6). Each axoneme contains about 3×10^7 tubulins, and the entire heliozoan contains 3×10^9 tubulins (Roth, Pihlaja, and Shigenaka 1970)— perhaps coincidentally, the precise quantity predicted by Orch OR for a 500-msec conscious event.

Allison and Nunn (1968) and Allison et al. (1970) studied living *Actinosphaerium* in the presence of the anesthetic gas halothane. They observed that the axoneme MT disassembled in the presence of halothane (although at anesthetic concentrations two to four times higher than that required for anesthetic effect).

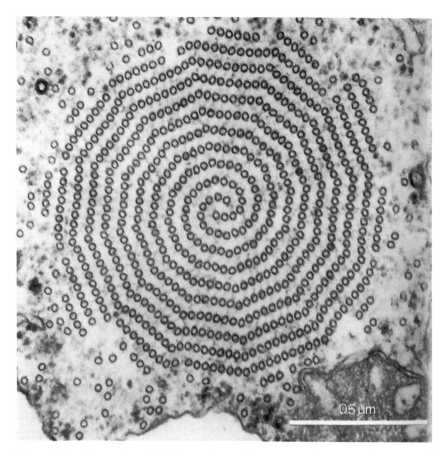

Figure 37.6 Cross-section of double spiral array of interconnected MTs in single axoneme of *Actinosphaerium*, a tiny heliozoan related to sea-urchin echinoderms present at the Cambrian evolutionary explosion (see Figure 37.1). Each cell has about 100 long and rigid axonemes, which are about 300 μm in length and are made up of a total of 3×10^9 molecules of tubulin. Scale bar: 500 nm. (From Roth 1970, with permission.)

Somewhat similar to axonemes are larger prehensile tentacles in suctorians such as *Akinetoposis* and *Heliophyra*. Small multicellular animals, suctorians (see Figure 37.3) have dozens of tiny, hollow tentacles that probe their environment and capture and ingest prey, such as *Paramecium*. The prehensile tentacles range from about 300 μm to 1 mm in length. Their internal structure comprises longitudinal arrays of about 150 MT in a ring around an inner gullet through which prey and food pass (see Figure 37.3). MT apparently slide over one another in a coordinated fashion to provide tentacle movement and contractile waves involved in food capture, ingestion, and other adaptive behaviors. The activity is interrupted by the anesthetic halothane (Hauser and Van Eys 1976). A single suctorian tentacle (150 MT, length of 500 μm) contains about 10^9 tubulins—the predicted requirement for a 500-msec Orch OR event. Perhaps consciousness arose in the probings of a Cambrian suctorian tentacle?

Would such primitive Orch OR experiences in a Cambrian worm, urchin, or suctorian be anything like experiences of humans? What would it be like to be a tentacle? A single, 10^9 tubulin, 500-msec Orch OR in a primitive system would have gravitational self-energy (and thus experiential intensity) perhaps equivalent to a human "touch lightly on the finger" experience. However, the human everyday coherent 40-Hz brain activity would correspond to 25 msec events involving 2×10^{10} tubulins, and so the typical human experience would be 20 times more intense. Humans also would have many more Orch OR events per second (40 vs. a maximum of 2) with extensive sensory processing and associative memory, which presumably, was lacking in Cambrian creatures. Nonetheless, by Orch OR criteria, a 10^9 tubulin, 500-msec Orch OR event in a Cambrian worm, urchin, or tentacle would have been a conscious experience—a smudge of awareness, a shuffle in funda-mental space-time.

CONCLUSION

The place of consciousness in evolution is unknown, but the actual course of evolution may offer a clue. Fossil records indicate that animal species as we know them today—including conscious humans—arose from a burst of evolutionary activity some 540 million years ago in the Cambrian explosion. Thus, I suggest that:

1. Occurrence of consciousness most likely accelerated the course of evolution.

2. Small worms, urchins, and comparable creatures reached critical biological complexity for emergence of primitive consciousness at the early Cambrian period 540 million years ago.

3. Cooperative dynamics of MT, cilia, centrioles, and axonemes were the critical biological factors for consciousness.

4. Cytoskeletal complexity available in early Cambrian animals closely matches criteria for the Penrose-Hameroff Orch OR model of consciousness.

5. Orch OR caused the Cambrian explosion.

REFERENCES

Albrecht-Buehler, G. 1994. Cellular infra-red detector appears to be contained in the centrosome. *Cell Motility and the Cytoskeleton* 27(3):262–271.

Allison, A. C., G. H. Hulands, J. F. Nunn, J. A. Kitching, and A. C. MacDonald. 1970. The effects of inhalational anaesthetics on the microtubular system in *Actinosphaerium* nucleofilm. *Journal of Cell Science* 7:483–499.

Allison, A. C., and J. F. Nunn. 1968. Effects of general anesthetics on microtubules. A possible mechanism of anesthesia. *Lancet* 2:1326–1329.

Barinaga, M. 1996. Neurons put the uncertainty into reaction times. *Science* 274:344.

Chalmers, D. J. 1996a. *The Conscious Mind—*In *Search of a Fundamental Theory*. New York: Oxford University Press.

Chalmers, D. J. 1996b. Facing up to the problem of consciousness. In S. R. Hameroff, A. Kaszniak, and A. C. Scott, eds., *Toward a Science of Consciousness—The First Tucson Discussions and Debates*. Cambridge: MIT Press, pp. 5–28.

Crick, F. H. C., and C. Koch. 1990. Towards a neurobiological theory of consciousness. *Seminars in the Neurosciences* 2:263–275.

Cronly-Dillon, J. R., and R. L. Gregory. 1991. *Evolution of the Eye and Visual System (Vision and Visual Dysfunction*, vol. II.) Boca Raton: CRC Press.

Dawkins, R. 1989. *The Selfish Gene*, rev. ed. Oxford: Oxford University Press.

Dayhoff, J. E., S. Hameroff, R. Lahoz-Beltra, and C. E. Swenberg. 1994. Cytoskeletal involvement in neuronal learning: A review. *European Biophysics Journal* 23:79–93.

Dennett, D. C. 1995. *Darwin's Dangerous Idea: Evolution and the Meanings of Life*. New York: Touchstone.

Eccles, J. C. 1992. Evolution of consciousness. *Proceedings of the National Academy of Sciences USA* 89:7320–7324.

Fröhlich, H. 1975. The extraordinary dielectric properties of biological materials and the action of enzymes. *Proceedings of the National Academy of Sciences USA* 72:4211–4215.

Fröhlich, H. 1970. Long-range coherence and the actions of enzymes. *Nature* 228:1093.

Fröhlich, H. 1968. Long-range coherence and energy storage in biological systems. *International Journal of Quantum Chemistry* 2:641–649.

Gould, S. J. 1989. *Wonderful Life—The Burgess Shale and the Nature of History*. New York: W. W. Norton.

Gelber, B. 1958. Retention in *Paramecium aurelia*. *Journal of Comparative and Physiological Psychogy* 51:110–115.

Hameroff, S. 1996. Cytoplasmic gel states and ordered water: Possible roles in biological quantum coherence. *Proceedings of the Second Advanced Water Symposium*, Dallas, Texas, October 4–6. http://www.u.arizona.edu/~hameroff.

Hameroff, S. 1997. Funda-mental geometry: The Penrose-Hameroff Orch OR model of consciousness. In N. Woodhouse, ed. *Geometry and the Foundations of Science: Contributions from an Oxford Conference Honoring Roger Penrose*. Oxford: Oxford University Press.

Hameroff, S. R., and R. Penrose. 1996a. Orchestrated reduction of quantum coherence in brain microtubules: A model for consciousness. In S. R. Hameroff, A. Kaszniak, and A. C. Scott eds., *Toward a Science of Consciousness—The First Tucson Discussions and Debates*. Cambridge: MIT Press.

Hameroff, S. R., and R. Penrose. 1996b. Conscious events as orchestrated spacetime selections. *Journal of Consciousness Studies* 3(1):36–53.

Hameroff, S. R., and R. C. Watt. 1982. Information processing in microtubules. *Journal of Theoretical Biology* 98:549–561.

Hauser, M., and H. Van Eys. 1976. Microtubules and associated microfilaments in the tentacles of the suctorian *Heliophyra erhardi* Matthes. *Journal of Cell Science* 20(3):589–617.

Jibu, M. 1990. On a heuristic model of the coherent mechanism of the global reaction process of a group of cells (in Japanese). *Bussei Kenkyuu (Material Physics Research)* 53(4):431–436.

Jibu M., K. H. Pribram and K. Yasue. 1995. From conscious experience to memory storage and retrieval: The role of quantum brain dynamics and Bose condensation of evanescent photons. *International Journal of Modern Physics B* 13 and 14:1735–1754.

Jibu, M., S. Hagan, S. R. Hameroff, K. H. Pribram, and K. Yasue. 1994. Quantum optical coherence in cytoskeletal microtubules: Implications for brain function. *BioSystems* 32:195–209.

Joliot, M., U. Ribary, and R. Llinas. 1994. Human oscillatory brain activity near 40 Hz coexists with cognitive temporal binding. *Proceedings of the National Academy of Sciences USA* 91(24):11748–11751.

Károlyházy, F. 1966. Gravitation and quantum mechanics of macroscopic bodies. *Nuova Chimica* 42:390–402.

Károlyházy, F., A. Frenkel, and B. Lukacs. 1986. On the possible role of gravity on the reduction of the wave function. In R. Penrose and C. J. Isham, eds., *Quantum Concepts in Space and Time*. New York: Oxford University Press.

Kauffman, S. 1995. *At Home in the Universe*. New York: Oxford University Press.

Lange, B. M. H., and K. Gull. 1996. Structure and function of the centriole in animal cells: Progress and questions. *Trends in Cell Biology* 6:348–352.

Leibniz, G. W. 1768. *Opera Omnia*. (L. Dutens, ed.) Geneva.

Leibovic, K. N. 1990. *Science of Vision*. New York: Springer-Verlag.

Libet, B., E. W. Wright, Jr., B. Feinstein, and D. K. Pearl. 1979. Subjective referral of the timing for a conscious sensory experience. *Brain* 102:193–224.

Llinas, R. R. 1985. Electrotonic transmission in the mammalian central nervous system. In M. V. L. Bennett and D. C. Spray, eds., *Gap Junctions*. Cold Spring Harbor, NY: Cold Spring Harbor Laboratory, pp. 337–353.

Lo, C. W. 1985. Communication compartmentation and pattern formation in development. In M. V. L. Bennett and D. C. Spray eds., *Gap Junctions*. Cold Spring Harbor, NY: Cold Spring Harbor Laboratory, pp. 251–263.

Margulis, L. 1975. *Origin of Eukaryotic Cells*. New Haven: Yale University Press.

Margulis, L., and D. Sagan. 1995. *What Is Life?* New York: Simon & Schuster.

Penrose, R. 1994. *Shadows of the Mind*. New York: Oxford University Press.

Penrose, R. 1989. *The Emperor's New Mind*. Oxford: Oxford University Press.

Penrose, R. 1971. In E. A. Bastin, ed., *Quantum Theory and Beyond*. Cambridge: Cambridge University Press.

Penrose, R. 1996. On gravity's role in quantum state reduction. *General Relativity and Gravitation Journal* 28(5):581–600.

Penrose, R., and S. R. Hameroff. 1995. What gaps? Reply to Grush and Churchland. *Journal of Consciousness Studies* 2(2):99–112.

Puck, T. T., and A. Krystosek. 1992. Role of the cytoskeleton in genome regulation and cancer. *International Review of Cytology* 132:74–108.

Rasmussen, S., H. Karampurwala, R. Vaidyanath, K. S. Jensen, and S. Hameroff. 1990. Computational connectionism within neurons: A model of cytoskeletal automata subserving neural networks. *Physica D* 42:428–449.

Roth, L. E., D. J. Pihlaja, and Y. Shigenaka. 1970. Microtubules in the heliozoan axopodium. I. The gradion hypothesis of allosterism in structural proteins. *Journal of Ultrastructural Research* 30:7–37.

Rovelli, C., and L. Smolin. 1995. Discreteness of area and volume in quantum gravity. *Nuclear Physics B* 442:593–619.

Rovelli, C., and L. Smolin. 1995. Spin networks in quantum gravity. *Physical Review D* 52(10):5743–5759.

Saubermann, A. J., and M. L. Gallagher. 1973. Mechanisms of general anesthesia: Failure of pentobarbital and halothane to depolymerize microtubules in mouse optic nerve. *Anesthesiology* 38:25–29.

Schrödinger, E. 1935. Die gegenwarten situation in der quantenmechanik. *Naturwissenschaften* 23:807–812, 823–828, 844–849. Translation: J. T. Trimmer (1980). *Proceedings of the American Philosophical Society* 124:323–338.

Schrödinger, E. 1958. *Mind and Matter*. Cambridge: Cambridge University Press.

Scott, A. 1995. *Stairway to the Mind*. Berlin: Springer-Verlag.

Scott, A. C. 1996. Book review: Lynn Margulis and Dorion Sagan, *What Is Life? Journal of Consciousness Studies* 3(3):286–287.

Tuszyński, J., S. Hameroff, M. V. Sataric, B. Trpisova, and M. L. A. Nip. 1995. Ferroelectric behavior in microtubule dipole lattices: Implications for information processing, signaling and assembly/disassembly. *Journal of Theoretical Biology* 174:371–380.

Vermeij, G. J. 1996. Animal origins. *Science* 274:525–526.

Wheatley, J. N. 1982. *The Centriole: A Central Enigma of Cell Biology*. Amsterdam: Elsevier.

Wray, G. A., J. S. Levinton, and L. H. Shapiro. 1996. Molecular evidence for deep precambrian divergences among metazoan phyla. *Science* 274:568–573.

VII Anesthesiology

OVERVIEW

Each year millions of people have their consciousness temporarily erased while they undergo general anesthesia for surgical procedures. Use of anesthesia is a recent luxury—surgery from ancient times until the nineteenth century was routinely performed only with sedation and partial pain relief from alcohol, alkaloids, hypnosis, or ice cooling. Modern anesthesia stems from the discovery of inhalational gas anesthetics—nitrous oxide, chloroform and ether—a little more than 100 years ago. When properly administered, these gases cause complete loss of consciousness and insensibility to pain, yet their effects are completely and rapidly reversible. The gases are delivered via the airway to the lungs, where they diffuse and dissolve in the blood and are then carried to the brain and other organs. Inside the brain, anesthetic gases leave the blood and dissolve by weak binding in a certain water-free hydrophobic environment.

Continuing improvements in anesthetics have led to modern gases such as isoflurane and sevoflurane and the ever-dependable nitrous oxide ("laughing gas," which played a supporting role in *The Little Shop of Horrors*). In addition to these vapors, anesthesiologists use intravenous drugs including opioids for pain relief, benzodiazepines for sedation and amnesia, sodium pentothal to induce loss of consciousness, and propofol for a combination of effects. But these drugs may also affect breathing, blood pressure, and heart and kidney function. Because such changes must be countered, anesthesiologists are obliged to administer minimal doses sufficient to prevent consciousness. Despite enormous advances in the technology of cardiovascular, respiratory and metabolic monitoring, however, there is still no way to directly detect consciousness.

Anesthesiologists determine adequate anesthesia—absence of consciousness—primarily by autonomic correlates that indicate indirectly the *depth* of anesthesia. For example, increased heart rate or blood pressure, changes in pupils, tearing, sweating, airway secretions, and so on may signify light anesthesia and a need to deepen the anesthetic. Decreases in these signs may indicate too deep anesthesia. Although electroencephalographic (EEG) monitoring also correlates with anesthetic depth—frequencies become slower with deep anesthesia—it is rarely used for monitoring anesthetic depth because it is no more predictive than autonomic signs. Other monitoring techniques include facial muscle microsensing, electroretinography, sensory-evoked potentials, and esophageal contractility (Hameroff, Polson, and Watt 1994), but, as with electoencephalograms, these monitors are rarely used because they appear no better than vigilant monitoring of autonomic signs.

Prevention of consciousness is an essential objective of every general anesthetic. Sadly, a few cases of recall of intraoperative events have been documented in patients presumed to have been unconscious. Many of these situations are relatively innocuous; for example, patients remember conversations but experience no pain or anxiety. In some very rare and disturbing cases, however, patients have reported remembering extreme pain and suffering. Causes of intraoperative awareness and recall include "pilot error" (anesthetic vaporizer running dry, insufficient dosing, enhanced patient metabolism, etc.), equipment malfunction, reduced dosing because of a tenuous condition (shock or hemorrhage), or unknown causes. (General anesthesia should not be confused with sedation, which is used in relatively minor procedures with local anesthesia. For sedation, patients are given amnestics; they may sleep lightly but are not intended to be—nor do they need to be—completely unconsicous.)

Intraoperative conscious awareness can be distinguished from postoperative recall; for example, it is theoretically possible for patients to have intraoperative awareness but no memory of the procedure. This possibility has led to a frightening conjecture that intraoperative awareness may be more common than has been realized—the patients have no postoperative recall of their awareness because of the amnestic effects of anesthetic drugs. Such a situation is extremely unlikely, however, because signs of light anesthesia are promptly treated before awareness can occur. There is also evidence that memory (implicit learning) of intraoperative events can occur without awareness; the information is processed subconsciously. Thus, recall could occur without intraoperative consciousness, which implies that in some circumstances subconscious or preconscious processes continue during anesthesia. Diethyl ether (no longer used) was often associated with bizarre dreams, and dreaming is occasionally reported following light anesthesia with intravenous propofol or ketamine, but these occurrences are rarely experienced under deep anesthesia with a potent modern gas. Nevertheless, the problem of intraoperative awareness is of great concern and is being carefully studied.

Anesthesiology provides a window into the phenomena of consciousness through the mechanism of action of anesthetic drugs. Part VII includes two chapters on the pharmacological actions of anesthetics.

The preeminent work in the study of anesthetic mechanisms during the past 15 years has been done by biophysicists Nicholas Franks and William

Lieb at Imperial College in London. They give an overview of the actions of the diverse group of anesthetics, which ranges from the inert gas xenon and other volatile gases to soluble barbiturates, alcohols, and steroids. It has been known since the seminal work of Meyer and Overton at the turn of the century that these disparate compounds share a common solubility in a particular lipidlike hydrophobic environment akin to olive oil. For most of this century, this observation was interpreted to mean that anesthetics exert their actions in lipid portions of neural membranes. Recognizing that intrinsic proteins (ion channels, receptors) are the essential, active components of neural membranes, Franks and Lieb looked critically at this interpretation in the early 1980s (as did Michael Halsey and a few others). Franks and Lieb showed that anesthetic effects in the lipid portions of membranes are inconsequential, but their effects on isolated proteins follow the Meyer-Overton correlation: The more potent an anesthetic, the more it dissolves in olive oil, the more it inhibits the protein. The anesthetics manage this by weakly binding in hydrophobic pockets within the sensitive proteins. (For a view that hydrophobic pockets harbor quantum effects essential for consciousness, see Hameroff, Chapter 18).

The identification of precisely which neural proteins are critically affected by anesthetics might identify key sites for consciousness. Franks and Lieb point out that most work has been done on either axonal presynaptic ion channels, or on postsynaptic receptor-gated channels. Among postsynaptic receptors, those responsive to glutamate (the principal excitatory neurotransmitter in mammalian brain) are surprisingly resistant to anesthetics. On the other hand, Franks and Lieb have found a genetically linked group extremely sensitive to anesthetics—gamma-aminobutyric acid (GABA), glycine, serotonin, and nicotinic acetylcholine receptors. Oddly, because GABA and glycine receptors are inhibitory, anesthetics appear to somehow promote their activation while inhibiting the excitatory action of serotonin and nicotinic receptors. Franks and Lieb also observe that other less sensitive proteins, such as presynaptic channels and cytoskeletal proteins, are far more prevalent; slight effects on a large number of critical sites could account for anesthesia, particularly if those sites are essential for consciousness.

The most common excitatory, postsynaptic receptors (e.g., N-methyl-D-aspartate [NMDA] receptors) respond to glutamate and are resistant to gaseous anesthetics. They are, however, markedly affected by intravenous *dissociative* drugs such as ketamine and the animal anesthetic—street hallucinogen phencyclidine (PCP). Hans Flohr discusses the pharmacology of NMDA receptors and argues that their activity is necessary for consciousness. He describes how these large receptor complexes interact with ion channels, other receptors like GABA, a variety of biomolecules, and with second-messenger and cytoskeletal factors. At low doses, ketamine and phencyclidine cause "sensory illusions, visual and auditory hallucinations, distortions of body image, and disorganized thought"; at high doses they cause anesthesia.

Sites of action of anesthetic drugs provide a map of consciousness, but the mechanism of anesthetic effect and the nature of consciousness remain unknown. The two may be closely related.

REFERENCES

Hameroff, S. R., J. S. Polson, and R. C. Watt 1994. Monitoring anesthetic depth. In C. Blitt and R. Hines, eds., *Monitoring in Anesthesia and Critical Care Medicine*, 3rd ed. New York: Churchill Livingstone, pp. 491–507.

38 The Molecular Basis of General Anesthesia: Current Ideas

Nicholas P. Franks and William R. Lieb

General anesthetics represent a most extraordinary and diverse collection of chemicals, ranging from the inert gas xenon to barbiturates and steroids. Although these chemicals are all, by definition, capable of inducing a state of loss of consciousness, they do much more. Anesthetics are capable of producing a wide spectrum of effects, and this spectrum differs considerably among the different agents. Nonetheless, despite the complexity, certain relatively arbitrary stages that characterize progressive anesthetic "depth" can be defined. The stages are listed in Table 38.1. (In clinical practice, the principal components of "anesthesia," namely, loss of consciousness and recall, analgesia, and muscle relaxation, are often achieved using a combination of different drugs to supplement the anesthetic agent.)

For the practicing anesthetist, the assessment of anesthetic depth is a matter of observation, experience, and common sense. For the neuropharmacologist interested in understanding how general anesthetics exert their effects, certain defined endpoints that can be precisely and reproducibly measured are needed. For humans, two measurements have particular value. The first measure, and the one of most surgical relevance, is the anesthetic concentration at which 50 percent of patients do not move purposefully in response to a painful stimulus (e.g., a surgical incision). For inhalational anesthetics this point is termed the minimum alveolar concentration (MAC) (Quasha, Eger, and Tinker 1980). MAC is usually expressed as a concentration in air, but it can also be expressed as a free aqueous concentration. For certain intravenous anesthetics, equivalent concentrations can also be determined but this is much more difficult because of their complex pharmacokinetics (e.g., intravenous anesthetics are continuously metabolized); measurement requires establishing known steady-state anesthetic concentrations in the blood.

The second measure is the anesthetic concentration at which 50 percent of patients fail to respond to a verbal command (e.g., "squeeze my hand"). This measure is often termed MAC awake. MAC awake values for humans appear to be equivalent to anesthetic concentrations needed to inhibit the righting reflex in laboratory animals (e.g., is a mouse placed on its back able to get to its feet); the painful stimulus applied for a determination of MAC is equivalent to the pain caused by a tail clamp in a dog or rodent.

Table 38.1 Stages of Anesthetic Depth (Rang, Dale, and Ritter 1995)

Stage	Description
Stage I	*Analgesia.* The patient is conscious, but drowsy. The degree of analgesia (if any) depends on the anesthetic.
Stage II	*Excitement.* The patient loses consciousness and does not respond to a nonpainful stimulus. The patient may move, talk incoherently, be hypotensive, or have other respiratory or cardiovascular irregularities.
Stage III	*Surgical anesthesia.* Spontaneous movement ceases and ventilation becomes regular. As anesthesia deepens, various reflexes are lost and the muscles relax.
Stage IV	*Medullary depression.* Respiration and vasomotor control cease, leading to death.

Although it seems obvious that failure to respond to a verbal command is some measure of loss of consciousness and that failure to respond to a surgical incision depends on both the loss of consciousness and the extent of anesthetic-induced analgesia, these endpoints are essentially arbitrary measures of anesthetic depth (albeit of great practical utility) and reflect a complex state in which numerous functions of the nervous system are affected. General anesthetics should not, therefore, be thought of as "magic bullets" that specifically ablate consciousness but as relatively blunt instruments whose most striking common property is to render a patient insensitive to pain.

How do these remarkable drugs work? Most progress has been made at the molecular level, and some simplifying themes have emerged. This chapter reviews current thinking in the field and emphasizes areas that promise most for the future.

PRIMARY SITES OF GENERAL ANESTHETIC ACTION

Almost a century ago, Meyer and Overton noted an excellent correlation between the potency of an anesthetic and its solubility in olive oil. A modern version (Franks and Lieb 1994) of this correlation is shown in Figure 38.1 in the plot of the logarithm of anesthetic potency (defined as the reciprocal of the aqueous molar EC_{50} concentration for general anesthesia) against the logarithm of the lipid bilayer–water partition coefficient. Despite some exceptions, this correlation is exceptionally good.

The observations of Meyer and Overton led to the idea that general anesthetics act by dissolving in lipid regions of the brain. When it was later discovered that neuronal membranes consist of lipid bilayers and associated proteins, attention focused on the effects of anesthetics on lipid bilayers. Until the late 1970s, the most widely accepted theory was that anesthetics so perturb the structural and dynamic properties of neuronal lipid bilayers (e.g., by acting like plasticizers and fluidizing the bilayers) that the functioning of membrane-associated proteins such as ion channels are affected. This

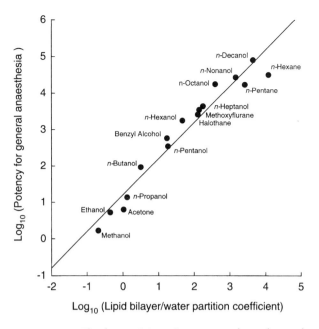

Figure 38.1 The famous Meyer-Overton correlation has traditionally been interpreted as meaning that the primary target sites are lipid portions of nerve membranes. In its modern form, shown here, a good correlation is seen to exist between the potency of an anesthetic (reciprocal of its molar EC_{50} concentration for anesthesia) and its lipid–water partition coefficient. (From Franks and Lieb 1994, with permission.)

was an attractive idea because it accounted for the Meyer-Overton correlation and also suggested specific molecular mechanisms of general anesthetic action.

However, in the late 1970s, quantitative structural studies using x-ray and neutron diffraction (Franks and Lieb 1978, 1979) showed that clinical concentrations of general anesthetics had little, if any, effect on the structure of lipid bilayer models of neuronal membranes. These studies were followed by dynamic investigations (e.g., use of laser Raman scattering by Lieb, Kovalycsik, and Mendelsohn 1982) showing barely measurable changes in the fluidity of lipid bilayers. Moreover, and perhaps most important, in almost all studies, changes reported at surgical concentrations of anesthetics could be mimicked by very small changes ($<1\,^{\circ}C$) in temperature (Franks and Lieb 1982). Because such temperature variations are well within the normal physiological range and do not result in anesthesia, it followed that changes in lipid bilayers caused by clinical concentrations of anesthetics were unlikely to be important in general anesthesia.

These negative experimental findings with lipid bilayers suggested that general anesthetics may instead act by binding directly to proteins. It is generally agreed that proteins are the ultimate targets in general anesthesia; could it be that proteins are also the primary targets to which anesthetics bind? Strong evidence in favor of this idea came from our finding that a purified, lipid-free enzyme (firefly luciferase) not only could bind a diverse

Nicholas P. Franks and William R. Lieb: Molecular Basis of General Anesthesia: Current Ideas

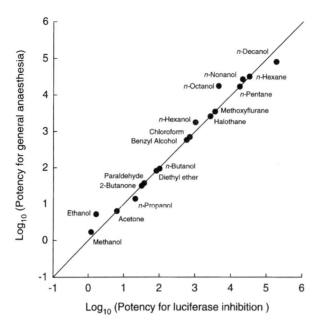

Figure 38.2 General anesthetic potencies for inhibiting the activity of the lipid-free enzyme firefly luciferase are essentially identical to their potencies for causing general anesthesia in animals. (From Franks and Lieb 1994, with permission.)

range of anesthetic agents but was inhibited at IC_{50} concentrations that were essentially identical to the EC_{50} concentrations that produce general anesthesia (Franks and Lieb 1984). Figure 38.2 plots the logarithm of potency for general anesthesia against the logarithm of the potency for inhibiting firefly luciferase; the straight line is the line of identity. These results showed that the observations of Meyer and Overton could be explained quantitatively by anesthetics binding to proteins. Together with the negative results for lipids, this result encouraged the view that most, if not all, the effects of clinical levels of general anesthetics are caused by direct interactions with proteins.

The strongest support for this new view has come from recent experiments with optical isomers (enantiomers) of general anesthetics. The recent availability of the two enantiomers of the inhalational agent isoflurane has been particularly important because, in contrast to intravenous agents, their EC_{50} concentrations (MACs) for mammalian general anesthesia can be determined very accurately. In the rat, the MAC for R(−) isoflurane is 50 percent greater than that for S(+) isoflurane; in other words, the S(+) isomer is 50 percent more potent than the R(−) isomer (Lysko, Robinson, Casto, and Ferrone 1994). Because the lipid bilayers of neuronal membranes are mainly composed of optically active phospholipids and cholesterol, it was, a priori, possible that they interact stereoselectively with the isoflurane enantiomers; this differential partitioning might have accounted for the observed stereoselectivity. However, we have now found that there is no differential partitioning of S(+) and R(−) isoflurane between lipid bilayers (with and without cholesterol) and water (Dickinson, Franks, and Lieb 1994). Thus, the stereoselectivity of general anesthetics is not ascribable to interactions with lipid bilayers; it most likely reflects chiral binding to proteins.

Overall, the available evidence strongly suggests that general anesthetics act by binding directly to proteins rather than to lipids. The properties of the protein-binding sites are discussed later in the chapter.

EFFECTS OF GENERAL ANESTHETICS ON ION CHANNELS

Because most workers agree that the ultimate targets are ion channels in neuronal membranes, ion channels have been the focus of recent research on the molecular mechanisms of general anesthesia. Many studies have been carried out on the effects of anesthetic agents on a variety of ion channels from diverse sources. On the basis of numerous positive reports in the literature, it might appear that all ion channels are affected by general anesthetics. However, this is only true at very high (often lethal) anesthetic levels; we believe that the likely number of anesthetic target sites has often been overstated because of lack of care with the concentrations of anesthetics used.

Most anesthetic studies have been on members of two of the major classes of ion channels directly involved in neural transmission: those opened and closed by changes in transmembrane electrical potential (voltage-gated channels) and those opened by direct binding of neurotransmitters (neuro-transmitter-gated channels).

Voltage-Gated Ion Channels

It has long been known that axonal conduction is much more refractory to anesthetic inhibition than is synaptic transmission (Larrabee and Posternak 1952); thus, it is perhaps not surprising that the voltage-gated Na^+ and K^+ channels involved in the generation of action potentials have been found to be insensitive to inhibition by general anesthetics (Elliott and Haydon 1989). However, it has recently been reported (Rehberg, Xiao, and Duch 1996) that recombinant rat brain Na^+ channel alpha subunits expressed in a mammalian cell line are, under depolarized conditions, sensitive to volatile anesthetics.

Voltage-gated Ca^{++} channels are probably the most sensitive of all voltage-gated channels and are, in addition, plausible presynaptic targets because neurotransmitter release is triggered by Ca^{++} entering presynaptic terminals via these channels. Hall, Lieb, and Franks (1994a) studied anesthetic inhibition of the P-type channel in rat cerebellar Purkinje neurons because this voltage-gated Ca^{++} channel subtype is thought to be the most important subtype involved in central synaptic transmission. These authors found that only small inhibitions ($\sim 10\%$) were produced by surgical EC_{50} concentrations of commonly used inhalational and intravenous general anesthetics. Similarly small degrees of inhibition have generally been found for other voltage-gated Ca^{++} channel subtypes at clinical concentrations of general anesthetics (Franks and Lieb 1993).

As a class, voltage-gated ion channels are relatively insensitive to anesthetics. However, although this makes them less attractive candidates as principal target sites underlying general anesthesia, it certainly does not rule them out. Because of their ubiquitous distributions and important roles in the central nervous system, it could be that small anesthetic effects on a large number of such channels can summate to produce major pharmacological consequences. Clearly, other criteria besides anesthetic sensitivity, such as the use of anesthetic optical isomers (discussed later in the chapter), are needed to assess relevance.

Neurotransmitter-Gated Ion Channels

Ion channels directly activated by the binding of neurotransmitters are critically important in the rapid transmission of neuronal signals across chemical synapses. The principal excitatory neurotransmitter in the mammalian central nervous system is glutamate, but glutamate-gated ion channels appear to be insensitive to most general anesthetics (except ketamine and barbiturates) (Franks and Lieb 1994).

However, an important structurally and genetically related superfamily of neurotransmitter-gated receptor channels is exceptionally sensitive to many general anesthetics (Franks and Lieb 1996). This superfamily includes gamma-aminobutyric acid (GABA)$_A$, glycine, serotonin 5-HT$_3$, and nicotinic acetylcholine receptor channels (but *not* glutamate receptor channels), all of which are found at central synapses. The amino-acid sequences of the subunits of this superfamily are homologous both within and between receptor channels. The proposed phylogenetic relationships between some of the receptor subunits are shown schematically in Figure 38.3, in which the distance between any two subunits is a measure of the similarity of their DNA base sequences. In mammalian brain, subunits on the far right (GABA and glycine receptor

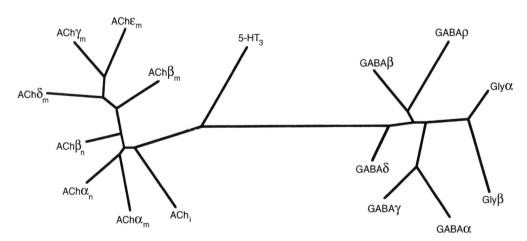

Figure 38.3 Simplified phylogenetic relationship between subunits of members of a superfamily of fast, neurotransmitter-gated receptor channels. Most members of this superfamily are unusually sensitive to general anesthetics. (From Downie et al. 1996, with permission.)

subunits) form ion channels selectively permeable to Cl⁻ ions; subunits on the left (nicotinic acetylcholine and serotonin 5-HT₃ receptor subunits) form channels permeable to Na⁺ and K⁺ ions. Under normal physiological conditions, neurotransmitter binding to GABA_A and glycine receptor channels tends to stabilize the membrane at hyperpolarized potentials, whereas binding to nicotinic acetylcholine and 5-HT₃ receptor channels depolarises the membrane.

Most general anesthetics have been found to potentiate the activities of the glycine and GABA_A receptor channels and to inhibit the activities of the nicotinic acetylcholine receptor channels; thus, in mammals, these agents tend to hyperpolarize the membranes in which the receptor channels are embedded, which makes these membranes less excitable. 5-HT₃ receptor channels, which occupy an intermediate position in the phylogenetic tree (see Figure 38.3), also appear to occupy an intermediate position with regard to the effects of general anesthetics—volatile agents potentiate channel activity, but intravenous agents appear to inhibit channel activity (Jenkins, Franks, and Lieb 1996).

What is the mechanism of potentiation? A clue comes from Figure 38.4, which plots the concentration–response curves for the neurotransmitter glycine activating the glycine receptor channel in the presence of different concentrations of the popular inhalational general anesthetic isoflurane (Downie, Hall, Lieb, and Franks 1996). Increasing the isoflurane concentration shifts the glycine concentration–response curves to the left in a dose-dependent manner. This behavior is consistent with anesthetic binding to the

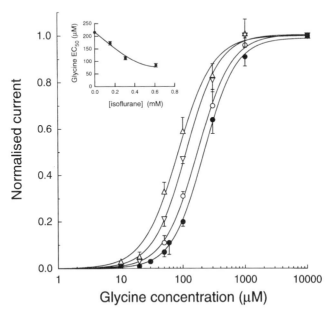

Figure 38.4 Glycine concentration-response curves are shifted to the left by increasing concentrations of the anesthetic isoflurane. This suggests that anesthetics enhance the binding of the neurotransmitter glycine. (From Downie et al. 1996, with permission.)

Nicholas P. Franks and William R. Lieb: Molecular Basis of General Anesthesia: Current Ideas

glycine receptor and increasing the association constant for the binding of glycine. The result can be generalized to other members of the superfamily; that is, when anesthetic potentiation occurs, it is consistent with anesthetic binding to the receptor channel at one site and increasing the apparent association constant for neurotransmitter binding at another (neurotransmitter-activating) site. Whether this involves a true, rather than only an apparent, increase in neurotransmitter-binding affinity or a change in gating properties (or a combination of these effects) remains to be seen. At synapses, where neurotransmitter concentrations often transiently rise to very high levels (before being rapidly reduced by reuptake or hydrolytic mechanisms), such an apparent anesthetic-induced increase in neurotransmitter affinity would have the effect of prolonging neurotransmitter binding and, thus, channel activity. Such anesthetic prolongation of channel activity has been often observed for postsynaptic currents at GABAergic synapses (MacIver, Tanelian, and Mody 1991).

The activities of neuronal nicotinic acetylcholine receptors, on the other hand, are almost always inhibited by general anesthetics (McKenzie, Franks, and Lieb 1995; Pocock and Richards 1993). To date, the most comprehensive study (McKenzie, Franks, and Lieb 1995) of the effects of a wide number of agents on any ion channel was carried out on a molluscan neuronal nicotinic acetylcholine receptor Cl^- channel. All 31 general anesthetics studied inhibited this receptor channel, and the IC_{50} concentrations needed to half-inhibit the channel were close to the EC_{50} concentrations for general anesthesia. This is shown graphically in Figure 38.5, in which the straight line is the line of identity. This graph is similar to that in Figure 38.2 for inhibition of the lipid-free protein firefly luciferase and shows that a neurotransmitter-gated receptor channel can have the same sensitivity to general anesthetics as that of whole animals.

Overall, as a class, members of the neurotransmitter-gated ion channel superfamily that includes the $GABA_A$, glycine, 5-HT_3, and neuronal nicotinic acetylcholine channels are generally much more sensitive to general anesthetics than are members of the class of voltage-gated ion channels and are at present the most promising candidates for primary anesthetic targets. Strategies for choosing among these receptor channels for biological relevance is discussed later.

Effects of General Anesthetics on Microtubules

The possible importance of microtubules in the fundamental mechanisms underlying the conscious state is discussed elsewhere in this volume (see Chapters 18, 37, and 54). Although Churchland in Chapter 8 argues the merits of this provocative proposal, it is worth noting that the involvement of microtubules in the actions of general anesthetics was postulated almost 30 years ago. Indeed, it was suggested by Allison and Nunn (1968) that anesthetics might act by reversibly depolymerizing neuronal microtubules. Subsequently, a variety of inhalational anesthetics were found (Allison et al.

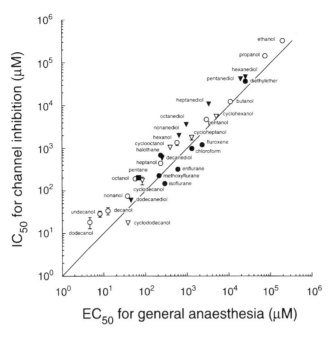

Figure 38.5 General anesthetic concentrations for inhibiting a molluscan neuronal nicotinic acetylcholine receptor are close to the concentrations that cause general anesthesia in animals. (From McKenzie et al. 1995, with permission.)

1970) to reversibly depolymerize microtubules in protozoan axopods, but (except for nitrous oxide) at aqueous concentrations much higher than those that produce general anesthesia in mammals. After the demonstration by Saubermann and Gallagher (1973) that axonal microtubules in mice anesthetized with halothane or pentobarbital were identical to those in control animals, interest in the microtubule theory waned and all but disappeared. Recently, however, there have been reliable reports (Delon and Legendre 1995; Whatley et al. 1994) of the activities of $GABA_A$ and glycine receptor channels being modulated by agents which affect microtubule polymerization. These observations suggest that, although general anesthetics at surgical EC_{50} concentrations probably do not affect microtubules directly, the involvement of microtubules in general anesthesia in a subsidiary role cannot be ruled out.

PROPERTIES OF ANESTHETIC-BINDING SITES

General anesthetics are small molecules, with molecular weights less than 400 gm/mol, which suggests that the relevant anesthetic binding sites are correspondingly small, consistent with their being pockets or clefts (rather than extended surfaces) on proteins. The size dependence for general anesthesia has been most thoroughly investigated for the homologous series of *n*-alcohols and tadpoles (Alifimoff, Firestone, and Miller 1989). As one ascends this series, potencies for producing general anesthesia increase until

Nicholas P. Franks and William R. Lieb: Molecular Basis of General Anesthesia: Current Ideas

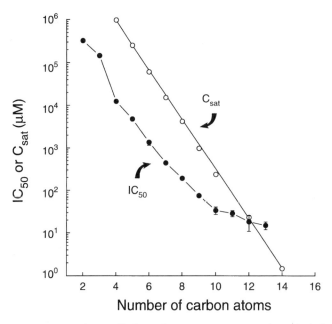

Figure 38.6 The cutoff effect. The IC_{50} concentrations for *n*-alcohols inhibiting a molluscan neuronal nicotinic acetylcholine receptor level out after decanol, which suggests the binding site has a volume of about $200 \, cm^3/mol$. C_{sat}, saturated aqueous solubility. (From McKenzie et al. 1995, with permission.)

a point is reached (the cutoff point) above which remaining members of the series can no longer produce general anesthesia on their own. For general anaesthesia, the cutoff point is at dodecanol (Alifimoff, Firestone, and Miller 1989). Similarly placed cutoff points (Jenkins, Franks, and Lieb 1996; McKenzie; Franks, and Lieb 1995; Nakahiro, Arakawa, Nishimura, and Narahash 1996) exist for the molluscan neuronal nicotinic acetylcholine receptor channel (also at dodecanol), the rat $GABA_A$ receptor channel (at undecanol), and for the mouse $5\text{-}HT_3$ receptor channel (at tridecanol).

Figure 38.6 plots (on a semilogarithmic scale) the aqueous solubility of the *n*-alcohols and their IC_{50} concentrations for inhibiting the molluscan neuronal nicotinic acetylcholine receptor as a function of alcohol chain length. Our interpretation of these data is that the binding affinities of the *n*-alcohols increase with increasing alcohol size until a point is reached (at about decanol) where the alcohol-binding pocket or cleft is effectively full, and additional methylene ($—CH_2—$) groups must remain in aqueous solution, and thus no longer contribute substantially to the binding energy. This accounts for the tendency of the IC_{50} concentrations to level off after decanol. Since aqueous solubility (C_{sat}) monotonically decreases with increasing alcohol size, eventually (in Figure 38.6 after dodecanol) it must become less than the alcohol concentration required for half-inhibiting the receptor channel. By this interpretation, the volume of the alcohol-binding pocket is roughly equal to the molar volume of decanol (approximately $200 \, cm^3/mol$).

What makes a binding site sensitive to general anesthetics? This is an important and intriguing question, especially because most proteins appear to be insensitive to these agents at EC_{50} concentrations for general anaesthesia. Although the answer to this question is not known, a number of important clues are now available. Potencies for general anaesthesia correlate much better with partition coefficients between the amphiphilic solvent n-octanol and water than with those between n-hexadecane and water (Franks and Lieb 1978), which suggests that the relevant target sites are both polar and apolar in nature.

Use of a multiple regression approach to quantify the importance of various physical properties of an anesthetic molecule for producing general anesthesia suggests (Abraham, Lieb, and Franks 1991) that the polar regions are excellent hydrogen-bond acceptors but poor hydrogen-bond donors; the reasons for this behavior are unclear. Temperature-variation studies of the potencies of volatile anesthetics for producing general anaesthesia, for inhibiting firefly luciferase (Dickinson, Franks, and Lieb 1993), and for inhibiting a molluscan neuronal nicotinic acetylcholine receptor channel (Dickinson, Lieb, and Franks 1995) indicate a strong interaction between the relevant binding sites and bound anesthetic. Because it seems unlikely that a protein site could have an intrinsically high affinity for a wide range of such agents, it is possible that anesthetics trigger an allosteric conformational change that effectively occludes the anesthetic molecule and reduces its rate of dissociation. Such a "Venus flytrap" mechanism is consistent with the recently determined crystal structure of firefly luciferase (Conti, Franks, and Brick 1996).

CRITERIA FOR IDENTIFYING TARGET SITES RELEVANT TO GENERAL ANESTHESIA

To identify target sites relevant to general anesthesia, the main criterion discussed thus far is sensitivity to anesthetics at concentrations that produce the state of general anesthesia in animals. Clearly, if a target site is found to be substantially affected (either inhibited or potentiated) by surgical levels of a general anesthetic, that target is likely to play a role in either general anesthesia or in side effects associated with general anesthesia. Just as clearly, if a putative target is found to be almost completely insensitive to surgical levels of a general anesthetic, it can probably be ruled out as a primary target. However, as discussed earlier, for voltage-gated ion channels, if a physiologically important and widely distributed putative target is only minimally but significantly affected by surgical concentrations of a general anesthetic, the situation is less clear cut. Clearly, other criteria are needed.

One criterion for assessing relevance relies on the observation that general anesthetics often act stereoselectively. Many general anesthetics are optically active and, although usually used clinically as racemic mixtures, actually exist in at least two optically active, mirror-image forms, optical isomers or enantiomers. When tested separately on mammals, enantiomers often display stereoselective effects; one enantiomer is more potent than another in producing general anesthesia (Franks and Lieb 1994). Once the rank order and potency ratio of the optical isomers of a given anesthetic are accurately known for general anesthesia, the same information can be obtained for selected ion channels and other potential anesthetic targets. If there are only a few major targets involved in general anesthesia (as we suspect), one might expect the rank order and potency ratios for the major targets to be comparable to those for general anesthesia.

Enantiomeric potency ratios for general anaesthesia are known most accurately for the popular volatile anesthetic isoflurane—in rats, the S(+) isomer is 50 percent more potent than the R(−) isomer (Lysko, Robinson, Casto, and Ferrone 1994). An identical rank order and similar potency ratios have been found for these enantiomers acting on a molluscan neuronal nicotinic acetylcholine receptor (Franks and Lieb 1991), mammalian GABA$_A$ receptor channels (Hall, Lieb, and Franks 1994b; Jones and Harrison 1993; Moody, Harris, and Skolnick 1993), and on a molluscan anesthetic-activated K$^+$ channel (Franks and Lieb 1991); however, virtually no stereoselectivity was found for inhibiting a molluscan voltage-gated K$^+$ channel (Franks and Lieb 1991) or a mouse voltage-gated (L-type) Ca^{++} channel (Moody, Harris, Hoehner, and Skolnick 1994) or for potentiating rat glycine receptor channels (Downie, Hall, Lieb, and Franks 1996). These early results provide provisional support for an important role in isoflurane general anesthesia of at least two members of the anesthetic-sensitive superfamily of neurotransmitter-gated receptor channels (though the molluscan neuronal nicotinic acetylcholine receptor results must be confirmed for mammalian receptors).

Another criterion is to look for exceptions to the Meyer-Overton rule for both general anesthesia and for specific potential targets. The use of the n-alcohol cutoff effect is an example of this approach. For example, the alcohol cutoffs for the neuronal nicotinic acetylcholine, 5-HT$_3$ and GABA$_A$ receptors are close to those for tadpole general anesthesia; Li, Peoples, and Weight (1994) reported that the cutoff for inhibiting a fast ATP-activated current in bullfrog neurons occurs much earlier (after propanol). This finding might be understood as supporting a role in alcohol general anesthesia for the three superfamily receptor channels but not for the ATP-gated channel. A recent example of this approach is that of Eger and colleagues (Koblin et al. 1994), who identified new halogenated compounds that are not anesthetic at concentrations predicted from the Meyer-Overton rule. The idea is to apply these compounds to potential anesthetic targets to see whether the compounds have the same effects as those of conventional agents; if they do, the targets are deemed to be irrelevant to general anesthesia.

No doubt the use of a combination of these, and other, criteria will be required before one can state unequivocally which molecular targets are important in general anesthesia and which are not.

CONCLUSION

General anesthetics produce a wide spectrum of pharmacological effects, including the reversible loss of consciousness. How loss of consciousness is achieved by these agents is completely unknown at the anatomical level, but substantial progress has recently been made at the molecular level. Contrary to the traditional view, it is now known that general anesthetics act by directly binding to neuronal proteins rather than to lipids. The most likely neuronal proteins belong to an anesthetic-sensitive superfamily of neurotransmitter-gated ion channels found at central synapses. In mammals, general anesthetics tend (with some exceptions) to block excitatory synaptic channels and to potentiate the activity of inhibitory synaptic channels.

The loss of consciousness produced by general anesthetics could, in principle, be caused by their actions at a highly localized site in the brain and the result of turning off some unknown but critical "switch" in the brain. However, although this idea cannot be dismissed, it seems unlikely in view of the importance and wide distribution in the brain of the most likely molecular targets of general anesthetics. Rather, the inhibitory modulation of synaptic channels by these agents may so interfere with and "scramble" brain signal processing that the conscious brain can no longer make coherent sense of its internal and external environments.

In the future, we anticipate that by using emerging techniques such as functional brain imaging (Alkire et al. 1995) along with the careful selection of anesthetic agents and an appreciation of the spectrum of effects that anesthetics have on higher brain function, the use of anesthetic drugs will provide a powerful tool to unlock some of the mysteries of consciousness.

REFERENCES

Abraham, M. H., W. R. Lieb, and N. P. Franks. 1991. Role of hydrogen bonding in general anesthesia. *Journal of Pharmaceutical Sciences* 80:719–724.

Alifimoff, J. K., L. L. Firestone, and K. W. Miller. 1989. Anaesthetic potencies of primary alkanols: Implications for the molecular dimensions of the anaesthetic site. *British Journal of Pharmacology*. 96:9–16.

Alkire, M. T., R. J. Haier, S. J. Barker, N. K. Shah, J. C. Wu, and Y. J. Kao. 1995. Cerebral metabolism during propofol anesthesia in humans studied with positron emission tomography. *Anesthesiology* 82:393–403.

Allison, A. C., G. H. Hulands, J. F. Nunn, J. A. Kitching, and A. C. Macdonald. 1970. The effect of inhalational anaesthetics on the microtubular system in *Actinosphaerium nucleofilum. Journal of Cell Science* 7:483–499.

Allison, A.C., and J. F. Nunn. 1968. Effects of general anaesthetics on microtubules. A possible mechanism of anaesthesia. *Lancet* 2:1326–1329.

Conti, E., N. P. Franks, and P. Brick. 1996. Crystal structure of firefly luciferase throws light on a superfamily of adenylate-forming enzymes. *Structure* 4:287–298.

Delon, J., and P. Legendre. 1995. Effects of nocodazole and taxol on glycine evoked currents on rat spinal-cord neurons in culture. *Neuroreport* 6:1932–1936.

Dickinson, R., N. P. Franks, and W. R. Lieb. 1993. Thermodynamics of anesthetic/protein interactions. Temperature studies on firefly luciferase. *Biophysical Journal* 64:1264–1271.

Dickinson, R., N. P. Franks, and W. R. Lieb. 1994. Can the stereoselective effects of the anesthetic isoflurane be accounted for by lipid solubility? *Biophysical Journal* 66:2019–2023.

Dickinson, R., W. R. Lieb, and N. P. Franks. 1995. The effects of temperature on the interactions between volatile general anaesthetics and a neuronal nicotinic acetylcholine receptor. *British Journal of Pharmacology* 116:2949–2956.

Downie, D. L., A. C. Hall, W. R. Lieb, and N. P. Franks. 1996. Effects of inhalational general anaesthetics on native glycine receptors in rat medullary neurones and recombinant glycine receptors in *Xenopus* oocytes. *British Journal of Pharmacology* 118:493–502.

Elliott, J. R., and D. A. Haydon. 1989. The actions of neutral anaesthetics on ion conductances of nerve membranes. *Biochimica et Biophysica Acta* 988:257–286.

Franks, N. P., and W. R. Lieb. 1978. Where do general anaesthetics act? *Nature* 274:339–342.

Franks, N. P., and W. R. Lieb. 1979. The structure of lipid bilayers and the effects of general anaesthetics. An X-ray and neutron diffraction study. *Journal of Molecular Biology* 133:469–500.

Franks, N. P., and W. R. Lieb. 1982. Molecular mechanisms of general anaesthesia. *Nature* 300:487–493.

Franks, N. P., and W. R. Lieb. 1984. Do general anaesthetics act by competitive binding to specific receptors? *Nature* 310:599–601.

Franks, N. P., and W. R. Lieb. 1991. Stereospecific effects of inhalational general anesthetic optical isomers on nerve ion channels. *Science* 254:427–430.

Franks, N. P., and W. R. Lieb. 1993. Selective actions of volatile general anaesthetics at molecular and cellular levels. *British Journal of Anaesthesia* 71:65–76.

Franks, N. P., and W. R. Lieb. 1994. Molecular and cellular mechanisms of general anaesthesia. *Nature* 367:607–614.

Franks, N. P., and W. R. Lieb 1996. An anesthetic-sensitive superfamily of neurotransmitter-gated ion channels. *Journal of Clinical Anesthesia* 8:S3–S7.

Hall, A. C., W. R. Lieb, and N. P. Franks. 1994a. Insensitivity of P-type calcium channels to inhalational and intravenous general anesthetics. *Anesthesiology* 81:117–123.

Hall, A. C., W. R. Lieb, and N. P. Franks. 1994b. Stereoselective and non-stereoselective actions of isoflurane on the GABA$_A$ receptor. *British Journal of Pharmacology* 112:906–910.

Jenkins, A., N. P. Franks, and W. R. Lieb. 1996. Actions of general anaesthetics on 5-HT$_3$ receptors in N1E-115 neuroblastoma cells. *British Journal of Pharmacology* 117:1507–1515.

Jones, M. V., and N. L. Harrison. 1993. Effects of volatile anesthetics on the kinetics of inhibitory postsynaptic currents in cultured rat hippocampal neurons. *Journal of Neurophysiology* 70:1339–1349.

Koblin, D. D., B. S. Chortkoff, M. J. Laster, E. I. Eger, M. J. Halsey, and P. Ionescu. 1994. Polyhalogenated and perfluorinated compounds that disobey the Meyer-Overton hypothesis. *Anesthesia and Analgesia* 79:1043–1048.

Larrabee, M. G., and J. M. Posternak. 1952. Selective action of anesthetics on synapses and axons in mammalian sympathetic ganglia. *Journal of Neurophysiology* 15:91–114.

Li, C., R. W. Peoples, and F. F. Weight. 1994. Alcohol action on a neuronal membrane receptor: Evidence for a direct interaction with the receptor protein. *Proceedings of the National Academy of Sciences USA* 91:8200–8204.

Lieb, W. R., M. Kovalycsik, and R. Mendelsohn. 1982. Do clinical levels of general anaesthetics affect lipid bilayers? Evidence from Raman scattering. *Biochimica et Biophysica Acta* 688:388–398.

Lysko, G. S., J. L. Robinson, R. Casto, and R. A. Ferrone. 1994. The stereospecific effects of isoflurane isomers in vivo. *European Journal of Pharmacology* 263:25–29.

MacIver, M. B., D. L. Tanelian, and I. Mody. 1991. Two mechanisms for anesthetic-induced enhancement of GABA$_A$ mediated neuronal inhibition. *Annals of the New York Academy of Sciences* 625:91–96.

McKenzie, D., N. P. Franks, and W. R. Lieb. 1995. Actions of general anaesthetics on a neuronal nicotinic acetylcholine receptor in isolated identified neurones of *Lymnaea stagnalis*. *British Journal of Pharmacology* 115:275–282.

Moody, E. J., B. Harris, P. Hoehner, and P. Skolnick. 1994. Inhibition of [3H]isradipine binding to L-type calcium channels by the optical isomers of isoflurane. Lack of stereospecificty. *Anesthesiology* 81:124–128.

Moody, E. J., B. D. Harris, and P. Skolnick. 1993. Stereospecific actions of the inhalation anesthetic isoflurane at the GABA$_A$ receptor complex. *Brain Research* 615:101–106.

Nakahiro, M., O. Arakawa, T. Nishimura, and T. Narahashi. 1996. Potentiation of GABA-induced Cl$^-$ current by a series of *n*-alcohols disappears at a cutoff point of a longer-chain *n*-alcohol in rat dorsal root ganglion neurons. *Neuroscience Letters* 205:127–130.

Pocock, G., and C. D. Richards. 1993. Excitatory and inhibitory synaptic mechanisms in anaesthesia. *British Journal of Anaesthesia* 71:134–147.

Quasha, A. L., E. I. Eger, and J. H. Tinker. 1980. Determination and applications of MAC. *Anesthesiology* 53:315–334.

Rang, H. P., M. M. Dale, and J. M. Ritter. 1995. *Pharmacology*. New York: Churchill Livingstone.

Rehberg, B., Y. Xiao, and D. S. Duch. 1996. Central nervous system sodium channels are significantly suppressed at clinical concentrations of volatile anesthetics. *Anesthesiology* 84:1223–1233.

Saubermann, A. J., and M. L. Gallagher. 1973. Mechanisms of general anesthesia: Failure of pentobarbital and halothane to depolymerize microtubules in mouse optic nerve. *Anesthesiology* 38:25–29.

Whatley, V. J., S. J. Mihic, A. M. Allan, S. J. McQuilkin, and R. A. Harris. 1994. γ-aminobutyric acid$_A$ receptor function is inhibited by microtubule depolymerization. *Journal of Biological Chemistry* 269:19546–19552.

39 On the Mechanism of Action of Anesthetic Agents

Hans Flohr

Dissociative anesthetics such as ketamine or phencyclidine are known to act as noncompetitive antagonists of the N-methyl-D-aspartate (NMDA) receptor. They bind to a recognition site within the receptor-operated cation channel and block the influx of Na^+ and Ca^{++} ions into neurons and thereby antagonize glutamate-evoked excitation and the induction of activity-dependent changes in synaptic efficacy, which are triggered by Ca^{++}.

Noncompetitive NMDA antagonists cause severe disturbances of consciousness. In low doses, they induce altered states of consciousness. Patients experience sensory illusions, visual and auditory hallucinations, distortions of body image, and disorganized thought. In high doses that lead to a large fractional occupancy of cortical NMDA receptors, they produce general anesthesia. The anesthetic state produced by noncompetitive NMDA antagonists is different from that produced by classic anesthetic gases such as halothane. The NMDA antagonist dissociative state is characterized by a rather selective loss of conscious functions in combination with relative maintenance of protective reflexes. Patients are in a trance-like state and do not appear to be asleep, but they seem "disconnected from the surroundings." On the basis of electroencephalographic studies, Corssen and Domino (1966) attributed the special features of this state to a depression of neuronal activity in cortical association areas and a selective blockade of higher associative functions.

Dissociative anesthetics also interact with other components of the central nervous system such as opioid receptors, monoaminergic, gamma-aminobutyric acid (GABA)ergic and cholinergic transmitter systems. But these actions are not able to fully account for the drugs' anesthetic and psychotomimetic properties. However there are good reasons to assume that both anesthetic and psychoactive effects are caused by their NMDA antagonism. First, all substances known so far that bind within the NMDA receptor-associated channel produce a similar anesthetic state. Among them is the selective, high-affinity antagonist MK-801 (Koek, Colpaert, Woods, and Kamenka 1989; Scheller et al. 1989; Daniell 1990; Löscher, Fredow, and Ganter 1991; Irifune, Shimizu, Nomoto, and Fukuda 1992; Perkins and Morrow 1992a). Second, the anesthetic potency of these compounds is highly correlated with their relative affinity for the binding site within the channel (Koek, Colpaert, Woods, and Kamenka 1989; Perkins and Morrow 1992b). The same is true for their subjective psychoactive effects, as indicated by animal discrimination studies (Martin and Lodge 1988). Third, the anesthetic effects can be modified by changing their binding kinetics. Agonists of the glutamate and glycine receptors increase the opening time of the NMDA receptor channel and enhance the dissociation of ligands bound within it. Both agonists reduce the anesthetic effects of the channel blockers (Irifune, Shimizu, Nomoto, and Fukuda 1992). The antianesthetic effect of glutamate and glycine can be reversed by selective glycine and glutamate antagonists. From these observations one can draw the following conclusions:

1. The normal functioning of the NMDA synapse is a *necessary condition* for the presence of states of consciousness.

2. All other physiological processes that remain intact after a selective blockade of the NMDA system—taken together—are *not sufficient* for the occurrence of states of consciousness.

3. If, however, the NMDA system is switched on again when the channel blockade is removed, a physiological state that is a *sufficient condition* for consciousness arises.

In this sense, processes mediated by the NMDA synapse are constitutive for the occurrence of consciousness.

States of unconsciousness are not necessarily accompanied by a global depression of neural activity throughout the central nervous system. Rather, consciousness is bound to a specific subset of physiological processes. If this hypothesis is correct, not only channel-blocking agents but all other drugs that directly interfere with the function of the NMDA receptor channel complex must possess anesthetic properties and the anesthetic efficacy of agents that do not directly act on the NMDA synapse but have other primary targets can be explained as an indirect action on this synapse.

The NMDA synapse is a target for many different drugs that bind to a number of modulatory sites that regulate the activity of the receptor channel complex. Included among these are:

1. The glutamate receptor, which can be blocked by specific so-called competitive NMDA antagonists

2. A strychnine-insensitive glycine binding site, the coactivation of which is necessary for receptor activation, which can be blocked by glycine antagonists

3. A binding site for *polyamines*, which can be blocked by polyamine antagonists

Downstream from the channel, the enzyme nitric oxide synthase (NOS) can be inactivated by various NOS inhibitors. The enzyme is activated by Ca^{++} ions and catalyzes the production of nitric oxide (NO) from arginine. Nitric oxide is an extremely labile gas and acts as a retrograde messenger that mediates postsynaptic to presynaptic communication. It stimulates the production of cyclic guanosine monophosphate (GMP) in the presynaptic terminal and thereby enhances presynaptic transmitter release. It thus modifies synaptic efficacy in an activity-dependent manner. Upstream from the channel, presynaptic transmitter release can be inhibited pharmacologically, for example, by riluzole.

The working conditions of the NMDA receptor channel complex can be influenced indirectly in various ways. The NMDA synapse is ligand-gated *and* voltage-dependent, which means that the receptor-operated channel opens under two conditions. First, the presynapse must release the transmitter glutamate, and, second, the postsynaptic membrane must be depolarized to about -35 mV. At membrane potentials around the resting potential, the channel is blocked by a magnesium ion that binds in a voltage-dependent manner to a site in the lumen of the channel (which is distinct from the phencyclidine binding site). This blockade will be removed if the postsynaptic membrane is depolarized to -35 mV, which means that the functioning of the receptor channel complex can be modulated by altering the postsynaptic membrane potential. In particular, it can be altered by inhibitory or excitatory synapses located in the vicinity of the NMDA receptor complex.

In fact, it appears that *any* of the possible direct or indirect interventions that block the activation of the NMDA receptor complex or the subsequent plastic processes triggered by Ca^{++} inevitably produce anesthetic effects. Figure 39.1 summarizes what is currently known about this process. This finding is not only true for the large number of channel blockers known so far, but also for competitive NMDA antagonists that block the glutamate receptor, such as AP5, CPP, CGS 19755 and D-CPP-ene (Koek, Colpaert, Woods, and Kamenka 1986; Boast and Pastor 1988; Woods 1989; France, and Woods 1990; Daniell 1991; Irifune, Shimizu, Nomoto, and Fukuda 1992; Perkins and Morrow 1992, Kuroda, Strebel, Raffecty, and Bullock 1993), for specific glycine antagonists such as ACEA (McFarlane, Warner, Nader, and Dexter 1995), and for polyamine antagonists such as spermidine and spermine (Daniell 1992). All these drugs have been shown to increase sleeping time in a standard barbiturate narcosis or decrease the minimum alveolar concentration (MAC) in a standard halothane narcosis.

Moreover, an increasing number of classic anesthetic agents, such as chloroform, diethylether, enflurane, isoflurane, halothane, methoxyflurane, and ethanol, have been shown to interact directly with the NMDA receptor complex (Martin et al. 1991, 1992; Aronstam, Martin, and Dennison 1994; Orser, Bertlik, Wang, and McDonald 1995). Thus, the anesthetic properties of classic gas anesthetics may possibly result, at least in part, from an interaction with the NMDA receptor.

Drugs acting upstream or downstream from the receptor complex also possess anesthetic properties. Riluzole, a recently discovered agent that blocks glutamate release from the presynaptic terminal, is a strong anesthetic

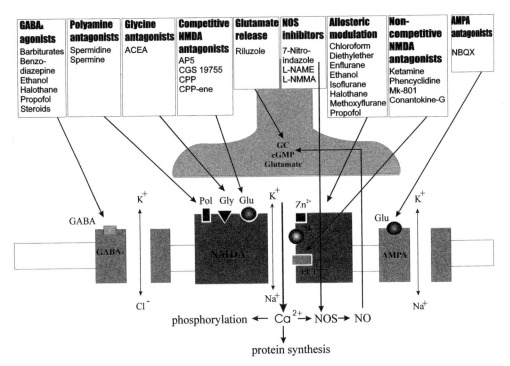

GABAᴀ agonists	Polyamine antagonists	Glycine antagonists	Competitive NMDA antagonists	Glutamate release	NOS inhibitors	Allosteric modulation	Non-competitive NMDA antagonists	AMPA antagonists
Barbiturates Benzo-diazepine Ethanol Halothane Propofol Steroids	Spermidine Spermine	ACEA	AP5 CGS 19755 CPP CPP-ene	Riluzole	7-Nitro-indazole L-NAME L-NMMA	Chloroform Diethylether Enflurane Ethanol Isoflurane Halothane Methoxyflurane Propofol	Ketamine Phencyclidine Mk-801 Conantokine-G	NBQX

Figure 39.1 The NMDA synapse as a target for anesthetics. Schematic representation of the NMDA receptor channel complex with its regulatory sites and of neighboring AMPA and GABA receptors by which the working conditions of the NMDA receptor channel complex can be influenced. All agents mentioned in this scheme have been shown to possess anesthetic properties. Arrows indicate possible interaction sites.

(Mantz et al. 1992; Martin, Thompson, and Nadler 1993). A possible role of NO in general anesthesia is suggested by several studies. Originally it was reported that NOS inhibition with N^G-nitro-L-arginine methyl ester (L-NAME) decreased the MAC of halothane in a dose-dependent manner. The effect could be reversed by L-arginine (Johns, Moscicki, and Difazio 1992). Adams, Meyer, Sewing, and Cicero (1994) found that L-NAME prolongs sleeping time in alcohol narcosis. However, these findings could not be confirmed by Adachi and colleagues (1994), and an explanation for these opposite findings was not offered. Recently, Glade, Motzko, Tober, and Flohr (1996) showed that administration of the brain-specific NOS inhibitor 7-nitroindazole prolongs barbituate sleeping time in rats. This effect could be reversed by L-arginine. Dzoljic, de Vries, and van Leeuwen (1996) arrived at similar results. Moreover, Dzoljic and de Vries (1994) found that N^G-mono-methyl-L-arginine (L-NMMA), another NOS inhibitor, reduces wakefulness in the rat. The assumption that interference with NO activity results in anesthesia is also supported by evidence that halothane and other inhalational anesthetics can interact with NO production or action (Tobin, Marzin, Breslow, and Traystman 1993; Blaise et al. 1994).

For a large number of intravenous anesthetics, such as barbiturates, benzodiazepines, steroids, etomidate, and propofol, the GABAₐ receptor is assumed to be the primary site of action. GABA receptors are typically located in the immediate vicinity of the NMDA receptor. Activation of the inhibitory GABA receptor results in hyperpolarization of the postsynaptic membrane and therefore in an alteration of the working conditions of the NMDA receptor. Thus, the anesthetic action of these agents could be explained as an indirect effect on the NMDA receptor. Antagonists of excitatory synapses in the vicinity of the NMDA receptor, such as the glutamatergic (AMPA) receptor, in theory should have similar effects. In fact, it has been shown that 2,3-dihydroxy-6-nitro-7-sulfamoylbenzo(F)quinoxaline (NBQX), a selective AMPA antagonist, possesses anesthetic properties. It reduces halothane MAC in a dose-dependent manner and increases the sleeping time for pentobarbital narcosis (McFarlane, Warner, Todd, and Nordholm 1992). These observations support two hypotheses: first, that states of consciousness critically depend on information processing mediated by the NMDA system (Flohr 1991, 1994, 1995b); second, that the direct or indirect inhibition of these processes is the common operative mechanism of anesthetic action (Flohr 1995a).

NMDA RECEPTOR-DEPENDENT PLASTICITY, ASSEMBLIES, AND MENTAL REPRESENTATIONS

The significance of the NMDA synapse for cortical information processing is not fully clear. It appears that the activation of the NMDA receptor is not required for fast, "normal," synaptic transmission. The fact that this synapse is both voltage-dependent and ligand-gated qualifies it as a Hebbian coincidence detector, that is, activation occurs if pre- *and* postsynaptic activities coincide. The relatively slow rate of dissociation of glutamate from its binding site and the long-time course of the NMDA receptor-mediated excitatory postsynaptic potential allows the possibility of detecting coincident inputs within a relatively long time window.

This synapse instantiates a repertoire of different mechanisms and distinct forms of synaptic plasticity. Removal of the Mg^{++} block suddenly changes the contribution of the NMDA receptor to the interaction between simultaneously active neurons. This action establishes positive feedback among the participating neurons, enhances their activity, and triggers various plastic processes, which strengthen the connections between the neurons belonging to the assembly. There is a gradual transition from reversible, short-term modifications to firmly established, long-term structural changes. Thus, this synapse may qualify as an implementation of the original Hebb synapse (Hebb 1949), which leads to the formation of an engram, and of the fast Malsburg synapse (von der Malsburg 1981), which is responsible for the formation of short-lived assemblies, essential for cognitive processes.

Hebb claimed that neuronal assemblies instantiate mental representations. In principle, such structures automatically generated by a mechanism that combines a coincidence detector with synaptic plasticity can represent all kinds of external events and lawlike relationships between events. Under certain conditions, nets containing Hebb synapses can also represent coincident internal events, such as the activity of different assemblies, and thus produce higher-order self-referential representations. Such systems can bind first-order representations and higher-order representations in a hierarchical representation system ("hyperstructure," Baas 1996).

Nets developing such representational hyperstructures may develop a sort of subjectivity—they are able to produce concepts and beliefs about their inner state. They would become what Rey (1983, 1988) called "recursive believer" systems or what Dennett (1978) called "an n-order intentional" system. These systems develop a model of themselves (i.e., a mental representation of the self as an agent or experiencer) and are able to bind other mental representations to it. In Nagel's (1986) terms such systems would *know* "what it is like to be such a system" and have a subjective perspective (Flohr 1994, 1995b).

I have argued elsewhere (Flohr 1991, 1995b) that the unique properties of the NMDA receptors define their role in the representational activity of the brain. In particular, I assume, they play a pivotal role in the production of higher-order representational states. The activation state of the NMDA synapse determines the rate at which such assemblies are built up and determines the size and complexity of the representational structures that emerge in a given period of time. Higher-order representational structures automatically develop whenever the plastic changes are accomplished at a critical rate. Thus, I assume that the essential difference between anesthetized brains and conscious brains consists in the capacity to produce higher-order representational structures.

METAREPRESENTATIONS AND PHENOMENAL CONSCIOUSNESS

Consciousness, according to this view, is a consequence of the brain's representational activity. A state of high representational activity is both necessary and sufficient for the occurrence of conscious states. Such assumptions are in line with philosophical theories that have been called higher-order representation theories of consciousness. Common to the various versions of this concept is the claim that consciousness is a sort of metarepresentation—either a higher-order perception or a higher-order thought. This line of thinking has a long tradition in philosophy and plays an important role among theories of consciousness today (Rosenthal 1986, 1990, 1993a,b). This approach now seems supportable by physiological arguments.

REFERENCES

Adachi, T., J. Kurata, S. Nakao, M. Murakawa, T. Shichino, and G. Shirakami. 1994. Nitric oxide synthase inhibitor does not reduce minimum alveolar anesthetic concentrations in rats. *Anesthesia and Analgesia* 78:1154–1157.

Adams, M. L., E. R. Meyer, B. N. Sewing, and T. J. Cicero. 1994. Effects of nitric oxide-related agents on alcohol narcosis. *Alcoholism, Clinical and Experimental Research* 18:969–975.

Aronstam, R. S., D. C. Martin, and R. L. Dennison. 1994. Volatile anesthetics inhibit NMDA-stimulated ^{45}Ca uptake by rat brain microvesicles. *Neurochemical Research* 19:1515–1520.

Baas, N. A. 1996. A framework for higher-order cognition and consciousness. In S. R. Hameroff, A. W. Kaszniak, and A. C. Scott, eds., *Toward a Science of Consciousness: The First Tucson Discussions and Debates*. Cambridge: MIT Press, pp. 633–648.

Blaise, G., Q. To, M. Parent, B. Laguide, F. Asenjo, and R. Sauve. 1994. Does halothane interfere with the release, action or stability of endothelium-derived releasing factor/nitric oxide? *Anesthesiology* 80:417–426.

Corssen, G., and E. F. Domino. 1966. Dissociative anesthesia: Further pharmacologic studies and first clinical experience with the phencyclidine derivative CI-581. *Anesthesia and Analgesia* 45:29–40.

Daniell, L. C. 1990. The non-competitive NMDA antagonists MK 801, phencyclidine and ketamine increase the potency of general anesthetics. *Pharmacology, Biochemistry and Behavior* 36:111–115.

Daniell, L. C. 1992. Alteration of general anesthetic potency by agonists and antagonists of the polyamine binding site of the N-methyl-D-aspartate receptor. *Journal of Pharmacology and Experimental Therapies* 261:304–310.

Dennett, D. C. 1978. Conditions of personhood. In D. C. Dennett, *Brainstorms*. Cambridge: Bradford Books, pp. 267–285.

Dzoljic, M. R., and R. de Vries. 1994. Nitric oxide synthase inhibition reduces wakefulness. *Neuropharmacology* 33:1505–1509.

Dzoljic, M. R., R. de Vries, and R. van Leeuwen. 1996. Sleep and nitric oxide: Effects of 7-nitro-indazole, inhibitor of brain nitric oxide synthase. *Brain Research* 78:145–150.

Flohr, H. 1991. Brain processes and phenomenal consciousness. A new and specific hypothesis. *Theory and Psychology* 1:245–262.

Flohr, H. 1994. Die physiologischen bedingungen des bewußtseins. In H. Lenk and H. Poser, eds., *Neue Realitäten—Herausforderung der Philosophie*. Berlin: Akademie Verlag, pp. 222–235.

Flohr, H. 1995a. An information processing theory of anaesthesia. *Neuropsychologia* 33:1169–1180.

Flohr, H. 1995b. Sensations and brain processes. *Behavioural Brain Research* 71:157–161.

France, C. P., and J. Woods. 1990. Analgesic, anesthetic, and respiratory effects of the competitive N-Methyl-D-aspartate (NMDA) antagonist CGS 19755, in rhesus monkeys. *Brain Research* 526: 355–358.

Glade, U., D. Motzko, C. Tober, and H. Flohr. 1996. Anaesthetic potency of the brain specific NOS inhibitor 7-nitro-indazole. In N. Elsner and H. U. Schnitzler, eds., *Göttingen Neurobiology Report*, vol. II. Stuttgart: Thieme, p. 652 (Abstract).

Hebb, D. O. 1949. *The Organization of Behavior*. New York: Wiley.

Irifune, M., T. Shimizu, M. Nomoto, and T. Fukuda. 1992. Ketamine-induced anesthesia involves the N-methyl-D-aspartate receptor-channel complex in mice. *Brain Research* 596:1–9.

Johns, R. A., J. C. Moscicki, and C. A. Difazio. 1992. Nitric oxide synthase inhibitor dose-dependently and reversibly reduces the threshold for halothane anesthesia. *Anesthesiology* 77:779–784.

Koek, W., F. C. Colpaert, J. H. Woods, and J. M. Kamenka. 1989. The phencyclidine (PCP) analog N-[1-(2-Benzo(B)thiophenyl)cyclohexyl] piperidine shares cocaine-like but not other characteristic behavioral effects with PCP, ketamine and MK 801. *Journal of Pharmacology and Experimental Therapies* 250:1019–1027.

Kuroda, Y., S. Strebel, C. Rafferty, and R. Bullock. 1993. Neuroprotective doses of N-Methyl-D-aspartate receptor antagonists profoundly reduce the minimum alveolar anesthetic concentration (MAC) for isoflurane in rats. *Anesthesia and Analgesia* 77:795–800.

Löscher, W., G. Fredow, and M. Ganter. 1991. Comparison of pharmacodynamic effects of the non-competitive NMDA receptor antagonists MK 801 and ketamine in pigs. *European Journal of Pharmacology* 192:377–382.

Mantz, J., A. Cheramy, A. M. Thierry, J. Glowinski, and J. M. Desmonts. 1992. Anesthetic properties of riluzole (54274 RP), a new inhibitor of glutamate neurotransmission. *Anesthesiology* 76:844–848.

Martin, D., and D. Lodge. 1988. Phencyclidine receptors and N-methyl-D-aspartate antagonism: Electrophysiologic data correlate with known behaviors. *Pharmacology, Biochemistry and Behavior* 31:279–286.

Martin, D., M. A. Thompson, and J. V. Nadler. 1993. The neuroprotective agent riluzole inhibits the release of glutamate and aspartate from slices of hippocampal area CA1. *European Journal of Pharmacology* 250:473–476.

Martin, D. C., J. E. Abraham, M. Plagenhoef, and R. S. Aronstam. 1991. Volatile anesthetics and NMDA receptors. Enflurane inhibition of glutamate-stimulated [^{3}H]MK-801 binding and reversal by glycine. *Neuroscience Letters* 132:73–76.

Martin, D. C., R. L. Dennison, and R. S. Aronstam. 1992. Barbiturate interactions with N-methyl-D-aspartate (NMDA) receptors in rat brain. *Molecular Neuropharmacology* 2:255–259.

McFarlane, C., D. S. Warner, A. Nader, and F. Dexter. 1995. Glycine receptor antagonism. Effects of ACEA 1021 on the minimum alveolar concentration for halothane in the rat. *Anesthesiology* 82:961–968.

McFarlane, C., D. S. Warner, M. M. Todd, and L. Nordholm. 1992. AMPA receptor competitive antagonism reduces halothane MAC in rats. *Anesthesiology* 77:1165–1170.

Nagel, T. 1986. *The View from Nowhere*. Oxford: Oxford University Press.

Orser, B. A., M. Bertlik, L. Y. Wang, and J. F. McDonald. 1995. Inhibition of propofol (2,6 di-isopropylphenol) of the N-methyl-D-aspartate subtype of glutamate receptor in cultured hippocampal cells. *British Journal of Pharmacology* 116:1761–1768.

Perkins, W. J., and D. R. Morrow. 1992a. A dose-dependent reduction in halothane MAC in rats with a competitive N-methyl-D-aspartate (NMDA) receptor antagonist. *Anesthesia and Analgesia* 74:233.

Perkins, W. J., and D. R. Morrow. 1992b. Correlation between anesthetic potency and receptor binding constant for non-competitive N-methyl-D-aspartate receptor antagonists. *Anesthesiology* 77:A742.

Rey, G. 1983. A reason for doubting the existence of consciousness. In R. J. Davidson, G. E. Schwartz, and D. Shapiro, eds., *Consciousness and Self-Regulation. Advances in Research and Theory*, vol. 3. New York: Plenum Press, pp. 1–39.

Rey, G. 1988. A question about consciousness. In H. R. Otto and J. A. Tuedio, eds., *Perspectives on Mind*. Dordrecht: Reidel, pp. 5–24.

Rosenthal, D. 1986. Two concepts of consciousness. *Philosophical Studies* 49:329–359.

Rosenthal, D. 1990. A theory of consciousness. *Mind and Brain, Perspectives in Theoretical Psychology and the Philosophy of Mind*, Report No. 40/1990. Zif: University of Bielefeld.

Rosenthal, D. 1993a. Thinking that one thinks. In M. Davies, and G. Humphreys, eds., *Consciousness*. Cambridge: Blackwell, pp. 197–223.

Rosenthal, D. 1993b. Higher-order thoughts and the appendage theory of consciousness. *Philosophical Psychology* 6:155–166.

Scheller, M. S., M. H. Zornow, J. E. Fleischer, G. T. Shearman, and T. F. Greber. 1989. The noncompetitive NMDA receptor antagonist, MK 801, profoundly reduces volatile anesthetic requirements in rabbits. *Neuropharmacology* 28:677–681.

Tobin, J. R., D. L. Marzin, M. J. Breslow, and R. J. Traystman. 1993. Anesthetic inhibition of brain nitric oxide synthase *FASEB Journal* 7:A257 (Abstract).

von der Malsburg, C. 1981. *The Correlation Theory of Brain Function, Internal Report 81–2.* Göttingen: Department of Neurobiology, Max-Planck-Institute for Biophysical Chemistry.

VIII Sleep, Dreaming, and Nonconscious Processes

OVERVIEW

Questions concerning the nature and correlates (neuronal and contextual) of altered states of consciousness (e.g., sleep and dreaming) and the nature and complexity of nonconscious mental process have been of long-standing interest to a wide range of writers, scholars, and scientists. Indeed, a comprehensive psychological theory and approach to treating psychological disorders (Freud 1933) grew mainly from observations concerning dream reports and other presumed reflections of unconscious processes. What accounts for the experiential differences between waking and dreaming consciousness? What are the neural correlates of these different states? What does the phenomenon of lucid dreaming tell us about consciousness? What and how much information can be processed and represented nonconsciously? What aspects of emotion are available to consciousness and what aspects are not? These are among the questions addressed by the authors of the following five chapters.

J. Allan Hobson contributes the first chapter of Part VIII, exploring whether global aspects of consciousness can be correlated with specific neurobiologic mechanisms by mapping changes in conscious states onto changes in brain states, such as those occurring in the transition from waking to dreaming. Hobson's chapter defines consciousness as an "integrated awareness of the world, the body, and the self," and notes that one of the most distinctive aspects of consciousness is its variability as the brain changes state during the course of each day and night. Hobson's "conscious states paradigm" holds that variation in an individual's consciousness over the course of the day reflects changes in the functional organization of higher order neuronal networks across waking, sleep onset, and rapid eye movement (REM) sleep.

Hobson reviews cross-species and human developmental research to outline a phylogeny of rest and sleep and provides a brief history of concepts related to the regulation of sleep and waking—the discovery of REM sleep, observations of the neural correlates of input and output gating during REM sleep, and discoveries concerning different brain chemical processes accompanying sleep onset and the transition from non-REM to REM sleep. This body of information is the basis for a three-dimensional, state-space model

(AIM model) for conscious states, in which each of the three dimensions of the state space can be quantified from physiological measures of activation, input–output gating, and neurochemical modulation. The chapter closes with a discussion of how the AIM model has explanatory and predictive utility for understanding lucid dreaming and proposes approaches to testing specific predictions of the model.

The consideration of dream sleep and waking experience is continued in the chapter contributed by Allan Combs and Stanley Krippner. These authors argue against the view presented by Hobson and other researchers that dream images are the product of intrinsic random cortical and subcortical activity during REM sleep, without significant meaning. Rather, Combs and Krippner suggest that the large neuronal impulses originating in the pontine reticular formation and traveling through the lateral geniculate body to the occipital cortex (PGO waves) serve as a perturbation to visual cortex, similar to tapping a drum head on which sand has been sprinkled. Seen as a complex nonlinear system, the sand forms complex patterns characteristic of the dynamics of the drum head and the rate of tapping.

Similarly, the effect of PGO waves on the visual cortex is seen as disrupting waking associations, knowledge, and memory structures and allowing the mind to "flow along the subtle channels of yearning, desire, obsession, and love." The authors close their chapter by noting that the dreaming mind, by being able to acquire the attractor basins of a wide range of states of consciousness, is able to give rise to the richness of meaning in dreams.

The third chapter of this section, authored by Stephen LaBerge, focuses specifically on the contributions of research on lucid dreaming for our understanding of dreaming and its relationship to waking consciousness. LaBerge asserts that waking and dreaming experiences are created by the same "world modeling" mechanism of the brain. According to this view, dream experience is determined by which schemas (organized mental representations) are activated above the threshold for consciousness, and which is determined by the same processes of expectation and motivation that influence waking perception. The experienced meaning of dreams thus reflects activation of story, or narrative, schema that are intimate personal creations.

LaBerge then describes the method he and others have independently developed for studying consciousness during lucid dreaming. The method is based on the reasoning that if lucid dreamers can, in fact, act voluntarily in their dreams, they should be able to demonstrate it by making a prearranged eye movement signal (eye movements being the exception to a general motor-output gating that occurs during REM sleep) to mark the exact time that they became lucid.

Extending this method in combination with the recording of electroencephalograms from multiple scalp sites, LaBerge and his colleagues discovered that different dreamed experiences (e.g., time estimation, singing, sexual activity) are correlated with brain (and to a lesser extent, body) activity that is quite similar to the physiological correlates of the actual experiences of the corresponding events while awake.

Moving away from research on sleep and dreaming to considerations of nonconscious knowledge information representation, the next chapter, by Timothy Hubbard, reviews a creative, informative series of experiments showing that the remembered position of a stimulus is typically displaced from the actual position of that stimulus in ways that are consistent with the operation of invariant physical principles. Thus, a representational system appears to act as if the internal mental model of the external physical world is subject to the same physical principles as the external physical world.

Hubbard argues that the observed displacements in spatial representation reflect largely nonconscious (or implicit) knowledge of environmentally invariant physical principles that have been incorporated into the functional architecture of the representational system. Hubbard goes on to speculate about the selective advantage conveyed to an organism that could anticipate or extrapolate effects of physical principles on stimuli (e.g., predator or prey).

The chapter concludes by noting that displacement does not result from purely nonconscious process, given evidence that the direction or magnitude of displacement may be modified by conscious expectations regarding the stimulus. On the basis of this observation, Hubbard suggests that displacement may provide a useful paradigm for investigating interaction between conscious and nonconscious knowledge.

The final chapter of Part VIII, written by Daniel Levine, begins with a brief review of evidence supporting his assertion that there is not a one-to-one relationship between emotions and conscious states. Rather, emotions are viewed as computational processes within neural networks, the operations of which are nonconscious. He reviews evidence for the unconscious biasing of behavior by emotion and for the lack of conscious control over most emotional expression and presents a discussion of candidate neural systems subserving the interplay of emotion and reason in problem solving.

Levine then describes the skeleton neural network that he introduced, which embodies Maslow's (1968) notion of self-actualization, or optimal cognitive functioning. The chapter closes with a discussion of potential developments of his network model of interactions among consciousness, emotion, and reason.

The five chapters of Part VIII provide theoretical perspectives and empirical evidence concerning the relationship between conscious and nonconscious processes and knowledge. Studies of dreaming mentation and physiology, displacement of remembered stimulus placement, and neural network models of emotion and decision making provide unique empirical windows to understanding these relationships.

REFERENCES

Freud, S. 1933. *New Introductory Lectures on Psycho-Analysis.* (W. J. Sprott, ed.) New York: Norton.

Maslow, A. H. 1968. *Toward a Psychology of Being.* New York: Van Nostrand.

40 The Conscious State Paradigm: A Neuropsychological Analysis of Waking, Sleeping, and Dreaming

J. Allan Hobson

Philosophical and experimental psychological approaches have failed in their efforts to clearly define, let alone to explain, human consciousness. Recently, a renewed interest in this ancient and obdurate problem has been inspired by the rapid growth in the power of the cognitive and brain sciences.

In the transition from wakefulness to dreaming, so dramatic and so synchronous are the alterations in mind and brain states that specific, identified brain processes simultaneously affect the entire constellation of psychological functions that together constitute consciousness.

Prominent among the psychological functions that shift dramatically in the transition from wakefulness to sleeping to dreaming are perception, memory, orientation, attention, and emotion. It is becoming increasingly clear that a series of events in the pontine brain stem initiates changes in the global physiology and chemistry of the limbic system and cortex, which, in turn, produce profound alterations in these components of our conscious experience.

Some cellular and molecular details of the pontine system are clear. In wakefulness, the noradrenergic locus coeruleus and the serotonergic raphe neurones fire regularly to bathe the brain in adequate levels of neuromodulators that support alertness, attentiveness, memory, orientation, directed logical thought, and emotional stability. When these two chemical systems diminish their output, drowsiness supervenes; when sleep commences, the output of the two systems reaches the nadir, and the pontine cholinergic system, whose activity has been gradually augmenting throughout nonrapid eye movement (NREM) sleep, increases its output exponentially. This chemical switch turns on the cholincergic brain activation and autostimulation of rapid eye movement (REM) sleep. Together with aminergic demodulation, the cholinergic overdrive accounts for the characteristic hallucinations, delusions, disorientation, memory loss, and emotional intensifications of dreaming.

By studying the physiology and phenomenology of waking, sleeping, and dreaming and by elucidating the mechanisms that shift the brain and mind from one state to another, one can learn much about the control and alteration of consciousness. By providing techniques for analyzing and altering conscious states, such studies provide powerful experimental tools with which one can learn more about consciousness itself. I call this set of facts, assumptions, and strategies the *conscious state paradigm*.

This chapter reviews the evidence for brain–mind state dependency and explores the mechanisms known to govern the changes in brain–mind state that occur during the course of a day as we wake, fall asleep, enter REM sleep, and dream. Waking and REM sleep–dreaming are both activated brain states but have very different conscious-state features. As a way of beginning to understand how the state of the brain determines the state of consciousness, the focus is on the neurophysiological mechanisms that could account for these differences.

Thus, the chapter explores the possibility that by mapping changes in conscious states onto changes in brain states global aspects of consciousness can be meaningfully correlated with precisely specified microscopic neurobiological mechanisms.

STATE-DEPENDENT FEATURES OF CONSCIOUSNESS

Consciousness may be defined as an integrated awareness of the world, the body, and the self. One of the most distinctive aspects of consciousness is its variability as the brain changes state during the course of each day and night (Arkin, Antrobus, and Ellman 1991; Foulkes 1985). This strict and reliable dependency of mental state on brain state encourages a view of the brain–mind as a unified system; the investigation of the details of this state dependency may finally allow us to construct a realistic and testable theory of consciousness (Antrobus 1991; Hobson, 1993, 1994b; Hobson and Stickgold 1994a).

The integrated nature of consciousness is another remarkable feature that demands that the many discrete components of the brain–mind function in a unified way to create our global awareness of the world, our bodies, and ourselves (Hobson 1994b). As shown in Table 40.1, these components include sensation, perception, attention, memory, cognition, language, emotion, instinct, volition, and action. I limit my analysis to the brain mechanisms that may function to help all these modules work together synchronously and in the same mode of processing. I believe that the temporal and modal

Table 40.1 Components of Consciousness

Component	Definition
Attention	Selection of input data
Perception	Representation of input data
Memory	Retrieval of stored representations
Orientation	Representation of time, place and person
Thought	Reflection on representations
Narrative	Linguistic symbolization of representations
Emotion	Feelings about representations
Instinct	Innate propensities to act
Intention	Representation of goals
Volition	Decisions to act

integration is accomplished by the modulatory neuronal systems in the brain stem core that can confer both the necessary synchrony and chemically consistent operating conditions for the whole brain because of their widespread projections (Aston-Jones and Bloom 1981a, b; Chu and Bloom 1974; Hobson, McCarley, and Qyzink 1975; Jouvet 1972).

The states of waking, NREM, and REM sleep can be objectively distinguished by use of a combination of behavioral, electrophysiological, and psychological measures. The data reveal an impressive global correlation between the changes that components of consciousness undergo as the brain changes states. Compared to waking, the dreaming brain is off-line with respect to inputs and outputs; it self-activates and self-stimulates to create a state of consciousness characterized by vivid internally generated precepts with illogical and bizarre cognition.

Conscious states are differentiated not only in a diurnal sense but also across and within species. Consciousness develops with age (Roffwarg, Muzio, and Dement 1996) and with evolution (Zepelin and Rechtschaffen 1974). By comparing ontogenetic data with phylogenetic data (Table 40.2), one can see that, in the case of sleep, ontogeny does not recapitulate phylogeny because REM sleep, which is very abundant in immature animals (and might be thought to be phylogenetically primitive because of its brainstem origin) is actually a relatively modern invention of evolution. Because NREM sleep is not seen in subreptilian species, we conclude that sleep is a function of highly evolved brains, particularly brains with large cortices, and that sleep may play an active role in the development of cortical function.

We may resolve the controversial issues in speculating about infant and animal consciousness by realizing that different levels or even different kinds of consciousness arise in different brains according to the level of development and complexity of the particular brain. For example, a brain that cannot represent information abstractly as language is unlikely to achieve the prepositional and self-reflective modes of consciousness that awake adult humans

Table 40.2 Phylogeny of Rest and Sleep

Subject	Rest	Sleep REM	Sleep
Mammals			
Adults	+	+	+
Neonates	+	+	++
Birds			
Adult	+	+	—
Neonates	+	+	+
Reptiles	+	+	—
Amphibians	+	—	—
Fish	+	++	—

REM, rapid eye movement; +, present; ++, ambiguously or inconsistently present; —, absent.

J. Allan Hobson: Neuropsychological Analysis of Waking, Sleeping, and Dreaming experience. But this statement does not imply that brains lacking language are not perceptually or emotionally aware. The fundamental features of human conscious experience strongly depend on the state of the brainstem modulatory neurons, thus making their study in nonspeaking animals relevant to the understanding of human experience.

HISTORICAL BACKGROUND

Philosophical speculation regarding the nature of consciousness is as old as recorded history, and many materialist philosophers including the Ionian Greeks anticipated the physicalistic models that only recently have assumed the specific articulation of modern neuroscience (Hobson 1988). The signal event that demarcates the modern scientific era was the discovery of the electrical nature of nervous activity and, more specifically, the 1928 discovery of the electroencephalogram (EEG) by the German psychiatrist, Adolf Berger.

The state-dependent nature of the EEG helped Berger convince his skeptical critics that the rhythmic oscillations he recorded across the human scalp and skull with his galvanometer were of brain origin, not artifacts of movement or of scalp-muscle activity. When his subjects relaxed, closed their eyes, or dozed off into drowsiness, the low-voltage, fast brain-wave activity associated with alertness gave way to higher-voltage, lower-frequency patterns. These patterns, in turn, were rapidly blocked when the subjects were aroused.

The Reticular Activation Concept

The intrinsic nature of brain activation in waking was clearly demonstrated in 1949 when Giuseppe Moruzzi and Horace Magoun (1949) discovered that EEG desynchronization and behavioral arousal could be produced by high-frequency electrical stimulation of the midbrain. To explain their observation, Moruzzi and Magoun advanced the concept of the nonspecific (i.e., nonsensory) reticular activating system operating in series and in parallel with the ascending sensory pathways. This concept allowed the translation of afferent stimuli into central activation and opened the door to the more radical idea of auto-activation of the brain–mind *sui generis*. Because the spontaneous activity of neurons and the continuity and elaboration of such activity in determining the several substages of sleep is now an accepted concept, it is difficult for us to appreciate how strong and persistent was its antecedent concept. However, we need only consult Ivan Pavlov (1960) and Charles Sherrington (1955), both of whom were so imbued with the reflex doctrine that they were convinced that brain activity and consciousness simply ceased in the absence of sensory input.

The Discovery of REM Sleep

In 1953, Eugene Aserinsky and Nathaniel Kleitman (1963), working in Chicago, discovered that the brain–mind indeed self-activates, especially during sleep. At regular intervals they observed the spontaneous emergence of EEG desynchronization accompanied by clusters of rapid, saccadic eye movements (REMs) along with acute accelerations of heart and respiration rates. Working with Kleitman, William Dement was able to show (Dement and Kleitman 1955, 1957) that these periods of spontaneous auto-activation of the brain–mind were associated with dreaming and that the auto-activation process was also found in cats (Dement 1958).

In adult humans, the intrinsic cycle of inactivation (NREM sleep) and activation (REM sleep) recurred with a period length of 90 to 100 min. REM sleep occupied 20 percent to 25 percent of the recording time and NREM the remaining 75 percent to 80 percent of the recording time. The NREM phases of the first two cycles were deep and long, but because REM sleep occupied more of the last two or three cycles, sleep lightened.

In the early days of EEG recording, brain waves with frequencies in excess of 25 Hz were either ignored or filtered out because of the problem of interference by 50-or 60-Hz artifacts from electrical power sources. Recently, research aimed at solving the "binding problem" (how consciousness can be unified if it arises in a multimodular system) has focused on the 35 to 40-Hz activity that is found in adjacent neuronal ensembles when animals attend to external stimuli (Singer 1979). It has been proposed that by synchronizing multiple and distant brain units, the spatiotemporal unity of conscious experience may be achieved.

Further, Rodolfo Llinas proposed that as the cortex is scanned by the thalamus, 40-Hz waves are propagated from the frontal to the occipital poles. Noting that 40-Hz activity is observed in REM sleep and in wakefulness, Llinas emphasized the importance of intrinsic neuronal oscillations in the genesis of all states of consciousness and suggested that the main difference between wakefulness and dreaming arises from input–output gating (Llinas and Pare 1991).

Demonstration of Input–Output Gating

The paradoxical preservation of sleep in the face of brain–mind activation during sleep began to be explained when Francois Michel and Michel Jouvet, working in Lyon in 1959, demonstrated that active muscle inhibition was a regular component of REM sleep in cats. Using transection, lesion, and stimulation techniques, the Jouvet team also discovered that the control system for REM sleep was localized to the pontine brain stem and that the pons was the source of the EEG activation and the REMs themselves. Muscle inhibition was mediated by pontine signals relayed via the bulbar inhibitory reticular formation to the spinal cord (Jouvet 1962).

Synchronous with each flurry of REMs, phasic activation signals or pontogeniculo-occipital (PGO) waves were sent from the pons up into the forebrain (and down into the spinal cord). Jouvet also discovered that the PGO waves triggered bursts of firing by geniculate and cortical neurones and that other signals of brainstem origin damped both sensory input (via presynaptic

Table 40.3 Physiological Basis of Differences Between Waking and Dreaming.

Function	Nature of Difference	Causal Hypothesis
Sensory input	Blocked	Presynaptic inhibition
Perception (external)	Diminished	Blockade of sensory input
Perception (internal)	Enhanced	Disinhibition of networks storing sensory representations
Attention	Lost	Decreased aminergic modulation causes a decrease in signal–noise ratio
Memory (recent)	Diminished	Because of aminergic demodulation, activated representations are not restored in memory
Memory (remote)	Enhanced	Disinhibition of networks storing mnemonic representations increases access to consciousness
Orientation	Unstable	Internally inconsistent orienting signals are generated by cholinergic system
Thought	Reasoning, ad hoc; logical rigor, weak; processing, hyperassociative	Loss of attention , memory, and volition leads to failure of sequencing and rule inconstancy; analogy replaces analysis
Insight	Self-reflection lost	Failures of attention, logic, and memory weaken second- and third-order representations
Language (internal)	Confabulatory	Aminergic demodulation frees narrative synthesis from logical restraints
Emotion	Episodically strong	Cholinergic hyperstimulation of amygdala and related temporal lobe structures triggers emotional storms unmodulated by aminergic restraint
Instinct	Episodically strong	Cholinergic hyperstimulation of hypothalamus and limbic forebrain triggers fixed-action motor programs experienced fictively but not enacted
Volition	Weak	Top-down motor control and frontal executive power cannot compete with disinhibited sub-cortical network activation
Output	Blocked	Postsynaptic inhibition

inhibition) and motor output (via postsynaptic inhibition) (Callaway, Lydic, Baghdoyan, and Hobson 1987). Thus, in REM sleep, the autoactivated brain–mind is effectively off-line with respect to external inputs and outputs, and it stimulates itself (Table 40.3).

The cellular and molecular basis of the dramatic changes in input–output gating mechanisms were detailed by use of Sherrington's reflex paradigm along with extracellular and intracellular recording techniques (Pompeiano 1967). For example, researchers showed that during REM sleep, each moto-neurone was subjected to 10 mV of tonic hyperpolarization, which blocked all but a few of the phasic activation signals generated by the REM–PGO system and that this inhibition was mediated by glycine (Morales and Chase 1981; Soja, Finch, and Chase 1987).

In cats, when the motor inhibition was experimentally disrupted by lesioning the pons, the animals—still in a REM-like sleep state but without the atonia—evinced stereotyped behaviors (such as fear–defense and aggression–attack postures) that expressed the activation (in REM) of the specific motor-pattern generators for these instinctual fixed acts (Jouvet and Delorme 1965; Henley and Morrison 1974). The clear implication was that in normal REM sleep the motor inhibiton contained the motor commands of the instinctual behavior pattern generators and rendered them virtual for the outside world and fictitious for the internal world of the brain–mind itself.

The strong significance of these findings for a theory of dream consciousness is their ability to explain the ubiquity of imagined movement in dreams (Porte and Hobson 1996). From a functional point of view, it may also be important to recognize that the autoactivation process of REM sleep is highly patterned (hence, nonrandom) from a sensorimotor point of view.

The recording of individual neurons in behaving animals was pioneered by Edward Evarts (1960) using the moveable microelectrode system of David Hubel (1959). Evarts was able to show that both the tonic EEG activation and the phasic PGO-wave activation signals of REM reflected the excitation of neurons throughout the forebrain, including the visual motor and association cortices (Adey, Kado, and Rhodes 1963) and the thalamic nuclei reciprocally connected to them (Steriade, Pare, Parent, and Smith 1988; Bizzi and Brooks 1963).

We now know more about the neurophysiology of REM sleep and dreaming than we know about wakefulness. This paradox is explained by the fact that in REM the animal is paralyzed and partially anesthetized by intrinsic modulation of its motor and sensory systems! REM sleep is therefore a natural state favoring deep neurophysiological analysis.

The picture that emerges is of global but specific alterations of neuronal activation and information flow throughout the brain. This picture is highly relevant to our understanding of the differences that distinguish the conscious states of wakefulness from states of NREM sleep and REM sleep with dreaming. In wakefulness the activated brain–mind gives priority to processing data from the outside world and acting on the world accordingly. (In NREM sleep the system is taken off-line passively via deactivation.) In REM sleep, in extreme contrast with wakefulness, the internal representations of the world become inputs; the action that is summoned (but not executed) is one of the inputs (Llinas and Pare 1991).

Demonstration of Modulation

The chemical means by which the dramatic changes in brain–mind state occur are mediated by the modulatory neuronal system of the brain stem (Jouvet 1972). In this regard, the noradrenergic locus coeruleus and the serotonergic raphe neurones of the pons are particularly critical. Both these aminergic populations contain pacemaker elements that fire spontaneously and tonically throughout wakefulness. They also phasically increase their output in response to salient stimuli and decrease their output during inter-stimulus lulls and at sleep onset (Aston-Jones and Bloom 1981a, b; Chu and Bloom 1974). In their phasic response to stimuli, they are joined by the cholinergic neurones of the far lateral pedunculopontine nucleus, but these cells are not pacemakers and tend to be otherwise quiescent in waking.

Thus, the wakeful brain is bathed in constant levels of norepinephrine and serotonin and receives pulsatile boosts of the two chemicals and acetylcholine when new input data call for them. These observations suggest that the chemistry of attentive, mnemonic wakefulness is an aminergic–cholinergic collaboration.

All three modulatory systems abate at sleep onset. As NREM sleep deepens, the activity of the two aminergic systems gradually and sponta-neously declines (Chu and Bloom 1974; Hobson, McCarley, and Qyzinki 1975; McGinty and Harper 1976), and the activity of the cholinergic neurones gradually and spontaneously increases (Hobson, McCarley, and Qyzink 1975). At REM sleep onset, the aminergic system is completely arrested, and the cholinergic system is unabatedly auto-active. The net effect, confirmed by measurements of transmitter release (Lydic, Baghdoyan, and Lorinc 1991), is a shift from an aminergic microclimate in wakefulness to a cholinergic microclimate in REM.

These physiological findings have inspired—and are strengthened by—the results of systemic and local pharmacological experiments showing that both antiaminergic and procholinergic drugs tend to increase REM and that both proaminergic and anticholinergic agents suppress it. As predicted by the physiological model (see below), these drugs have reciprocal effects on waking and NREM sleep.

Among the wealth of pharmacological studies yielding these conclusions (Hobson and Steriade 1986), two are particularly impressive and both reveal dramatic REM sleep enhancement. When the cholinergic agonist carbachol or the anticholinesterase neostigmine are injected into the paramedian pon-tine brain stem, they cause immediate, intense, and prolonged REM sleep episodes (Baghdoyan et al. 1984; Baghdoyan, Rodrigo-Angulo, McCarley, and Hobson 1984; 1987). This effect, which wanes in about six hours, is called *short-term REM sleep enhancement*. When the agents are injected into the far lateral peribrachial pons, they cause immediate but only unilateral PGO-wave enhancement and delayed (24–48 hr) enhancement of REM sleep episodes of normal lengths for six to ten days; this effect is called *long-term REM sleep enhancement* (Calvo, Datta, Quattrochi, and Hobson 1992; Datta, Calvo, Quattrochi, and Hobson 1992).

EXPLANATORY MODELS

Two models, one neurobiological (McCarley and Hobson 1975) and the other neuropsychological (Hobson and McCarley 1977), were advanced to organize these findings and their implication for a theory of consciousness. A third model linking the two models is the psychophysiological model, AIM (Hobson 1990).

The Neurobiological Model

The neurobiological model of reciprocal interaction between aminergic and cholinergic systems has stimulated extensive hypothesis testing, including the studies described above. According to this model, the activation and open input–output gates of waking are the result of tonic aminergic and phasic aminergic–cholinergic modulation. The electrical activation, the closed input–output gates, and the intense phasic autostimulation of REM sleep are the result of tonic aminergic demodulation and phasic cholinergic modulation of the brain.

The Neuropsychological Model

The physiological differences between waking, NREM, and REM sleep that have been described can now be linked in a tentative way to the changes in conscious state that are correlated with them (see Table 40.3). In the domain of sensation and perception, responsiveness to the external world is progressively lost with the cortical deactivation of sleep onset; responsiveness declines further as NREM sleep deepens. During REM sleep, the brain reactivates but presynaptic inhibition blocks the exteroception of sensory signals and the phasic sensorimotor activation embodied by the REMs and their associated PGO waves come to constitute internal stimuli. These endogenous signals send specific information about the eye movements from the brain stem to the thalamocortical visual system, which may account for the intense visual hallucinations of dreams. Furthermore, the PGO signals cholinergically also drive the amygdala (perhaps accounting for dream emotions such as anxiety and surprise).

Cognition also undergoes a reliable shift from the wakeful state as attention, orientation, and logically directed thought give way, first, to the nonprogressive ruminations of NREM sleep (Foulkes 1985; Hobson, Lydic, and Baghdoyan 1986; Arkin, Antrobus, and Ellman 1991) and, next, to the disoriented, undirected, and illogical cognition of dreaming. In addition to the loss of the temporal and spatial constancies conferred by the sleep-dependent sensorimotor deafferentation, the brain in REM sleep is aminergically demodulated, which may contribute to the failures of attention, orientation, memory, and logic that characterize dreaming itself and that make dreams so hard to remember (McCarley and Hobson 1975; Hobson 1993, 1994b, c; Hobson and Stickgold 1994a).

The AIM Model

The simple neuropsychological model first called the activation-synthesis hypothesis of dreaming (Hobson and McCarley 1977), has recently been

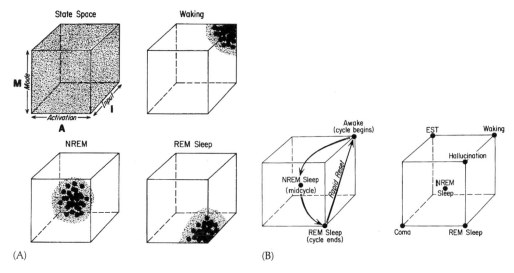

Figure 40.1 AIM: A three-dimensional, state-space model. (A) Three-dimensional state space defined by the values for brain activation [A], input source and strength [I], and mode of processing [M]. It is theoretically possible for the system to be at any point in the state space and an infinite number of state conditions is conceivable. In practice, the system is normally constrained to a boomerang-like path from the back upper right in wakefulness (high A, I, and M), through the center in NREM (intermediate A, I, and M) to the front lower right in REM sleep (high A, low I, and M). (B) [A] Movement through the state space during the sleep cycle. [B] Segments of the state space associated with some normal, pathological, and artificial conditions of the brain.

developed into a comprehensive, three-dimensional, state-space model for conscious states (Hobson 1990). In this model, each dimension of state space—A, activation; I, input–output gating; M, modulation—can be quantified from physiological measurements (Figure 40.1).

To appreciate the explanatory and predictive utility of the AIM model, consider lucid dreaming (Hobson 1988)—an unusual, but not rare, state of consciousness in which the dreamer correctly diagnoses his own conscious state as dreaming (instead of making the usual error of supposing he or she is awake). Lucid dreaming occurs spontaneously in late childhood and early adolescence and can be cultivated by performing presleep autosuggestion (Hobson 1988). Because lucid dreaming combines features of wakefulness with features of REM, it is a hybrid, dissociated condition that is both pleasurable and instructive. The pleasure derives from one's emergent ability in lucid dreams to control the dream's "plot" and, hence, to indulge in otherwise impossible or forbidden behaviors, such as flying or sexual adventure.

Because of the anomalous copresence of dream hallucinosis and insight about the conscious state in which these features arise, the lucid dreaming state is also instructive. I believe that lucid dreaming must be situated on the right sidewall of the AIM state space between the normally widely separated domains of REM and wakefulness. This part of the state space is a "no-man's land" because of the unidirectional, rapid reset mechanism that switches the brain to waking. This finding fits with the fact that lucid dreaming is both rare and evanescent—the lucid dreamer is either pulled up from the ecstasy of his controlled dream to a waking state or pulled back down into a dream over which he or she no longer exerts control.

Two physiological hypotheses immediately suggest themselves. The first is that the frontal cortex, thought to be responsible for controlled and deviated thought, will be found to be relatively inactivated in REM with non-lucid dreaming, but the pontine cholinergic PGO system will be found to be highly active. The second hypothesis is that, in lucid dreaming, the frontal cortex will be relatively activated and the pontine PGO system suppressed.

Both predictions are now testable by taking advantage of imaging techniques such as positron-emission tomography (PET), single-photon-emission computed tomography (SPECT), and magnetic resonance imaging (MRI). Other testable predictions that follow from the AIM model include the probability that the lucid state is unstable because top-down messages from the frontal cortex to the brain stem not only suppress the cholinergic system but also turn on the aminergic system and thus cause awakening. This set of predictions specifies the cerebral mechanics by which the nature of conscious experience is biochemically determined and moves us one important step closer to specifying the biochemical substance of consciousness itself.

CONCLUSION

The conscious states paradigm holds that an individual's experience of consciousness varies during the course of the day as the functional organization of higher-order neuronal networks changes. We have begun to develop this strategy by tracking how the modular components of conscious experience change when one first falls asleep and when one later enters REM sleep and dreams most intensely.

The basic assumption is that the phenomenological changes that differentiate, for example, dreaming from waking, can be understood at the level of the brain. By detailing the specific physiological and biochemical changes that underlie this stereotyped shift in conscious state, some organizational rules controlling the large, populous neuronal networks that together generate full, unified conscious experience may be deduced. By observing how consciousness breaks down with the natural changes in brain state, we may also be able to deduce causes of the diminished conscious unity experienced in mental illness.

REFERENCES

Adey, W. R., R. T. Kado, and J. M. Rhodes. 1963. Sleep: Cortical and subcortical recordings in the chimpanzee. *Science* 141:932.

Antrobus, J. 1991. Dreaming: Cognitive processes during cortical activation and high afferent thresholds. *Psychological Review* 98:96–121.

Arkin, A., J. Antrobus, and S. Ellman, eds. 1991. *The Mind in Sleep*, 2nd ed. Hillsdale, NJ: Erlbaum.

Aserinsky, E., and N. Kleitman 1963. Regularly occurring periods of ocular mobility and concomitant phenomena during sleep. *Science* 118:361–375.

Aston-Jones, G., and F. E. Bloom. 1981a. Activity of norepinephrine-containing locus coeruleus neurons in behaving rats anticipates fluctuations in the sleep-waking cycle. *Journal of Neuroscience* 1:876–886.

Aston-Jones, G., and F. E. Bloom. 1981b. Norepinephrine-containing locus coeruleus neurons in behaving rats exhibit pronounced responses to nonnoxious environmental stimuli. *Journal of Neuroscience.* 1:887–900.

Baghdoyan, H. A., A. P. Monaco, M. L. Rodrigo-Angulo, F. Assens, R. W. McCarley, and J. A. Hobson. 1984. Microinjection of neostigmine into the pontine reticular formation of cats enhances desynchronized sleep signs. *Journal of Pharmacology and Experimental Therapies* 231:173–180.

Baghdoyan, H. A., M. L. Rodrigo-Angulo, R. W. McCarley, and J. A. Hobson. 1984. Site-specific enhancement and suppression of desynchronized sleep signs following cholinergic stimulation of three brainstem regions. *Brain Research.* 306:39–52.

Baghdoyan, H. A., M. L. Rodrigo-Angulo, R. W. McCarley, and J. A. Hobson. 1987. A neuro-anatomical gradient in the pontine tegmentum for the cholinoceptive induction of desynchronized sleep signs. *Brain Research.* 414:245–261.

Bizzi, E., and D. C. Brooks. 1963. Functional connections between pontine reticular formation and lateral geniculate nucleus during deep sleep. *Archives Italiennes de Biologie* 101:666–680.

Callaway, C. W., R. Lydic, H. A. Baghdoyan, and J. A. Hobson. 1987. Ponto-geniculo-occipital waves: Spontaneous visual system activation occurring in REM sleep. *Cellular and Molecular Neurobiology* 7:105–149.

Calvo, J., S. Datta, J. J. Quattrochi, and J. A. Hobson. 1992. Cholinergic microstimulation of the peribrachial nucleus in the cat. II. Delayed and prolonged increases in REM Sleep. *Archives Italiennes de Biologie* 130:285–301.

Chu, N. S., and F. E. Bloom. 1974. Activity patterns of catecholamine-containing pontine neurons in the dorsolateral tegmentum of unrestrained cats. *Journal of Neurobiology* 5:527–544.

Datta, S., J. Calvo, J. J. Quattrochi, and J. A. Hobson. 1992. Cholinergic microstimulation of the peribrachial nucleus in the cat. I. Immediate and prolonged increases in ponto-geniculo-occipital waves. *Archives Italiennes de Biologie* 130:263–284.

Dement, W. 1958. The occurrence of low voltage, fast, electroencephalogram patterns during behavioral sleep in the cat. *Electroencephalography in Clinical Neurophysiology* 10:291–296.

Dement, W., and N. Kleitman. 1955. Cyclic variations in EEG during sleep and their relation to eye movements, body mobility and dreaming. *Electroencephalography in Clinical Neurophysiology* 9:673–690.

Dement, W., and N. Kleitman. 1957. The relation of eye movements during sleep to dream activity: An objective method for the study of dreaming. *Journal of Experimental Psychology* 53:89–97.

Evarts, E. V. 1960. Effects of sleep and waking on spontaneous and evoked discharge of single units in visual cortex. *Federation Proceedings Supplement* 4:828–837.

Foulkes, D. 1985. *Dreaming: A Cognitive-Psychological Analysis*. Hillsdale, NJ: Erlbaum.

Henley, K., and A. R. Morrison. 1974. A re-evaluation of the effects of lesions of the pontine tegmentum and locus coeruleus on phenomena of paradoxical sleep in the cat. *Acta Neurobiologiae Experimentalis* 34:215–232.

Hobson, J. A. 1988. *The Dreaming Brain*. New York: Basic Books.

Hobson, J. A. 1990. Activation, input source, and modulation: A neurocognitive model of the state of the brain-mind. In R. Bootzin, J. Kihlstrom, and D. Schacter, eds., *Sleep and Cognition*. Washington, DC: American Psychological Association, pp. 25–40.

Hobson, J. A. 1994b. Consciousness as a state-dependent phenomenon. In J. Cohen and J. Schooler, eds., *Scientific Approaches to the Question of Consciousness*.

Hobson, J. A. 1994c. Consciousness: Lessons for anesthesia from sleep research. In J. F. Biebuyck, ed., *Anaesthesia: Biologic Foundations*. New York: Raven Press.

Hobson, J. A., R. Lydic, and H. A. Baghdoyan. 1986. Evolving concepts of sleep cycle generation: From brain centers to neuronal populations (with commentaries). *Behavioral Brain Science* 9:371–448.

Hobson, J. A., and R. McCarley. 1977. The brain as a dream state generator: An activation-synthesis hypothesis of the dream process. *American Journal of Psychiatry* 134:1335–1348.

Hobson, J. A., R. W. McCarley, and P. W. Qyzinki. 1975. Sleep cycle oscillation: Reciprocal discharge by two brainstem neuronal groups. *Science* 189:55–58.

Hobson, J. A., and M. Steriade. 1986. The neuronal basis of behavioral state control. In F. E. Bloom, ed., *Intrinsic Regulatory Systems of the Brain*, vol. IV, sec. I. Bethesda: American Physiological Society, pp. 701–823.

Hobson, J. A., and R. Stickgold. 1994a. The conscious state paradigm: A neurocognitive approach to waking, sleeping and dreaming. In M. Gazzaniga ed., *The Cognitive Neurosciences*, pp. 1373–1389.

Hubel, D. H. 1959. Single unit activity in striate cortex of unrestrained cats. *Journal of Physiology* (London) 147:226–238.

Jouvet, M. 1962. Recherche sur les structures nerveuses et les mecanismes responsables des differentes phases du sommeil physiologique. *Archives Italiennes de Biologie* 100:125–206.

Jouvet, M. 1972. The role of monoamines and acetylcholine-containing neurons in the regulation of the sleep-waking cycle. *Ergebnisse der Physiologie, Biologischen Chemie und Experimentellen Pharmakologie* 64:166–307.

Jouvet, M., and F. Delorme. 1965. Locus coeruleus et sommeil paradoxal. *Societe de Biologies* 159:895.

Llinas, R. R., and D. Pare. 1991. Of dreaming and wakefulness. *Neuroscience* 44:521–535.

Lydic, R., H. A. Baghdoyan, and Z. Lorinc. 1991. Microdialysis of cat pons reveals enhanced acetylcholine release during state-dependent respiratory depression. *American Journal of Physiology* 261:766–770.

McCarley, R. W., and J. A. Hobson. 1975. Neuronal excitability modulation over the sleep cycle: A structural and mathematical model. *Science* 189:58–60.

McGinty, D. J. and R. M. Harper. 1976. Dorsal raphe neurons: Depression of firing during sleep in cats. *Brain Research* 101:569–575.

Morales, F. R., and M. H. Chase. 1981. Postsynaptic control of lumbar motoneuron excitability during active sleep in the chronic cat. *Brain Research* 225:279–295.

Moruzzi, G., and H. W. Magoun. 1949. Brainstem reticular formation and activation of the EEG. *Electroencephalography in Clinical Neurophysiology* 1:455–473.

Pavlov, I. P. 1960. *Conditioned Reflexes: An Investigation of the Physiological Activity of the Cerebral Cortex*, G. V. Anrep, trans. New York: Dover.

Pompeiano, O. 1967. The neurophysiological mechanisms of the postural and motor events during desynchronized sleep. *Proceedings of the Association for Research in Nervous and Mental Disease* 45:351–423.

Porte, H. S., and J. A. Hobson. 1996. Physical motion in dreams: One measure of three theories. *Journal of Abnormal Psychology* 105:329–335.

Roffwarg, J. P., J. M. Muzio, and W. C. Dement. 1966. Ontogenetic development of the human sleep-dream cycle. *Science* 152:604–619.

Sherrington, C. 1955. *Man on His Nature.* New York: Doubleday.

Singer, W. 1979. Central-core control of visual cortex functions. In R. F. O. Schmitt and F. G. Worden, eds., *The Neurosciences: Fourth Study Program.* Cambridge: MIT Press, pp. 1093–1110.

Soja, P. J., D. M. Finch, and M. H. Chase. 1987. Effect of inhibitory amino acid antagonists on masseteric reflex suppression during active sleep. *Experimental Neurology* 96(1):178–193.

Steriade, M., D. Pare, A. Parent, and Y. Smith. 1988. Projections of cholinergic and non-cholinergic neurons of the brainstem core to relay and associational thalamic nuclei in the cat and macaque monkey. *Neuroscience* 25:47–67.

Zepelin, H., and A. Rechtschaffen. 1974. Mammalian sleep longevity and energy metabolism. *Brain, Behavior and Evolution* 10:425–470.

41 Dream Sleep and Waking Reality: A Dynamical View

Allan Combs and Stanley Krippner

If dreams are anything, they are fluid. Images, thoughts, and feelings flow as if seen through water. There is an elastic quality to the progression of events, which emerge as if through doorways from the past or from unknown landscapes. Sometimes a dream is shrouded in an atmosphere of joy or grief. Occasionally, if we are fortunate, our dreams are visited by epiphany. Waking life, on the other hand, is characterized by fixed objects and events that come and go across an essentially Cartesian terrain and that proceed one another in ordered steps. In both situations, experience is processual; that is, it is characterized more by motion than by rest and more by transformation than by stasis.

Process perspectives are very old and widespread. No English-speaking thinker, however, has written more lucidly about the process nature of human experience than William James, who coined the phrase "stream of thought" to characterize the process nature of the mind, an expression suggestive of the older image of the Heraclitean river. His word "thought" can be a bit deceptive for the modern reader because by "thought" James considered all aspects of the mental life—memory, perceptions, emotion, and the flow of ideas.

Process thinking recently entered the scientific mainstream through developments in systems theory (e.g., Laszlo 1972). Beginning in biology, systems theory has developed during the past few decades as a perspective that sees a wide range of phenomena in terms of the complex and fluid interactions of small processes that cooperatively blend to form hierarchically larger process structures (Laszlo 1987; Jantsch 1980). An example is a living cell, in which many chemical reactions combine in the formation of cycles and hypercycles that comprise the overall activity of the cell. Like other systems of this variety, a living cell is an autopoietic system; in other words, it is self-creating (Maturana and Varela 1975, 1987). The product of the entire set of interactions is nothing less than the cell itself.

We view consciousness, or at least the many psychological processes that constitute its content, as an autopoietic event not unlike a living cell. Psychological processes include thoughts, memories, feelings, and perceptions that weave themselves together to form the living fabric of moment-to-moment reality. They arise from relatively pure mental activity and from physiological states in the body. Such processes are subject to continuous flux and never appear more than once in exactly the same configuration. Moreover, as James also observed, each individual's stream of thought is unique; it is the defining feature of the person's personality.

Hence, each person's subjective life is constantly changing, never exactly repeating itself, and forming a unique, recognizable pattern that, in the Jamesian view, is the earmark of the individual. In systems theory, this set of qualities identifies a particular process pattern called a *chaotic attractor*. Another example of such a pattern is the weather, which is comprised of elements such as heat, humidity, barometric pressure, and wind velocity that constantly interact in a complex, fluid fashion. The result is a process configuration that is globally recognizable over long periods of time but generally unpredictable from day to day. Moreover, the configuration is never precisely the same on two different days. As the term itself suggests, attractors have a certain tenacity, a natural tendency to hold their own form. In the case of chaotic attractors, the pattern is not regular and does not precisely repeat itself; nevertheless, the pattern is usually apparent when observed long enough.

The elements that make up a complex chaotic system are often themselves chaotic. Moods, for example, fluctuate from hour to hour and day to day, never quite repeating themselves, but following a pattern that can be recognized in each particular individual. This has been shown in several empirical investigations (Combs, Winkler, and Daley 1994). Although less obvious, other elements of conscious experience appear to follow a similar course. These elements include the moment-to-moment, day-to-day, month-to-month ebb and flow of thoughts, memories, fantasies, and desires. There also seems to be a roughly rhythmic alteration of general arousal, which has been studied by Ernest Rossi (1986, 1996). Consistent with the empirical findings of Combs (Winkler and Combs 1993), Rossi believes that general arousal follows a chaotic pattern. The idea that many of the elements of experience may be chaotic is not surprising, given the considerable evidence that the brain itself in many respects is a chaotic system (Basar, 1990; Freeman, 1992; Pribram, 1995; Rapp et al. 1990).

As a practical note, it is difficult to rigorously demonstrate that any biological system is chaotic in the strict mathematical sense because such demonstrations require that very large data sets be obtained under unchanging conditions of observation (Rapp 1993). This stipulation is all but impossible to meet in studies of living organisms. We use the term chaos in speaking of systems that are chaos-like as far as can be ascertained.

STATES OF MIND–BODY AND STATES OF CONSCIOUSNESS

An important feature of many complex chaotic systems is that their processual elements conspire to support each other and the overall fabric of the system. This would seem to be the case with consciousness, in which feelings, thoughts, memories, and perceptions tend to unite into single, overall patterns that we term *states of mind–body* because these states often involve mental processes, such as thought and memory, and bodily aspects, such as general arousal and the physiological aspects of emotions, desires, and the like. (The term mind–body is an effort to express more precisely the common phrase, "state of mind," which is an informal reference to many different, coherent, daily experiential states.)

A temporary depression, for example, is a state of mind–body that is accompanied by feelings of sadness or hopelessness, a loss of physical energy, perhaps changes in appetite, and a variety of thoughts, perceptions, and overt behaviors, all of which support the overall state. A depressed person thinks unhappy thoughts, and memory becomes biased in favor of depressing recollections (Bower 1981). A depressed person may choose sad music, withdraw from the supportive company of others, and become physically inactive. Everything pulls together to support the depression. Each state of mind–body, whether sadness, joy, enthusiasm, curiosity, boredom, or anticipation, is not only supported by all its parts but the parts conspire in its continuous creation.

The process elements of consciousness configure themselves into states of mind–body and into larger holistic structures, *states of consciousness* (Combs 1995, 1996a). Some decades ago, Charles Tart (1975) described states of consciousness as built up of psychological functions much like the elements mentioned above—memory, thought, feelings, sensory perceptions, sense of self, and so on. Tart presented a substantial case, both theoretical and empirical, that states of consciousness such as ordinary wakefulness, dream states, shamanic experiences, and meditative states are each formed by particular patterns of psychological functions. In each state of consciousness these functions configure themselves in a particular pattern or *gestalt*. In other words, there is a natural resonance to each state of consciousness; its elements conspire in a unique way to produce the overall pattern of that state.

From a contemporary point of view, it is apparent that what Tart was describing were complex, chaotic-like attractors. We believe that consciousness can be understood as a three-tiered structure in which basic process elements (psychological functions) self-organize into states of mind–body that, in turn, are supported by particular states of consciousness (Combs 1996a, b; Combs and Krippner 1996). The entire process structure, in fact, can be viewed as a set of attractors nested within attractors, each flowing forward along chaotic trajectories. This general picture has also been developed in a mathematical model by Goertzel (1994). From this perspective, we can explore two types of consciousness, ordinary waking reality and dreaming consciousness.

Waking Consciousness

There are several salient features of ordinary waking consciousness. The most evident characteristic of the ordinary waking state of consciousness is its direct interaction with the consensual world. In the waking state, experience is structured significantly by sensory input from the eyes, ears, skin, and so on, and by interoceptive stimulation such as hunger, thirst, proprioception, and temperature sense from the body. Along with this input, behavioral output leads to reafferentation at the bodily level and feedback through the external senses, all of which tend to shape the processes of consciousness in the direction of effective interaction with the consensual environment.

As required for survival, the mechanisms of consciousness have become very skilled at calibrating themselves to the consensual world. Structures such as a working sense of self are built up hierarchically of process elements (Schwalbe 1991). Other processes of a largely cognitive nature provide the individual an understanding of events in the consensual world. As Piaget and many others (Eysenck and Keane 1990; Flavell 1963) have shown, mature knowledge structures are both sophisticated and flexible; they are able to modify themselves to compensate for changes in the material and social environments.

In addition, an insistent pull within the mind to organize information about life events in terms of stories seems to exist. This characteristic is seen in the functional organization of memory (Eysenck and Keane 1990) and in the tendency for people to make narrations of the circumstances of their own lives (Feinstein and Krippner 1988), a tendency that seems vital for coming to terms with the facts of existence. Harvy and Weber (1990), for instance, interviewed men and women about past romantic breakups. The researchers found that the subjects were unable to come to a sense of completion until they had formed their own personal stories about what had happened to them.

Dream Consciousness

Dreams belong to a class of forms of consciousness that are essentially disconnected from the external world. Consciousness is freed from the powerful patterning forces of consensual reality, and is thereby able to relax into intrinsically comfortable patterns of activity.

Research on sensory deprivation demonstrates that a dramatic reduction in sensory input is sufficient to cause the brain to produce imagery (Zubek 1969). During REM sleep dreaming, however, sensory input to higher brain centers is actively inhibited by the reticular formation, and other powerful physiological changes are also initiated. There is a shift of the brain's neuro-modulatory balance from aminergic dominance, characteristic of waking, to cholinergic dominance (Hobson and Stickgold 1994). Activity in important centers of the brain-stem reticular formation is redistributed, and large electrical pontogeniculo-occipital (PGO) waves originate in the pontine reticular formation and travel through the lateral geniculate bodies to the occipital cortex.

These changes are sufficiently impressive to have persuaded many researchers that dreaming can be accounted for entirely in terms of physiology. In this spirit, Allan Hobson proposed the activation-synthesis hypothesis, which explained dream imagery in terms of the misinterpretation of PGO stimulation as sensory input (Hobson 1988; Chapter 40 in this volume).

Although we hold Hobson's empirical work in the highest regard, we do not agree with the notion that the optical cortex "misinterprets" the PGO bombardment as visual stimulation. It seems unlikely that the brain mechanisms of vision and dream sleep, both products of millions of years of coevolution, would misfunction in this way. We suggest that the hail of PGO activity serves as a perturbation to visual cortex, much like tapping a drum head on which sand has been sprinkled. The sand forms complex patterns characteristic of the dynamics of the drum-head itself and the rate of the tapping. In a sense, the induced vibration allows the system of the sand on the drum head to "relax" into its own unique configuration.

This way of thinking is consistent with ideas inspired by neural network models of the dreaming brain. Goertzel (1994), for instance, speculated that during dreams the intrinsic networks of the brain relax into their own optimal, or most "comfortable" configurations; inherent emotional patterns, belief systems, and memory complexes have free reign. Goertzel (1996) states:

In dreams, we can get exactly what we want ... something that very rarely happens in reality. And we can also get precisely what we most fear.

The effect of the PGO bombardment is to increase the noise level ("temperature") of the cortical process, which disrupts waking associations, knowledge, and memory structures and allows the mind to flow along the subtle channels of yearning, desire, obsession, love, and so forth. In technical terms, the added noise of the PGO waves keeps the system of consciousness from getting caught in small depressions, or minima, in its state space by seeking larger patterns of wide attractor basins. Such basins are related to what Carl Jung discovered and named "complexes" in his word-association experiments in the late 1800s.

Like a collection of oddly shaped objects put into a jar and shaken gently, the emotional and cognitive aspects of the mental life settle down side by side in comfortable patterns. These elements, however, are process patterns in which psychological process elements interact in the continuous creation of new and creative configurations. Writing in terms of general systems theory, mathematician Ben Goertzel (1994) and systems theorist Georg Kampis (1991) have shown in detail how process elements in any complex system can join together in creative syntheses to yield new and original process elements. Their ideas follow in the tradition of Henri Bergson, who believed that the interactive play of events during evolution engenders new creative process structures which he termed "emergents."

This dynamic flow of creativity is evidently an important aspect of waking life but is amplified in dream consciousness, in which entire patterns of experience emerge with astonishing novelty. Not surprisingly, an important aspect of the patterns is that they form stories.

Brain researchers such as Hobson have argued for decades that dream images are the product of intrinsic, random, cortical and subcortical activity during REM sleep and have concluded that the images have no significant meaning. If the present theory is true, however, the intrinsic chaotic randomness of the dreaming brain is what spawns the richness of meaning that has been noted in dreams since time immemorial.

Interestingly, although REM sleep identifies a specific pattern of activity in the brain, dreaming itself does not seem to be a specific state of consciousness (Combs and Krippner 1996; Goertzel 1996). Aside from the fact that certain dream activity evidently occurs during both non-REM and REM sleep, the creative psychological processes, especially processes amplified by the physiology of REM sleep, lead to the emergence of both a wealth of mind–body states during dreaming and a variety of states of consciousness. Observed evidence supports this view. Dream experiences range across a wide phenomenal landscape that includes episodes much like ordinary wakefulness and powerful visionary experiences, mystical states, full-blown flashbacks to previous psychedelic experiences, and shamanic journeys (Van de Castle 1994), which suggests that the dreaming mind is able to acquire the attractor basins of a wide range of states of consciousness and play them in undeniable fidelity. Thus, the dreaming mind is more the vehicle than the message, more the stage than the play.

REFERENCES

Basar, E., ed. 1990. *Chaos in Brain Function*. Berlin: Springer-Verlag.

Bower, G. H. 1981. Mood and memory. *American Psychologist* 36, 129–148.

Combs, A. 1995. Psychology, chaos, and the process nature of consciousness. In F. Abraham and A. Gilgen, eds., *Chaos Theory in Psychology*. Westport, CT: Greenwood.

Combs, A. 1996a. *The radiance of Being: Complexity, Chaos, and the Evolution of Consciousness*. New York: Paragon House.

Combs, A. 1996b. Consciousness: Chaotic and strangely attractive. In W. Sulis and A. Combs, eds., *Nonlinear Dynamics in Human Behavior*. London: World Scientific.

Combs, A. 1996. The dynamical mind: Process and the collective unconscious. *World Futures: The Journal of General Evolution* 48:127–140.

Combs, A., and S. Krippner. 1996. Jung and the evolution of consciousness. *Psychological Perspectives* 33:60–76.

Combs, A., M. Winkler, and C. Daley. 1994. A chaotic systems analysis of circadian rhythms in feeling states. *Psychological Record* 44:359–368.

Eysenck, M. W., and M. T. Keane. 1990. *Cognitive Psychology*. Hillsdale, NJ: Erlbaum.

Feinstein, D., and S. Krippner. 1988. *Personal Mythology*. Los Angeles: Jeremy P. Tarcher.

Flavell, J. H. 1963. *The Developmental Psychology of Jean Piaget*. New York: Van Nostrand.

Freeman, W. J. 1992. Tutorial in neurobiology: From single neurons to brain chaos. *International Journal of Bifurcation and Chaos* 2:451–482.

Goertzel, B. 1994. *Chaotic Logic: Language, Mind and Reality from the Perspective of Complex Systems Science*. New York: Plenum.

Goertzel, B. 1996. *Form Complexity to Creativity*. New York: Plenum.

Harvy, J. H., and A. L. Weber. 1990. *Interpersonal Accounts: A Social Psychological Perspective*. Cambridge: Blackwell.

Hobson, J. A. 1988. *The Dreaming Brain*. New York: Basic Books.

Hobson, J. A., and R. Stickgold. 1994. Dreaming: A neurocognitive approach. *Consciousness and Cognition* 3:1–15.

Jantsch, E. 1980. *The Self-Organizing Universe*. New York: Pergamon.

Kampis, G. 1991. *Self-Modifying Systems in Biology and Cognitive Science*. New York: Pergamon.

Laszlo, E. 1972. *Introduction to Systems Philosophy: Toward a new Paradigm of Contemporary Thought*. New York: Gordon & Breach.

Laszlo, E. 1987. *Evolution: The Grand Synthesis*. Boston: Shambhala.

Maturana, H. R., and F. J. Varela. 1975. *Autopoietic Systems*. Urbana, IL: Biological Computer Laboratory, University of Ilinois.

Maturana, H. R., and F. J. Varela. 1987. *The Tree of Knowledge: the Biological Roots of Human Understanding*. Boston: Shambhala.

Pribram, K. H., ed. 1995. *Proceedings of the Second Appalachian Conference on Behavioral Neurodynamics; Origins: Brain and Self-Organization*. Hillsdale, NJ: Erlbaum.

Rapp. E. E., T. R. Bashore, I. D. Zimmerman, J. M. Martinerie, A. M. Albano, and A. I. Mees. 1990. Dynamical characterization of brain electrical activity. In S. Krasner, ed., *The Ubiquity of Chaos*. Washington, DC: American Association for the Advancement of Science, pp. 10–22.

Rapp, P. 1993. Chaos in the neurosciences: Cautionary tales from the frontier. *Biologist* 40(2):89–94.

Rescher, N. 1996. Process metaphysics: *An Introduction to Process Philosophy*. Albany: State University of New York Press.

Rossi, E. 1986. Altered states of consciousness in everyday life. In B. B. Wolman and M. Ullman, eds., *Handbook of Altered States of Consciousness*. New York: Van Nostrand Reinhold, pp. 97–132.

Rossi, E. 1996. *The Symptom Path to Enlightenment*. Palisades, CA: Palisades Gateway.

Schwalbe, M. L. 1991. The autogenesis of the self. *Journal of the Theory of Social Behavior.* 21(3):269–295.

Skarda, C. A., and W. J. Freeman. 1987. How brains make chaos in order to make sense of the world. *Behavioral and Brain Sciences* 10:161–195.

Tart, C. T. 1975. *States of Consciousness*. New York: E. P. Dutton.

Van de Castle, R. 1994. *Our Dreaming Mind*. New York: Ballantine.

Winkler, M., and A. Combs. 1993, July. *A Chaotic Systems Analysis of Individual Differences in Affect*. Paper presented at the 24th Interamerican Congress of Psychology, Santiago, Chile.

Zubek, J. P. 1969. *Sensory Deprivation: Fifteen Years of Research*. New York: Appleton-Century-Crofts.

42 Dreaming and Consciousness

Stephen LaBerge

Dreaming is commonly considered an unconscious mental process. However, if we use the criterion of *reportability* to distinguish unconscious from conscious processes, we must accept that dreams are conscious experiences. Indeed, they are the purest instances of consciousness we experience on a daily basis.

From the biological perspective, the basic task of an organism's brain is to predict the results of the organism's actions and control those actions to achieve optimal outcomes (in terms of survival and reproduction). To accomplish this task the brain internally "models" the world. The waking brain bases the features of its world model primarily on current information received from the senses and secondarily on expectations derived from past experience.

In contrast, the sleeping brain acquires little information from the senses. Therefore, in sleep, the primary sources of information available to the brain are past experience and the current state of the organism—memories, expectations, fears, desires, and so on. I believe dreams result from brains using internal information to create a simulation of the world in a manner directly parallel to the process of waking perception minus sensory input. Thus, by this theory, dreaming results from the same perceptual and mental processes used to comprehend the world when awake.

To understand dreaming we need to understand perception and vice versa. In short, dreaming can be viewed as the special case of perception without the constraints of external sensory input. Conversely, perception can be viewed as the special case of dreaming constrained by sensory input (LaBerge 1985; LaBerge and Rheingold 1990; Llinas and Pare 1991) Whichever way one looks at it, understanding dreaming is central to understanding consciousness.

Therefore, theories of consciousness that do not account for dreaming must be regarded as incomplete, and theories that are contradicted by the findings of phenomenological and psychophysiological studies on dreaming must be incorrect. For example, the behaviorist assumption that "the brain is stimulated always and only from the outside by a sense organ process" (Watson 1928) cannot explain dreams, nor can the assumption that consciousness is the direct or exclusive product of sensory input. Rather, the perceptual experiences of consciousness appear to arise from a complex and unconscious process of inference. This constructive process utilizes a variety of factors beyond simple sensory input, and these fall into two major classes: expectations and motivations.

Perception (what we see, hear, feel, etc.) depends to a great extent on expectation because the sensory information available in the world is often ambiguous. For example, suppose you see something round and try to guess what it is. If I were to tell you that the round thing is in a tree, what would it likely be? Or if it were in the middle of a tennis court? In a certain sense, what we perceive is what we most expect, consistent with sensory information. There are many sources of expectation: context, past, and especially, recent experience, familiarity, emotional states, and personality.

There are also many different kinds of motivation, the second class of internal processes bearing a strong influence on perception, ranging from the most basic drives such as hunger, thirst, and sex to psychological needs such as affection, recognition, and self-esteem to higher motives such as altruism and perhaps Maslow's self-actualization. It is likely that all of these levels of motivation can affect perceptual processes.

The influence of the lower levels of motivation is easiest to study. In one experiment in which school children were shown ambiguous figures before and after meals, the children were twice as likely to interpret the figures as referring to food when they were hungry than they were after they had eaten. As the proverb says, "What bread looks like depends upon whether you are hungry or not."

Strong emotions also motivate behavior and influence perception. For instance, it is well known that angry people are ready to see others as hostile; the fearful tend to see what they fear, even if it means mistaking a bush for a bear; and, on a more positive note, lovers tend to see their beloved mistakenly.

If perception involves analyzing and evaluating sensory information, the brain must use some kind of matching process to identify what is perceived. Suppose, for example, you are presented with an ambiguous pattern of light. What are you seeing? Is it a bush or a bear? A rock or a pear? To identify any of these things, you must already have mental models of bushes, bears, rocks, pears, or whatever, to which you can compare the information from your senses. The best match is what you see. In a highly ambiguous case, ample room exists for the influence of expectations and motivations.

The same process applies to more abstract levels of the mind, such as language, reasoning, and memory. For example, you cannot judge whether, in a given situation, someone has spoken tactfully or truthfully unless you have mental models of tact and truth. These mental models, also known as schemas, frames, or scripts, comprise the building blocks of perception and thought.

New schemas are created by adapting or combining old schemas, some of which may be inherited genetically. Schemas capture essential regularities about how the world has worked in the past and how we assume it will work in the future. In David Rumelhart's words (Goleman 1985), a schema is a kind of informal, private unarticulated theory about the nature of events, objects, or situations which we face. The total set of schemas we have available for interpreting our world in a sense constitutes our private theory of the nature of reality (p.76).

Schemas help organize experience by grouping together typical sets of features or attributes of objects, people, or situations. These sets of assumptions allow us to go beyond the partial information available to our senses and perceive a whole. We are not usually conscious of the schemas we are employing, for example, the particular rules we are following in a given social situation. We simply perceive what kind of situation we are in (formal, friendly, intimate, business meeting, church, competitive sport, cinema or theater, etc.) and act accordingly.

To this point, I have discussed schemas in purely psychological terms, but schemas are presumably embodied in the brain by networks of neurons. Current theory favors the idea that the extent to which a schema is active in organizing current experience is determined by the degree of activity in its respective neural network.

DREAMING AND PERCEPTION

Waking and dreaming experiences are created by the same mechanism: the brain's world-modeling function. Its output is our perception. To understand how dreaming affects the contents of our consciousness, first consider how sleep modifies the process of perception. During rapid eye movement (REM) sleep, sensory input from both the outside world and body movement are suppressed, but the entire brain, including the areas devoted to perception, is highly active. As a result of neural activation, certain schemas become activated above their perceptual thresholds. The schemas enter consciousness and cause the dreamer to see, feel, hear, and experience things not present in the external environment.

Ordinarily, if one were to perceive something not really there, contradictory sensory input would rapidly correct the mistaken impression. Why does the same thing not happen during dreaming? The answer is that there is little or no sensory input from the outside world available to the brain for correcting such mistakes.

Experience in dreams is determined by which schemas are activated above the threshold for consciousness. But what determines which schemas are activated? I believe it is the same processes that influence waking perception: expectation and motivation.

Expectation shows itself in dreams in many ways. Dream worlds tend to resemble past worlds we have experienced because they are what we have learned to expect. Thus, dream worlds are almost always equipped with gravity, space, time, and air. Personal interests, preoccupations, and concerns influence dreaming as they do waking perception and bias what is perceived and how it is interpreted.

Likewise, recent experience (Freud's "day-residue") influences dreaming in a manner similar to its influence on waking perception. However, as Gordon Globus has emphasized (Globus 1987), this does not mean that dreams are a patchwork made solely of past experiences. It is just as easy to dream things we have never experienced as it is to imagine them. (Think of a purple winged rabbit.)

Motivation and emotions strongly influence waking perception, and we would expect an even stronger effect in dreams, which lack grounding by external influence. In particular, one is likely to dream about what one desires—wish-fulfillment dreams. Suppose, for example, that you have gone to bed without supper. Like the hungry school children who were likely to interpret ambiguous figures as food, you are likely to dream about food. Freud was so impressed by the prevalence of wish-fulfillment in dreams that he made it the cornerstone of his entire theory of dreams (Freud 1900). According to Freud, *every* dream is the fulfillment of a wish. However, this view appears to overstate the case—nightmares are an obvious counterexample.

Indeed, just as fear makes a person more "jumpy," that is, ready to interpret ambiguous stimuli as danger while awake, fear has the same effect in dreams. This is probably why people dream about unpleasant and even horrible situations—not, as Freud believed, because people are masochistic and unconsciously wish to be frightened, but because they are afraid of certain events, and therefore, in a sense expect that the events may happen. One cannot be afraid of ghosts if one does not believe in ghosts.

By this account, one might expect that dreams would be sequences of disconnected images, ideas, feelings, and sensations, rather than the intricately detailed and dramatic story-like sequences that they often are. However, I believe that schema activation can also account for the complexity and meaningfulness of dreams. Thus, a few general-purpose schemas can generate a vast amount of meaningful detail—give a schema a dot, and it sees a fly; give a sleeping brain an activated schema or two and it makes a dream.

Some dreams have plots as coherent, funny, dramatic, and profound as the best stories, myths, and plays. After one awakens from such dreams, it sometimes seems as if the significance of characters or events set up early in the dream became clear only in the final climactic denouement; one is left with the impression of a complete dream plot worked out in advance.

It is probably this sort of dream that gives people the notion that their unconscious minds have put together a "dream film" with a message for their conscious minds to watch and interpret. However, I think a simpler explanation is that a story schema has been activated continuously throughout the dream.

The story, or narrative schema, is a basic and universally understood part of our culture. Stories most typically occur as sequences of episodes, which are typically divided into three parts: the exposition, the complication, and the resolution. The exposition introduces the characters and settings, who typically then encounter a complication or problem that is finally resolved at the end of the story.

Carl Jung described the dream as being like a drama in three acts. Story schemas can prespecify the sequences of events, the timing of character introductions, the patterns of dramatic tension and release, the surprise endings, and so on. Reifying the unconscious mind in the role of "dream director" is not necessary.

The view of dreams as world models is far from the traditional notion of dreams as messages from the gods or from the unconscious mind. (I have presented arguments against the "letters-to-yourself" view of dreams elsewhere.) Nonetheless, the interpretation of dreams can be very revealing of personality and can be a rewarding, valuable practice. For instance, think about the inkblot projection test. Why does what people see in inkblots tell something about the viewers? The answer is because their interpretations inform us about their personal interests, concerns, experiences, preoccupations and personality. Dreams contain much more personal information than do inkblots because the images in them are created by us, from the contents of our minds. Dreams may not be messages, but they are our own most intimately personal creations; they are unmistakably colored by who and what we are and by whom we would become.

Whether conscious or preconscious, expectations and assumptions about what dreams are like determine to a remarkable extent the precise form dreams take. This view applies in much the same way to waking life. Consider the myth of the four-minute mile. For many years it was believed impossible to run that fast—until someone did it—and the impossible became possible. Almost immediately, many others were able to do the same. It is easy to see why assumptions play a more important role during dreaming than during waking perception. In the physical world actual limitations are built into our bodies, not to mention the constraints of the laws of physics.

SIMILARITIES AND DIFFERENCES IN DREAMING AND WAKING EXPERIENCES

Dreaming experience is commonly viewed as qualitatively distinct from waking experience. Dreams are often believed to be characterized by lack of reflection and inability to act deliberately and with intention (Rechtschaffen 1978). However, this view has not been based on equivalent measurements of waking and dreaming state experiences. To achieve equivalence it is necessary to evaluate waking experience retrospectively, in the same way that dreams are evaluated.

Lynne Levitan, Tracey Kahan, and I recently conducted such a study examining cognition in dreaming and waking by sampling recall of recent experience from both conditions and collecting responses to questions pertaining to thought processes during the period recalled (LaBerge, Kahan, and Levitan 1995). Subjects were either undergraduates or from a high-dream-interest group. Each of 167 subjects contributed one waking and one dreaming sample.

Recent dream experience was sampled by having the subject record in writing as much detail as possible about the last (approximately) 15 minutes of the dream occurring just before awakening. Recent waking experience was sampled in a similar way by having the subjects record, at an arbitrary time in the day, as much detail as possible about the experiences of the last (approximately) 15 minutes of waking. After recording each sample, the subjects answered a series of questions about the experience described to assess whether they had engaged in certain cognitive and other activities such as deliberate choice between alternatives, reflection. sudden distraction of attention, focused intention, public self-consciousness, emotion, private self-consciousness, difficulty with achieving goals, task-irrelevant thought, and unusual action or experience. For each activity that subjects reported recalling, an example was requested for verification.

Differences appeared between waking and dreaming samples for several variables. For deliberate choice, 49 percent of subjects reported experiences from dreams and 74 percent of subjects reported experiences from wakefulness; for public self-consciousness, 41 percent of subjects reported experiences from dreams and 30 percent reported experiences from wakefulness; for emotion, 86 percent reported experiences from dreams and 74 percent reported experiences from wakefulness. Of note, significant differences between dreaming and waking were not evident for other cognitive activities, and none of the measured cognitive functions were absent or rare in dreams. Typically, waking and dreaming experiences have much in common, with dreams characterized by somewhat more emotionality and somewhat less choice.

However, less typical examples reveal a wider range of qualities of consciousness in dreaming than in the normal waking state. For example, at one end of the spectrum, dreams at times exhibit cognitive and perceptual errors similar to those produced by brain damage. However, one man's brain damage may be another's creativity, and dream bizarreness also shows the creative recombinatory potential of the dreaming brain (Hunt 1989). Moreover, as illustrated by lucid dreams, dreaming consciousness can also be as volitional and rational as that of waking consciousness.

REFLECTIVE CONSCIOUSNESS DURING REM SLEEP

Typically, we are not explicitly aware of the fact that we are dreaming while we are dreaming, but at times a remarkable exception occurs, and we become reflective enough to become conscious that we are dreaming. During such "lucid" dreams, it is possible to freely remember the circumstances of waking life, to think clearly, and to act deliberately on reflection or in accordance with plans decided upon before sleep while simultaneously experiencing a dream world that seems vividly real (LaBerge 1985; LaBerge 1990).

Although accounts of lucid dreaming exist at least as far back as Aristotle, until recently, dream reports of this sort were received with considerable skepticism. Because the concept of conscious sleep can seem so paradoxical to certain ways of thinking, some philosophers have written books claiming to show that lucid dreaming is an impossible absurdity (Malcolm 1959). In the absence of objective proof, sleep researchers doubted that the dreaming brain was capable of such a high degree of mental functioning and consciousness.

A new technique involving eye-movement signals, developed independently by researchers in the United States and in England in the late 1970s, proved the reality of lucid dreaming (Hearne 1978; LaBerge 1980). The technique was based on earlier studies (Roffwarg, Dement, Muzio, and Fisher, 1962) that found that the directions of eye movements recorded during REM sleep sometimes exactly corresponded to the directions in which subjects reported they had been looking in their dreams. I reasoned that if lucid dreamers could, in fact, act volitionally, they should be able to prove it by making a prearranged eye movement signal marking the exact time they became lucid. Using this approach, my colleagues and I at Stanford verified reports of lucid dreams from five subjects by eye-movement signals (LaBerge 1980; LaBerge, Nagel, Dement, and Zarcone 1981). All the signals (and, therefore, the lucid dreams) had occurred during uninterrupted REM sleep. This result has been replicated in a number of laboratories (Dane 1984; Fenwick et al., 1984; Ogilvie, et al. 1982).

LUCID DREAMING TO STUDY CONSCIOUSNESS

The eye-movement signaling experiment illustrates an important approach to the study of consciousness. The attempt to apply rigorous scientific methodology to the study of phenomena such as mental imagery, hallucinations, dreaming, and conscious processes in general faces a major challenge: The most direct account available of the private events occurring in a person's mind is that individual's subjective report. However, subjective reports are difficult to verify objectively, and introspection is far from being an unbiased or direct process of observation.

Two strategies are likely to increase the reliability of subjective reports: (1) the use of highly trained subjects (in the context of dream research, this is best achieved with lucid dreamers) who are skillful reporters of consciousness; (2) the use of a psychophysiological approach to provide validation of subjective reports by correlating the reports with physiological measures (Stoyva and Kamiya 1968).

Using these approaches in a series of studies (summarized below), my colleagues and I discovered that various dreamed experiences (e.g., time estimation, breathing, singing, counting, and sexual activity) produce effects on the dreamer's brain (and to a lesser extent, on the body) remarkably similar to the physiological effects that are produced by actual experiences of the corresponding events when the subject is awake.

We found a very high degree of correlation between the direction of gaze shift reported in lucid dreams and the corresponding polygraphically recorded eye movements. Thus, we now make routine use of employing eye

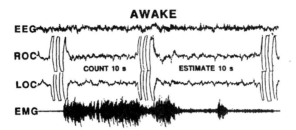

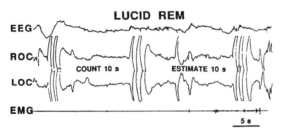

Figure 42.1 Estimation of 10-sec time duration in one subject while awake (top) and lucid dreaming (bottom). EEG, electroencephalogram; ROC, right outer canthus; LOC, left outer canthus; EMG, electromyogram; REM, rapid eye movement.

movements as markers in all our experiments (LaBerge 1985; LaBerge, Nagel, Dement, and Zarcone 1981). For example, to answer the question of how long dreams last we asked lucid dreamers to estimate various intervals of time while dreaming. The dreamers marked the beginning and end of estimated dream-time intervals with eye-movement signals, which allowed comparison of subjective dream time with objective time (Figure 42.1). In each case, the intervals of time estimated during the lucid dreams were very close in length to actual elapsed time (LaBerge 1985; LaBerge, Nagel, Dement, and Zarcone 1981).

In another experiment, we recorded the physiology of three lucid dreamers who had been asked either to breathe rapidly or to hold their breath in their lucid dreams and mark the interval of altered respiration with eye-movement signals. The subjects reported successfully carrying out the agreed-on tasks nine times. In each case, a judge was able to correctly predict from the physiological records which of the two breathing patterns had been executed (LaBerge and Dement 1982b).

In a study of task-dependent lateralization of electroencephalographic activity during dreaming, we recorded from four subjects' right and left temporal locations while they sang and counted in their lucid dreams. The results indicated that in each subject the right hemisphere was more activated than the left during singing; the reverse was true during counting. The shifts were similar to those during actual singing and counting (LaBerge and Dement 1982a).

A pilot study with two lucid dreamers (one man and one woman) who reported experiencing sexual arousal and orgasm in lucid dreams revealed patterns of physiological activity during dream sex closely resembling patterns accompanying corresponding experiences in the waking state (LaBerge, Greenleaf, and Kedzierski 1983).

All the studies support the conclusion that during REM dreaming, the events we consciously experience (or seem to) are the results of patterns of central nervous system activity that produce effects on the autonomic nervous system and the body that are to some extent modified by the specific conditions of active sleep but are still homomorphic to the effects that would occur if we had actually experienced the corresponding events while awake. This explains, in part, why we regularly mistake dreams for reality: To the functional systems of neuronal activity that construct the experiential world model of our consciousness, dreaming of perceiving or doing something is equivalent to actually perceiving or doing it (LaBerge 1990).

REFERENCES

Dane, J. 1984. An empirical evaluation of two techniques for lucid dream induction. Unpublished Ph.D. dissertation, Georgia State University.

Fenwick, P., M. Schatzman, A. Worsley, J. Adams, S. Stone, and A. Baker. 1984. Lucid dreaming: Correspondence between dreamed and actual events in one subject during REM sleep. *Biological Psychology* 18:243–252.

Freud, S. 1900. *The Interpretation of Dreams*. Reprinted (1965). New York: Avon.

Globus, G. 1987. *Dream Life, Wake Life*. Albany: State University of New York Press.

Goleman, D. 1985. *Vital Lies, Simple Truths*. New York: Simon & Schuster.

Hearne, K. M. T. 1978. Lucid dreams: An electrophysiological and psychological study. Unpublished Ph.D. dissertation, University of Liverpool.

Hunt, H. T. 1989. *The Multiplicity of Dreams*. New Haven: Yale University Press.

LaBerge, S. 1980. Lucid dreaming: An exploratory study of consciousness during sleep. Unpublished Ph.D. dissertation, Stanford University.

LaBerge, S. 1985. *Lucid Dreaming*. Los Angeles: J. P. Tarcher.

LaBerge, S. 1990. Lucid dreaming: Psychophysiological studies of consciousness during REM sleep. In R. R. Bootzin, J. F. Kihlstrom, and D. L. Schacter, eds., *Sleep and Cognition* Washington, D. C: American Psychological Association, pp. 109–126.

LaBerge, S., and W. Dement. 1982a. Lateralization of alpha activity for dreamed singing and counting during REM sleep. *Psychophysiology* 19:331–332.

LaBerge, S., and W. Dement. 1982b. Voluntary control of respiration during REM sleep. *Sleep Research* 11:107.

LaBerge, S., W. Greenleaf, and B. Kedzierski. 1983. Physiological responses to dreamed sexual activity during lucid REM sleep. *Psychophysiology* 20:454–455.

LaBerge, S., T. Kahan, and L. Levitan. 1995. Cognition in dreaming and waking. *Sleep Research* 24A:239.

LaBerge, S., L. Nagel, W. C. Dement, and V. Zarcone. 1981. Lucid dreaming verified by volitional communication during REM sleep. *Perceptual and Motor Skills* 52:727–732.

LaBerge, S., and H. Rheingold. 1990. *Exploring the World of Lucid Dreaming*. New York: Ballantine.

Llinas, R., and D. Pare. 1991. Of dreaming and wakefulness. *Neuroscience* 44:521–535.

Malcolm, N. 1959. *Dreaming*. London: Routledge.

Ogilvie, R., H. Hunt, P. D. Tyson, M. L. Lucescu, and D. B. Jeakins. 1982. Lucid dreaming and alpha activity: A preliminary report. *Perceptual and Motor Skills* 55:795–808.

Rechtschaffen, A. 1978. The single-mindedness and isolation of dreams. *Sleep* 1:97–109.

Roffwarg, H., W. C. Dement, J. Muzio, and C. Fisher. 1962. Dream imagery: Relationship to rapid eye movements of sleep. *Archives of General Psychiatry* 7:235–238.

Stoyva, J., and J. Kamiya. 1968. Electrophysiological studies of dreaming as the prototype of a new strategy in the study of consciousness. *Psychological Review* 75:192–205.

Watson, J. 1928. *The Ways of Behaviorism*. New York: Harper.

43 Representational Momentum and Other Displacements in Memory as Evidence for Nonconscious Knowledge of Physical Principles

Timothy L. Hubbard

The remembered position of a stimulus is often displaced from the actual position of that stimulus in ways consistent with the operation of invariant physical principles; in other words, the representational system acts as if the internal mental model of the external physical world is subject to the same invariant physical principles as the external physical world. For example, the remembered position of a horizontally moving target is usually displaced in front of and below the actual position of the target, and this pattern is consistent with influences of momentum and gravitational attraction on such a target. Even though mental representations per se are not similarly influenced by such physical forces (e.g., the mental representation of a falling object is not itself falling), mental representations nonetheless often respond as if they are similarly influenced by physical forces. The resultant displacements in spatial representation appear to reflect nonconscious or implicit knowledge of environmentally invariant physical principles that has been incorporated into the functional architecture of the representational system.

TYPES OF DISPLACEMENT

Representational Momentum

If an observer views a moving target, memory for the final position of that target is usually displaced forward in the direction of motion (Figure 43.1); faster target velocities usually produce larger displacements (Hubbard 1995b). Freyd and Finke (1984) and Finke, Freyd, and Shyi (1986) referred to this displacement as *representational momentum*. They suggested it resulted from an internalization of the principles of physical momentum by the representational system; in other words, much as a moving physical object cannot be immediately halted because of its momentum, the mental representation of that motion cannot be immediately halted because of an analogous momentum within the representational system. More recently, Freyd (1987, 1993) suggested that representational momentum reflects spatiotemporal coherence between the represented and representing worlds, and Hubbard (1995b) suggested that representational momentum (and related displacements) reflects internalization of environmentally invariant physical principles into the representational system.

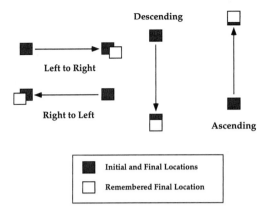

Figure 43.1 The relationship between actual and remembered final location of horizontally and vertically moving targets. Targets move smoothly from initial to final location. After targets vanish, observers indicate remembered final location by positioning a computer mouse. Representational momentum is shown by the forward displacement of remembered location; representational gravity is shown by the downward displacement in remembered location of horizontally moving targets and by the larger forward displacement for descending motion than for ascending motion. Arrows indicate direction of motion. (Adapted from Hubbard and Bharucha 1988; Hubbard 1990).

Representational Gravity

Hubbard and Bharucha (1988) and Hubbard (1990) measured displacement in remembered location along both the axis aligned with motion and the axis orthogonal to motion for targets that moved either horizontally or vertically. The direction of target motion influenced displacement along the axis of motion; horizontally moving targets produced greater representational momentum than did vertically moving targets, and descending targets produced greater representational momentum that did ascending targets. In addition, memory for horizontally moving targets was displaced downward below the axis of motion (see Figure 43.1). Larger forward displacements for descending motion and downward displacements for horizontally moving targets are consistent with the effects of gravity on a moving target (i.e., descending targets accelerate, ascending targets decelerate, and unpowered horizontally moving targets fall along a parabola). Thus, these data appear to demonstrate influences of *representational gravity*. The existence of representational gravity is also consistent with the hypothesis that observers internalize the effects of mass as effects of weight (Hubbard 1995b, in press).

Representational Friction

Hubbard (1995a) presented horizontally moving targets in isolation; crashing through a stationary barrier; sliding along a single, larger stationary surface; or sliding between two larger stationary surfaces. When targets crashed through a barrier, forward displacement decreased. When targets slid across

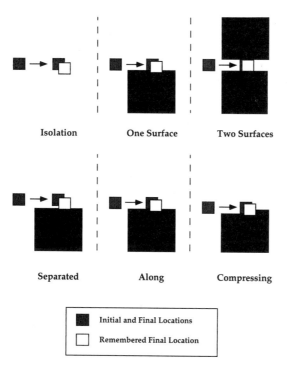

Isolation   One Surface   Two Surfaces

Separated   Along   Compressing

Initial and Final Locations

Remembered Final Location

Figure 43.2 The top panel illustrates effects of implied friction on displacement for targets presented in isolation, sliding along one surface, or sliding between two surfaces. The bottom panel illustrates effects of implied friction for targets separated from a surface, sliding along a surface, or compressing a surface. Targets move smoothly from initial to final location, and after targets and surfaces simultaneously vanish, observers indicate remembered final location by positioning a computer mouse. Representational friction is shown by decreases in the forward displacement with increases in the number of surfaces contacted by the target and implied contact with (and pressure on) a surface. Arrows indicate direction of motion. (Adapted from Hubbard 1995a).

one or two larger stationary surfaces, forward displacement decreased as the number of surfaces increased (Figure 43.2, top). When targets moved along a surface and compressed the surface behind them, forward displacement decreased even more (Figure 43.2, bottom). Given that increases in physical friction produce decreases in physical momentum, the patterns are consistent with the existence of *representational friction*. Of importance, target velocity within the experiments remained constant within each trial, but observers responded as if targets encountering more implied friction decelerated more than targets encountering less implied friction. Such decreases in forward displacement in the absence of decreases in actual velocity demonstrate the robustness of representational friction.

The existence of representational friction and an interaction of representational friction and representational gravity may also account for Bertamini's (1993) findings regarding memory for the location of a stationary circular target placed midway along an inclined plane. When the slope of the inclined plane was relatively shallow, memory for the target was not displaced along the inclined plane; when the slope of the inclined plane was relatively steep, memory for the target was displaced downward along the inclined plane. Just as a physical object becomes more likely to slide down an inclined plane as the slope of the plane increases (and effects of gravity become stronger than effects of friction), memory for an object on an inclined plane is also more likely to be displaced down the inclined plane as the slope of the plane increases (and effects of representational gravity become stronger than effects of representational friction).

Representational Centripetal Force

Hubbard (1996) presented targets moving along circular orbits. Displacement for remembered location was measured along both the axis aligned with the tangent and the axis aligned with the radius. Memory for the target was displaced forward and inward (Figure 43.3), and the magnitude of displacement (in pixels) increased with increases in angular velocity and increases in radius length. Because circular motion is specified by forward velocity along the tangent and by inward centripetal acceleration toward the focus of the orbit, this pattern is consistent with the existence of both repre-

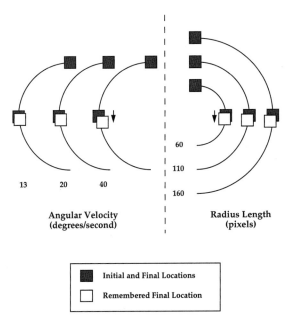

Angular Velocity
(degrees/second)

Radius Length
(pixels)

Initial and Final Locations

Remembered Final Location

Figure 43.3 The left panel illustrates effects of angular velocity on representational momentum and representational centripetal force for targets orbiting in a counterclockwise direction. The right panel illustrates effects of radius length on representational momentum and representational centripetal force for targets orbiting in a clockwise direction. Targets move smoothly from initial to final location. After targets vanish, observers indicate remembered location by positioning a computer mouse. Representational friction and representational centripetal force are shown by the forward and inward displacements. Arcs and arrows indicate path and direction of motion. (Adapted from Hubbard 1996).

sentational momentum and *representational centripetal force*. Freyd and Jones (1994) presented targets that traveled through a spiral tube and followed either a spiral, curvilinear, or straight path after exiting the tube. Displacement along the path of motion was largest along the spiral path and smallest along the straight path. Although Freyd and Jones did not propose such an explanation, their data are also consistent with an interaction of representational momentum and representational centripetal force.

THE ENVIRONMENTAL INVARIANTS HYPOTHESIS

The results of numerous studies of displacement are consistent with the *environmental invariants hypothesis*, which states that laws specifying environmentally invariant physical principles (e.g., momentum, gravitational attraction, friction, centripetal force) have become incorporated into our representational system (Hubbard 1995b). In other words, our representational system appears to respond as if mental representations were subject to the same physical principles that influence physical objects.[1] Of course, mental representations of physical objects would not actually be displaced within the three-dimensional coordinates of the brain; rather, the "as if" nature of displacement is suggestive of a second-order isomorphism between mental representations and the physical world in which functional properties of the physical world are recreated within mental representations. Much as visual imagery has been suggested to reflect a second-order isomorphism between physical objects and visual images of those objects (Shepard and Chipman 1970), incorporated invariants might also reflect a second-order isomorphism between physical and mental realms.

Although previous investigators have discussed possible roles of environmental invariants in perceptual or cognitive processing, the environmental invariants hypothesis goes beyond previous theories. For example, the environmental invariants hypothesis goes beyond Gibson (1979) in proposing that our representational system has been shaped by the influence of environmentally invariant physical principles, beyond Shepard (1984, 1994) in proposing that information regarding forces (as well as information regarding geometry and kinematics) has been incorporated into our representational system, and beyond Freyd (1987, 1993) in broadening the reach of spatiotemporal coherence to include all principles invariant across human experience. Finally, the environmental invariants hypothesis goes beyond previous theories in proposing that displacement in spatial memory is also influenced by noninvariant factors (e.g., observers' expectations, memory averaging) (Hubbard 1995b).

One consequence of the incorporation of environmentally invariant physical principles into the representational system is that memory for spatial position is displaced in ways consistent with those principles. In essence, mental representation does not portray the world-as-it-is-right-now, but rather mental representation portrays an extrapolated world-as-it-soon-will-be. Simple and binary choice reaction time in humans is on the order of a few hundred milliseconds, a processing time remarkably consistent with Freyd and Johnson's (1987) finding that representational momentum peaks after a few hundred milliseconds and then declines. If the response to a stimulus is to be maximally effective, the response should be tailored to the stimulus as that stimulus will be at the moment of response, not as the stimulus was when the decision-and-response process began. Thus, an extrapolation consistent with environmentally invariant principles could potentially offer a selective or survival advantage. The human representational system may have been "shaped" or "biologically prepared" to incorporate such environmentally invariant principles and extrapolate spatial position accordingly.

The environmental invariants hypothesis suggests that veridical knowledge of physical principles has been incorporated into the representational system; however, studies in so-called "naive physics" initially appear to challenge this notion. For example, when untutored observers predict the path of a ball ejected from a spiral tube, many observers predict a trajectory in which the ball continues to follow a curved path after exiting the tube, but the ball would actually follow a straight path after exiting the tube. McCloskey and Kohl (1983) and McCloskey (1983) interpreted these results as suggesting that untutored observers do not have veridical knowledge of physical principles and might instead believe the tube imparted a "curvilinear impetus" to the ball. However, Hubbard (1996) suggested the choice of an inward trajectory might reflect the averaging of a constant forward representational momentum and a gradually diminishing inward representational centripetal force.[2] Thus, the pattern typically interpreted as suggesting that untutored observers do not have veridical physical knowledge might actually reflect an interaction of two accurately internalized physical principles.

IMPLICATIONS FOR THE STUDY OF CONSCIOUSNESS

The environmental invariants hypothesis suggests that humans (and, on the basis of phylogenetic similarity, other organisms) extrapolate effects of physical principles on physical stimuli and that this extrapolation results in the displacement of spatial representation. An organism that could anticipate or extrapolate effects of physical principles on stimuli (e.g., predator or prey) would presumably have a selective advantage. To maximize this advantage, the results of such extrapolation should be available rapidly and without use of limited attentional resources; that is, extrapolation should occur automatically. This automaticity could best be accomplished by nonconscious processes (Posner and Snyder 1974); indeed, conscious access to extrapolations would probably interfere with the extrapolation process and thereby make extrapolation less adaptive. Thus, the extrapolations that produce displacement in spatial representation may result from nonconscious knowledge of environmentally invariant physical principles.

For the possession of nonconscious knowledge of physical principles to be maximally adaptive, the organism would need a strategy for coping with cases in which a stimulus did not behave as initially expected. If a stimulus did not behave in accordance with environmentally invariant physical principles, displacement could lead to errors in perception that would not be advantageous. A mismatch between an automatically extrapolated position and a subsequent perceptually sampled position could evoke more effortful conscious processing. Thus, one possible function of consciousness is to compensate for errors produced by nonconscious extrapolation when a stimulus does not behave as extrapolated (e.g., prey that changes its direction of movement). Such correction would presumably be less effortful than if conscious processing were used continually. A second, and related, possible function of consciousness is to prime particular representational pathways corresponding to the most likely pathways suggested by explicit knowledge of a target's characteristics and expectations regarding the target's future behavior.

Displacement does not result from purely implicit or nonconscious processes because the direction and magnitude of displacement may be modified by conscious expectations regarding the stimulus (Hubbard 1994, 1995b). However, displacement does not result from purely explicit or conscious processes because representational momentum is not eliminated by error feedback (Freyd 1987). Therefore, spatial representation may be composed of (1) conscious and explicit knowledge regarding the stimulus and (2) nonconscious and implicit knowledge regarding environmentally invariant physical principles. This conclusion is consistent with findings that the magnitude of representational momentum and observers' explicit physical knowledge are uncorrelated (Freyd and Jones 1994) and with claims that only some aspects of displacement are modular or cognitively impenetrable (Hubbard 1995b). Displacement may thus provide a paradigm case of an interaction between conscious and nonconscious knowledge, and adaptation of the displacement paradigm may be helpful in dissociating conscious and nonconscious cognition in other domains.

NOTES

1. The claim that metal representations respond "as if" influenced by physical forces should not be taken as suggestive of dualism; mental representations are created within the brain, and the brain is a physical device subject to physical laws. Rather, the point is more subtle: The nature of representation (both mental and nonmental) is such that factors influencing a given object need not similarly influence a representation or be literally present within a representation (e.g., a videotape depiction of a moving physical target does not experience the same momentum as the actual physical target). Thus, findings that mental representations respond as if influenced by physical forces reveals something interesting about mental representation.

2. Such averaging would occur only in observers relying on perceptual knowledge (e.g., visualization) and would not occur in observers relying on conceptual or semantic knowledge.

REFERENCES

Bertamini, M. 1993. Memory for position and dynamic representations. *Memory and Cognition* 21:449–457.

Finke, R. A., J. J., Freyd, and G. C. W. Shyi. 1986. Implied velocity and acceleration induce transformations of visual memory. *Journal of Experimental Psychology: General* 115:175–188.

Freyd, J. J. 1987. Dynamic mental representations. *Psychological Review* 94:427–438.

Freyd, J. J. 1993. Five hunches about perceptual processes and dynamic representations. In D. Meyer and S. Kornblum, eds., *Attention and Performance XIV: Synergies in Experimental Psychology, Artificial Intelligence, and Cognitive Neuroscience.* Cambridge: MIT Press, pp. 99–119.

Freyd, J. J., and R. A. Finke. 1984. Representational momentum. *Journal of Experimental Psychology: Learning, Memory, and Cognition* 10:126–132.

Freyd, J. J., and J. Q. Johnson. 1987. Probing the time course of representational momentum. *Journal of Experimental Psychology: Learning, Memory, and Cognition* 13:259–269.

Freyd, J. J., and K. T. Jones. 1994. Representational momentum for a spiral path. *Journal of Experimental Psychology: Learning, Memory, and Cognition* 20:968–976.

Gibson, J. J. 1979. *The Ecological Approach to Visual Perception.* Boston: Houghton Mifflin.

Hubbard, T. L. 1990. Cognitive representation of linear motion: Possible direction and gravity effects in judged displacement. *Memory and Cognition* 18:299–309.

Hubbard, T. L. 1994. Judged displacement: A modular process? *American Journal of Psychology* 107:359–373.

Hubbard, T. L. 1995a. Cognitive representation of motion: Evidence for friction and gravity analogues. *Journal of Experimental Psychology: Learning, Memory, and Cognition* 21:241–254.

Hubbard, T. L. 1995b. Environmental invariants in the representation of motion: Implied dynamics and representational momentum, gravity, friction, and centripetal force. *Psychonomic Bulletin and Review* 2:322–338.

Hubbard, T. L. 1996. Representational momentum, centripetal force, and curvilinear impetus. *Journal of Experimental Psychology: Learning, Memory, and Cognition* 22:1049–1060.

Hubbard, T. L. In press. Target size and displacement along the axis of implied gravitational attraction: Effects of implied weight and evidence of representational gravity. *Journal of Experimental Psychology: Learning, Memory, and Cognition.*

Hubbard, T. L., and J. J. Bharucha. 1988. Judged displacement in apparent vertical and horizontal motion. *Perception and Psychophysics* 44:211–221.

McCloskey, M. 1983. Naive theories of motion. In D. Gentner and A. L. Stevens, eds., *Mental Models.* Hillsdale, NJ: Erlbaum, pp. 299–324.

McCloskey, M., and D. Kohl. 1983. Naive physics: The curvilinear impetus principle and its role in interactions with moving objects. *Journal of Experimental Psychology: Learning, Memory, and Cognition* 9:146–156.

Posner, M. I., and C. R. R. Snyder. 1974. Attention and cognitive control. In R. L. Solso, ed., *Information Processing and Cognition: The Loyola Symposium.* Hillsdale, NJ: Erlbaum, pp. 55–85.

Shepard, R. N. 1984. Ecological constraints on internal representation: Resonant kinematics of perceiving, imaging, thinking, and dreaming. *Psychological Review* 91:417–447.

Shepard, R. N. 1994. Perceptual-cognitive universals as reflections of the world. *Psychonomic Bulletin and Review* 1:2–28.

Shepard, R. N. and S. Chipman. 1970. Second-order isomorphism of internal representations: Shapes of states. *Cognitive Psychology* 1:1–17.

44 Emotion and Consciousness: A Shotgun Marriage?

Daniel S. Levine

ARE EMOTIONS CONSCIOUSLY FELT?

Recall an aesthetic experience, such as a concert, that you found intensely pleasurable. When you were at the concert, in all probability you were focused on the music: what the different instruments or voices were doing, what effects they generated, and perhaps at times the expressions on the musicians' faces. During the time that you listened to the music, there may have been two minutes in which you said to yourself, "I'm really enjoying this!" Yet when you recall the experience, you do not say, "I enjoyed the concert for two minutes, and didn't feel anything for the other fifty-eight." Instead, you simply say, "I enjoyed the concert." Thus, although a considerable amount of conscious experience of emotions such as joy, fear, anger, disgust, and sadness exists, a one-to-one relationship between emotions and conscious states does not exist.

Joseph LeDoux, a neuroscientist who has done extensive research on the neural basis for emotions (especially fear), came to the same conclusion (LeDoux 1989; Rogan and LeDoux 1996). LeDoux saw emotions as amenable to the same set of methods that can be used to study other cognitive phenomena because, like all cognitive phenomena, emotions can be thought of in terms of computational processes. Specifically, Rogan and LeDoux (1996) stated:

at least some emotions can be thought of as reflecting the operation of evolutionarily old brain systems that control behaviors necessary for the survival of the individual or its species (p. 469)

This idea goes back at least to Paul MacLean's and Karl Pribram's early work on the limbic system (MacLean 1952; Pribram and Kruger 1954).

Treating emotions as computational processes suggests the fruitfulness of neural network models of emotion (Watt 1995). It is now fashionable in artificial intelligence, robotics, and connectionist circles to talk about including emotions in intelligent machines to provide a basis for valuation of potential sensory events or motor acts. This idea is not as new as many people believe. The idea was central to some neural network models propounded in the 1970s by researchers such as Stephen Grossberg (1971), Paul Werbos (1974),

Harry Klopf (1972), and Gershom-Zvi Rosenstein (1991). A review of recent work, both theoretical and experimental, on neural networks for emotion appeared in Levine and Leven (1992). Although the research still falls short of a neural theory for the specific emotions, it includes drive representations and affective evaluation areas as key components of the decision circuitry. There is no reason to believe this methodology will not ultimately yield theories for specific emotions, such as fear, anger, joy, disgust, and sadness.

EVIDENCE FOR UNCONSCIOUS BIASES

Even when emotions *are* consciously felt, are we conscious of all the ways they influence behavior? There is abundant evidence from many fields (e.g., economics, linguistics, psychology) that we are not always conscious of their influence. Doeringer and Piore (1971) studied hiring decisions made by Boston-area white employers who did not show conscious race prejudice. The researchers discovered that in spite of the employers' sincerity about lack of prejudice, they still tended to hire a white person instead of an African American with the same measurable qualifications. The reason, Doeringer and Piore found, was that the hiring personnel had unconscious standards for "good employee behavior" that were subtly influenced by white culture; African Americans tended to be less likely than whites to fulfill these standards.

Unconscious biases can also be reinforced by positive feedback between beliefs and language. Lakoff and Johnson (1980) illustrated many unconscious metaphors in language, for example, the metaphor that argument is war. This metaphor leads to common American phrases such as "your claims are indefensible," "He attacked every weak point in my argument," "His criticisms were right on target," and "I've never won an argument with him." Because such phrases are embedded in unconscious American usage, it is natural that they influence behavior. For example, they could lead the speaker unintentionally to treat someone with a differing political or religious or scientific viewpoint as an enemy, rather than as a partner, as some other cultures (e.g., Native Americans) might.

Tversky and Kahneman (1974) discussed the heuristics by which most of us make decisions. The heuristics included *representativeness* (i.e., whether a person or thing exhibits the behavior we intuitively feel is typical for a class) and *availability* (how we focus on the aspect of something that is most eye-catching or that "grabs our attention"). These heuristics operate even when we are consciously trying to make decisions using more rational criteria, such as in making professional judgments.

Moreover, decisions are often made by weighting attributes or aspects of a situation. Changes in external contest or internal mood can shift the relative weighting of different attributes. Leven and Levine (1996) introduced a neural network model of this process and applied it to a consumer preference situation ("Old Coke" versus "New Coke").

Taylor (1992) reviewed neuroanatomical evidence for lack of conscious control over most emotional expression. Specifically, the nucleus reticularis of the thalamus (NRT), which is often considered the major site of attentional influence on cortical activity, does not have a similar influence on limbic system structures. The amygdala and Papez circuit project on the medio-dorsal thalamus, which in turn projects to NRT, giving an "emotional color" to consciousness, but there is no direct return connection from the NRT or from the mediodorsal thalamus.

Yet people can and do develop conscious attention to their own emotions, even if not control of their feelings. Because the prefrontal cortex is a seat of integration of lower-level systems (Damasio 1994; Levine, Leven, and Prueitt 1992) and seems to contain "copies" of various subcortical circuits (Levine 1994), it may be that the frontal copy of the NRT may be able with sufficient priming to exert influence on the frontal copy of the amygdala. This mechanism has remained the subject of speculation, however, because little is known about the functions of circuits connecting different subregions of the prefrontal cortex (Bates 1995).

NEURAL SYSTEMS FOR GENERATING AND SELECTING ALTERNATIVES

Most previous network models of decision making, including that of Leven and Levine (1996), involve a relatively passive evaluation of known alternative courses of action. To mimic decision making by the actual brain, the capacity for actively exploring the environment, the conceptual database, also needs to be included. A few network models have begun to include exploratory capacities (Öğmen and Prakash 1997). To be useful for real-time tasks, exploratory search should not be entirely random but guided by the needs of the task. For example, in the Verbal Fluency Test used by clinical neuropsychologists (Parks and Levine, in press), the subject needs to search his or her database for words that begin with a specified letter of the alphabet, or that belong to a particular category (animals, supermarket items, etc.). The requirements of the task, whether directed from the outside (e.g., by an experimenter) or from the subject's internal priority-setting apparatus, generate the *episode* that organizes and biases the search. Thus, the conscious biases in the exploration seem to be influenced by the hippocampus, which is involved in episodic memory (Cohen and Eichenbaum 1993) and in orienting the organism toward new stimuli or situations (Teyler and DiScenna 1986).

The hippocampus is strongly connected to the dorsolateral part of the frontal cortex. On the basis of these connections and hippocampal functions, Pribram (1991) suggested that

the dorsal far frontal system controls the ordering of priorities to ensure effective action. (p. 242)

As noted by results on the Wisconsin Card Sorting Test (Milner 1964), damage to this frontal region prevents shifting of attentional biases as reinforcement contingencies change. On this basis, various neural network models (Parks and Levine, in press); Sloman and Rumelhart 1992) suggest that the frontal lobes perform *episodic gating* (i.e., filtering out the previously stored representations that are most relevant to the current episode). This process may be performed by a modulation of connections from hippocampus to semantic storage areas in other parts of the association cortex.

The role of episodic memory in consciousness, through connections between the hippocampus and thalamus, was discussed in Taylor (1992). But I suspect that emotional biases, conscious or unconscious, may go through a different brain system. Because the amygdala monitors emotional values of sensory events (Pribram 1991; Rogan and LeDoux 1996), it should play a role in this system. So should the orbital region of the prefrontal cortex, which has strong reciprocal connections with the amygdala. Damasio (1994) noted that orbital damage prevents people from having the usual types of emotional reactions to events or decisions and therefore distorts the normal process by which people decide between alternative courses of action.

In the exploratory search for rules to govern a situation, one might posit complementary roles for these two parts of the prefrontal cortex. The dorsolateral area is involved in the generation of alternative courses of action, selectively activating mental images of possible action appropriate for the current episode through its hippocampal connections. In their model for the Wisconsin Card Sorting Test (on which performance is impaired by dorsolateral lesion), Dehaene and Changeux (1991) proposed that one function of a frontal-like area in their network is to be a "generator of diversity," which means it generates alternative rules to the ones currently in force. The orbitomedial area is involved in limiting the choices among the generated courses of action, based on emotional factors as measured by the orbitoamygdalar system. Damasio (1994) discussed orbitally damaged patients who endlessly and obsessively develop alternative ways for solving problems and cannot decide between them.

Damasio also discussed the interplay of emotion and reason in problem solving and assigned emotions to the central role to which modern science has been loath to ascribe them. However, he also suggested that once emotions (through the orbitoamygdalar system) have limited the choices to a few acceptable ones, reason "takes over" to make the optimal choice. I believe the time distinction between these processes is less sharp than Damasio made it. Both rational biases through the hippocampal–dorsolateral system and emotional biases through the orbital–amygdalar system are more likely to operate simultaneously in real time, and both have conscious and unconscious components. Also, unconscious effects can influence the processing done by the conscious system, and vice versa. Moreover, both emotional and rational arguments are sometimes used to generate alternatives and sometimes to reject them. The resulting decisions might be optimal by any of several criteria or by none of them! Levine (1995) considered speculative mathematical dynamics for interactions among all these processes.

SELF-ACTUALIZATION AND OPTIMIZATION

Levine (1994) introduced a skeleton neural network embodying the notion of *self-actualization* or optimal cognitive function, introduced by Maslow (1968). The basic idea is that a competitive network (Cohen and Grossberg 1983) representing "needs" has a Lyapunov or system-energy function, called V; the optimal state is the global minimum of V. However, the state could approach another equilibrium that is not a global minimum but a local minimum of the same Lyapunov function. A "negative affect" signal, possibly from the amygdala, detects nonoptimality of such a state by comparing the value of V at the current state with its value at alternative states of the needs module imagined by a prefrontal "world modeler" that imagines other states.

The Lyapunov function V is likely to be encoded in the same frontolimbic connections mentioned above, probably in the amygdalar—orbital system for emotional valuation. The exact value of V could have both a hard-wired and a learned component. The hard-wired part reflects a certain element of intrinsic human needs, including self-actualization (what the American Declaration of Independence calls "inalienable rights"). The learned part could be based on a sort of error-correcting neural network, such as back propagation (Werbos 1993) or vector-associative map (VAM) (Gaudiano and Grossberg 1991). Also, Levine's (1994) self-actualization network could be influenced by chaotic mechanisms (discussed in Levine 1995). Perhaps a chaotically biased or perturbed competitive network of alternatives (actions, plans, percepts, representations, etc.) could connect with the competitive needs module by means of a bidiretional connection, so that alternatives could be evaluated for how well they satisfy basic needs.

Levine's (1994) network allowed tremendous variation in the amount to which an optimal state is approached. Humans can act, for example, according to our deepest desires (optimal actions) or to suboptimal actions we choose because we believe they are possible. Choosing optimal actions corresponds roughly to a global minimum of the Lyapunov function V for the needs system; choosing suboptimal actions corresponds roughly to a local minimum of V, to what economists call *satisficing* (Simon 1979). Both optimizing and satisficing decisions are influenced by unconscious as well as conscious mechanisms. Levine (1994) further elaborated part of the self-actualization network to include an arousal input. Nonspecific arousal corresponding to possible functions of the neurotransmitter noradrenalin (NA) could influence how many needs the network is motivated to satisfy, and therefore how hard the network tries to reach a global optimum.

In an interdisciplinary social science dissertation, Leven (1987) posited three prevailing human-decision styles named for three mathematicians whose major research was isomorphic to each style. These styles are Dantzig solvers, who try to achieve an available solution by a repeatable method; the Bayesian solvers, who play the percentages and try to maximize a measurable criterion; and the Godelians, who use both intuition and reason to arrive at innovative solutions. Godelians are more likely than the other two types to accept temporary discomfort to achieve long-term understanding. They are also more sensitive than the other types to affective mismatches at high levels of complexity. A good example was Albert Einstein, who noted that some (seemingly minor) results on light and radiation mismatched the Newtonian paradigms for physics; instead of glossing over the data, Einstein changed the paradigms.

Leven's three decision styles could reflect three attractors for a system like Levine's (1995), perhaps adding influence from a chaotic system. Parameter differences, such as those involving the strength of negative affect—which might also be called "creative discontent"—and noradrenalin levels (Levine, in preparation), can lead to dynamic bifurcations between regimes approaching one of these styles. Leven suggested that different styles are more appropriate for different types of work (e.g., Dantzig for managing a basic service such as highway construction, Bayesian for applying advanced economic decision tools, Godelian for forming goals for a company). Analysis of conflicting biases suggests conclusions that amplify Leven's. Because the Dantzig, Bayesian, and Godelian solvers each have different personal, mostly unconscious, biases, the interaction between a personal style and a task that she or he is not well fitted for could lead to unintended, or even chaotic, consequences.

A coherent network model incorporating all these effects is still to come. Nevertheless, I believe the ideas yield myth-defying (not mystifying!) suggestions about how consciousness, emotion, and reason interact.

REFERENCES

Bates, J. F. 1995. Multiple information processing domains in prefrontal cortex of rhesus monkey. Unpublished Ph. D. dissertation, Yale University.

Cohen, M. A., and S. Grossberg. 1983. Absolute stability of global pattern formation and parallel memory storage by competitive neural networks. *IEEE Transactions on Systems, Man, and Cybernetics* 13:815–826.

Cohen, N. J., and H. Eichenbaum. 1993. *Memory, Amnesia, and the Hippocampal System.* Cambridge: MIT Press.

Damasio, A. 1994. *Descartes' Error.* New York: Grosset/Putnam.

Dehaene, S., and J.-P. Changeux. 1991. The Wisconsin Card Sorting Test: Theoretical analysis and modeling in a neuronal network. *Cerebral Cortex* 1:62–79.

Doeringer, P. B., and M. J. Piore. 1971. *Internal Labor Markets and Manpower Analysis.* Lexington, MA: D. C. Heath.

Gaudiano, P., and S. Grossberg. 1991. Vector associative maps: Unsupervised real-time error-based learning and control of movement trajectories. *Neural Networks* 4:147–184.

Grossberg, S. 1971. On the dynamics of operant conditioning. *Journal of Theoretical Biology* 33:225–225.

Grossberg, S., and D. S. Levine. 1975. Some developmental and attentional biases in the contrast enhancement and short-term memory of recurrent neural networks. *Journal of Theoretical Biology* 53:341–380.

Klopf, A. H. 1972. Brain function and adaptive systems: a heterostatic theory. Bedford, MA: U.S. Air Force Cambridge Research Laboratories Research Report AFCRL-72-01-64.

Lakoff, G., and M. Johnson. 1980. *Metaphors We Live By*. Chicago: University of Chicago Press.

LeDoux, J. E. 1989. Cognitive-emotional interactions in the brain. *Cognition and Emotion* 3:267–289.

Leven, S. J. 1987. Choice and neural process. Unpublished Ph.D. dissertation, University of Texas at Arlington.

Leven, S. J., and D. S. Levine. 1996. Multiattribute decision making in context: A dynamic neural network methodology. *Cognitive Science* 20:271–299.

Levine, D. S. 1994. Steps toward a neural network theory of self-actualization. *World Congress on Neural Networks*, vol. 1. Mahwah, NJ: Erlbaum, pp. 215–220.

Levine, D. S. 1995. Do we know what we want? *World Congress on Neural Networks*, vol. II. Mahwah, NJ: Erlbaum, pp. 955–962.

Levine, D. S. In preparation. Common sense and common nonsense. New York: Oxford University Press.

Levine, D. S., S. J. Leven, and P. S. Prueitt. 1992. Integration, disintegration, and the frontal lobes. In D. S. Levine and S. J. Leven, eds., *Mtivation, Emotion, and Goal Direction in Neural Networks*. Hillsdale, NJ: Erlbaum, pp. 301–335.

MacLean, P. D. 1952. Some psychiatric implications of physiological studies on frontotemporal portion of limbic system (visceral brain). *Electroencephalography and Clinical Neurophysiology* 4:407–418.

Maslow, A. H. 1968. *Toward a Psychology of Being*. New York: Van Nostrand.

Milner, B. 1964. Some effects of frontal lobectomy in man. In J. M. Warren and K. Akert, eds., *The Frontal Granular Cortex and Behavior*. New York: McGraw-Hill.

Ögmen, H., and R. V. Prakash. 1997. A developmental perspective to neural models of intelligence and learning. In D. S. Levine and W. R. Elsberry, eds., *Optimality in Biological and Artificial Networks?* Mahwah, NJ: Erlbaum, pp. 363–395.

Parks, R. W., and D. S. Levine. In press. Neural network modeling of The Wisconsin card sorting and verbal fluency tests. In R. W. Parks, D. S. Levine, and D. L. Long, eds., *Fundamentals of Neural Network Modeling for Neuropsychology*. Cambridge, MA: MIT Press.

Pribram, K. H. 1991. *Brain and Perception*. Hillsdale, NJ: Erlbaum.

Pribram, K. H., and L. Kruger. 1954. Function of the "olfactory" brain. *Annals of the New York Academy of Sciences* 54:109–138.

Rogan, M. T., and J. E. LeDoux. 1996. Emotion: Systems, cells, synaptic plasticity. *Cell* 35:469–475.

Rosenstein, G.-Z. 1991. *Income and Choice in Biological Systems*. Hillsdale, NJ: Erlbaum.

Simon, H. A. 1979. *Models of Thought*. New Haven: Yale University Press.

Sloman, S. A., and D. E. Rumelhart. 1992. Reducing interference in distributed memories through episodic gating. In H. Healy, S. Kosslyn, and R. Shiffrin, eds., *From Learning Theory to Connectionist Modeling*. Hillsdale, NJ: Erlbaum.

Taylor, J. G. 1992. Towards a neural network model of the mind. *Neural Network World* 6:797–812.

Teyler, T. J., and P. DiScenna. 1986. The hippocampal memory indexing theory. *Neuroscience* 100:147–154.

Tversky, A., and D. Kahneman. 1974. Judgment under uncertainty: Heuristics and biases. *Science* 185:1124–1131.

Watt, D. F. 1995. Neurodevelopmental and limbic network issues for neural network theories of consciousness. *World Congress on Neural Networks*, vol. II. Mahwah, NJ: Erlbaum, pp. 973–991.

Werbos, P. J. 1974. Beyond regression: new tools for prediction and analysis in the behavioral sciences. Unpublished Ph. D. dissertation, Harvard University.

Werbos, P. J. 1993. *The Roots of Backpropagation*. New York: John Wiley and Sons.

IX Language, Animals, and Consciousness

OVERVIEW

Are animals conscious? Do animals such as apes, parrots, and dolphins utilize language? Is language the sine qua non of consciousness?

These questions were the core of a popular session chaired by Colin Beer at Tucson II. To begin Part IX, Beer presents the history and current understanding of animal language, which serves as an extended overview of this topic. Sue Savage-Rumbaugh and Duane Rumbaugh describe cognition and communication in bonobo apes, and Diana Reiss discusses the question of consciousness in dolphins. In the final chapter in Part IX, Paul Bloom tackles the tangled relationship between language and mental life.

45 King Solomon's Ring Redivivus: Cross-Species Communication and Cognition

Colin G. Beer

Descartes is notorious for having regarded nonhuman animals as automata; hence, he denied that they entertain thought or experience feeling. In his correspondence with the Cambridge Platonist Henry More, Descartes said that his main reason for holding this view was that animals other than ourselves lack "real speech ... such speech [being] the only certain sign of thought hidden in a body" (Kenny 1970).

Three hundred years later, the Cornell philosopher Norman Malcolm returned to the subject of "thoughtless brutes," the title of his Presidential Address to the American Philosophical Association in 1972. Malcolm agreed with Descartes that, without speech, animals are incapable of thought with propositional content—hence, of thinking *about* something—but he argued that this limitation did not apply to their thinking that something *might be a fact*. Just as humans often judge what other people think (believe) from what they do, one can reasonably infer an animal's beliefs from the way it behaves. Malcolm took the common-sense position that some animals share with humans some kinds of thought-free consciousness. He ended his address (Malcolm 1973) by saying:

It is the prejudice of philosophers that only propositional thoughts belong to consciousness, that stands in the way of our perceiving the continuity of consciousness between human and animal life. (p. 86)

Thus, there is continuity of consciousness but discontinuity of thought. Thought is tied to language both for its formulation and for its expression. Hence the complaint that an old lady made to E.M. Forster (Auden 1962): "How can I know what I think till I see what I say?" Malcolm and others who think like him, for example, Matthews (1978) and Vendler (1972), take for granted, like Descartes, that animals lack anything like linguistic capacity and must therefore be truly dumb—thoughtless brutes.

Donald Griffin took issue with this position in 1975 in a lecture entitled "A New King Solomon's Ring." The title alludes to an ancient legend in which King Solomon possessed a magic ring that gave him the power to converse with animals in their own tongues (Lorenz 1952). In the lecture, and in his book, *The Question of Animal Awareness* (1976), Griffin argued that evolutionary continuity implies that whatever cognitive equipment underlies human language must have ancestral and cognate forms in species phyloge-netically connected to humans—the differences are of degree, not of kind. Even for phylogenetically remote species, such as arthropods, Griffin pro-posed that their communication systems offer a "window on the minds of animals," a way to "eavesdrop" on what the signals say about an animal's mental states and its beliefs about things in the outside world.

THE ANIMAL LANGUAGE PROJECTS

Although study of and experiments on animal communication systems have revealed much information about what the signals are used for and the nature of the information they encode (Smith 1977), Griffin's hope that such inves-tigation might lead to the understanding of what it might be like to be a bee, a bat, or a bonobo chimpanzee (Nagel 1974) has yet to be realized. An alternative, reverse approach is thought to hold a more promising prospect for breaking through to a purchase on animal cognition and awareness—teaching animals a language-like sign system so that they can tell us what they think in something like human terms.

The first attempts involved trying to get apes to talk with vocal utterance (Furness 1916; Kellog and Kellog 1933; Hayes 1951; Laidler 1978). The results were pitiful; no responses in one study, and no more than four indis-tinctly pronounced words in any of the other studies, even after the animals had years of intensive training. The failure was blamed on the animals' lack of adequate vocal equipment and lack of adequate cognitive capacity.

However, a different mode of communication offered a means of adjudicat-ing between these two possibilities. Yerkes (1929) remarked that chimpan-zees use many hand gestures in their social interactions, which suggested that they might be capable of learning a sign language like that used by deaf and mute people. Beatrice and Allen Gardner tried this approach with a young female chimpanzee they called Washoe (Gardner and Gardner 1969; Gardner and Gardner 1975). They trained the animal on a simplified version of the American Sign Language (ASL) by rewarding her when she made appropriate hand gestures and responded appropriately to signs presented to her. To teach the signs, the Gardners sometimes had to shape Washoe's hands manually into the right positions.

After years of such training, the Gardners claimed that Washoe had mas-tered over 130 signs, often in combinations perceived as having syntactic order, which she used in communicating with her trainers. There were even instances of purported originality—the most publicized was Washoe's sign-ing "water bird" when she saw a swimming swan. Roger Fouts took over training Washoe from the Gardners and continued to study her use of ASL and its use with other chimpanzees. He reported signing by the chimps to one another and Washoe's teaching signs to a juvenile chimp with which she had been placed (Fouts, Hirsch, and Fouts 1982). In separate projects (Terrace 1979), ASL was taught to another chimpanzee, Nim Chimpsky, to gorillas (Patterson 1978a), and to an orangutan (Miles 1983).

In addition, chimpanzees have been the subjects of other approaches to quasilinguistic interactions with people. For instance, David Premack (1976) and associates used magnetized plastic chips of differing shapes and colors to stand for objects, actions, and attributes. The animals were rewarded for selecting the correct chips and placing them in the right order on a board when presented with the objects they had been trained on, and for responding appropriately to requests made in the chip "language" on the board. The brightest ape in the project was called Sarah.

Duane Rumbaugh (1977) and Sue Savage-Rumbaugh (1986) adapted a computer keyboard as a means of using symbols to communicate with a number of common chimpanzees (*Pan troglodytes*) and pigmy chimpanzees (bonobos, *Pan paniscus*). Each key of the keyboard carried a "lexigram"—a geometrical symbol representing an object, a location, an action, or a part of speech. The apes readily learned to get the computer or caretaker to furnish food, drink, tools, or access to some desired location by pressing the right keys in the right order to make the requests. The lexigram technology has also been used in the study of chimpanzees' ability to label colors and work with numbers (Matsuzawa 1985a, b; Boysen 1992, 1993).

Other projects have involved nonprimate species. For instance, Louis Herman (Herman and Morrel-Samuels 1996) experimented with bottlenosed dolphins (*Turciops truncatus*) by training them to respond to sequences of computer-generated whistles or human gestures by performing a specific action such as bringing a ball to a hoop. Similarly, Ron Schusterman used gestural signing to explore the capacity of California sea lions to comprehend combinations of symbols (Schusterman 1988; Schusterman and Kneger 1984). The ventures with marine mammals emphasize receptivity to signaled commands, not the production of symbolic communication. However, work with an African gray parrot (*Psittacus erithacus*) involved two-way vocal communication. Since 1977 Irene Pepperberg has been training her parrot Alex to use English words to answer questions put to him in English about the shape, color, material, and number of objects presented to him (Pepperberg 1991).

DISSENSION AND DEFENSE

News of the animal language projects created great public interest. Media coverage encouraged exaggerated claims for what had been revealed about animal mentality and linguistic ability, and, in turn, led to what Dan Dennett (1983) called the "kill-joy" reaction. Skeptics and critics were dubious of aspects of the earlier ape language work on various grounds. Some argued that conventional learning paradigms, such as conditional discrimination and paired-associate conditioning, without recourse to linguistic capacities, could account for at least some of the performances (Petitto and Seidenberg 1979; Thompson and Church 1980). Nonpartisan observers of apes "signing" in ASL contended that the number of "words" learned and their frequency of production were highly inflated and overinterpreted because many movements recorded as signs appeared to belong to the animals' natural repertoire of gestures and that other signs approximated what they were supposed to be in ASL so tenuously that the connection appeared to be confined to the eye of the beholder (Pinker 1994).

Perhaps the most damaging case against the cause came from Herbert Terrace, who had started out as a believer. Terrace had trained his chimpanzee Nim in much the same way that the Gardners had trained Washoe, except that Terrace had videotaped large portions of the training and testing sequences. When he subjected the tapes to sequential analysis, Terrace found that what he expected to be evidence of syntactic order in the strings of signs was nothing of the sort. Instead, the ape was revealed as having haphazardly repeated movements for which it had been rewarded (e.g., "Give orange me give eat orange me eat orange give me eat orange give me you") (Pinker 1994), as though the "words" had come out of a hat rather than a head. Nim's occasional signing of something that looked grammatical was no more significant than that a stopped clock tells the right time twice a day.

Furthermore, in one sample of tapes Terrace found that 40 percent of Nim's signings copied those that the trainer had just given, often before the trainer had finished (Terrace 1979; Terrace, Pettito, Sanders, and Bever 1979, 1980). Evidence that the ape had been cueing its behavior on that of its human attendants led to assertion that the entire animal language movement should be dismissed as "sleight of Clever Hans" (Umiker-Sebeok and Sebeok 1980; Sebeok and Rosenthal 1981).[1]

Because trainers were usually present during times when symbolic exchanges between people and the apes and other animals was supposed to be occurring, the specter of Clever Hans haunted the precincts. Even double-blind procedures, as used in formal testing of the animals, were thought to be no guarantee against the possibility of giving the show away by subtle signs (Umiker-Sebeok and Sebeok 1980; Wilder, 1996).

Raising the specter led to more careful designs in testing procedures and to counter arguments for situations in which the specter's presence is implausible (Ristau and Robbins 1982). Moreover, recognition that cueing of a sort is a legitimate training technique, as exemplified by its prevalence in the communicative interactions leading to language acquisition by children, has also happened.

In the work of Sue Savage-Rumbaugh with the pigmy chimpanzee Kanzi (Savage-Rumbaugh and Brakke 1996; Savage-Rumbaugh and Lewin 1994), communication with Kanzi involved spoken English words and lexigrams via the portable keyboard and computer screen. To test Kanzi's comprehension strict, double-blind procedures were followed; for instance, when the ape heard the spoken words through headphones, it was impossible for the tester to know what the words were. Although food was available to the animal during testing, food was never given as a reward for being right or withheld as a consequence of being wrong. Thus Kanzi had no need to attend to cues because nothing tangible depended on correct performance.

On the other hand, in learning contexts apart from test situations, a teacher does serve as a model and uses cueing and prompting in the service of education. Savage-Rumbaugh and Brakke (1996) stressed that

This is an essential process in language acquisition for the child and there is no reason to deny it to animals attempting to learn a language. (p. 284)

The comparison to children also shows how the project with Kanzi differed from other animal language projects. Instead of laborious drilling, shaping, and reinforcement regimens standardly used to instill symbolic communication capacity in an animal, Kanzi was left to construct on his own ways of conversing with his caretakers. Apparently, he began by attending his mother's training on lexigrams and, through observational learning and spontaneous performance, acquired sufficient facility at the keyboard for interchange with his keepers and for them to build on without their needing to resort to drilling and conventional reinforcement.

The process was much more like the way in which children learn to talk and understand speech, and the results with Kanzi came closest (of all the animal language projects) to the frequently claimed comparability with human performance at ages 18 to 30 months. For instance, on blind testing of responses to spoken requests such as "Take the rock outdoors" or "Fetch the rock that's outdoors," Kanzi did what was asked in 74 percent of the trials—a child's score at age 18 to 30 months is 65 percent on the same set. Such performance has led Ristau (1996), one of the most acute critics of the animal language work, to comment:

Kanzi apprehends order information, and does so in a wide array of contexts. He understands simple English, and understands it more quickly than he learns lexigrams." (p. 654)

However, Wallman (1992) and Pinker (1994) expressed deflating views.

In Chapter 46, Sue Savage-Rumbaugh discusses her work with Kanzi in the light of the view that true language is possessed only by human beings. Savage-Rumbaugh maintains that Kanzi's accomplishments reveal that an ape can spontaneously acquire a human language system if exposed to it at an early age; hence, conscious use of language is clearly within the cognitive reach of the ape mind. She believes that the natural communication system of these animals utilizes their capacity for conscious use of language. In support of this view, she presents evidence of symbolic transmission of information among wild bonobos.

One of the few generally agreed-upon judgments of the animal language projects is that comprehension of symbols comes more easily than production of symbols. This conclusion has proved to be especially true in work with marine mammals (Herman 1996; Herman, Richards, and Wolz 1984; Schusterman 1988; Schusterman and Gisiner 1988; Schusterman and Kneger 1984 1986). Yet for dolphins, the natural behavior comprises a rich, complex repertoire of vocal and visual signals, which suggests the give and take of social dialogue. Diana Reiss (Chapter 47) examined vocal development in bottlenosed dolphins, thus far the only nonhuman mammals for which there is good evidence of vocal learning. Reiss found much that is comparable to linguistic development in humans and to song acquisition in songbirds, including influences of heard vocalizations, acoustic feedback, and social interaction on vocal development, and developmental progression through stages of overproduction, selective attrition, and a parallel to babbling or subsong. In work with adult dolphins, Reiss observed spontaneous mimicry of computer-generated simulations of dolphin whistles and of sounds that are not species specific, which the animals produced spontaneously in behaviorally appropriate contexts.

Along with the evidence of comprehension of artificial gestural and acoustic signals, Reiss's work suggests that dolphins are capable of simple, two-way communication with people. Observations of reactions to their mirror images and of social play further suggest that there may be conscious and even self-conscious dimensions to the dolphins' communication behavior.

Irene Pepperberg presented information at the Tucson II conference, Toward a Science of Consciousness 1996, about her African gray parrot, Alex.

Pepperberg's parrot learned to comprehend and use English labels for seven different colors, five different shapes, and various materials such as cork, wood, and paper. He can say how many objects are in a group (up to six) even and whether the objects are novel, heterogeneous, or randomly arranged. He can use his repertoire of labels to accurately identify, request, refuse, categorize, and count more than 100 different objects, including objects that differ somewhat from the ones on which he was trained. In response to the questions "What color?" or "What shape?" he answers correctly for objects having both colors and shapes with which he is familiar. He makes accurate judgments of same–different and bigger–smaller comparisons and appropriately uses phrases such as "Come here," "I want X," and "Wanna go Y," when X and Y refer to objects or places. If Alex's requests are responded to inappropriately, he usually utters "Nah" and asks again. If presented with an array of objects, Alex can, when asked, identify something that is uniquely defined by conjunction of color and shape, even though other items share the color or the shape.

Although Alex's performances on these cognitive exercises are the result of training involving reinforcement and social modeling and during which trainers were always present, the range and flexibility of Alex's responses make implausible the possibility that they can be reduced to conventional operant learning or the effects of cueing. The possibility of cueing was further countered in formal tests because the people scoring the tests were unfamiliar to Alex; he had no opportunity to learn their body language. This bird (and presumably others, if they were exposed to similar experience) seems to possess cognitive capacities once thought to be restricted to humans.

To what extent does mental life depend on possession of language? Descartes thought there could be no thought without language. Paul Bloom disagrees. Nevertheless, Bloom concedes that language makes an enormous difference. The contrasting richness of human mental life compared with the undoubted lack of most of what humans think about, imagine, conjecture, devise, invent, and so forth, in the minds of even our closest relatives, speaks to that difference. In Chapter 48, Bloom discusses evidence of how use of language has been thought to give rise "to novel concepts, to new ways of categorizing entities and construing the world."

On the other hand, Bloom argues against the strong version of Benjamin Lee Whorf's (1956) thesis that all human concepts derive from language, which also determines how humans carve up reality into categories and kinds. Bloom posits that language learning would occur if there were no prior ideas in our heads to attach words to and that linguistically impaired people, such as aphasics, prelinguistic children, and otherwise normal adult linguistic isolates, lead mental lives as fully conscious as those of the linguistically endowed. From such evidence Bloom concludes that "at least some of the unique aspects of human mental life exist independently of language."

What of the aspects of human mental life that humans might share with other animals? So far, attempts to use communication as a window into animal mentality have revealed cognitive capacities once thought exclusive to humans, but the attempts have yet to provide any clear access to what it is like to be a creature of another sort in the subjectivity of its being. No doubt attempts to find a linguistic point of entry—a new King Solomon's ring—will continue. But if language is neither a necessary condition for consciousness, nor sufficient to reveal consciousness, cognitive ethology will have to go on trying other ways of putting the question of animal awareness (Griffin 1992; Dawkins 1993; Bekoff and Jamieson 1996). In the meantime, consideration of this question will have to be included in any fully realized science of consciousness.

NOTES

1. Clever Hans was a famous German performing horse in the early 1900s and was reputed for ability to do arithmetic, understand spoken and written German, and carry out other intellectual feats. When asked a question, the horse would repeatedly tap a foot or shake its head until it arrived at the number corresponding to the right answer. However, if the questioner was hidden from view or did not know the answer to the question, Hans failed to perform, which encouraged the suspicion that all was not as it appeared. Oskar Pfungst (1911) and Rosenthal (1965) established that the questioners were unwittingly telling the horse when to stop by making slight movements such as raising their eyebrows or inclining their heads.

REFERENCES

Auden, W. H. 1962. *The Dyer's Hand*. New York: Vintage.

Bekoff, M., and D. Jamieson, eds. 1996. *Readings in Animal Cognition*. Cambridge: MIT Press.

Boysen, S. T. 1992. Counting as the chimpanzee views it. In W. K. Honig and J. G. Fetterman, eds., *Complex Extended Stimuli in Animals*. Hillsdale, NJ: Erlbaum.

Dawkins, M. S. 1993. *Through Our Eyes Only—The Search for Animal Consciousness*. New York: Freeman.

Dennett, D. C. 1983. Intentional systems in cognitive ethology: The "Panglossian Paradigm" defended. *Behavioral and Brain Sciences* 6:343–390.

Fouts, R. S., A. Hirsch, and D. H. Fouts. 1982. Cultural transmission of a human language in a chimpanzee mother/infant relationship. In H. E. Fitzgerald, J. A. Mullins, and P. Page, eds., *Psychobiological Perspectives: Child Nurturance Series*, vol. III. New York: Plenum Press.

Furness, W. 1916. Observations on the mentality of chimpanzees and orangutans. *Proceedings of the American Philosophical Society* 65:281–290.

Gardner, B. T., and R. A. Gardner. 1975. Evidence for sentence constituents in the early utterances of child and chimpanzee. *Journal of Experimental Psychology: General* 104:244–267.

Gardner, R. A., and B. T. Gardner. 1969. Teaching sign language to a chimpanzee. *Science* 165:664–672.

Griffin, D. R. 1976. *The Question of Animal Awareness: Evolutionary Continuity of Mental Experience*. New York: Rockefeller University Press.

Griffin, D. R. 1992. *Animal Minds*. Chicago: Chicago University Press.

Hayes, C. 1951. *The Ape in Our House*. New York: Harper.

Herman, L. M., and P. Morrel-Samuels. 1996. Knowledge acquisition and asymmetry between language comprehension and production: Dolphins and apes as general models for animals. In M. Bekoff and D. Jamieson, eds., *Readings in Animal Cognition*. Cambridge: MIT Press.

Herman, L. M., D. B. Richards, and J. P. Wolz. 1984. Comprehension of sentences by bottlenosed dolphins. *Cognition* 16:129–219.

Kellog, W. N., and L. A. Kellog. 1933. *The Ape and the Child: A Study of Environmental Influence upon Early Behavior*. New York: Whittlesey House.

Kenny, A., ed. 1970. *Descartes. Philosophical Letters*. Oxford: Oxford University Press.

Laidler, K. 1978. Language in the orang-utan. In A. Lock, ed., *Action, Gesture and Symbol: The Emergence of Language*. New York: Academic Press.

Lorenz, K. Z. 1952. *King Solomon's Ring*. London: Methuen.

Malcolm, N. 1973. Thoughtless brutes. *American Philosophical Association* 46:5–20.

Matsuzawa, T. 1985a. Use of numbers by chimpanzee. *Nature* 315:57–59.

Matsuzawa, T. 1985b. Color naming and classification in a chimpanzee (*Pan troglodytes*). *Journal of Human Evolution* 14:283–291.

Matthews, G. A. 1978. Animals and the unity of psychology. *Philosophy* 53:437–454.

Miles, H. L. 1983. Apes and language: The search for communicative competence. In J. de Luce and H. T. Wilder, eds., *Language in Primates: Perspectives and Implications*. New York: Springer-Verlag.

Nagel, T. 1974. What is it like to be a bat? *Philosophical Review* 83:435–450.

Patterson, F. G. 1978a. The gestures of a gorilla: Language acquisition in another pongid. *Brain and Language* 5:72–97.

Patterson, F. G. 1978b. Linguistic abilities of a young lowland gorilla. In F. C. Peng, ed., *Sign Language and Language Acquisition in Man and Ape: New Dimensions in Pedolinguistics*. Boulder, CO: Westview Press.

Pepperberg, I. M. 1991. A communicative approach to animal cognition: A study of conceptual abilities of an African gray parrot. In C. A. Ristau, ed., *Cognitive Ethology—The Minds of Other Animals*. Hillsdale, NJ: Erlbaum.

Petitto, O., and M. S. Seidenberg. 1979. On the evidence for linguistic abilities in signing apes. *Brain and Language* 8:162–183.

Pfungst, O. 1911. *Clever Hans, the Horse of Otto von Osten*, C. L. Rahn, trans. New York: Holt, Rinehart and Winston.

Pinker, S. 1994. *The Language Instinct—How the Mind Creates Language*. New York: William Morrow.

Premack, D. 1976. *Intelligence in Ape and Man*. Hillsdale, NJ: Erlbaum.

Ristau, C. A. 1996. Animal language and cognition projects. In A. Lock and C. R. Peters, eds., *Handbook of Human Symbolic Evolution*. London: Oxford University Press.

Ristau, C. A., and D. Robbins. 1982. Language in the great apes: A critical review. *Advances in the Study of Behavior* 12: 142–255.

Rosenthal, R., ed. 1965. *Clever Hans, The Horse of Mr. von Osten*. New York: Holt, Rinehart and Windton.

Rumbaugh, D. M., ed. 1977 *Language Learning by a Chimpanzee: The Lana Project*. New York: Academic Press.

Savage-Rumbaugh, E. S. 1986. *Ape Language: From Conditioned Response to Symbol*. New York: Columbia University Press.

Savage-Rumbaugh, E. S., and K. E. Brakke. 1996. Animal language: Methodological and interpretive issues. In M. Bekoff and D. Jamieson, eds., *Readings in Animal Cognition*. Cambridge: MIT Press.

Savage-Rumbaugh, E. S., and R. Lewin. 1994. *Kanzi: The Ape at the Brink of the Human Mind*. New York: Wiley/Doubleday.

Schusterman, R. J. 1988. Artificial language comprehension in dolphins and sea lions: The essential cognitive skills. *The Psychological Record* 38:311–348.

Schusterman, R. J., and R. C. Gisiner. 1988. Animal language research: Marine mammals re-enter the controversy. In H. J. Jerison and I. Jerison, eds., *Intelligence and Evolutionary Biology*. Berlin: Springer-Verlag.

Schusterman, R. J., and K. Kneger. 1984. California sea lions are capable of semantic comprehension. *Psychological Record* 39:3–23.

Sebeok, T. A., and R. Rosenthal, eds. 1981. The Clever Hans Phenomenon: Communications with horses, whales, apes, and people. *Annals of the New York Academy of Sciences* 364:1–311.

Smith, W. J. 1977. *The Behavior of Communicating*. Cambridge: Harvard University Press.

Terrace, H. S. 1979. *Nim*. New York: Knopf.

Terrace, H. S., L. A. Pettito, R. J. Sanders, and T. G. Bever. 1979. Can an ape create a sentence? *Science* 206:891–902.

Terrace, H. S., L. A. Pettito, R. J. Sanders, and T. G. Bever. 1980. On the grammatical capacity of apes. In K. Nelson, ed., *Children's Language*, vol. 2. New York: Gardner.

Thompson, C. R., and R. M. Church. 1980. An explanation of the language of a chimpanzee. *Science* 206:313–314.

Umiker-Sebeok, J., and T. A. Sebeok. 1980. Introduction: Questioning apes. In T. A. Sebeok and J. Umiker-Sebeok, eds., *Speaking of Apes: A Critical Anthology of Two-Way Communication with Man*. New York: Plenum.

Vendler, Z. 1972. *Res Cogitans*. Ithaca: Cornell University Press.

Wallman, J. 1992. *Aping Language*. Cambridge: Cambridge University Press.

Whorf, B. L. 1956. *Language, Thought and Reality*. Cambridge: MIT Press.

Wilder, H. 1996. Interpretive cognitive ethology. In M. Bekoff and D. Jamieson, eds., *Readings in Animal Cognition*. Cambridge: MIT Press.

Yerkes, R. M. and A. Yerkes. 1929. *The Great Apes: A Study of Anthropoid Life*. New Haven: Yale University Press.

46 Perspectives on Consciousness, Language, and Other Emergent Processes in Apes and Humans

E. Sue Savage-Rumbaugh and Duane M. Rumbaugh

DO ANIMALS AND HUMANS SHARE "MIND"?

Scholars have debated the mental competencies of animals relative to man since antiquity. Some have been Animists, who believed in the immortality and transmigration of souls from animals to human beings; others have been Mechanists, who proclaimed that neither animals nor humans are anything more than protoplasmic machines acted on by mechanical forces beyond their control or understanding. There were the Vitalists, who eschewed these debates in favor of the view that a continuity of some fashion existed between animals and humans. Vitalism was accepted by church doctrine, and from it emerged the metaphoric Great Chain of Being in which the designer of the world is said to have created all in finely graded scale from barely alive to sentient to intelligent to wholly spiritual, in the case of humans. A human being was the supreme creation; although a human's assent to spirituality was possible, it was not assured (Wise 1995, 1996).

The basic sentiments of these positions have resisted change and are very much alive today. The views were modified by Descartes, who kept both the mechanist and the animist position but drew a distinction between the mind and body of man. For Descartes (1956), the body behaved in a mechanistic manner not substantially different from that of animals, but the human mind operated according to "rational thought"—a capacity denied to animals because they lacked souls. Since Descartes, science has set about defining a "rational" view of the construction of mind.

Darwin (1859) challenged the accepted wisdom further with his concept of evolution as process shaped by numbers of offspring rather than by Divine will. For Darwin, both man and animals existed because of random sets of events, which their forebears had negotiated sufficiently successfully to leave offspring behind. Unlike Descartes, Darwin was willing to attribute mind to animals. He suggested that the display of emotions in humans could be traced directly to similar displays in animals, and he believed that many, if not all, higher cognitive processes could be demonstrated among animals. Nevertheless, the question of how to demonstrate this belief in a scientific manner remained open.

Romanes (1898) attempted to put together a group of behavioral accounts that would reveal the evolution of behavior in the same manner that Darwin had revealed the evolution of anatomy. But behavior, and the intent behind the behavior, could not be dissected in the same manner as the liver or the spleen. An organ can be laid open for all to see, but the intent behind a set of actions remains hidden to the optical eye. For example, a fox might outwit a carefully laid trap by biting through the string and thus free the bait, but was this mindless habit or did the fox understand what it was doing? Descartes's view that only humans could behave with deliberate intent was buttressed by the observation that only humans could *describe* intent. Only a human being could *say*, "I cut the rope to spoil the trap."

The need to prove, in an indisputable manner, that intent existed, led directly to language and the self-expression of intent as the sole determinant of mind. No other criterion was acceptable. Because a creature could not state the intent behind an action, it was assumed that the action stemmed from a mechanistic plane that was not grounded in reason or understanding. This solution seemed simple enough—if a creature had language and could make its intentions known, its behavior was not mechanistic. Lacking language, there was no other option. Behaviors, no matter how complex or intelligent they might appear, were not the product of intentional planned actions. They were only complex chains of reactions to external stimuli and, as such, were not under the volitional control of the animal organism.

The attempts of modern neuroscience to explain the construction of mind have relied heavily on experimental work with animals as human surrogates and with brain-damaged human subjects. Underlying the work is the basic assumption that "mind" emerges from matter in a completely predictable, understandable fashion. The more the basic architecture underlying brain function in an animal is similar to that of humans, the more probable it becomes that the mental states experienced by the animal are similar to those experienced by humans. Animals such as apes, who share more than 98 percent of human DNA and an anatomy nearly identical to that of humans (Sibley and Ahlquist 1987) may have mental states that are complex and intentional. It seems nearly inconceivable that intentionality and language has arisen only once in evolutionary history. It also seems inconceivable that such complex behavior requires only a slight genetic alteration (Churchland 1986, 1995).

THE CENTRALITY OF GRAMMAR

The idea that humans and animals live in completely different mental worlds does not die an easy death; the idea has become ingrained in our way of life. Because the biological similarity between ape and man makes it unlikely that any organ within the brain will be found to account for all the differences between humans and animals we perceive as we look around. Linguists have postulated the existence of a grammatical parser hidden within the connective neural tissue of the brain (Chomsky 1988; Pinker 1994). So powerful is this parser that it acts as a key for each human being, a key that permits the child to unlock the language that he hears from birth.

Lacking this key, the world is but a jumble of unrelated sound, and one can only react, not act with plan and intent. But with the key, the world of understanding and reason opens up, through the structure of language itself. The capacity to analyze an "if-then" conditional structure into its components, the capacity to determine what is the agent and recipient of action in a sentence—and other such logical structures—are made visible to the mind through this key. It is not only that the key enables the child to learn language, but that through language, the key enables the child to think in a logically reasoned form. Without such a key, the linguist posits that reasoning, as humans know it, cannot occur.

The key is a sort of mathematical device that enables us to divide sentences properly and understand the relationships between various parts of them, even before we know the meaning of all the words. Thus, a new human–animal dichotomy is constructed on the basis of an innate linguistic processor hidden deep within the brain—a device that permits the arranging and organizing of symbols to real-world events in specific ways. So efficient is this device that it does not take up much space or require any dramatic restructuring of the brain.

The human child needs only a normal upbringing with customary exposure to the activities of others to enable this device to become effective. Animals, held to be devoid of language, are said to lack this module of "innate intelligence." Thus, they are viewed as constrained to learning complex response chains. Though the chains can become elaborate, animals are held to remain, nonetheless, under the specific influence of environmental stimuli and are therefore incapable of contemplating the existence of self and nature.

By positing the existence of a bit of critical (though unidentifiable) neural tissue that is said to contain something akin to the elements and rules of thought, linguists have been satisfied that they can incorporate Descartes, Darwin, and DNA into their cosmology without altering the central basic tenet that only a human being is capable of conscious, rational thought.

Although this view resurrects the familiar human–animal dichotomy, it nonetheless seems to have an increasingly hollow note. We find that we must ignore increasing amounts of evidence from all different fields suggesting that man and animals do share similar mental worlds.

Humans clearly perceive that some animals, particularly mammals, are psychologically like themselves in many ways. Many animals appear to have facial expressions and behaviors not unlike those that humans display when they are sad, hungry, tired, lonely, frightened, or angry. Animals take action not unlike those humans take to deal with such states and circumstances. Many animals appear to be as bonded to their young, their mates, and their homes as humans are. However, although we infer that animals can share with us many major perceptual aspects of varied contexts, it is also clear animals differ and can have, for example, sensory and perceptual capacities that are keener or different from ours. Many appear to share complex communication systems that currently are all but impossible to decipher (McFarland 1984). Many animals and birds build complex shelters and modify objects to use as tools.

In spite of acknowledging these similarities between animals and humans, many scholars have no difficulty stating with great assurance that humans and animals live in different mental worlds. Could this duality of thought be related to the fact that animals are very useful to us? We use animals as important sources of food, clothing, and labor for our lives. Some major industries are economically dependent on animals. Might it be reassuring to regard animals as different and humans as superior so that we can control every aspect of their existence and lives with a clear conscience?

The debate regarding the presence of mind in animals has continued since the dawn of recorded history (Griffin 1976). The controversy has assumed many guises, but all can be seen as different ways of dealing with the basic fact that humans alone have been viewed as being endowed with the gift of speech (Rumbaugh and Savage-Rumbaugh 1994; Savage-Rumbaugh, Shanker, and Taylor 1997).

IMPACT OF DISCOVERING LINGUISTIC CAPACITY IN APES

Given our history of hunting, eating, and domesticating animals, our conceptual and legal separation from all lesser creatures probably would have continued had it not been for a chimpanzee named Washoe. Washoe, according to Allen and Beatrice Gardner (1971), could "talk." Washoe could not actually speak, but she nonetheless learned to use a natural human language. The language was American Sign Language for the Deaf—widely used in deaf communities. Washoe was not fluent in this language, but she was able to express simple desires and needs. This report, at odds with assumptions regarding animals accepted since before the Greeks, created a maelstrom of controversy (Wallman 1992).

Given the history of thought and the economic forces at play underlying the human concept of self as the only rational agent on Earth and empowered with unquestioned dominion over animals, it is no surprise that initial claims that apes could learn human language were met with skepticism and cries of fraud (Sebeok and Rosenthal 1981). The first debates centered on attempts to determine whether what Washoe was doing was "really" language.

Students of language began to realize that no consensus existed regarding what was meant by "language." Had Washoe simply begun speaking in scholarly terms, no one would have contested the Gardners' claims for her ability. Instead, when Washoe did sign, her signs were often repetitive. Successive signs seemed to lack structure common to sentences, and what she was trying to say was not always obvious.

Nevertheless, this event marked the first time another species had been taught the use of a human language. Admittedly, the articulations of American Sign Language were not especially appropriate for a chimpanzee's hand to produce. Neither was Washoe's vocal tract fashioned for the articulation of human speech. But not infrequently, new scientific endeavors are clumsy, and it was concluded that Washoe's performance reflected not only her own limitations but our ability to understand.

Clearly Washoe could produce different signs when shown a wide variety of objects. She could name them. It also was impressive that she generalized her signs to new objects of similar form or conceptual class. For instance, the sign for meat was applied accurately to hamburger, steak, chicken, and so forth (Gardner and Gardner 1971). Soon other laboratories reported that their chimpanzees also could designate objects and could do so using plastic tokens or geometric symbols.

THE DEBATE SHIFTS AGAIN

Since it could not be argued that Washoe did not know the names of things, the debate about human–animal mind shifted to a new plane—determining when a behavior that appeared to be language was actually "linguistic."

For the first time the question "What is naming?" was raised. Behaviorists argued that Washoe's naming ability was merely "paired-associate learning." In other words, she simply learned which gesture to make when presented with each object but she did not *know in her mind* that the sign was a "name" for an object. From this perspective, names for Washoe were without meaning other than that inherent in her signing.

This problematic point presented a unique challenge because, at the time, there was no way of asking Washoe whether she had learned paired associates or whether she really knew that her signs were symbols for objects. It was suggested, however, that the way in which Washoe used her signs interactively with other signs might tell how she viewed them. If her combinations exhibited a syntax, Washoe might possess a grammar module similar to our own.

Although at times Washoe signed to herself when she was alone, she most frequently used her signs when humans "talked" to her with signs. Sometimes, her combinations contained components of the combinations that her caretakers had employed. How much of what Washoe signed was imitation of others and how much was her effort to communicate (Terrace, Pettito, Sanders, and Bever 1979; Seidenberg and Pettito 1979)?

At first these issues seemed simple, but it soon became clear that there were major challenges to overcome because the issues drove straight to the heart of what humans call "language." What does it mean to say, "What is on your mind?" What is a mind, and how can it have something "on" it? How can it be known what is "on" someone's mind other than by what the person says or does? Even more problematic is the question whether one might "say something" without having a mind.

Even with young children it is taken for granted that speech is a reflection of the mind—the intentions and information of the speaker. But with Washoe, the question was: Did she have a mind that her language signs could reflect?

If she did not have such a mind, how could her attempts to sign be explained? The behaviorists offered the concept of "instrumental conditioning." Washoe used signs, they said, because of rewards received for so doing. She "spoke" not to express her mind but to get a reward.

As simple and attractive as this explanation seemed, there is something profoundly wrong with it. When we humans speak to express what is on our minds, we do so with the expectation that someone else will understand, and that is rewarding to us. If we did not receive this reward, we would cease to talk. Why should we demand more of an ape?

Humans speak so that they will be understood. If Washoe wanted a banana and she signed to convey this want, did she also want to be understood? Are we risking a double standard—allowing things to be on our minds, but not on Washoe's?

The attempts to determine whether Washoe signed for different reasons than the reasons humans communicate were destined to fail because intent is not an externally observable behavior; it is something one infers on the basis of the purposeful nature of the person speaking. Critics, who opposed the idea that apes could talk, argued that Washoe had no intent to communicate. Researchers who favored the idea argued that intent was self-evident. But no one could pull up a piece of intent and measure it—for Washoe or for a human being. Human beings, of course, could express "meta-intent"—that is, they could say they had intent, and they could describe it. This is a high-level process that does not appear in children until they are approximately four years of age. Thus, the issue of whether Washoe indeed knew what she was saying focused on the presence or absence of syntactical constructions in her utterances.

The willingness to debate the issues of syntactical competency placed the ape-language researchers squarely in the camp of the linguists. By default, linguists assumed that the existence of a grammar module was more than a theoretical construct designed to erect a boundary between ape and man. They assumed that it was a real thing, and they searched for its imprint in the behavior of an ape.

Looking for the elusive grammar module sent animal language down a slippery slope. From the outset, the basic idea was that an essential difference existed in the reasoning capacities of man and animal. The idea that because human beings "taught language" to an animal they could then endow the animal with a reasoning grammatical processor was almost a laughable proposition to the linguist. The kinds of competencies demanded for mind of any sort became the complex embedded and convoluted competencies displayed by the adult human speaker. The animal was not to be admitted to the club of humans unless it behaved precisely as a human. The issue was no longer one of science, but of a human being's self-definition.

LANGUAGE UNDERSTANDING

However, an important difference between Washoe's use of language and human use was ignored in the early rush to determine whether Washoe was producing her utterances with intent. The difference lay not in what Washoe wanted, what she signed, or what she otherwise did; it lay in what she *understood*.

Language is a two-way street, as humans use it. We tell people what is on our minds, and we listen to what is on others' minds. We confirm our understandings by our language and actions. If there is little or no indication that a listener is understanding what we are trying to say, we soon move on to another activity or listener. Thus, if someone tells us they want a banana (or a hug, love, understanding, sympathy, or that they want us to change an opinion), we respond with an action in kind. In the simplest case, if someone straightforwardly asks for a banana and we have one, we might offer it—or sell it.

In this way Washoe's use of language differed from that of humans, and to this area, rather than to syntax, is where the debate should have turned. Washoe was adept at asking for a banana, but unable to give one on request. Indeed, she was not accomplished in listening or giving anything on specific request. Her language was that of production only—an announcer, a requester, a speaker—not someone who listened to the needs others. For Washoe, language had one function—requesting others to do what she wanted. Thus, half of human language communication, *listening* or *comprehending*, was missing. Washoe had learned to speak, but not to listen.

Studies of child language, prior to the work with Washoe, had focused on what children said, not on their understanding. Understanding, if considered at all, was considered merely a reliable companion of competence in speaking.

The problem of understanding and responding was not limited to Washoe; it characterized two other chimpanzees, Sarah (Premack 1976) and Lana (Rumbaugh 1977). Premack ascribed comprehension as something that predates language and then dismissed need for its further study.

But comprehension is complex because it requires assumptions regarding the perspectives of others, notably by the speaker. The speaker talks with the assumption that the listeners want to learn about what the speaker has to say. The listener attends on the assumption that the speaker has something to offer that they do not know and that they want to know. In brief, comprehension requires a "theory of mind."

Not only does language as humans know it require comprehension, it is through comprehension that language is acquired (Bates 1993). One hears what is said, and one begins to match sounds with the meaning and intent that is inherent in the mind of the speaker. To do this, one must learn to separate the speech stream into words and syllables, to determine the relationship between strings of these units, and to determine what meaning is being attached to the words by the utterer. Because statements can be said in many different ways, and generally are, it is not clear how a child comes to discern the meaning of the utterances of others. What is known is that the capacity is not systematically taught by the parents or caretakers.

APES LEARN TO LISTEN

Recognition that the capacity to comprehend utterances of others was central to the development of true linguistic skills came with the first attempts to get two chimpanzees to communicate with one another (Savage-Rumbaugh 1986). The studies initially involved two male chimpanzees, Sherman and Austin, who had learned lexical symbols.

Sherman and Austin, like Washoe and Lana, could "speak their minds" in that they had learned to ask for bananas, soft drinks, candy, tickling, trips outdoors, and so forth. As long as their utterances were directed to humans their language functioned very well. Humans listened and responded by giving the foods or other events the chimps requested.

But the situation was quite different when the chimpanzees were encouraged to request foods or other activities from each other. Suddenly, it became clear that language entailed a lot more than simply speaking. "Talking" on the part of one ape did not entail listening and responding on the part of the other. Communication with a another chimpanzee was a one-way street.

Learning to "talk" did not lead to language-like interactions between apes. Training had to begin anew to foster comprehension rather than production. Sherman and Austin had to learn not only to interpret what another ape said, but to intuit why he/she had said it and to cooperate with the utterance. To precipitate language between apes we had to bring about an understanding of the reasons for language as well as the capacity for language.

We quickly found that instruction became successful only to the degree that language coordinated behaviors between individuals. Language began to manifest itself through a complex process of exchange actions punctuated by speech. We saw that successful language wove a fabric of expectancies and constraints set up by patterns of coordination actions and reactions concerning a theme.

Efforts to generate linguistic communication between apes made it possible to peer through the veil that had shrouded a proper understanding of language for centuries. Language, it appeared, was not about talking or about expressing ourselves; it was about joining actions and attention between speakers. Perhaps the salience of speech had led us to think that language expressed the mind, but, in effect, it patterned inter-individual action.

From attempting to establish language between apes, we realized that words were not linked to things but to the coordination of actions on things. The nature of the linkage lay not in teaching "talking," but in engendering the expected forms of responses to the "talk of others." Because understanding the speech of others was the true key to language, the "conditioning argument" was doomed to fall by the wayside. It is not possible to condition comprehension—because one does not know when comprehension occurs—to reinforce it. Comprehension, like intent, is often silent. We only know that comprehension exists when the recipient of our utterances responds as we expect or anticipate. Nevertheless, we are also aware that comprehension can exist independently of such responses.

The critics had been partly correct because, although Washoe, Sarah, and Lana had mastered various pieces of the language pie, persons who interacted with the apes were still left with the unsettled feeling that the overall effect of the apes' capacities fell painfully short of what happens when humans converse. The feelings of "falling short" were generated because Sarah, Washoe, and Lana failed to comprehend and respond to the language of others; they succeeded only in conveying their own desires. This result was not the apes' failing, but a failure of the people who taught them because comprehension had been taken for granted, assumed a by-product of production, rather than the key to language itself. Never understanding what others were doing with language left Sarah, Washoe, and Lana in a communicative vacuum. They could express their desires, but they could not learn more language by listening to others. They could learn only if new words were rewarded by designed consequences.

Sherman and Austin were different. They could talk to each other because they learned to incorporate comprehension into their symbol cosmology. Sherman could listen and respond when Austin requested things or assistance, and Austin could do the same. The effectiveness of their communications on one another were astutely monitored, and misunderstandings were corrected by restatement. For example, when Austin did not understand the food or tool Sherman requested, Sherman "read" his puzzled expression and clarified his intent by pointing to the object. If Austin gave him other than the requested tool, Sherman discarded it and clarified his request.

However, their exchanges had limits. Sherman and Austin did not discuss the "state of the world" or past events. Their exchanges were generally focused on immediate needs. Yet they clearly understood the basic power of symbols to communicate with each other and how to use the symbols to convey information of relevance to them. Thus, when Sherman saw and heard a partially anesthetized ape moaning as it was transported on a gurney, past the building, he rushed inside to the keyboard and announced to people and to Austin, "Scare outdoors."

Such events are often dismissed by critics as anecdotes because they have not been planned by the experimenter and are not repeated. However, the criticism misses the mark. To expect that Sherman would run in with obvious fear and say, "Scare outdoors," each time in which a moaning chimpanzee is carried past the building is no more reasonable than to expect that humans would make an identical exclamation in response to recurrent events. The need for communication would vanish because when an utterance is predictable, it has little information value.

LANGUAGE WITHOUT TRAINING

Work with additional apes has taken language research even further, not because the other apes have been more intelligent, but because the realization that the key to language lay in comprehension led to a new way of permitting language transactions to occur.

Because language is about learning to comprehend the connections between the behaviors, the expectancies, and the utterances generated by others, not the establishment of large vocabularies; four additional apes (Kanzi, Mulika, Panbanisha, and Panzee) were introduced to symbols by an entirely different route. These apes received no formal instruction in language. Instead, the language they acquired came through being reared in a language-rich environment (Savage-Rumbaugh et al. 1993). Each ape was spoken to, in English, in a manner intended to encourage an understanding and anticipation of daily events, such as trips in the forest to locate food caches, and of general daily activities, such as feeding, playing, grooming, cleaning, and watching television. Coordinated with speech was use of a keyboard with keys embossed with colorful geometric word symbols (lexigrams) (Rumbaugh 1977). Whenever possible, a spoken word was coupled with the speaker's pointing to its lexigram equivalent on the keyboard.

These conditions are all that is needed for apes to acquire an understanding of spoken language, and they are far superior to methods that entail discrete training trials, such as the methods used with Lana. Notably, by this kind of rearing (essentially from birth) the ability to comprehend spoken words becomes established—a skill never instated in Sherman and Austin despite their capacity to comprehend and employ lexigrams in a communicative way.

The consequence of the method of cultivating language through rearing is that the ape comes to understand speech at a level comparable to that of a two- to three-year-old child. The understanding includes past and future verb tenses, syntactical constructions that entail embedded phrases, and word order. This kind of rearing also enables the apes to spontaneously learn to discriminate among hundreds of word symbols (lexigrams) on the keyboard, learn the equivalence between those symbols and spoken words, and to use lexigrams to communicate information about their desires for food, drink, specific companions, and places to visit.

As in normal language acquisition by human children, this type of rearing causes the apes' language comprehension to far outpace language production. New four- to eight-word sentences can be accurately understood. On the other hand, the constructions made by the ape are generally limited to a single word plus a gesture and sometimes a vocal sound (Greenfield and Savage-Rumbaugh 1991, 1993). Their language construction is limited, in part, by limitations imposed by the keyboard (e.g., it takes time to locate each symbol, which interferes with the capacity to use multiple symbols in rapid sequence—for both humans and apes).

REALIZING THAT OTHERS "THINK"

Apes reared with exposure to spoken language and printed symbols are able to follow and easily participate in three- and four-way conversations that deal with the intentions, actions, and knowledge states of different agents. The apes constantly impute states of mind to others and recognize the value of communication in altering the perceptions of others. They instigate games of pretend, and they hide objects and themselves from others.

In a formal test for "theory of mind" (Premack and Woodruff 1978), the bonobo, Panbanisha, demonstrated that she could answer questions about what another agent (person or ape) thought was hidden in a box. She could say what another party thought even though she knew that the person's thinking was not an accurate reflection of the actual contents of the box. That is, she could evaluate the contents of another's mind independently of the contents of reality. She could also manipulate the contents of other minds. For example, she scared Kanzi by telling him that there was a snake close by, when there was no snake.

Not only can Panbanisha understand and answer questions appropriately, but she can also understand and comment on the fact that one party played a deceitful trick on another. When Sue took candy out of a box and put a bug in its place and then gave a caretaker the box supposedly filled with candy, Panbanisha informed Sue that she was being "bad."

This level of understanding requires far more complex capacities than a syntactical processor. For example, one can decode the relationship between the words in a question such as "What does party A think is in the box?", with a processor. However, one cannot answer the question without an awareness that "think" refers to party A and that the question is not referring to what *actually* is in the box, but to what party A observed in the box at an earlier time and failed to observe being removed. That is, the question is dealing with party A's state of mind, which is different from that of the ape who is observing party A and the events occurring. The capacity to understand that the perceptions and knowledge states of different agents may differ and that the word "think" refers to nonobservable perceptions requires a complex understanding that far surpasses the syntactical structure of the sentence itself.

The structure of a question such as, "What does A think is in the box?" is similar in terms of syntactical structure to a question used by Premack: "What Mary give Sarah?" To solve the question, Sarah needed only to select one token when Mary gave her a banana and another when Mary gave her an apple. However, to answer a question about what party A thinks is in a box, Panbanisha must realize that she needs to differentiate between the caretaker's knowledge and that of her own. Nothing to reveal the necessity of this understanding is present in the syntactical construction of the question. Sytactically, the structure of "What does X think is in the box?" is identical with that of the question "What does X see that is in the box? Yet these

E. Sue Savage-Rumbaugh and Duane M. Rumbaugh: Emergent Processes in Apes and Humans questions call for completely different answers—answers not based on syntax, but on the previously observed experiences of X and the proper inferences drawn about the thoughts of X as a result of the experiences. There is no adequate method for instructing an ape or child with regard to forming speculations regarding the contents of others' minds as a function of their observed experiences. Such sophisticated judgments cannot emerge from "trial and error" learning. Syntactical explanations of the question and/or the answer can never satisfactorily characterize the true complexity of a language task such as the one Panbanisha coped with.

It is astonishing that apes can do these things easily, even when their language production skills are typically limited to the use of one or two symbols at a time. An ape that does not understand language cannot do these things so far as we know. Do apes without language know that different people can have different perceptions and experiences of events? We do not even know whether apes are able to view groups of activities (e.g., hiding something in a box, taking it out while party A is not looking, replacing it with something else, then asking a question about party A's state of mind) as related events, much less events that are connected differently in party A's mind than in their own.

Language leads to the formation of a consensual interpretation by a group, which results in a psychological "connectedness" concerning such events. Perhaps simply by saying, "Ok, let's do this while Party A is not watching," a connectedness occurs between what Party A is now doing (i.e., not watching) and what events are now happening. Does the connectedness enable inferences that might not otherwise occur? For an ape that cannot understand spoken sentences, we currently have no straightforward means to ascertain what connectedness they assign to events and no means to query them about their interpretation.

WINDOWS TO OTHERS' MINDS

Language-competent apes *can* be asked such complex questions. The fact that we do not need to train them to understand human questions reveals that their language competence functions to structure a joint perception and interpretation of the world. Coordinated action thus becomes an option. Such events are windows to the basic function, power, and value of language. That apes who have been exposed every day to language in their early rearing can peer through the windows in the same way humans do tells us that, in measure, apes and humans can share a common world (Rumbaugh, Savage-Rumbaugh, and Washburn 1996).

It is no longer reasonable to view the communications among such creatures in nature as "instinctive" and necessarily devoid of meaning or intentionality. It is quite likely the focus has been so exclusively on syntax and human speech that we may have missed the natural origins and evolution of language and, thus, failed to realize its existence in other species. By defining language by the human standard of speech and writing, we have risked misunderstanding the essence and function of communication in other animals.

Animal language research has taken us a long way toward understanding who we are and what language is. Names are more than instrumental responses or paired-associate members for things and agents. Once a name is given to something, it can begin to carve the world into the divisions of the name giver. Thus, we may identify different sorts of cheeses, different sorts of animals, or different sorts of snow. Once we have "named" these things, we may then begin to ask "causative" questions that can generate detailed knowledge. "Why did this type of snow fall?" "Why did this sort of grass grow in this climate and ground?" "Why are these birds and plants different from those?" Names can encourage distinctions and similarities among things of the world and encourage the systematic building of knowledge.

Even by giving a name such as "thought" to a state we experience but cannot see, we have, in a sense, changed the experience from an intangible to a tangible entity. We can then proceed to differentiate periods of "thought" and "nonthought" even though we have no real means of ascertaining whether "nonthought" actually exists. By inventing a word such as "think," we are encouraged to determine why, how, and when we "think." In due course, we might then ask whether thought as a process is shared with at least some kinds of animals.

Naming is a core principle of language and of mathematics. We invent a word, such as "indivisible" to describe things we cannot reduce. We then apply this concept to another concept, such as to a line, and find how it applies. We even learn that language permits us to formulate questions that cannot be answered if we apply concepts or names beyond the domain they were intended to embrace. For example, the concept of "one" and the concept of "plus one," leads inevitably to the concept of infinity. The concept of infinity did not occur initially, but eventually was derived through the application of the concept of addition. We cannot know infinity in a first-hand manner, but we benefit in our everyday lives by having it as a construction, even though we might not understand its mathematics. Thus, linguistically, we can construct abstract concepts from simpler ones that map everyday distinctions.

TOWARD A SCIENCE OF ANIMAL CONSCIOUSNESS

Thus, language is nothing more and nothing less than the uses to which it is applied. As humans, we are particularly proud of the embedded and recursive structures that characterize the syntax of our language and we have assumed that such structures exist *only* in our language. Until we allow the possibility that other creatures have the ability to learn to communicate complex messages, we will be ill equipped ever to discern similar syntactical complexities, if, indeed, they exist. That Kanzi and Panbanisha so readily came to understand the use of syntactic devices reveals that these facets of the human linguistic system are not beyond the reach of apes. Possibly these linguistic facets exist in their natural communications too, as is strongly suggested by the evidence that bonobo groups traveling through the brush systematically bend vegetation in an obvious manner at junctures or chosen points to leave a message, for following groups, regarding which trail has been taken (Savage-Rumbaugh, Williams, Furuichi, and Kano 1996).

If we are to understand the possible language skills of animals in nature, we should not assume that animal language must be exactly like that of humans and encode the kinds of things that are of special interest to humans. Animal language may be expressed in media apart from vocalizations and gestures; it may use natural materials, such as vegetation, to communicate topics that are germane to the cohesiveness of the community.

Animals likely classify the world in ways that are substantially different from ways that humans use. For instance, humans recognize a relationship between the movement of the moon and the tide. By contrast, animals may sense a relationship between the patterns of movement of insects and the ripening of fruit in a remote location, a relationship that humans may not notice. Because we do not sense this relationship, the animals' encoding system may have little or no meaning for us.

There has been a readiness to conclude that because animals do not typically point at and name objects, they have no language. What we may have overlooked is that there are other sorts of things that are much more complicated and more important to convey linguistically and that many of these other things are not "point-at-able."

Given what we have now learned from apes such as Kanzi and Panbanisha, we should no longer assume that other species lack language and conscious thought. We should extent to animals the possibility that their existence includes living, thinking, and experiencing events. The nature of experiencing can vary between species, between individuals, and between groups within a species. Understanding the nature and parameters of the variation is central to the study of animal consciousness.

CONCLUSION

The basic premise of the new paradigm must be that animal consciousness is extant, that for some species, consciousness may be similar to the consciousness that humans experience. Consciousness may be an emergent characteristic[1] of many life-forms. Unless we allow that consciousness may be present in animals, we will never take the critical steps of considering how and under what circumstances consciousness is manifested in behavior.

We also should recognize that the researcher who studies consciousness in animals cannot not necessarily work in the traditional stance, that is, as a detached observer. No two observers can be expected to achieve complete agreement or to infer precisely the same dimensions or processes. In addition, no one observer will see the same reality at two different times.

Consciousness is surely ever changing, whether the consciousness of humans or others. But questions pertaining to consciousness are far too important to say, as others have traditionally said, "Consciousness? We won't study that, ever, because we currently can't do so with scientific precision."

"Minds" do not have "things in them" to be discovered; minds are compositions of the experiences of interactions across time. The experiences of Kanzi, for instance, were not his alone. Rather, they were also part of all who have interacted with him. Others' perceptions and inferences shaped his awareness and knowledge states, and his shaped theirs.

From joint interactions, on the basis of communication and the building of consensual perceptions of events with Kanzi, Panbanisha, and others, we have been able to obtain many means to verify that the understanding of one party can indeed be valid for another. The methods of this new science remain to be developed, but the essence of what the methods will be lies in the situations which give rise to the learning of a human language by a bonobo. The understanding and use of communication is *central* to achieving shared perspectives and constructions of a presumed real world.

We should anticipate that there are no final answers to questions that pertain to animal consciousness. If that point is acknowledged, even partial answers will provide helpful steps along the way to understanding consciousness in comparative perspective.

ACKNOWLEDGMENTS

Supported by grants from the National Institute of Child Health and Human Development (HD-06016), from the National Aeronautics and Space Administration (NAG2-438), and by the College of Arts and Sciences, Georgia State University. Special appreciation is extended to Mr. and Mrs. Steve Woodruff and to Dr. Stephen Draper for their commitment to the future of the Language Research Center.

NOTE

1. See Rumbaugh et al. (1996) for a definition of emergents.

REFERENCES

Bates, E. 1993. Comprehension and production in early language environment: A commentary on Savage-Rumbaugh, Murphy, Sevcik, Brakke, Williams, and Rumbaugh, "Language comprehension in ape and child." *Monographs of the Society for Research in Child Development* 58(3–4):222–242.

Churchland, P. S. 1986. *Neurophilosology: Toward a Unified Science of the Mind/Brain*. Cambridge: MIT Press.

Churchland, P. 1995. *The Engine of Reason, the Seat of the Soul*. Cambridge: MIT Press.

Chomsky, N. 1988. *Language and Problems of Knowledge: The Managua Lectures*. Cambridge: MIT Press.

Darwin, C. 1859. *The Origin of the Species*. London: Murray.

Descartes, R. 1956. *Discourse on Method*. (1637). Reprinted, New York: Liberal Arts Press.

Gardner, B. T., and R. A. Gardner. 1971. Two-way communication with an infant chimpanzee. In A. M. Schrier and F. Stollnitz, eds., *Behavior of Non-Human Primates*, vol. 4. New York: Academic.

Greenfield, P., and E. S. Savage-Rumbaugh. 1991. Imitation, grammatical development and the invention of protogrammar by an ape. In N. A. Krasnegor, D. M. Rumbaugh, R. L. Schiefelbusch, and M. Studdert-Kennedy, eds., *Biological and Behavior Determinants of Language Development*. Hillsdale, NJ: Erlbaum, pp. 235–258.

Greenfield, P., and E. S. Savage-Rumbaugh. (1993). Comparing communicative competence in child and chimp: The pragmatics of repetition. *Journal of Child Language* 20:1–26.

Griffin, D. 1976. *The Question of Animal Awareness*. New York: Rockefeller University Press.

McFarland, D. 1984. *The Oxford Companion to Animal Behavior*. New York: Oxford University Press.

Pinker, S. 1994. *The Language Instinct: How the Mind Creates Language*. New York: Harper-Collins.

Premack, D., 1976. *Intelligence in Ape and Man*. Hillsdale, NJ: Erlbaum.

Premack, D., and G. Woodruff. 1978. Does the chimpanzee have a theory of mind? *The Behavioral and Brain Sciences* 4, 515–526.

Romanes, G. J. 1898. *Mental Evolution in Animals*. New York: Appleton-Century-Crofts.

Rumbaugh, D. M. 1977. *Language Learning by a Chimpanzee*. New York: Academic.

Rumbaugh, D. M., and E. S. Savage-Rumbaugh. 1994. Language in comparative perspective. In N. J. Mackintosh, ed, *Animal Language and Cognition*. New York: Academic Press, pp. 307–333.

Rumbaugh, D. M., E. S., Savage-Rumbaugh, and D. A. Washburn. 1996. Toward a new outlook on primate learning and behavior: Complex learning and emergent processes in comparative perspective. *Japanese Psychological Research*. 3(3):113–125.

Rumbaugh, D. M., D. A. Washburn, and W. Hillix. 1996. Respondents, operants, and emergents: Toward an integrated perspective on behavior. In K. Pribram and J. King, eds., *Learning as a Self-Organizing Process*. Hillsdale, NJ: Erlbaum.

Savage-Rumbaugh, E. S. 1986. *Ape Language: From Conditioned Response to Symbol*. New York: Columbia University Press.

Savage-Rumbaugh, E. S., and R. Lewin. 1994. *Kanzi: An Ape at the Brink of Human Mind*. New York: Wiley.

Savage-Rumbaugh, E. S., J. Murphy, R. Sevcik, K. E. Brakke, S. L. Williams, and D. M. Rumbaugh, 1993. Language comprehension in ape and child. *Monographs of the Society for Research in Child Development* 58(3 and 4):1–221.

Savage-Rumbaugh, E. S., S. Shanker, and T. Taylor. 1997. *Philosophical Primatology: Apes and Language*. New York: Oxford University Press.

Savage-Rumbaugh, E. S., S. L. Williams, T. Furuichi, and T. Kano. 1996. Paniscus branches out. In B. McGrew, L. Marchant, and T. Nishida, eds., *Great Ape Societies*. London: Cambridge University Press.

Sebeok, T. A., and R. Rosenthal. 1981. The Clever Hans phenomenon: Communication with horses, whales, apes, and people. *Annals of the New York Academy of Sciences* 364.

Seidenberg, M. S., and L. A. Pettito. 1979. Signing behavior in apes: A critical review. *Cognition* 7:177–215.

Sibley, C. G., and J. E. Ahlquist. 1987. DNA hybridization evidence of hominoid phylogeny: Results from an expanded data set. *Journal of Molecular Evolution* 26:99–121.

Terrace, H. S., L. A. Pettito, R. J. Sanders, and T. G. Bever. 1979. Can an ape create a sentence? *Science* 206:891–900.

Wallman, J. 1992. *Aping Language*. New York: Cambridge University Press.

Wise, S. M. 1995. How non-human animals were trapped in a nonexistent universe. *Animal Law* 15:15–43.

Wise, S. M. 1996. How a nonexistent universe created then sustained the perpetual legal thinghood of non-human animals. *Boston College Environmental Affairs Law Review* 23:471–546.

FURTHER READING

Corbey, R. and B. Theunissen. 1995. *Ape, Man, Apeman: Changing Views since 1600*. Leiden: Department of Prehistory, Leiden University.

Rogoff, R. 1990. *Apprenticeship in Thinking*. New York: Oxford University Press.

Tuttle, R. H. 1986. *Apes of the World: Their Social Behavior, Communication, Mentality and Ecology*. Park Ridge, NJ: Noyes.

Wrangham, R. W., W. C. McGrew, F. B. M. de Waal, and P. G. Heltne. 1994. *Chimpanzee Cultures*. Cambridge: Harvard University Press.

47 Cognition and Communication in Dolphins: A Question of Consciousness

Diana Reiss

Are dolphins conscious? They must be. Some degree of consciousness must be operating for dolphins to survive and function in their physical and social environment.

Rather than asking whether dolphins are conscious, instead, we need to investigate the nature of their conscious awareness. Consciousness can be defined as a state of being aware of what is happening around oneself, and thus according to this definition, dolphins demonstrate a certain level of consciousness.

Numerous studies of sensation and perception in dolphins have documented their abilities in avoiding, detecting, discriminating, and reporting the presence or absence of sensory stimuli (Herman 1988). On a kinesthetic level, dolphins demonstrate an awareness of the location and position of their bodies relative to objects and events in the external world. However, when we question whether dolphins or any other species show evidence of consciousness, we are implicitly referring to other degrees of consciousness, but what these other degrees entail is unclear even for human processes.

Although we all experience consciousness, formalizing a working definition of it is difficult. Armstrong (1981), Bunge (1980), and others made a useful distinction between awareness and consciousness to address levels of consciousness beyond sensory, kinesthetic, and perceptual awareness. Awareness, these authors claim, involves sensation and perception of an object or an event remembered from the past, perceived in the present, or anticipated in the future and requires a special level of self-awareness beyond the sensory or kinesthetic level. Awareness involves self-reflection: the knowledge that an organism knows that it is doing something, the knowledge that it is thinking and feeling something. This is close to Ryle's (1949) distinction between an organism's "knowing how" to do something and "knowing that" it is doing something.

This view of consciousness is helpful to cognitive ethologists in formulating criteria for evaluating animal behavior, but it still leaves the problem of determining intentionality in another species. Because we do not have access to the mental states of other species, how do we know whether a member of another species really "knows" what it is doing or why? We infer that other humans are conscious because we believe from our own subjective experiences that we are conscious and we share languages that enable us to communicate about our perceptions.

As early as the fourth century B.C., Greek philosophers viewed the processes of rational thought (*ratio*) and language (*oratio*) as inextricably linked; thus, species devoid of language were considered to be without thought. The Cartesian view of animals as unconscious automata further bolstered the idea of "unconscious animals." The behaviorists effectively argued that consciousness was far too vague to be investigated scientifically, which led them to reject studies of mental states in all animals (Griffin 1992).

With the emergence of the cognitive revolution in the 1950s and a growing interest in attention, memory, language, problem solving, and concept formation, it became increasingly apparent that the behavior of humans and other animals could not be adequately explained solely by traditional behaviorist learning theory.

Comparative neurophysiology shows that basic neural mechanisms are similar in all mammals, which suggests continuity in basic information processing and the reality of cognitive states in other animals (Griffin 1992). However, finding evidence of conscious behavior in nonhuman animals remains difficult because contemporary cognitive ethologists must work with what can be empirically observed in an animal's behavior and are thus challenged to find appropriate measures and frameworks for assessing an animal's information processing and mental states.

Innovative ethological and laboratory studies are now providing compelling evidence for a high degree of complexity and versatility in the communication and behavior of diverse species. Past views that humans are unique as a symbol-and-tool-using species are currently being challenged by reports that highly divergent species such as chimpanzees (Gardner and Gardner 1969; Fouts 1973, Savage-Rumbaugh 1986), African grey parrots (Pepperberg 1981), California sea lions (Schusterman and Krieger 1984), and bottlenose dolphins (Reiss and McCowan 1993; Richards, Woltz and Herman 1984; Herman 1988) can comprehend and produce symbolic codes. Several species have shown varying degrees of tool use (Griffin 1992), and there is increasing evidence for the use of semantic communication in the natural communication systems of nonhuman species (Seyfarth, Cheney and Marler 1980; Owings and Leger 1980). Evidence for conceptual quantitative abilities has been reported in the African grey parrot (Pepperberg 1987) and the chimpanzee (Boysen and Berntson 1989).

Although our longitudinal research program—investigating the cognitive and communicative abilities of bottlenose dolphins (*Tursiops truncatus*)—does not directly address dolphin consciousness, it has provided data supporting the view that the large-brained dolphin shows behavioral characteristics of perceptual awareness, spontaneous learning, versatile behavior, anticipatory behavior, and methodological testing of contingencies.

Bottlenose dolphins are highly social mammals widely distributed throughout the world in temperate and tropical waters. Longitudinal field studies have indicated a fission–fusion type of social structure that shows social complexity rivaling that found in chimpanzee societies (Wells, Scott, and Irvine 1987; Wursig 1979; Connor, Smolker, and Richards 1992). Although variations in demographics, social structure, and behavioral ecology may vary in different populations, the formation and maintenance of social relationships and coalitions seems critical in the lives of these mammals.

Dolphins have demonstrated many cognitive abilities, such as memory capacity and the comprehension of artificial codes (Richards, Wolz, and Herman 1984; Herman 1988), comparable to those of chimpanzees. Bottlenose dolphins have a rich vocal repertoire that has been broadly categorized into three classes of signals: broadband, short duration clicks (used in echolocation), wide-band pulsed sounds, and narrow-band, frequency-modulated whistles (Herman and Tavolga 1988). Dolphins are the only nonhuman mammals that have shown strong evidence of vocal learning and vocal mimicry (Richards, Wolz, and Herman 1984; Tyack 1986; Reiss and McCowan 1993; McCowan and Reiss 1995). Under experimental conditions dolphins have demonstrated a proclivity for vocal mimicry of both conspecific whistles and nonspecies-specific sounds (Richards, Wolz, and Herman 1984; Reiss and McCowan 1993).

Although dolphins have a rich vocal repertoire, whether they use a referential communication system is unclear. In an experimental study conducted at our laboratory with four dolphins, we reported their spontaneous acquisition of new vocalizations and the subsequent use of these signals in behaviorally appropriate contexts. The results of the study provide evidence for perceptual awareness in this species.

SPONTANEOUS VOCAL MIMICRY AND LEARNING THROUGH USE OF KEYBOARDS

An interactive underwater keyboard system was designed to investigate the functional and developmental aspects of dolphin vocal learning and to provide dolphins with an environmental enrichment activity in which they could gain rudimentary control over certain aspects of their environment.[1] The use of an interactive keyboard system to train chimpanzees in artificial language skills was pioneered by Rumbaugh, Gill, and Von Glaserfeld (1973).

In the course of a two-year study, four captive bottlenose dolphins, two adult females, and their one-year-old male offspring were presented with an underwater keyboard that displayed visual forms that could be used to obtain specific items (e.g., balls, rings, rubs from humans). The dolphins' use of specific keys resulted in a systematic chain of events—a specific, computer-generated whistle followed immediately after use of specific keys, which was followed by the presentation of a particular object or activity.

Although most investigators train dolphins to make forced-choice discriminations through food reinforcement, our approach provided animals with a free-choice system, which allowed them to freely interact with a self-reinforcing system without explicit training procedures other than the temporal chain of events described above. The keyboard was designed to provide

Diana Reiss: Cognition and Communication in Dolphins: A Question of Consciousness the dolphins with keys that the dolphins could physically manipulate and with computer-generated whistles that they could vocally reproduce. By observing and recording their behavior while they interacted with this system, we were able to elucidate more clearly the role and process of mimicry in dolphin vocal learning.

Although this system was not designed to elicit vocal mimicry, the whistles could be easily perceived and reproduced by the dolphins, which facilitated their ability to process, produce, and remember the signals. The computer-generated whistles were designed to be similar to the frequency and temporal parameters of natural dolphin whistles but different from the actual frequency modulation (the actual whistle contours) of the whistles in the repertoires of the dolphins in the study. This precaution was deemed necessary because vocal mimicry has been operationally defined as copying an otherwise improbable act or utterance (Thorpe 1963; Richards, Wolz, and Herman 1984) rather than a mere elicitation of species-specific whistles (Andrew 1962).

MIMICRY AND PRODUCTIVE USE OF WHISTLES

Our analysis of audio and video recordings of experimental sessions revealed that the dolphins had begun to spontaneously mimic and produce facsimiles of the computer-generated model sounds, which provided strong evidence for vocal learning in this species. The term "mimicry" was designated to represent facsimiles of the model sounds emitted by dolphins immediately after the model sound, and the term "production" was used to indicate when facsimiles were emitted by dolphins in other contexts and at times not immediately after the model sound.

After only 19 exposures to the "ball" whistle, an interesting pattern of vocal mimicry was recorded. In three successive trials, one young male dolphin reproduced different aspects of the model sound; he first mimicked the end of the ball whistle, then the beginning of the whistle, and finally the entire harmonic structure of the whistle. From the onset of mimicry, the dolphins showed a tendency to mimic and reproduce the absolute frequency and temporal parameters of the model sounds and to compress or expand the temporal parameters of their whistled versions.

Similar patterns were observed in the initial mimicry of other model sounds, and far fewer acoustic exposures were required prior to the onset of initial mimicry in these cases. For example, the "rub" whistle was mimicked after nine exposures and the "ring" whistle after two exposures. In addition, the dolphins began to spontaneously produce facsimiles of the model sounds before they used the corresponding key. The first instance of productive use occurred in the same session in which vocal mimicry began. This session was marked by a multiplicity of contexts in which the facsimiles were emitted. For example, during this session, the following sequence was recorded. One young male used the "ball" key and immediately mimicked the model sound. The dolphin remained at the keyboard and interacted with the ball it obtained. The dolphin produced two instances of the ball whistle while it pushed the ball about in the vicinity of the keyboard. The dolphin then reapproached the keyboard, produced the ball whistle, immediately used the ball key on the keyboard, and swam away with the ball that it subsequently received.

During the first year of this study, the amount of vocal mimicry in relation to production followed a consistent relation across keyboard sessions (simple regression, $R^2 = 0.539$, F test, $P = 0.0118$). Across all sessions, vocal mimicry ($N = 165$) was about 19 percent higher than production ($N = 139$). In contrast, during the second year, the occurrence of vocal mimicry in relation to production showed no consistent relation across sessions (simple regression, $R^2 = 0.047$, F test, $p = 0.8777$). However, in this later stage of the research program, vocal production ($N = 210$) was slightly higher than vocal mimicry ($N = 19$). This was a significant increase in the ratio of productions to vocal mimicry (χ^2 test, $p = 0.0001$), and productions were 13.2 times more likely to occur in year 2 than in year 1 (odds ratio, 13.2; range, 10.1–17.1, 95 percent confidence interval).

NEW COMBINATION WHISTLES

Analysis of keyboard sessions during the second year of the study revealed that the dolphins had spontaneously begun to produce a new sound that appeared to be a combination of the ball- and ring-model sounds combined into one continuous whistle. A minimal delay of 0.3 sec between successive computer-generated whistles precluded the possibility of more than one model sound being produced in a continuous manner. Thus, the emergence of this apparent combination could not have been acquired through vocal mimicry. Producing the new combination persisted during the second year, and a total of 28 such whistle types were recorded, primarily in the context of a new pattern of interaction with balls and rings that also emerged during the same time period. The new behavior involved the dolphins holding both objects in their mouths or interacting with a ball and ring simultaneously in various manners.

CONTEXTUALLY APPROPRIATE USE OF WHISTLES

Analysis of behavioral narratives recorded during keyboard sessions during the second year enabled us to determine the contextual use of the whistle production and mimicry. As noted above, the dolphins were producing whistles much more often than they were mimicking during the second year. Our analysis revealed that they were also using whistle facsimiles in behaviorally appropriate contexts:

1. In a total of 92 ball productions, 74 (80 percent) were emitted in contexts of ball play

2. Of 64 ring productions, 47 (73 percent) were emitted during ring play

3. Of 5 rub productions, all (100 percent) were produced during contexts of physical rubbing between the dolphin and investigators

4. Of 28 instances of productions of the novel ring-ball combination whistle, 23 (82 percent) were emitted during simultaneous ring and ball play

The results of this study provide compelling evidence for vocal learning by this species and for the ability of dolphins to spontaneously acquire new vocal signals, to learn associations between new acoustic signals and specific objects or actions, and to use these signals in new, appropriate behavioral contexts in the absence of explicit training. The contexts in which the dolphins interpolated instances of mimicry and production—as evidenced by facsimiles preceding, following, and often overlapping the model sounds— can be viewed as the model sounds providing auditory input and feedback in comparison with the dolphins' own renditions of the model sounds.

Furthermore, results of our study are inconsistent with results reported in previous studies of vocal learning (Richards, Wolz, and Herman 1984; Sigurdson 1989) in which dolphins were trained to reproduce and acquire new vocal signals by traditional shaping procedures and food reinforcement. In these studies, the investigators selectively reinforced and shaped the acoustic parameters (e.g., duration and frequency modulation) that the dolphins were to imitate, and their subjects required approximately 1000 exposures to model sounds before vocal mimicry was achieved. In contrast, the dolphins in our study determined the type of input, the frequency of input, and the acoustic parameters they would imitate and acquired the signals much more rapidly, appearing to incorporate the signals into their repertoire. Our methodology may more closely simulate learning processes in a social environment and thus produce more rapid and effective learning by this species. By having more degrees of freedom than are given in a traditional training approach, the dolphins seemed to take an active role in the learning process.

The results of this study provide behavioral evidence that dolphins are aware of acoustic and visual stimuli in their environment and that they have a proclivity to develop associations between stimuli that occur in consistent and temporally related patterns. The dolphins' use of new whistles in new behaviorally appropriate contexts provides suggestive evidence that dolphins are aware of relationships among various stimuli. The apparent development and awareness of relationships among environmental stimuli without explicit training is suggestive but inconclusive evidence of a level of consciousness in this species.

We focused on the productive skills of the dolphins, but other investigators have studied receptive skills of dolphins and have reported semantic comprehension and "sentence comprehension" of artificial codes in the same species (Richards, Wolz, and Herman 1984; Herman 1987). Further research is needed to determine whether the strong associations between stimuli are referential.

MANIPULATIVE PLAY BY DOLPHINS: AN INDICATOR OF CONSCIOUSNESS?

Although nonhanded, dolphins show manipulative abilities in using their mouths, pectoral fins, or tail flukes to carry, move, or interact with objects in their environment. Several years ago, the head dolphin trainer at Marine World Africa USA in Vallejo, California (where our research laboratory is located) described an interesting behavioral pattern he had observed in one of the exhibition dolphins. Occasionally, paper or plastic debris blew into the dolphin pools, and he had trained a dolphin to retrieve the items for a food reward. On one occasion he noticed that the dolphin continuously retrieved small pieces of brown paper, each time receiving a food reward. Suspecting something odd, the trainer subsequently discovered that a brown paper bag was lodged in a crevice in the pool and the dolphin was ripping off small pieces, retrieving them one at a time. The trainer speculated that the dolphin was aware of what it was doing and was intentionally bringing back small pieces to maximize its rewards.

Such cases fill the dolphin folklore, but more parsimonious explanations can be offered to explain the behavior. First, perhaps only small pieces could be pulled away one at a time or perhaps the trainer had inadvertently reinforced the behavior after the dolphin unintentionally retrieved just part of the bag. I relate this anecdote to stress that without complete knowledge of the environmental history of a particular animal, it is difficult to argue that this was an intentional act. Even if the dolphin continued to display this behavior, it could be argued that it had been inadvertently trained to do so. It is difficult to demonstrate univocal intentionality and conscious thought from complex-looking behaviors.

In contrast to this scenario, we have previously described and reported a behavior pattern of manipulative play by dolphins that seems clear evidence for dolphins exhibiting conscious acts (Reiss 1988). During systematic observations of dolphins, we observed numerous behavioral sequences in which dolphins demonstrated anticipatory actions, an awareness of the contingencies of their past actions, and an awareness of the contingencies of future acts.

Several dolphins at the exhibition and research pools were quite proficient in producing their own objects of play, called "bubble rings." It has been well documented that dolphins play with objects in their environment, and other reports of manipulative bubble ring production have recently been reported and described (Marten, Shariff, Psarakos, and White 1996). We have observed and documented numerous instances in which individual dolphins swim to the bottom of the pool, stop, and assume a horizontal position. With a sharp upward jerk of the head, they expel a ring of air through their blowhole (the external opening of the nasal passages). This action results in a silvery bubble ring that slowly rises to the water surface. The action closely resembles a person blowing a smoke ring of cigarette smoke. After producing a bubble ring, dolphins show a rich variety of behaviors. For example, they often follow the rings to the surface, sometimes attempting to catch or bite the ring with their mouths just as they reach the surface. Dolphins also rotate their rostrums in a circular motion in the interior of the ring as it rises.

We have also observed many occasions in which a dolphin produces an ill-formed or irregular ring, quickly destroys it with a swipe of the tail flukes, and then quickly returns to the pool bottom and subsequently produces a well-formed ring that is not destroyed. Another observed variation is for a dolphin to blow one ring and then a second ring that rises and intersects with the first ring to form a larger, hoop-sized ring. The dolphin follows the second ring and, when the hoop is formed, swims through it.

On another occasion, we observed several dolphins and a large pilot whale (*Globicephala malaena*) playing. One dolphin in the group produced bubble rings, and the other animals followed the rings to the surface. During a particular sequence, one observing dolphin swam to the pool bottom, retrieved a piece of fish, and placed it in the rising torus. The fish spun violently in the ascending turbulence while the dolphins and pilot whale closely watched the rising objects.

The act of putting pieces of fish in a rising bubble ring requires a sense of timing and planning in advance. As my colleagues and I observed this behavior, we noted that the animals repeated the act several times and they exhibited an intense and prolonged focus of attention to the stimuli. The animals appeared to be testing the contingencies of their behavior and repeating their tests.

The production of a bubble ring itself provides evidence of anticipating and planning a future event. Prior to the stimulus of the ring, the dolphin assumes a specific physical position and voluntarily expels air from its blowhole. It is important to note that breathing in the dolphin, unlike in other mammals, is under voluntary control. The dolphin has to think to breathe, a crucial feature in its adaptation to a totally marine existence. Thus, the act of expelling the air provides evidence of a conscious act. Furthermore, it is not clear how the dolphin forms the ring, but dolphins also release air in different forms, such as bubble streams or bubble bursts. In the case of ring production, the dolphin appears to control both the form and the timing of the release of air. Therefore, the positioning assumed prior to bubble ring production, the production of the bubble ring or sequence of rings, and the testing of contingencies provide evidence of intentionality and awareness of behavior.

CONCLUSION

Clearly, much more complexity and plasticity can be found in the behavior and communication systems of nonhuman animals than was previously thought. More research is needed with diverse species to properly assess the extent to which complex information processing has developed throughout the biological world and to clarify the nature of consciousness in nonhuman minds. The marriage of innovative laboratory studies of animal cognitive abilities with evaluations of animal cognitive abilities in the natural ecological situation seems imperative to promote our understanding of other minds in nature and address the issue of consciousness in the biological world.

NOTE

1. See Reiss and McCowan (1993) for a detailed description of the apparatus, procedures and results.

REFERENCES

Andrew, R. J. 1962. Evolution of intelligence and vocal mimicking. *Science* 137:585–589.

Armstrong, D. M. 1981. *The Nature of Mind and Other Essays*. Ithaca: Cornell University Press.

Boysen, S. T., and G. G. Berntson. 1989. Numerical competence in a chimpanzee (*Pan troglodytes*). *Journal of Comparative Psychology* 103(1):23–30.

Bunge, M. A. 1980. *The Nature of Mind, and Other Essays*. Ithaca: Cornell University Press.

Connor, R. C., R. A. Smolker, and A. F. Richards. 1992. Dolphin alliances and coalitions. In A. H. Harcourt and F. B. M. de Waal, eds., *Coalitions and Alliances in Humans and Other Animals*. Oxford: Oxford University Press, pp. 415–443.

Fouts, R. S. 1973. Acquisition and testing of gestural signs in four young chimpanzees. *Science* 180:978–980.

Gardner, R. A., and B. T. Gardner. 1969. Teaching sign language to a chimpanzee. *Science* 165:664–672.

Herman, L. M. 1987. Receptive competencies of language-trained animals. In J. S. Rosenblatt, C. Beer, M. C. Busnel, and P. J. B. Slater, eds., *Advances in the Study of Behavior*, vol. 17. Petaluma, CA: Academic Press.

Herman, L. M. 1988. Cognitive characteristics of dolphins. In L. M. Herman, ed. *Cetacean Behavior: Mechanisms and Functions*. New York: John Wiley and Sons, pp. 149–210.

Herman, L. M., and W. N. Tavolga. 1988. The communication system of cetaceans. In L. M. Herman, ed. *Cetacean Behavior: Mechanisms and Functions*. New York: John Wiley and Sons, pp. 149–210.

Griffin, D. 1992. *Animal Minds*. Chicago: University of Chicago Press.

Marten, K., K. Shariff, S. Psarakos, and D. White. 1996. Ring bubbles of dolphins. *Scientific American* (August) pp. 83–87.

McCowan, B., and D. Reiss. 1995. Whistle contour development in captive-born infant bottlenose dolphins: A role for learning? *Journal of Comparative Psychology* 109(3):242–260.

Owings, D. H., and D. W. Lager. 1980. Chatter vocalizations of California ground squirrels: Predator and social role-specificity. *Zeitschrift fur Tierpsychologie* 54:163–184.

Pepperberg, I. M. 1981. Functional vocalizations by an African grey parrot (*Psittacus erithacus*). *Zeitschrift fur Tierpsychologie* 55:139–160.

Pepperberg, I. M. 1987. Evidence for conceptual quantitative abilities in the African grey parrot: Labeling cardinal sets. *Ethology* 75:37–61.

Reiss, D. 1988. Can we communicate with other species on this planet: Pragmatics of communication between humanoid and nonhumanoid species. In G. Marx, ed., *Bioastronomy—The Next Steps*. Norwell, MA: Kluwer Academic, pp. 253–264.

Reiss, D., and B. McCowan. 1993. Spontaneous vocal mimicry and evidence for vocal learning. *Journal of Comparative Psychology* 107(3):301–312.

Richards, D. G., J. P. Wolz, and L. M. Herman. 1984. Vocal mimicry of computer-generated sounds and vocal labeling of objects by a bottlenose dolphin. *Journal of Comparative Psychology* 98:10–28.

Rumbaugh, D. M., T. V. Gill, and E. C. Von Glaserfeld. 1973. Reading and sentence completion by a chimpanzee (*Pan*). *Science* 182:731–733.

Ryle, G. 1949. *The Concept of Mind.* New York: Barnes and Noble.

Savage-Rumbaugh, E. S. 1986. *Ape Language: From Conditioned Response to Symbol.* New York: Columbia University Press.

Schusterman, R. J., and K. Krieger. 1984. California sea lions are capable of semantic comprehension. *Psychological Record* 34:3–23.

Seyfarth, R. M., D. L. Cheney, and P. Marler. 1980. Vervet monkey alarm calls: Semantic communication in a free-ranging primate. *Animal Behavior* 28:1070–1094.

Sigurdson, J. 1989. Frequency-modulated whistles as a medium for communication with the bottlenose dolphin (*Tursiops truncatus*). Paper presented at the Animal Language Workshop, Honolulu, HI.

Thorpe, W. H. 1963. *Learning and Instinct in Animals,* 2nd ed. Cambridge: Harvard Unviersity Press.

Tyack, P. L. 1986. Whistle repertoires of two bottlenose dolphins, *Tursiops truncatus*: Mimicry of signature whistles? *Behavioral Ecology and Sociobiology* 18:251–257.

Wells, R. S., M. D. Scott, and B. A. Irvine. 1987. The social structure of free-ranging bottlenose dolphins. In H. Genoways, ed. *Current Mammalogy*, vol. I. New York: Plenum Press, pp. 274–305.

Wursig, B. 1979. Dolphins. *Scientific American* 240:136–148.

48 Language and Mental Life

Paul Bloom

If it could be proved that certain high mental powers, such as the formation of general concepts, self-consciousness, etc., were absolutely peculiar to man ... it is not improbable that these qualities are merely the incidental results of other highly-advanced intellectual faculties; and these again mainly the result of the continued use of a perfect language.
—Charles Darwin, 1871

Perhaps the kind of mind you get when you add language to it is so different from the kind of mind you can have without language that calling them both minds is a mistake.
—Daniel Dennett, 1996

There are two striking facts about the minds of humans. First, compared to all other species, humans have a rich mental life. Like other animals, humans can think about material entities, such as rocks, and about actions, such as kicking. But humans are not limited to these types of thoughts. Humans can also consciously consider abstract entities, such as arguments, alimony, jokes, conferences, consciousness, and pension plans. Humans can imagine the future, can think about situations from the perspective of other people, and can create and appreciate fictional worlds. Although other primates may exhibit rudimentary forms of these abilities (e.g., the ability to appreciate certain abstract relationships), their mental life is nevertheless qualitatively poorer than that of humans.

Second, humans not only think deep thoughts, we can express them to others. A normal human adult knows tens of thousands of words referring to objects, actions, spatial relations, social entities, and so forth, and unconsciously commands syntactic rules that combine the words into a potential infinity of sentences. This capability enables humans to produce and understand ideas that nobody has ever thought of before. In this regard, human language is so much more powerful than the communication systems of other primates that they seem to differ in kind, not merely in degree.

How can we explain these two facts about humans? Could they be caused by a single capacity? One well-known theory is that humans have evolved an enhanced general intelligence from which all other cognitive capacities derive. If this theory were true, it would vastly simplify psychology. We would not need a separate theory of the evolution and nature of language, for instance, or of the ability to anticipate and understand the actions of others. We would only have to explain the nature and origin of the general intelligence.

But the theory is not true. There is considerable evidence from studies of language development, processing, and pathology to show that the ability to learn and use language results from neural mechanisms that cannot be entirely derived from the systems of thought underlying reasoning in general (Bloom 1997; Pinker 1994).

The quotations that begin this chapter suggest an alternative. Perhaps language first evolved through natural selection as an adaptation for communication (Pinker and Bloom 1990) and then, as an accidental by-product of language, much of the richness of our mental life emerged. According to this hypothesis, being smart does not, as many have assumed, give language. Instead, having language makes one smart.

This is an intriguing hypothesis because it entails not needing multiple evolutionary accounts for self-consciousness, for abstraction, for language, and so on. We need only to explain how language evolved. This hypothesis also implies that the sole important cognitive difference between humans and other primates is *linguistic*. Thus, if we could give chimpanzees the ability to learn a language such as English or ASL, they soon would be playing chess, planning bank robberies, debating the nature of consciousness, and doing whatever humans can do. Similarly, if we could strip language away from a human, we would end up with someone who has the mental life of a chimp. These are striking claims.

In one sense language has clearly had a profound influence on the mental life of humans. Language is a superb mechanism for the transmission and accumulation of information. Without language, most human culture, from scientific inquiry to professional football, would not exist. As Pinker (1994) said:

A common language connects the members of a community into an information-sharing network with formidable collective powers.

But there is an important difference between saying that language is an excellent tool for information transfer, which is obviously true, and the much stronger (and more controversial) claim that language explains a person's ability to understand and generate the information in the first place.

There are several different versions of the proposal that language is causally responsible for the richness of human mental life. One is that, in the course of human evolution, certain "generative" properties of language extended to nonlinguistic domains, such as music and formal logic (Corballis 1992). Another is that language provides us with the capacity for complex reasoning. As Darwin (1871) said:

A long and complex train of thought can no more be carried on without the aid of words, whether spoken or silent, than a long calculation without the use of figures or algebra.

Dennett (1996) and Jackendoff (in press) echo this view. A third version is Bickerton's (1995) suggestion that language evolved, not as a communication system, but as an enhanced internal system of mental representation and that inherent in linguistic structure itself is a system for richer and more abstract thought.

I have considered these proposals elsewhere (Bloom 1994, 1997), but in this chapter I focus on a different claim—that language gives rise to new concepts and new ways of categorizing entities and construing the world. Whorf (1956) provides the most famous formulation of this view:

We dissect nature along lines laid down by our native languages ... The world is presented as a kaleidoscopic flux of impressions which has to be organized by our minds—and this means largely by the linguistic systems in our minds.

Few scholars currently adopt a position as radical as that of Whorf. From studies of prelinguistic infants and nonhuman primates abundant evidence now exists to show that the mind is capable of imposing considerable structure on the world without the aid of language (Premack 1983; Spelke 1994). However, there are more plausible versions of Whorf's position. Some developmental psychologists, such as Gentner and Boroditsky (in press), argue that Whorf's hypothesis is true for *abstract* concepts; that is, although our notions of middle-sized objects exist before language, our abstract concepts emerge only after we learn to speak. Others defend this view for concepts that are consciously apprehended, concepts that are the objects of our experience, but not for concepts involved in unconscious mental processes. This version of the hypothesis has been most articulately defended by Dennett (1996).

The argument I will make has three parts. First, these proposals make sense; it is not incompatible with the way the mind works that language could help to create new concepts. Second, there is some evidence suggesting that an effect of language does in fact occur in some conceptual domains. Third, the strong position that one can explain the origin of all concepts, or even all abstract concepts or all concepts that are consciously apprehended, is nevertheless false. Diverse and abstract concepts exist independently from linguistic experience, and hence the origin of this aspect of our mental life cannot be the result of language.

Is the Whorfian proposal coherent? Suppose someone said that a person does not have the mental capacity to think about dogs until after the person has learned the word "dog." This view makes no sense. How could one learn the word "dog" without the capacity to think about dogs? As Fodor (1975) puts said:

Nothing can be expressed in a natural language that can't be expressed in the language of thought. For if something could, we couldn't learn the natural language [word] that expresses it.

Nevertheless, there are other ways of couching the Whorfian proposal that are perfectly coherent. Fodor himself notes that although language cannot cause previously unthinkable concepts to emerge, it may affect the sorts of concepts one can consciously entertain. For instance, one might be able to unconsciously distinguish different types of dogs, but only consciously make the distinction on hearing the types of dogs described with different words. To take another example, suppose one uses a language in which verbs differ according to the shape of the object that is acted on (e.g., the Navajo language, in which one verb is used to describe giving a long, thin object such as a stick, but a different verb is used to describe giving a spherical object such as a rock). Continued use of this type of language might lead the language user to consciously consider object shape more than would a person who used a language such as English that does not usually make such distinctions. Making distinctions in these ways can be called an "attentional" effect of language.

Another way in which language can lead to the creation of new concepts is by bringing to mind combinations of preexisting concepts. For instance, we may possess the concepts MALE and CHILD before learning language, but only by hearing the word "boy" can the concepts be brought together into a new complex concept. In fact, the orthodox view in psychology is that new concepts come to exist through the combination of old ones. We are not born with concepts such as BOY, TRUMPET, and PROTON, it is argued; the concepts come into existence as the result of combining our innate atoms of thought in new ways, as prototypes, definitions, and so on (Smith and Medin 1981; but see Fodor 1981). If this view were valid and if language were an indispensable tool for composing new concepts from old ones, then language would have a profound effect on human mental life. Forming new concepts in this way can be called a "compositional" effect of language.

Do these processes actually occur? Do languages actually have these effects on human mental life? Whorf (1956) made his case in terms of cross-linguistic comparisons. He argued that speakers of distinct languages think in important, different ways. Specifically, he argued that Hopi speakers do not think about time and space in the same way as do speakers of languages such as English because Hopi speakers express these notions differently than English speakers do. But this claim has had little support. For one thing, Whorf never presented evidence that the Hopi think any differently about time and space than do English speakers. In addition, Whorf's linguistic claims about the Hopi language were inaccurate; on careful scrutiny, the two languages are not really as dissimilar as Whorf suggested (Malotki 1983).

Subsequent psychological research has provided little support for the Whorfian hypothesis. Studies in domains as disparate as color memory and counterfactual reasoning have found either that speakers of different language have identical nonlinguistic capacities (e.g. Au 1983; Brown 1958) or that the expression differs only in tasks that are themselves language-dependent, such as explicit recall memory (e.g. Kay and Kempton 1984). As a result, many psychologists view the Whorfian claim as having been decisively refuted (e.g. Pinker 1994).

Nevertheless, to a limited extent, some recent studies in the domain of spatial cognition provide support for the Whorfian theory. Languages differ in how they carve up space. Bowerman (1996) considered a cup on a table, a handle on a door, and an apple in a bowl. In English, the first two items are deemed to be in the same relationship (contact and support), which is expressed with the spatial preposition "on"; the third item has the relationship of containment, expressed by "in." Other languages work differently. For instance, the Finnish language treats the handle on the door and the apple in the bowl as instantiating the same relationship (Finnish collapses containment and attachment as both highly "intimate"), distinct from the support relationship present in the cup on the table; Dutch treats each relationship with a different expression; Spanish collapses all the relationships into a single expression.

Despite these differences, Bowerman (1996) found that children have little difficulty acquiring the spatial system present in the language that they are exposed to, and they acquire the system before age three. Bowerman (1996) concludes:

We have to appeal to a process of learning in which children *build* spatial semantic categories in response to the distribution of spatial morphemes across contexts in the languages that they hear.

Is this evidence for the Whorfian position? Only if acquisition of these lexical differences affects categorization and conceptualization outside language. As Bowerman is careful to note, the linguistic differences may have no influence on nonlinguistic mental life. There might be a profound psychological difference between the "semantic structure" of language and the "conceptual structure" that underlies human nonlinguistic thought and action (Pinker 1989). If so, the existence of cross-linguistic semantic differences and the early acquisition of these differences may have no direct implications for the question of how language affects other modes of cognition.

Levinson's (1996) research is perhaps the strongest evidence for a Whorfian effect. Languages typically use multiple frames of reference and choose the frame according to the situation, but within a given language, some frames of reference are more predominant than others. For objects in proximity, the Dutch language, like English, uses a *relative* system of reference based on spatial properties relative to the speaker or to the objects being described (e.g., "in front of" or "to the left of"). Other languages, such as Tzeltal, use an *absolute* system, roughly akin to "north," "south," "east," or "west." As a result, the situation that is described by a Dutch speaker as "the boy is in front of me" is described by a Tzeltal speaker as "The boy is to the north of me." In fact, Levinson noted that phrases such as "take the first right turn" are simply untranslatable into the Tzeltal language.

Levinson tested the hypothesis that speakers of different languages encode their spatial experience of the world in different ways and predicted that, even in tasks that have nothing to do with language, Dutch speakers will think about objects in close proximity in terms of relative notions such as right and left and that Tzeltal speakers will think about them in terms of absolute notions such as north and south. Levinson's hypothesis was confirmed—Dutch speakers differed substantially from Tzeltal speakers both in nonlinguistic tasks requiring spatial inference and in their visual recall and gesture. These differences were not due to the use of linguistic coding, either overtly or implicitly. Levinson (1996) concluded:

The frame of reference dominant in the language, whether relative or absolute, comes to bias the choice of frame of reference in various kinds of nonlinguistic conceptual representation.

These are impressive findings, although for them to be a conclusive demonstration of the role of language in spatial cognition, one would have to rule out the possibility that a third nonlinguistic factor—such as differences in early spatial experience—explains both the linguistic and the cognitive differences between members of the radically different cultures. More convincing would be studies that look at the cognitive effects of linguistic differences between people raised in the same type of physical and cultural environment, such as between English and Japanese speakers in Japan or between English and Spanish speakers in the United States. Levinson and others are currently involved in such research.

Assume, however, that Levinson's analysis of the effects is correct—language, not culture, causes the effects. To accept this analysis as showing that language somehow *creates* systems of spatial thought would be a mistake. Both relative and absolute systems are encoded in brain mechanisms that underlie the navigation of species other than humans; hence, these systems are independent of language (O'Keefe and Nadel 1978; Peterson, Nadel, Bloom, and Garrett 1996). Furthermore, Dutch speakers can think in absolute terms, and Tzeltal speakers can think in relative terms—they simply tend not to. Perhaps the best way to make sense of Levinson's finding is to accept that use of language can *exercise* certain preexisting ways of thinking about the world and thereby affect what Whorf (1956) called "habitual thought and behavior." That is, one's language affects one's spatial thought in the "attentional" fashion.

A similar effect occurs in the course of word learning. The presence of a new word serves to draw a child's attention to a category. Markman and Hutchinson (1984), for instance, found that if one shows a two-year-old a new object and says, "See this one; find another one," the child typically reaches for something that had a spatial or thematic relationship to the original object (e.g., finding a bone to go with a dog). But if one uses a new word, "See this fendle; find another fendle," the child typically looks for something from the same category (e.g., finding another dog to go with the first dog). In this sense, the presence of a word can motivate categorization. Note that in this situation the child already knows, before the word was presented, that the two dogs belong to the same category; the concept DOG existed before the child heard the new word. The role of the word is attentional; it tells the child that the category, not a spatial or thematic relationship, is relevant in this context.

Is there any evidence that language can affect thought in the "compositional" way, creating new concepts by signaling new ways of combining old concepts? One domain in which this might happen is that of perceptual learning (Bedford 1993). In wine tasting, for instance, linguistic labeling can give rise to both conceptual and phenomenological distinctions. For the wine novice, all wines may taste the same. But because of the linguistic cues repeatedly provided in the context of a wine-tasting class ("this is a Merlot, this is a Beaujolais, this is dry, this is sweet") one can begin to organize the "flux of impressions" into discrete categories and to appreciate the ways in which wines differ. As a result, one can acquire the functional ability to distinguish the wines and have a different, richer, phenomenal experience of the tastes of the wines. This experience is different from the examples with the children (Markman and Hutchinson 1984) because the categories "Merlot," "Beaujolais," and so on are not present, not even unconsciously, before one has exposure to their names, the concepts come to exist solely through linguistic cues.

Linguistic labeling can also affect inductive reasoning. Gelman (1996) carried out experiments in which children were shown a target object and two other objects, one that looked very much like the target object and another that did not. Children who were told that the target object had a new property (e.g., that it contained a certain type of substance) generalized the property to the perceptually similar object. But children who were also told that the target object and the dissimilar object had the same name (e.g., "This is a blicket, and this is a blicket"), generalized the new fact to the dissimilar object, which suggests that linguistic cues alone can lead children to form a new category for inductive inference.

Thus, language can sometimes drive concept formation. Is, therefore, the possession of language *responsible for* the existence of the rich mental life of humans? There are reasons to believe that the answer is no. One source of evidence comes from studies of congenitally deaf adults who grew up without any exposure to sign language. As Sacks (1988) described, the cognitive abilities of such linguistic isolates was a central topic of debate in the nineteenth century. One classic case study was that of Theophilus d'Estrella, who did not acquire a formal sign language until age nine. After he had acquired language, he wrote an autobiographical account of his early experience in which he described elaborate ruminations about religion and other matters. His discussion profoundly impressed William James (1893), who wrote:

His narrative tends to discountenance the notion that no abstract thought is possible without words. Abstract thought of a decidedly subtle kind, both scientific and moral, went on here in advance of the means of expressing it to others.

D'Estrella's account is hardly decisive; one should be skeptical of autobiographical reports (and many of James's contemporaries rejected his conclusion for this reason). Nevertheless there is recent support for James's conclusion. Schaller (1991), who studied contemporary deaf isolates in the United States and Mexico, observed that they show all signs of possessing a rich mental life. Her subjects have elaborate spatial knowledge and skills, including the ability to repair complicated machinery, and they can handle money; some can even live on their own. Furthermore, they can actively describe events from the past by using pantomimed narratives (Pinker 1994).

A second source of evidence concerns language learning by young children. Preschoolers are extremely good at learning the meanings of words, even with limited and sporadic experience, a phenomenon described as "fast mapping" (Carey 1978). From about 18 months of age, children learn an average of five new words a day; with the onset of schooling, the rate of word learning increases to about 20 new words a day (Anglin 1993; Carey 1978). The vocabularies of young children include many names for middle-sized objects (e.g., "dog" and "truck"). But they also know words that refer to events, times, spatial relations, mental states, and many types of abstract entities. In fact, by the time a child is about two years of age, roughly half the child's words refer to entities that are not middle-sized objects (Bloom, in press).

An analysis of word learning is one way to discover which concepts exist prior to language capability and which need the shaping power of language to emerge. If a concept is already present, the word for the concept should be quickly learnable as long as the child can perform the correct mapping. If the concept is not present, multiple trials in different contexts may be necessary to establish the nature and boundaries of the concept in the child's mind.

Many words, particularly scientific terms, seem to require a lengthy shaping process. But many words do not. There is striking experimental evidence that some abstract expressions can be fast mapped by young children. For instance, after being given only a few exposures to a new word in a single context, children can learn new names for actions, for collections (e.g., "family"), and for social institutions (e.g., "church") (see Bloom, in press, for a review). Although the meanings of such words might not precisely map to the adult meanings and further shaping might be the result of linguistic cues, such findings give no support to the view that abstract concepts do not exist before word learning.

Finally, infants have a surprisingly rich mental life. They expect objects to continue to exist after the objects go out of sight (Baillargeon 1987); they can predict the trajectories of moving objects (Spelke 1994); they can determine the numerosities of small arrays of objects (Starkey, Spelke, and Gelman 1990); they can even compute the results of simple additions and subtractions performed over these arrays (Wynn 1992). But the conceptual abilities of infants are not limited to objects. For instance, they can also determine the numerosities of sequences of distinct sounds (Starkey, Spelke, and Gelman 1990) and can individuate and enumerate distinct actions, such as the jumps of a continuously moving puppet (Wynn 1996). Infants also show an ability to recall spatial location (Wilcox, Rosser, and Nadel 1994), make simple causal inferences (Leslie 1982), and predict the actions of an agent on the basis of its previous intentional behavior (Premack 1990).

Of course, infants have a lot to learn. Their mental life is limited in many ways; many concepts emerge only after considerable conceptual development. In many instances, this development is facilitated by language (Bloom 1996). Nevertheless, research with infants provides further evidence that even abstract conceptualization exists before language is acquired.

CONCLUSION

This chapter considers one variant of the claim made by Darwin, Dennett, and others—that the richness of human mental life is the result of our capacity for language. Although linguistic cues can sometimes lead to the existence of new concepts, their claim is mistaken. At least some unique aspects of human mental life exist independently of language. The nature and origin of these aspects must be explained in another way.

ACKNOWLEDGMENTS

I am grateful to Karen Wynn for very helpful comments on an earlier draft of this manuscript.

REFERENCES

Anglin, J. 1993. Vocabulary development: A morphological analysis. *Monographs of the Society for Research in Child Development* 238:1–166.

Au, T. K.-F. 1983. Chinese and English counterfactuals: The Sapir-Whorf hypothesis revisited. *Cognition* 15:155–187.

Baillargeon, R. 1987. Object permanence in 3.5- and 4.5- month-old infants. *Child Development* 23:655–664.

Bedford, F. 1993. Perceptual learning. In D. Medin, ed., *The Psychology of Learning and Motivation*. San Diego: Academic Press, pp. 1–60.

Bickerton, D. 1995. *Language and Human Behavior*. Seattle: University of Washington Press.

Bloom, P. 1994. Generativity within language and other cognitive domains. *Cognition* 51:177–189.

Bloom, P. 1996. Possible individuals in language and cognition. *Current Directions in Psychological Science* 5:90–94.

Bloom, P. 1997. Some issues in the evolution of language and thought. In D. Cummins and C. Allen, eds., *Evolution of Language*. Oxford: Oxford University Press, pp. 344–375.

Bloom, P. in press. Roots of word learning. In M. Bowerman and S. Levinson, eds., *Conceptual development and Language Acquisition*. Cambridge: Cambridge University Press.

Bowerman, M. 1996. Learning how to structure space for language. In P. Bloom, M. Peterson, L. Nadel, and M. Garrett, eds., *Language and Space*. Cambridge: MIT Press, pp. 385–436.

Brown, R. 1958. *Words and Things*. New York: Free Press.

Carey, S. 1978. The child as word-learner. In M. Halle, J. Bresnan, and G. A. Miller, eds., *Linguistic Theory and Psychological Reality*. Cambridge: MIT Press, pp. 264–293.

Corballis, M. 1992. On the evolution of language and generativity. *Cognition* 44:197–226.

Darwin, C. R. 1871. *The Descent of Man and Selection in Relation to Sex*. New York: Hurst.

Dennett, D. C. 1995. *Darwin's Dangerous Idea*. New York: Simon & Schuster.

Dennett, D. C. 1996. *Kinds of Minds*. New York: Basic Books.

Fodor, J. A. 1975. *The Language of Thought*. New York: Crowell.

Fodor, J. A. 1981. The current status of the innateness controversy. In J. A. Fodor, ed., *Representations*. Cambridge: MIT Press, pp. 257–321.

Gelman, S. 1996. Concepts and theories. In R. Gelman and T. Au, eds., *Perceptual and Cognitive Development*. San Diego: Academic Press, pp. 117–150.

Gentner, D., and L. Boroditsky. In press. Individuation, relativity and early word learning. In M. Bowerman and S. Levinson, eds., *Conceptual Development and Language Acquisition*. Cambridge: Cambridge University Press.

Jackendoff, R. In press. How language helps us think. *Pragmatics and Cognition*.

James, W. 1893. Thought before language: A deaf-mute's recollections. *American Annals of the Deaf* 38:135–145.

Kay, P., and W. Kempton. 1984. What is the Sapir-Whorf hypothesis? *American Anthropologist* 86:65–79.

Leslie, A. M. 1982. The perception of causality in infants. *Perception* 11:173–186.

Levinson, S. C. 1996. Frames of reference and Molyneux's question: Crosslinguistic evidence. In P. Bloom, M. Peterson, L. Nadel, and M. Garrett, eds., *Language and Space*. Cambridge: MIT Press, pp. 109–169.

Malotki, E. 1983. *Hopi Time: A Linguistic Analysis of the Temporal Concepts in the Hopi Language*. New York: Mouton.

Markman, E. M., and J. E. Hutchinson. 1984. Children's sensitivity to constraints in word meaning: Taxonomic versus thematic relations. *Cognitive Psychology* 16:1–27.

O'Keefe, J., and L. Nadel. 1978. *The Hippocampus as a Cognitive Map*. Oxford: Clarendon Press.

Peterson, M., L. Nadel, P. Bloom, and M. Garrett. 1996. *Space and Language*. In P. Bloom, M. Peterson, L. Nadel, and M. Garrett, eds., *Language and Space*. Cambridge: MIT Press, pp. 553–577.

Pinker, S. 1989. *Learnability and Cognition*. Cambridge: MIT Press.

Pinker, S. 1994. *The Language Instinct*. New York: Morrow.

Pinker, S., and P. Bloom. 1990. Natural language and natural selection. *Behavioral and Brain Sciences* 13:585–642.

Premack, D. 1983. The codes of man and beasts. *Behavioral and Brain Sciences* 6:125–167.

Premack, D. 1990. The infant's theory of self-propelled objects. *Cognition* 36:1–16.

Sacks, O. 1988. *Seeing Voices: A Journey into the World of the Deaf*. Berkeley: University of California Press.

Schaller, S. 1991. *A Man without Words*. New York: Summit Press.

Smith, E. E., and D. L. Medin. 1981. *Categories and Concepts*. Cambridge: MIT Press.

Spelke, E. S. 1994. Initial knowledge: Six suggestions. *Cognition* 50:431–445.

Starkey, P., E. S. Spelke, and R. Gelman. 1990. Numerical abstraction by human infants. *Cognition* 36:97–127.

Whorf, B. L. 1956. *Language, Thought, and Reality*. Cambridge: MIT Press.

Wilcox, T., R. Rosser, and L. Nadel. 1994. Representation of object location in 6.5-month-old infants. *Cognitive Development* 9:193–209.

Wynn, K. 1992. Addition and subtraction by human infants. *Nature* 358:749–750.

Wynn, K. 1995. Infants' individuation and enumeration of actions. *Psychological Science* 7:164–169.

X   Emergent and Hierarchical Systems

OVERVIEW

Academics face a peculiar professional hazard. Being funded to formulate and paid to preach, we are wont to confuse our learned descriptions of reality—whatever that might be—with the real thing. And we happily project our confusions on all who are willing to listen.

How can you know when you are being conned by the cognoscenti? Ask a question about something important. Is there such a thing as free will? May one speak of a human soul? As academics start to answer, watch our eyes. Do they quickly flick to a formula written in curious distortions of Greek letters, sometimes extending on for pages and transparent only to perhaps five minds in the universe? Check our frames of reference. Do we immediately turn the discussion back to some out-of-date doctrine that was quite properly discarded a generation ago? Do we parrot what we learned as graduate students? Such are the telltale signs of what classical German scholars have called "Mist."

Do we look inward for our answers, or do we look outward? That is a key question. Do we confine our concepts of consciousness within mended walls, or do we recognize with Robert Frost that there is something in nature that does not like a wall? Do we propose formulations—if formulations we must have—that are closed or formulations that are open, welcoming by the nature of their structures the new facts and insights that tomorrow will surely bring?

Members of the scientific community who grow uncomfortable with talk of the soul should remember that the fundamental aim of science is to describe reality, without fear or favor, bowing to none in the endless quest for truth. Thus, an open approach to the unknown lies within the highest traditions of science (Scott 1995). On the other hand, the person who claims that free will does not exist because it is not included in a certain set of assumptions carries on the medieval traditions of the Church.

At this point, the reader may be asking: What is an "open formulation" of knowledge? Is this phrase not a contradiction in terms? An oxymoron? One answer to these questions is provided by the title of Section X; "emergent and hierarchical systems" are open by their very nature. Organized in a hierarchical structure, knowledge is a tree, and trees grow. In the course of evolution, new forms of life are ever emerging. As a human mind experiences, new ideas are ever appearing. As a human culture struggles from decade to decade, new configurations of personal interactions are constantly developing. Hierarchical structures are expressly tailored to represent such emergent dynamics.

In the first chapter of this section, Andrew Bailey reviews the taxonomy of hierarchies, the "geography of levels." Some higher levels are defined for convenience, others because the theoretical space of a lower level is not sufficiently capacious. (A numerical example of theoretical irreducibility is given in Chapter 63 by King and Scott.) Finally, there are constraints that arise from the very nature of explanation. An explanation of human interaction in terms of "quarks, gluons, and weak forces," Bailey observes, "would at best be an extremely poor explanation, if we were even to count it as an explanation."

Beyond such pragmatic classifications, Bailey discusses ontological classifications. Can one assign distinctly different "levels of being"? Are there higher levels of description that are irreducible to those at lower levels of the hierarchy but necessary for a full description of the universe? Inflation, Bailey suggests, is a phenomenon that "does not exist at the level of quantum mechanics." These considerations get to the heart of certain themes of the second Tucson conference.

The second chapter of Section X, by Syed Mustafa Ali and Robert Zimmer, presents a mathematical framework for describing the phenomenon of emergence in the context of states that are defined in discrete space-time, which thereby makes explicit several concepts introduced by Bailey. A key feature of the Ali and Zimmer description is the notion that organizational rules (dynamic laws) at one level of description play the role of states in an adjacent level. Because initial conditions can be specified arbitrarily at each level of description, the model is an open system. Ontological duality, which is of concern to Bailey, arises readily in the Ali-Zimmer formulation if one assumes neither lowest nor highest level of description.

In dealing with discrete space-time systems such as those proposed by Ali and Zimmer, it is important to remain aware that there are many sets of possibilities (e.g., the number of possible games of chess) that, although finite in number, are so large that to consider ever looking at all of them is impossible. This seemingly simple observation raises serious problems with numerical investigations of hierarchical models that are sometimes ignored by computer enthusiasts.

Computational difficulties contribute to another problematic aspect of hierarchical models of emergent phenomena—we do not know what the hierarchical systems can do. Of course the usual suspects (fixed-point attractors, cyclic attractors, chaotic attractors, complex attractors that can compute, etc.) are brought in, and rightly so, but can we be sure that they are all? Chaotic attractors, for instance, were unknown to mathematics a generation ago.

The generally accepted notion is that some atomistic entity emerges from the nonlinear dynamics of a particular hierarchical level (e.g., a molecule of benzene from the atomic elements or a tornado from atmospheric equations) to provide a basis for the dynamics of an adjacent level. But life may be a phenomenon that emerges from many levels of biological organization, ranging from the biochemistry of proteins and nucleic acids to the physiology of a fully developed organism. Similarly, mind may emerge from many levels of the brain's organization, ranging from the dynamics of intrinsic membrane proteins to the configurations of a human culture. If these ideas are correct, twentieth-century science is not even close to comprehending the nature of such phenomena.

REFERENCES

Scott, A. 1995. *Stairway to the Mind*. New York: Springer-Verlag.

49   The Five Kinds of Levels of Description

Andrew Bailey

THE NEED FOR A GEOGRAPHY OF LEVELS

The phrase "levels of description" is usually understood as denoting the various positions of descriptions in some vertical scale of possible descriptions, in which levels correspond to different degrees of generality or detail. Very often this spectrum is implicitly understood as relative to an absolute bottom level of full causal description, with higher levels of description giving increasingly less close approximations to the full description.

These notions are simplistic. I believe the analytic technique of invoking levels of description, despite the way it uncritically tends to be treated in the literature, is not a monolithic phenomenon. Hierarchies of levels of description may vary significantly in their function and in the degree of reducibility or eliminability of higher levels in favor of lower ones. In fact, at least five distinct breeds of hierarchy of levels of description exist. They can be sorted as a function of the reason why ascent to a higher level is made: three sorts of epistemic (or perhaps pragmatic) use, and two ontological uses.

The multiplicity of levels is not widely recognized. For example, in the philosophy of mind, if the diversity is acknowledged at all, it is primarily and merely when one draws a contrast between epistemological or pragmatic reasons to ascend to higher levels and reasons of ontology. Writers tend to exclude such ascent when it applies to reasons of ontology, but they feel perfectly comfortable with such ascent when it applies to epistemological or pragmatic reasons.[1] Their assumptions need to be examined more critically.

EPISTEMOLOGICAL AND PRAGMATIC LEVELS

Three sorts of levels of hierarchy within the epistemological (pragmatic) camp are sufficiently distinct to count as different types: hierarchies of epistemological convenience, modeling hierarchies, and explanatorily pragmatic hierarchies.

Levels of Convenience

Levels of convenience are the most evident type of levels of description. These are higher levels used because it is in some way too cumbersome to give full descriptions at the more fundamental levels. Examples of this kind of use of levels are commonplace. For instance, a complete historical account of the battle of Agincourt would not give the description in terms of the physical equations that governed the flight of each arrow.

The ascent to higher levels of convenience may be for reasons of mere convenience—it is quicker, less irritating, or less tiring to work at the higher level, although one could descend to lower levels if one were not so lazy. In other cases, however, levels of convenience are used because work at lower levels is a practical impossibility. There are situations in which one cannot at the lower levels hold everything in memory or compute things fast enough to produce results in a human life span. In addition, one may find it impossible to work at lower levels because of a constraint contingent on current technological development or because of a basic principle impossible to overcome.

Ascent to higher levels for reasons of convenience is sometimes not dismissible as "in principle eliminable," as some have labeled it, for it need not be "in principle eliminable" by any human being or even any finite describer no matter how conscientious. However, this kind of use of levels of description is fully consistent with (though it does not entail) the view that only one fundamental and complete description of the physical universe exists and that descriptions at the higher levels are ontologically fully reducible to, or even eliminable in favor of, descriptions at the bottom level.

Model Levels

Some authors[2] move from one level to a higher level when they apply a model to the phenomenon under consideration. The model explains or describes the phenomenon in a particularly helpful way that for some reason is not available at the lower level. For example, artificial intelligence (AI)-like computer programs can be (and often are) treated as providing models of human cognitive processes; other examples are the planetary model of the atom or the person as agent model of human action.

The reducibility of models to lower levels is a complex issue. It is consistent with model-style levels of description that, at a particular time, they need not be ontologically reducible to lower levels, and they need not be eliminated if they are not so reducible. Further, that two models within the same theoretical space are inconsistent with each other is not itself reason to reject one of the models. The nature of the irreducibility or incliminability in these cases is simply a function of the fact that the goal of the modeling is not directly the representation of any reality but the search for an instrumentally fruitful structure for information about the domain.

Explanatory Pragmatics

Explanatory pragmatics is the most interesting and underrecognized of the varieties of epistemological levels of description. It does not arise directly from pragmatic descriptive limitations, but from the nature of explanation itself. That certain patterns in the world must be picked out in performing certain explanatory tasks and that these patterns are only visible at certain levels of description has generally been misinterpreted in the literature. Authors tend to implicitly assume that the patterns themselves are irreducibly higher level or that the reason for using the higher-level predicates is solely for convenience. I contend that the patterns are not necessarily irreducible to lower levels (indeed, they are unlikely to be so) and that use of higher-level predicates is necessary to successfully make certain worthwhile explanations.

Consider Pylyshyn's well-known 9-1-1 example in which a pedestrian witnesses a car crash, runs to a nearby telephone booth, and dials the numbers 9, 1, and 1.[3] What physical explanation could be given of these events? Pylyshyn (among others) uses examples such as this to encourage the intuition that intentional terms are somehow irreducible. But what the example really shows is that any explanation using low-level predicates would simply be a poor explanation. It lacks many epistemic and pragmatic virtues required of good explanation, not only for psychological explanation but for most other high-level explanatory projects, such as economics and epidemiology.

The reason is that the explanation relation is not wholly a semantic relation, but a substantially pragmatic one. First, a function of explanation is to increase understanding; pragmatic, contextual factors (not semantic ones) operate to determine the "epistemic gaps" that need "filling."[4] Second, the explanation relation has a particular kind of asymmetry that renders it non-equivalent with logical or semantic relations such as constant conjunction and deduction (e.g., falling barometers are constantly conjoined with approaching storms, but the explanatory relationship runs only one way).[5] Third, explanation is not a transitive relation; therefore, much information supplied by low-level descriptions is not relevant to the explanation. For example, a complete explanation for the fact that a peg will not pass through a round hole is supplied by the fact that the hole is smaller than a section through the peg (further information may also explain why the peg and board are rigid, but this is extra).[6]

There are, then, certain virtues that a good explanation must have (relevance, brevity, and understandability), and these virtues are frequently unavailable to one working at lower levels of description. Therefore, to explain effectively one must necessarily often use higher levels of description; one cannot, for example, replace folk psychological explanations with adequate neurophysiological explanations. To respond to a request for an explanation of why the pedestrian dialed 9 and then 1 and 1 with a story about quarks, gluons, and weak atomic forces would be at best an extremely poor explanation, if we were even to count it as an explanation at all (quite likely, the explanation would utterly fail to fill the relevant epistemic gaps in the listener's cognitive structures).

Though superficially similar to the levels of convenience species of levels, this kind of level is importantly different. A sufficiently powerful, godlike being would have no need to construct a hierarchy of levels of epistemological convenience, but even such a god would be in principle unable to provide, at the bottom level, a good explanation of many perfectly real phenomena. Similarly, suppose that, by some mysterious and implausible chance, we had developed no vocabulary at the level of folk psychology (only, let us imagine, Newtonian physics), but we wanted to construct a science dealing with human action. In such a case, we would find it in principle impossible to give good explanations of human behavior without inventing new predicates at the folk psychological level.

Further, explanatory pragmatics give rise to a different kind of structure of levels of description. Levels of epistemological convenience are hierarchically nested. Presumably, they form a series of levels from more complex to less complex, and the degree of complexity of any one level can reasonably be compared to that of any other level of description. By contrast, explanatorily pragmatic levels often do not appear to be above or below each other—the levels of economic explanation and species-level biological explanation differ, but it is a fundamentally moot point which level is the higher level.

ONTOLOGICAL LEVELS

Within the roughly ontological group of varieties of levels of description there are two distinct varieties: group-level properties and (if they exist) levels of being.

Group-Level Properties

It is a logical commonplace that groups may have properties that are not properties of any of their components. For example, a soccer team has the quality of comprising exactly 11 human beings, but none of the team's components have that property. For group-level properties or patterns, a higher level of description must be adopted; it is necessary to consider the group as a mereological whole—to stand back and treat certain blocks of basic materials as property holders in their own right.

However, this kind of ontological level making, in itself, is rarely seen as a serious motivation for belief in levels of being—the belief, roughly, that the universe compartmentalizes itself ontologically or metaphysically into different levels—because mereological levels are consistent with one or both of the following moves: denial that particular group-level properties are ontologically serious, or indication that group-level properties are fully describable at the bottom level. For example, denial would say that "being a soccer team" is not a scientific property—the fact that such a property would not feature in a full description of the universe is then not a problem because the full description is supposed to be a scientific one. An example of indicating full describability would be to proffer a promissory note to the effect that the predicate "being a soccer team" is fully describable at the base level in terms of, perhaps, the physical makeup of the players in combination with the bottom-level physical descriptions of all the relevant societal beliefs, attitudes, and institutional structures.

As a tactic, I prefer the second move; the first seems to raise too many difficulties in dividing the properties in the world into "real" and "nonreal" in a non-ad hoc way. Note that adopting such a reductionist picture shows how deflated are the ontological claims of group-level hierarchies. It makes some intuitive sense to continue thinking of group-level properties as being at a higher level than the properties of their components, but, in fact, they are really just very complex concatenations of so-called bottom-level properties.

Levels of Being

What would it be to assert the existence of levels of being, that is, to assert that something exists at a higher level but not a lower one? A starting point, in terms of levels of description, might be that there are two conditions:

1. Descriptions at some higher level must be irreducible, capturing patterns or generalities which in principle cannot be captured by lower-level descriptions.

2. The higher-level descriptions must be ineliminable, that is, necessary for a full description of the universe.

One common approach to the irreducibility of high-level regularities has been to talk about patterns describable only at "the right level of detail," in which what is salient about a range of cases can be picked out. For example, Pylyshyn argues that the level of functional architecture is "the right level of specificity (or level of aggregation) at which to view mental processes."[7] What usually seems to be alluded to here as the reason that particular patterns are visible only at certain levels is the fact of multiple realizability. However, multiple realizability by itself is not enough to produce any strong form of irreducibility, hence, levels of being. Although higher levels may be multiply instantiated, they can still be explained by, and described in terms of, whatever structure does realize them. Complex predicates, including statements of initial and boundary conditions, can in principle be constructed at the bottom level, which correspond to upper-level predicates.[8]

As far as I know, it has not previously been noticed that multiple realizability can be tinkered with in such a way that it *does* bring about strong irreducibility of higher-level patterns, but this happens if one insists that no relevant similarity or regularity exists between, and only between, the group of token physical instantiations of an upper-level pattern (i.e., that there is no lower-level pattern corresponding to the upper-level pattern). This little-noted stipulation is very powerful. By this stipulation, the upper-level regularity (qua regularity) is not reducible to the lower level of description; the regularity (indeed *any* regularity, no matter how complex) does not exist at that level.

This view seems to be a moderate, convenient, clear notion of a pattern being instantiated by lower-level elements but not reducible to them. Indeed, the claim that such patterns may actually exist has some prima facie plausibility. The patterns would be of lower-level entities, not floating metaphysically free, and they need not violate causal closure. Further, one can describe actual patterns that seem to be good candidates for this kind of irreducibility. For instance, the pattern representing inflation, it seems prima facie reasonable to say, does not exist at the level of quantum mechanics.[9]

However, there are also strong reasons to think that no serious ontological patterns *will* turn out to be irreducible in this way. In particular, the assertion of this sort of ontological irreducibility for a pattern Φ would commit one to the claim that the token instantiations of that pattern do not have anything uniquely in common. Thus, either some tokens that are utterly different from other Φ-tokens must themselves also instantiate Φ, or others that are qualitatively identical with some Φ-tokens must fail to instantiate it, or both.

The latter situation is usually understood as violating supervenience and becomes quite implausible if one seriously considers all the properties of the instantiating tokens of a pattern, including all their manifest and nonmanifest (but still actual) interrelatednesses and interreactivities. It then becomes much harder to imagine plausible situations in which tokens with these properties could have instantiated another pattern or no pattern. Consider again the example of inflation. Imagine the vastly complex combination of basic properties that make up this pattern, including the (physical) instantiations of beliefs and attitudes toward money, the changes over time in the purchasing power of fiscal tokens (described in physicocausal terms), the (physical instantiations of the) beliefs governments and people have that this is inflation, and so on. If it were possible to give such a bottom-level description, it is difficult to imagine that the description could be of anything other than inflation.

Similar considerations also weigh, though less forcefully, against the other possibility—that some of the different token instantiations of the same pattern could have nothing relevantly in common. Any instantiation of inflation would surely bear some significant resemblance to any other instantiation, for example, with respect to basic physical instantiations of the subpatterns of certain societal attitudes towards money and certain changes in purchasing power.

CONCLUSION

Four conclusions seem to follow from this discussion. First, an important and underrecognized fact is that no unified notion of level of description really exists and that talk of such levels can operate in different ways. Second, there is an interesting and little-emphasized, nonontological motivation for ineliminable levels of description, which follows from the very nature of explanation itself and its pragmatic virtues. Third, levels of being may consist of an absence of correspondence between the reference of ontologically serious predicates at the higher-level and any identifiable pattern or regularity at the lower level. Finally, the assertion that there are corresponding levels of being is less plausible than it might appear at first sight.

NOTES

1. A representative selection of a few users of levels in this area might include Dennett (1978, 1991), Fodor (1980), Putnam (1973), Pylyshyn (1984), and Smolensky (1988).

2. Such as Smolensky (1988) and Churchland and Sejnowski (1992).

3. See Pylyshyn (1984), pp. 3ff.

4. See, for example, Scriven (1975) and Van Fraassen (1977).

5. See, for example, Putnam (1973).

6. See Putnam (1973).

7. See Pylyshyn (1984) p. 92. See Hooker (1981) for more on reduction.

8. See Fodor (1974).

9. See Owens (1989).

REFERENCES

Churchland, P. S., and T. Sejnowski. 1992. *The Computational Brain.* Cambridge: MIT Press.

Dennett, D. C. 1978. *Brainstorms.* Cambridge: MIT Press.

Dennett, D. C. 1991. Real patterns. *Journal of Philosophy* 88:27–51.

Fodor, J. 1974. Special sciences. *Synthese* 28:77–115.

Fodor, J. 1980. *Representations.* Cambridge: MIT Press.

Hooker, C. A. 1981. Towards a general theory of reduction. Parts I, II, III. *Dialogue* 20:38–59, 201–236, 496–529.

Owens, D. 1989. Levels of explanation. *Mind* 98:59–79.

Putnam, H. 1973. Reductionism and the nature of psychology. In J. Haugeland, ed. *Mind Design.* Cambridge: MIT Press pp. 205–219.

Pylyshyn, Z. W. 1984. *Computation and Cognition.* Cambridge: MIT Press.

Scriven, M. 1975. Causation as explanation. *Nous* 9:3–10.

Smolensky, P. 1988. On the proper treatment of connectionism. *Behavioral and Brain Sciences* 11:1–23.

Van Fraassen, B. C. 1977. The pragmatics of explanation. *American Philosophical Quarterly* 14:217–227.

50 Beyond Substance and Process: A New Framework for Emergence

Syed Mustafa Ali and Robert M. Zimmer

Determining the conditions under which a spatially extended finite system can support potentially unbounded emergence would offer emergentism the status of a universal phenomenon. Determining the conditions for the system is possible if an infinite hierarchy of laws governing the behavior of such a system is admitted. We believe this condition is necessary for open or unbounded emergence in spatially extended finite systems. The ways in which one "cuts" the ontological hierarchy determine what counts as global physics and local atoms in our models of nature. Hence, we advocate an epistemology that is relativistic and motivated by intentional (i.e., conscious) concerns.

The earliest articulation of the essence of emergence may be the ancient Greek maxim "the whole is more than the sum of the parts." However, the first serious attempt at investigating the concept of emergence was not made until the middle of the nineteenth century when George Henry Lewes distinguished between resultants and emergents. In resultants, the sequence of steps that produce a phenomenon is traceable; in emergence, the sequence is not traceable. Thus, Lewes may be interpreted as believing that emergence merely indicates the epistemological limitations of an observer.

The concept was further described in C. Lloyd Morgan's *Emergent Evolution* (1923) and J. C. Smuts' *Holism and Evolution* (1926), but it was in Samuel Alexander's *Space, Time and Deity* (1920) that the first attempt at a comprehensive explanatory framework for emergence was made. Alexander identified emergence with the tendency for things to arrange themselves into new patterns that, as organized wholes, possess new types of structure and new qualities (i.e., properties). Recently, attempts have been made to define the concept in computational and information theoretical terms (Baas 1993; Darley 1994).

THE EMERGENT THEORY OF MIND

The concept of emergence finds application in the context of the mind–body problem. Proponents of the emergent theory of mind (ETM), such as Searle (1992), follow Alexander by adopting an evolutionary perspective, which holds that the mind (consciousness) emerges from the body (brain) as a consequence of bottom-up causal processes. The ETM describes the mind–body relation in terms of a two-level systemic hierarchy—the pattern of neuronal "firings" in the brain (lower, local, or substrate level) gives rise to mental phenomena, including the subjective experience of consciousness (higher, global, or emergent level).

Proponents of computational ETM (CETM) go further and assert that the formal aspect of bottom-up causation provides the necessary and sufficient conditions for the emergence of consciousness. This view is consistent with functionalism, which supports the possibility of artificial consciousness. Alexander's ontology is particularly appealing to proponents of CETM because CETM maps isomorphically onto the class of mathematical formalisms known as cellular automata. According to Alexander's view, space-time is the primordial ground of matter, life, mind, and so forth. Cellular automata are highly suitable for representing space-time and pattern formation within a spatiotemporal framework.

CELLULAR AUTOMATA

A cellular automaton (CA) is a D-dimensional lattice of K cells where each cell is a finite state automaton defined by the triplet S, N_S, r where S is a set of states, N_S is a state-vector given by the states of cells in the neighborhood of a central cell C, and $r : N_S \rightarrow S$ is a state-transition rule applied to each cell in parallel; hence, the global state of the lattice is updated at each time interval. An example of the space-time evolution of a $1 - D$ CA from an initial state is shown in Figure 50.1.

New kinds of functional behavior, such as billiard-ball mechanics (matter), self-reproduction (life), and universal computation (mind), emerge as a consequence of the spatiotemporal dynamics of certain types of CA. Feedback

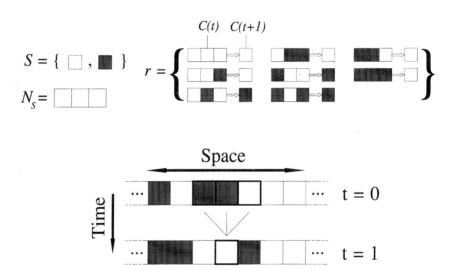

Figure 50.1 Space-time evolution of elementary one-dimensional cellular automata.

between the dynamics of the global (emergent) level constraining the dynamics of the local (substrate) level that gives rise to the global dynamics provides a kind of downwards causation. The nature of this constraint is best understood in system dynamical terms, namely, trajectories (sequences of global system states), attractors (the end state or sequence of end states in a given trajectory), and basins of attraction (the set of all trajectories converging on a given attractor). The existence of a set of basins of attraction, which constitutes the basin-of-attraction field, is a necessary condition for emergence in CA. A state-space portrait of a basin-of-attraction field for a CA has the topology of a "landscape" of branching transient trees rooted on attractors; nodes represent states, and arcs represent state-transitions.

Problems with Emergence in Cellular Automata

Cariani (1991) argued that CA with finite lattices, finite states, and finite rules have basin-of-attraction fields that are finite, hence, describable. Cariani maintains that, as a result, finite CA are examples of closed systems supporting a finite or bounded potential for emergence. For CA of this type, what appears as emergence actually indicates incomplete knowledge of the basin-of-attraction field at a particular instant in time by an observer. Once the field has been "mapped," no further emergence is possible.

CA with infinite lattices (but finite states and rules) have basin-of-attraction fields that are infinite and possibly nondescribable. Consequently, some infinite lattice CA are examples of open systems supporting an unbounded potential for emergence. Emergence as a *universal* phenomenon, unconstrained to only finitely many phenomenal levels, necessitates emergence without limit, and infinite-lattice CA meet this requirement. However, this scheme is inconsistent with current cosmological views regarding the closure (i.e., finitude) of the physical universe.

An alternative scheme that meets the requirement for unbounded emergence and is consistent with the idea of a closed universe (lattice in the CA model) necessitates introducing the potential for openness via an extension of the standard definition of CA.

Metarules

Metarule CAs introduce the required openness by postulating a hierarchy of CA rules. Each CA at a particular level in the hierarchy has a finite lattice, a finite number of states, and a finite number of rules. However, there are two ways in which metarule CAs extend the standard CA definition:

1. rules at level p are states at level $p + 1$ in the hierarchy, where $p \geq 0$.

2. initial conditions are independently specifiable at each level p in the metarule hierarchy.

The scheme may be expressed formally as follows:

Syed Mustafa Ali and Robert M. Zimmer: A New Framework for Emergence

Level 0 rule (r^0)

$$r^0 : N_{S^0} \rightarrow S^0, \quad r^0 \in R^1$$

$$S^0 = \{s_i^0 | i = 0 \ldots \alpha - 1, s_i^0 \in 0 \ldots \alpha - 1, i \neq j \Rightarrow s_i^0 \neq s_j^0\}$$

Level 1 metarule (r^1)

$$r^1 : N_{R^1} \rightarrow R^1, \quad r^1 \in R^2$$

$$R^1 = \{r_i^0 | i = 0 \ldots \beta - 1, r_i^0 \in 0 \ldots |S^0|^{|S^0|^{|N_{S^0}|}} - 1, i \neq j \Rightarrow r_i^0 \neq r_j^0\}$$

Level 2 metarule (r^2)

$$r^2 : N_{R^2} \rightarrow R^2, \quad r^2 \in R^3$$

$$R^2 = \{r_i^1 | i = 0 \ldots \gamma - 1, r_i^1 \in 0 \ldots |R^1|^{|R^1|^{|N_{R^1}|}} - 1, i \neq j \Rightarrow r_i^1 \neq r_j^1\}$$

Level m metarule (r^m)

$$r^m : N_{R^m} \rightarrow R^m, \quad r^m \in R^{m+1}$$

$$R^m = \{r_i^{m-1} | i = 0 \ldots \Omega - 1, r_i^{m-1} \in 0 \ldots |R^{m-1}|^{|R^{m-1}|^{|N_{R^{m-1}}|}} - 1, i \neq j \Rightarrow r_i^{m-1} \neq r_j^{m-1}\}$$

$$m \in \text{Nat}_+, \quad m \geq 1, \quad \alpha, \beta, \gamma, \Omega \in \text{Nat}_+$$

Rules r^p are numbered at each level p where $p \geq 0$ using the binary coding scheme described by Wolfram (1984).

The number of possible metarule configurations at level m in the metarule hierarchy is given by:

$$\prod_{k=1}^{m} \binom{|R^{m-k}|^{|R^{m-k}|^{|N_{R^{m-k}}|}}}{|R^m|} \left(|R^m|^{|R^m|^{|N_{R^m}|}} \right) \quad m \in \text{Nat}_+, \quad m \geq 1$$

For example, $m = 1$ (single level of metarules)

$$|R^{m-1}| = |R^m| = 2, \quad |N_{R^{m-1}}| = |N_{R^m}| = 3$$

That is, a cell can be in one of two states with three contiguous cells comprising a cell neighborhood. For such a CA with a single level of metarules, more than 8 million possible metarule configurations must be considered. Hence, empirical investigations have necessarily been restricted to small regions of the space of possible configurations.

EXPERIMENTS

In our experiments, we used Wolfram's (1984) classification scheme, which identifies four classes of CA behavior: class I (fixed-point attractors), class II (cyclic attractors), class III (chaotic attractors), and class IV (complex attractors supporting universal construction and computation).

Elementary 1-D CA (i.e., $|S| = 2$, $|N| = 3$) or binary automata with a neighborhood of three cells support behavior only in classes I, II, and II. However, it may be possible to generate class IV behavior at the "edge of chaos"

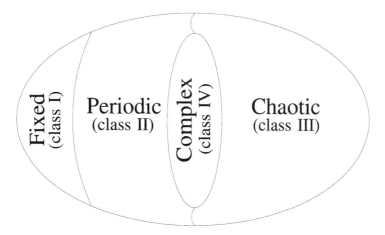

Figure 50.2 Cellular automata behavior profile (From Langton 1991, with permission).

(Langton 1991) by using rules that generate behaviors in classes II and III under a metarule scheme (Figure 50.2).

A small range of the possible metarule configuration space has been investigated in which $|S| = 2$, $|N| = 3$, $r^1 = 190$ and $R^1 = (x, 131)$ where $x \in$ {18, 22, 54, 60, 86, 90, 101, 102, 109, 120, 124, 129, 134, 135, 146, 150, 151, 165, 193, 195, 225}. x generates class III behavior; rule 131 generates class II behavior.

Preliminary results indicate that incorporating a single level of metarules into a 1-D elementary CA may allow behavior in class IV to be generated. Hence, universal computation, postulated as a necessary condition for mind in the CETM, is possible for elementary 1-D CA. Figure 50.3 is the space-time evolution for the metarule CA described above. Figure 50.4 is the space-time evolution of a 1-D CA (rule 906663673) generating class IV behavior.

BEYOND SUBSTANCE AND PROCESS

One possible objection to this scheme is that the scheme is ontologically dualistic at the lowest level in the hierarchy (states and rules) and ontologically monistic at all other levels (rules and metarules). This problem may be overcome by extending the framework to a bidirectionally infinite hierarchy in which states at level m are rules at level $m - 1$ and rules at level m are states at level $m + 1$ where $-\infty \geq m \geq +\infty$. Such a framework replaces the dualistic ontology of state and rule, and their corresponding physical counterparts, substance and process, with a monistic ontology based on an instance of a more general kind:

$$\zeta^m : N_{H^m} \rightarrow H^m, \quad \zeta^m \in H^{m+1}$$

$$H^m = \{\zeta_i^{m-1} | i = 0 \ldots \Phi - 1, \zeta_i^{m-1} \in 0 \ldots |H^{m-1}|^{|H^{m-1}||N_{H^{m-1}}|} - 1, i \neq j \Rightarrow \zeta_i^{m-1} \neq \zeta_j^{m-1}\}$$

$$m \in \text{Nat}, \Phi \in \text{Nat}_+$$

Syed Mustafa Ali and Robert M. Zimmer: A New Framework for Emergence

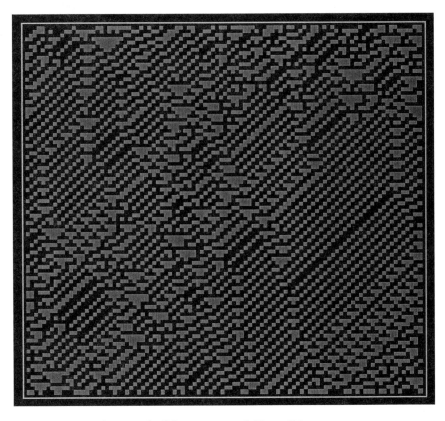

Figure 50.3 One-dimensional cellular automata with $|S| = 2$, $|N| = 3$.

CONCLUSION

An important epistemological result follows from adopting the hierarchy described above as the underlying ontology of nature. In the act of observation of a natural phenomenon, we cut (identify as separate) the levels in the hierarchy and thereby determine global physics (ς^m) and local atomic substrate (ς^{m-w} where w is the number of levels between cuts) (Figure 50.5).

Consequently, substrate atomism is epistemologically relativistic depending on where the cut is made in the hierarchy. The position of the cut affects (1) the extent to which emergence is possible (i.e., emergence relative to a model) (Cariani 1991), and (2) the types of phenomena (i.e., behavioral classes) that can emerge, given the global physics and atomic substrate. The idea of "cutting" the world was anticipated in an earlier work by Spencer-Brown (1969)—"a universe comes into being when a space is severed." However, the problem in that scheme and in the one presented here is the source or agency responsible for the cut. The fact that the problem of subjectivity remains (Nagel 1979) provides an indication as to where a possible solution may lie. We see the solution in an intentionalistic self-cutting ontological hierarchy based on a variant of panexperientialism. Such a scheme allows downwards causation via what Polanyi (1968) calls "higher principles." These

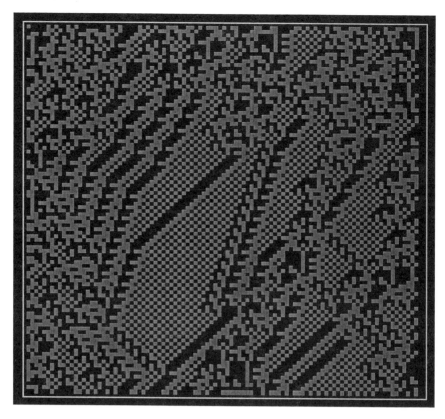

Figure 50.4 One-dimensional cellular automata with $|S| = 2$, $|N| = 5$.

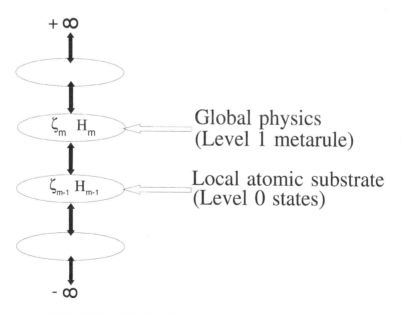

Figure 50.5 "Cutting" the hierarchy.

Syed Mustafa Ali and Robert M. Zimmer: A New Framework for Emergence

principles are boundary conditions imposed in the selective act of cutting by an intentional observer, that is, the subjective component of the hierarchy described in this chapter.

REFERENCES

Baas, N. A. 1993. Emergence, hierarchies and hyperstructures. In C. G. Langton, ed., *Artificial Life III*. Reading, MA: Addison-Wesley, pp. 515–537.

Cariani, P. 1991. Emergence and artificial life. In C. G. Langton, C. Taylor, J. D. Farmer, and S. Rasmussen, eds., *Artificial Life II*. Reading, MA: Addison-Wesley, pp. 775–797.

Darley, V. 1994. Emergent phenomena and complexity. In R. A. Brooks and P. Maes, eds., *Artificial Life IV*. Cambridge: MIT Press, pp. 411–416.

Langton, C. 1991. Life at the Edge of Chaos. In C. G. Langton, C. Taylor, J. D. Farmer, and S. Rasmussen, eds., *Artificial Life II*. Reading, MA: Addison-Wesley, pp. 41–91.

Nagel, T. 1979. *Mortal Questions*. Oxford: Cambridge University Press.

Polanyi, M. 1968. Life's irreducible structure. *Science* 160(6):1308–1312.

Searle, J. R. 1992. *The Rediscovery of the Mind*. Cambridge: MIT Press.

Spencer-Brown, G. 1969. *Laws of Form*. London: George Allen and Unwin, Ltd.

Wolfram, S. 1984. Universality and complexity in cellular automata. *Physica D* 10:1–35.

XI Quantum Theory, Space-Time, and Consciousness

OVERVIEW

Viewing the brain as a hierarchical system, one may ask: At which level in scale and complexity does consciousness critically depend? (Notice that this is not necessarily the same level at which consciousness emerges.) In other words: What is the hierarchical level below which neural components could in principle be replaced by silicon or other functional material while preserving consciousness?[1] Many would say that consciousness depends on neural-level electrochemical activities, claiming that consciousness emerges from higher-order functions whose fundamental component is a neuron either firing or not firing. Others contend that subneural activities are also relevant. For example, Pribram's dendritic microprocessing and various models of information dynamics in membranes, proteins, ions, and cell water may support cognitive functions and be involved in conscious experience.

Some suggest that consciousness may extend further down the brain's organizational hierarchy to the quantum level, or even to the fundamental Planck scale of space-time geometry. Because quantum theory and space-time are almost as enigmatic as consciousness, critics often deride juxtaposing the problems as a mere "minimization of mysteries" or "marriage of convenience." Insights from quantum theory and space-time geometry, however, may offer specific advantages in understanding consciousness, including potential solutions to: the binding problem, the "hard problem" of experience, noncomputability, free will, and the transition from preconscious processes to consciousness itself.

Quantum theory was developed in an attempt to describe the nature of reality at the atomic-structure scale, where experiments have confirmed the *wave–particle duality* of both atomic particles and light waves. Thus isolated atomic and subatomic-scale systems can exist in a *quantum superposition* of different states simultaneously, and experiments show that certain quantum systems manage to remain connected over surprisingly great distances. In the macroscopic world of our everyday experience, on the other hand, physical objects (like footballs and planet Earth) have well-defined positions and speeds and are decidedly nonwavelike.

Thus it is important to know why and how microscopic quantum systems correspond to the macroscopic classical systems in normal human experience. In the minds of some, the transition from possibility to concreteness is considered the "collapse" (or reduction) of a quantum-wave packet, which—according to the Copenhagen interpretation of quantum theory—occurs when the quantum system is measured or observed by a conscious observer. To illustrate the apparent absurdity of this notion in the biological realm, Erwin Schrödinger (1935) famously described his "cat-in-a-box" experiment (in which the poor beast would be simultaneously both dead and alive until the box is opened) as a "burlesque example" of the Copenhagen perspective misapplied. Nonetheless, the cat paradox continues to rankle many minds, and some deny that collapse occurs at all, holding our naive perceptions about the classical world to be at odds with reality in a wavelike universe. Others recall that when the ordinary rules in Schrödinger's wave mechanics are appropriately applied—as Born and Oppenheimer (1927) did to provide a quantum basis for molecular structures—classical nonlinear dynamics may be smoothly recovered at the biochemistry level (Scott 1995). Proposals such as the Fröhlich mechanism, however (e.g., Fröhlich 1968) suggest that coherent quantum states *can* possibly occur in protein assemblies such as membrane channels and microtubule subunits.

What if macroscopic quantum states *do* occur in the brain? Are they any more explanatory than neural-level correlates of consciousness? Several attributes of quantum states indicate that they *could* be:

1. Quantum-coherent states do have a unity, or "oneness," suggested as an explanation for "binding" in conscious vision, and self (e.g., Marshall 1989).

2. Like consciousness, quantum states cannot be directly observed.

3. Quantum states seem to involve some rearrangement of fundamental reality. What *is* reality?

How can we confidently judge our awareness of what's "out there" in the world without knowing what the "world" is? Such questions are especially important because some philosophers and physicists (e.g., Leibniz, Whitehead, Wheeler, Chalmers) suggest that the substrate for conscious experience (or *qualia*) is fundamental—like mass, spin, or electrical charge. Thus "fundamental" experience may be characterized by Planck-scale space-time geometry. Consciousness and the physics of reality are related.

The chapter authors in this section address various aspects in the relationships between the nature of mind and physical theories.

In "The Evolution of Consciousness," Henry Stapp argues that classical physics is ill equipped to deal with consciousness, treating it only as an epiphenomenon and thus unable to confer survival advantage on an evolving organism. It is quantum physics, according to Stapp, which provides a natural setting for conscious experience. Unlike classical physics, in which atomic particles are imagined as tiny billiard balls, quantum theory sees them as "nonlocalized elements of … a knowledge structure." Observing that the

Copenhagen interpretation of quantum theory made no attempt to describe collapse or its implications for the dynamics of the universe, Stapp reviews three major approaches to the collapse problem: Everett's "many-worlds" picture, the nonlinear "pilot-wave" theory of de Broglie and Bohm, and the more orthodox wave-function collapse view associated with Bohr, Heisenberg, von Neumann, and Wigner. The latter is most credible, according to Stapp, because wave-packet collapses (or quantum jumps) have been widely observed in nature. Conscious events are seen as special cases of collapse that are causally effective in choosing patterns of neurological activity.

"What are quantum theorists doing at a conference on consciousness?" asks Euan Squires in Chapter 52, and his answer is: Not because quantum theory can explain consciousness, but because consciousness can explain quantum theory.[2] Squires describes a simple superposition of two states and an observer, "Melinda," who consciously experiences one of them. Although quantum theory predicts the statistical probabilities, Squires argues that eventhough both states are in physics, the unique conscious result occurs only in Melinda's brain. Thus the statistical quantum rules do not tell us anything about physics, but they do say something about consciousness. To understand what that might be, Squires claims that the simplest explanation is this: after an observation, we have two Melinda minds, each experiencing one of the states. This is a "many-minds" view (notice that each mind would be unaware that any others existed), a refinement of Everett's original "many-worlds" view. Squires points out two defects in this approach: First, the experienced world is not identical to the physical world, and second, the explanation has no room for quantum probabilities. To rectify the quandary, Squires introduces his own "one-mind" interpretation, in which consciousness selects one experienced state among many possibilities. The same procedure could also select actions to take: choosing or deciding, thus giving consciousness an essential function and requiring that superpositions occur in the brain. But it also asks that different observers select the same experience, implying, according to Squires, that consciousness is nonlocal and actually universal.

Friedrich Beck next considers how and where quantum processes relevant to consciousness could occur in the brain. He investigates conditions under which coherent quantum states could be robust against the thermal fluctuations expected to be present in a warm and noisy brain, concluding that microscopic quantum jumps can occur only on very fast time scales (picoseconds to femtoseconds), corresponding to electronic transitions like electron transfer or breaking hydrogen bonds in neuronal structures. Macroscopic neural and synaptic processes, on the other hand, occur in the much-slower millisecond to nanosecond regime. The large difference in time scales decouples quantum processes from neural-level dynamics, except in the special circumstance that Beck calls a "quantum trigger." As an example, he identifies neurotransmitter exocytosis—the release of synaptic vesicles from axon terminals. Referring to earlier collaborations with John Eccles, Beck describes vesicle release as probabilistic, suggesting that it is the site and process at which quantum indeterminacy influences neural function.

In Chapter 53, we transcribe an informal discussion (accidentally recorded in the Sonoran Desert) between Alwyn Scott and Stuart Hameroff on quantum theory's relevance to consciousness studies. Scott contends that consciousness is an emergent property of classical nonlinear dynamics generated by the brain's hierarchical organization. Classical nonlinear states can be global and coherent, and sufficient for consciousness. Hameroff defends the quantum view, specifically the Penrose-Hameroff model involving quantum-coherent superposition and orchestrated self-collapse events in neuronal microtubules. Experience *is* "funda-mental," he argues, embedded in Planck-scale geometry and accessed and selected by quantum brain processes.

The debate goes on.

NOTES

1. Chalmers (1996) has addressed this question differently by asking if and when consciousness is lost as the brain's neurons are replaced "one by one" with functionally equivalent silicon devices. Whether or not a silicon device can be functionally equivalent to a neuron as far as consciousness goes is an open question, because we have imperfect knowledge about what neurons actually do (Scott 1995). In the present thought experiment, the natural brain is not replaced neuron by neuron, but from the bottom up.

2. Sadly, Euan Squires died in summer 1996. He was a kind and effervescent man of great intellect who will be sorely missed by his many friends and colleagues.

REFERENCES

Born, M., and J. R. Oppenheimer. 1927. Zur Quantentheorie der Molekeln. *Annalen der Physik* 84:457–484.

Chalmers, D. J. 1996. *The Conscious Mind: In Search of a Fundamental Theory*. New York: Oxford University Press.

Fröhlich, H. 1968. Long-range coherence and energy storage in biological systems. *International Journal of Quantum Chemistry* 2:641–649.

Marshall, I. N. 1989. Consciousness and Bose-Einstein condensates. *New Ideas in Psychology* 7:73–83.

Schrödinger, E. 1935. Die gegenwärtige Situation der Quantenmechanik. *Naturwissenschaften* 23:807–812, 823–828, and 844–849.

Scott, A. 1995. *Stairway to the Mind*. New York: Springer-Verlag (Copernicus).

51 The Evolution of Consciousness

Henry P. Stapp

INADEQUACY OF CLASSICAL MECHANICS AS THE BASIS FOR A SCIENCE OF CONSCIOUSNESS

Every major advance in science has involved an important conceptual development, and incorporating consciousness into physics should be no exception. Mapping out the empirical correlations between brain activity and consciousness will certainly contribute vitally to our understanding of the mind/brain system, but we must also achieve conceptual progress on the theoretical problem: how to bring consciousness into concordance with the principles of physics.

Rational analysis of this problem hinges on one fact: classical mechanics does not entail the existence of consciousness. Classical mechanics does not require, demand, or allow one to predict with certainty, the existence of (phenomenal) experience. The full content of nature, as represented in classical mechanics, resides in the locations and motions of particles, and the values and rates of change in local fields. Nothing in classical physical principles provides a basis for deducing how a physical system "feels"—for deducing whether it is happy or sad, or feels agony or delight. No phenomenal hook or toehold in classical mechanics itself can permit one to deduce, logically, simply from the principles of classical mechanics alone, the assured validity of assertions about the experiential aspects of nature. This is not a matter of lacking imagination, or inability to conceive new possibilities. It is a matter of basic principle. The principles of classical mechanics provide no basis for logically proving that a "feeling" exists because classical mechanics is a rationally closed conceptual system whose principles supply no more than is needed to determine the motions of particles and fields from the prior dispositions of these same variables. This dynamical connection is established within a narrow mathematical framework that never refers to any phenomenal (i.e., psychological or experiential) quality.

Classical mechanics is dynamically complete in all the variables with which it deals, namely the so-called physical variables, and so one has, for the phenomenal elements of nature, four options: (1) identify the phenomenal elements with certain properties or activities of the physical quantities; (2) say that these phenomenal elements are not identical to any physical property or activity, but are companions to certain physical properties or activities, and that their presence in no way disrupts the classical dynamics; (3) accept some combination of (1) and (2); or (4) accept that phenomenal elements do affect the dynamics, rendering classical dynamics invalid.

The first three options are scientifically indistinguishable, and they share this feature, that the classical dynamical principles do not logically determine whether the proposed connection of the physical variables to our felt experiences, or to the analogous feelings in members of other species, is valid or not. Thus the connection to physical parameters of something so basic to science as our experienced knowledge of what is going on about us is not logically entailed by the basic dynamical laws. Consequently, the feelings that we experience become appendages whose existence could, from a logical point of view, be denied without violating the posited classical laws. The phenomenal aspects of nature would be, in this sense, epiphenomenal: the classical dynamical principles could be completely valid without the feelings that we experience being present in nature at all.

It is very likely to be true that any physical system that is built and behaves in certain ways will also be conscious, and that this tight relationship between behavior and felt experience arises naturally out of the essential nature of the actual physical substrate. But such a connection would not mean that this tight relationship is a logical consequence of the principles of classical mechanics. On the contrary, it would mean that the principles of classical mechanics are incomplete because they fail to entail the existence of this naturally occurring aspect of nature, and are, moreover, necessarily false unless consciousness is epiphenomenal.

The epiphenomenal character of consciousness implied by classical mechanics cannot be reconciled with the naturalistic notion that consciousness evolved because of the survival advantage it conferred: epiphenomenal properties confer no survival advantage. Hence if the classical principles were taken to govern the dynamical process of nature, then the presence in human beings of highly developed consciousness would be a double mystery: the basic dynamical principles would neither entail the existence of the phenomenal realities that populate our experiential realms, nor, given their existence, allow any natural dynamical explanation of how they could have evolved to this high state from simpler forms.

These considerations would be very destructive for science's naturalistic program had classical mechanics not already been found, by purely physical considerations, to be basically incorrect: it does not describe correctly the empirically observed properties of physical systems. This failing is not merely a slight inaccuracy. To get an adequate theoretical foundation for a description of physical processes, the entire logical structure of classical mechanics had to be abandoned at the foundational level. It was replaced by a radically different logical structure that allows our experiences to play a key logical and dynamical role.

QUANTUM MECHANICS AND CONSCIOUSNESS

The successor to classical mechanics is called quantum mechanics. The basic change is to a mathematical description that effectively converts the atomic particles to something of a radically different ontological type. In the new theory, the "particles" can no longer be imagined to be tiny material objects of the kind encountered in everyday life, but merely smaller. They become more like nonlocalized elements in an information network, or in a knowledge structure. This ontological change infects everything made up of atomic constituents (and fields), hence the entire physical world. Thus the basic conceptual problem that the founders of quantum theory had to solve was how, facing this dissolution of the substantive classical-mechanics universe, to find some new foundational structure upon which to base an adequate new physics.

Their solution was pragmatic and epistemological. No matter what the world "out there" is really like, our direct experiences of it are just what they were before nature's quantum character was discovered: they are of the same kind that they were when classical mechanics seemed adequate. Given this empirical fact, that "our experiences of the world" are "classically describable," in that we can describe them as if they were experiences of a world that accords at the macroscopic level with the concepts of classical physics, one can take experiences of this kind to be the foundational elements upon which to build the new science. Thus the founders of quantum theory constructed the new physics as a theory of statistical correlations between experiences of this kind: the basic realities of the new physical science became these "classically describable" experiences, and the physical world became an information network that connected these classically describable experiential realities to each other in a mathematically specified statistical way.

The important thing about this new conception of basic physical theory, in the context of the mind/brain problem, is that the experiential things are no longer left out. Rather they have moved to a central position. Thus we are no longer forced to graft the experiential aspects of nature onto a physical theory which has no natural place for them, and which moreover excludes from the outset any possibility of their playing an irreducible dynamical role. Furthermore, because the theory's elemental ingredients are information and knowledge, rather than material objects resembling little rocks, we are no longer faced with the ontological puzzle of how to build consciousness out of something so seemingly unsuited to the task as a collection of tiny rocks hurtling through space. On the contrary, in quantum theory the rocklike aspects of nature arise from mathematical features that inhere in idealike qualities.

QUANTUM ONTOLOGIES

The original "Copenhagen" interpretation of quantum theory eschewed ontology: it made no attempt to provide a description of nature itself, but settled for a system of rules describing statistical correlations between our experiences (i.e., between our classically describable experiences of the world). Physicists have, by now, devised essentially three ontological pictures that could produce the same statistical connections as the earlier pragmatic system of rules. These ontologies are Everett's One-World/Many-Minds ontology, Bohm's Pilot-Wave Ontology, and the more orthodox Wave-Function-Collapse ontology associated with the names of Heisenberg, von Neumann, and Wigner. To get to the essential point of what consciousness can do, I will describe briefly the essential features of these three ontologies.

In all three ontologies a key component in nature is the quantum-state vector. This is a basic element in the quantum theory, and it can be represented in various equivalent ways. In the simplest way, one decomposes it into components corresponding to various numbers of "particles" of various kinds, where the word "particle" initially means just that there is a set of three variables x, y, and z, and a "mass," and perhaps a few other (spin) variables for each such "particle." Then, for example, the component of the state vector corresponding to N spinless particles would be a function of $3N$ variables, namely the three variables x, y, and z for each of the N particles. This function is called the "wave function" of the N particles: it can be imagined as something like a wave, or set of ripples, on a pond, where the different locations on the "pond" are specified now not by just two variables, as for an ordinary pond, but rather by $3N$ variables. This "wave," or set of ripples, evolves in time controlled by the Schrödinger equation, which causes the wave to propagate over this $3N$-dimensional "pond." This propagation's essential feature is the tendency for the wave continually to divide further and further into ever-finer separate branches that are narrowly focused and move off in different directions in the $3N$-dimensional space. Each such branch corresponds, roughly, to a different classically describable possibility. One such branch might correspond to the dead version of Schrödinger's notorious cat, whereas another branch would describe the alive version. The various separate branches become far apart on the $3N$-dimensional pond, hence evolving independently of one another: each branch quickly evolves almost exactly as it would if the various branches from which it is diverging were not present at all. On the other hand, various branches that are far apart and independently evolving in $3N$-dimensional space could be sitting right on top of each other if one were to project these branches down onto the ordinary 3-dimensional space that we seem to inhabit: the independently evolving dead and alive cats could be confined, for all appearances, to the same small 3D cage.

The basic interpretational question in quantum theory is how to comprehend these many coexisting "branches" of the universe, only one of which we ever observe.

I think almost every physicist who starts to think diligently about this question is led first (on our own if we have not already heard about it) to a natural interpretation that Everett (1957) first described in detail. This is the idea that, because the Schrödinger equation is the quantum-mechanical analogue of Newton's equations, which were supposed to govern the evolution of the universe itself, the physical world should have a really existing component corresponding to each of the branches generated by the Schrödinger equation. Because each of these branches essentially evolves independently of every other one, the realm of consciousness associated with each branch of the wave function in a person's brain must be dynamically independent of the realms of consciousness associated with every other branch. Thus each conscious observer should be aware only of the classically describable world that corresponds to the branch of the universe (as specified by the wave function) that includes the corresponding branch of our brain: the branches of the wave function of our brain that are parts of other branches of the universe should correspond to different, independently evolving realms of experience, namely to realms of experience corresponding to these other "classically describable" branches of the universe.

The existence of these branches of the wave function essentially evolving independently follows directly from the basic equations of quantum mechanics, and thus seems reasonable from a physicist's point of view, even though it leads to the strange idea that the complete reality is a superworld that is populated by a plethora of really existing ordinary worlds, only one of which is represented in any individual realm of consciousness.

The logical simplicity of this model is undermined, however, by a logical difficulty. It has to do with the statistical predictions that are the heart of quantum theory. The quantum evolution in accordance with the Schrödinger equation causes each branch generally to divide into subbranches, and quantum theory assigns to each subbranch a relative statistical weight, to which it gives an empirical meaning. This meaning entails that if I find myself to be on a branch then the probability that I will subsequently find myself to be on a specific subbranch will be specified by the aforementioned relative statistical weight of that subbranch. Thus if a subbranch has a very low relative statistical weight, according to the theory, then quantum theory predicts that the chance is very small that if I experience myself at one moment to be on the original branch then I will later experience myself to be on that subbranch.

To provide a basis for this notion of probability, one must have something that can belong to one branch *or* another. In this discussion this something was a realm of consciousness: each realm of consciousness is considered to belong to some one branch, not to all branches together. In the state vector, however, or its representation by a wave function, all the branches are conjunctively present: a toy boat might be sitting on one branch *or* another, but the pond itself has this ripple *and* that ripple, *and* that other ripple, and so on. Thus to deal with probabilities one is forced to introduce something that is logically different from the quantum state or wave function provided by the basic principles of quantum mechanics. This move introduces a new kind of ontological element: the theory becomes essentially dualistic, in contrast to the monistic structure of classical mechanics. Consciousness is a new kind of thing that, quite apart from its phenomenal character, has mathematical properties different from those of the "physical" part of nature represented by the wave function.

Once it is recognized that the realms of consciousness are not simply direct carryovers from the quantum state, but must have essentially different logical properties, it would seem more parsimonious and natural to have, for each person, one realm of consciousness that goes into one branch rather than having to introduce this new kind of ontological structure that, unlike the wave function, divides *disjunctively* into the various branches. This option produces a one-mind variation of Everett's many-minds interpretation. The one-mind version has been promoted by Euan Squires (1990).

David Bohm (1952, 1993) solves this *"and versus or"* problem by introducing in addition to the quantum state, or wave function, not consciousness but rather a classical universe, which is represented by a moving point in the $3N$-dimensional space. Bohm gives equations of motion for this point that cause it to move into one of the branches *or* another in concordance with the quantum-statistical rules, for a suitable random distribution of initial positions of this point. Thus Bohm's theory is also dualistic in the sense of having two ontological types, one of which, the quantum state, combines the branches conjunctively; the other, the classical world, specifies one branch *or* another.

The great seeming virtue of Bohm's model is that, like classical mechanics, it is logically complete without bringing in consciousness. But then, any later introduction of consciousness into the model would, from a logical point of view, be gratuitous, just as it is for classical mechanics: consciousness is not an integral and logically necessary part of the theory, but is rather a dangling epiphenomenal appendage to a theory whose chief virtue was that, like classical mechanics, it was logically and dynamically complete without consciousness.

Bohm's model is, moreover, nonparsimonious: it is burdened with a plethora of empty branches that evolve for all eternity even though they have no influence on the motion of the classical world. Squires's model has a similar defect: it has a plethora of empty (of consciousness) branches that evolve for all eternity, but have no effect on anyone's experiences. Everett's many-minds interpretation is nonparsimonious for the opposite reason: it has for each individual human being, Joe Doe, a plethora of minds only one of which is needed to account for the empirical facts. It is the presence of these superfluous elements in each of these interpretations that causes many physicists to turn away from these "unorthodox" interpretations.

The most parsimonious theory is the Bohr/Heisenberg/von Neumann/Wigner wave-function-collapse model. This model: (1) accepts Bohr's view that our experienced knowledge is an appropriate reality upon which to build physical theory; (2) accepts Heisenberg's view that transitions from potentiality to actuality are a basic component of nature; (3) accepts von Neumann's identification of these transitions with abrupt changes in the quantum state of the universe; and (4) accepts Wigner's proposal (attributed by Wigner to von Neumann) that our conscious experiences are associated with brain events that actualize new quantum states. This association of the experiential events (upon which Bohr based the whole theory) with brain events that are just special cases of the general collapse events of Heisenberg and von Neumann brings closure to the theory, and produces a natural basis for a science of consciousness.

This model is more parsimonious than the others because the state of the universe becomes a representation of a set of potentialities for an event to occur, and this event reconfigures the potentialities, hence the state vector, bringing them into concordance with the new knowledge actualized by the event. The experienced knowledge that an adequate physical theory must accommodate and explain is thus brought explicitly into the theory, rather than being left in some ineffable limbo, and the quantum state remains always in concordance with the potentialities for the next event, rather than being burdened with "empty branches" that no longer have any bearing on our experiences. The theory thus retains much of the pragmatism of the original Copenhagen interpretation, but brings into the theoretical description the brains that are the physical substrates of our experienced knowledge.

Large physical objects are at the same time both entities in their own right, parts of the world that envelops them, and also constructs fabricated from their atomic constituents. In a naturalistic science one expects thoughts and other experiences to have analogous properties. Therefore a primary problem is to understand, in the context of our basic physical theory (namely quantum mechanics) how our thoughts and other experiences can be both whole entities and yet also constructs built of elemental components.

How do our complex thoughts come to be part of nature? According to the notion of Platonic ideals the ideal forms are somehow eternal. But it is more in line with the naturalistic program of science to try to understand complex thoughts as constructed by some natural process out of more elemental forms. Indeed, the naturalistic program leads us to try to explain how our complex thoughts are built up by natural processes associated with our complex brains.

In any proof, or theorem, or theory, one can only get out what one puts in, in some form or another. Consciousness then cannot come out of a theoretical or computational model of the mind/brain unless at least the seeds of consciousness are put in. It would be contrary to science's naturalistic program to put full-blown complex thoughts or experiences directly into the conception of the mind/brain at the outset. But one must put in seeds that can bloom into our conscious thoughts in the physical environment of our brains. Classical mechanics has no such seeds, but the foregoing description of the Bohr/Heisenberg/von Neumann/Wigner collapse interpretation of quantum mechanics suggests that an appropriately constituted informational model that implements the mathematical structures that quantum phenomena have revealed to us could contain the requisite seeds of consciousness.

SEEDS OF CONSCIOUSNESS

I have argued above that classical mechanics does not entail the existence of consciousness. The reason was that classical mechanics has no reference to psychological qualities, hence one cannot deduce from the principles of classical mechanics alone that any activity that classical mechanics entails is necessarily accompanied by a psychological activity. But what is it that causes some scientists to resist the temptation to sweep away the problem of consciousness by asserting baldly that certain functional physical activities simply *are* psychological activities.

One reason to resist is that this is a bald assertion: it is a claim that is not entailed by the dynamical principles. One can define a thundercloud to be angry when its electrical potential is high relative to the earth, or nearby clouds, and justify this definition by pointing out that an angry cloud is, by virtue of the dynamic principles, likely to have a destructive outburst, which is a sign of anger. But making this definition does not mean that an angry thundercloud feels like you feel when you are angry. We cannot deduce from the classical dynamical principles anything about how a thundercloud feels, even though one can deduce, from this definition, that it is angry.

The question is entirely different if one accepts that quantum mechanics is the appropriate physical theory for explaining natural phenomena. As I have pointed out, the most parsimonious quantum ontology is the Bohr/Heisenberg/von Neumann/Wigner wave-function-collapse model, and conscious experiences are already woven into that theory's fabric. They were placed there to provide the basis not for a theory of consciousness, but for a rationally coherent and practically useful physical theory that accommodates the experimental evidence pertaining to the basic qualities of the physical stuff of nature. The core insight of Bohr and his colleagues was that because the key mathematical elements in the practical calculations were representations of structures that seemed more akin to ideas than to material substance, the theory should be pragmatic and epistemological, and built around our experienced knowledge, rather than around the classical notion of matter. This idea is retained: conscious events, and their images in the mathematical representation of nature, become key logical, dynamical, and epistemological elements in the theory. An experience is neither a companion of, nor claimed to be identical to, a physical activity that seems profoundly different from itself—namely a collection of tiny rocklike objects hurtling through space in some way. Rather it is identified as a contraction of an idealike structure to a more compact and cohesive structure. Such a contraction is naturally akin to a thought in these respects: it selects and brings into being a cohesive idealike reality, and it grasps as an integral unit an information structure that is extended over a large spatial region.

COLLAPSE CONDITIONS AND EVOLUTION OF CONSCIOUSNESS

My purpose in this section is to bring out some conditions that are imposed by the demand that consciousness evolve naturally in accordance with the principles of natural selection, hence in coordination with the survival advantage that consciousness can confer upon organisms that possess it.

Within the Bohr/Heisenberg/von Neumann/Wigner framework, conscious process has an image in the physicist's description of nature. This process is represented by a sequence of collapse events that directly controls evolution of the physical system. The basic problem in tying this causally efficacious conscious process to survival advantage is that in a first approximation quantum mechanics and classical mechanics, though conceptually very different, give essentially the same predictions about many physical quantities: it takes well-controlled experiments to establish the corpuscular character of light, or the wave character of atomic particles. But to the extent that classical mechanics is adequate to explain our physical behavior, consciousness can be regarded as unnecessary, hence unable to confer survival advantage. Thus to study the survival advantages conferred by consciousness it is necessary to consider behavioral features which cannot be accounted for by classical mechanics, but which depend critically upon effects of the collapse events that are, in this theory, physical images of conscious events.

Most of the extant analyses bearing on this problem have been carried out within the context laid down by von Neumann in his study of the measurement problem. The main condition in these studies is that the process being studied correspond to a "good measurement." This condition entails that the wave function of the full system divide during the "measurement" into several well-separated branches, so that within each branch some macroscopic variable, dubbed the "pointer," will be confined to a small region, and so that the various small regions associated with the various branches will be nonoverlapping. The collapse is supposed to occur after this separation has occurred, and is achieved by restricting the pointer variable to the region corresponding to some selected one of these branches, with the relative frequencies of the branches—selected in a long run of similar experiments—conforming to a specified statistical rule, namely the Born rule.

Within this "good-measurement" context, the predictions derived from the Bohr/Heisenberg/von Neumann/Wigner-collapse model will be no different from those derived from David Bohm's deterministic model, which has no collapses, hence no effect of consciousness. The point is that Bohm's model is designed to give the same predictions as the orthodox Copenhagen rules in these "good-measurement" cases, and it does so without bringing in either collapses or efficacious consciousness.

This is a key point: insofar as the collapses in the brain occur only under "good-measurement" conditions, and in accordance with the Born rule, it will be difficult if not impossible to obtain any effect of consciousness per se upon the organism's survival prospects. It is difficult because the evolution would not differ significantly from Bohm's statistical model, which gives the same statistical results without involving or invoking the notion of consciousness.

Conversely, however, if the collapses in the brain occur under conditions other than those of a "good measurement," then the collapses, which in this theory are images of thoughts and feelings, can in principle enter into the dynamics in ways that would lead to a natural evolution of consciousness.

Notice that the pertinent point here is not a difference between classical mechanics and quantum mechanics, *per se*. The issue is the role of consciousness. No one doubts that quantum theory should be used where it differs from classical mechanics, but that fact is not directly relevant to the consciousness issue. For the Bohm model can account for much of quantum phenomena without ever mentioning either consciousness or collapses. The Bohr/Heisenberg/von Neumann/Wigner formulation does bring consciousness *per se* into the dynamics in a natural and dynamically efficacious way. But if this dynamical effect does not produce, regarding prospects for survival, departures from what the Bohm formulation predicts, then one cannot rationally assert that consciousness *per se* is having any effect on survival.

The only way I can see to make the predictions of the collapse model depart from the predictions of the Bohm model is to say either that the collapses in brains occur sometimes under conditions that do not conform to "good measurements," or that under these conditions the Born rule can sometimes fail, or to say that the Bohm model does not apply to the real world, which may involve complexities such as "strings," or supersymmetries, or quantum gravity, and so on, which could render Bohm's model inapplicable.

The situation, therefore, is this. Naturalistic science requires the existence of our complex human consciousness to be explained, in the sense that we should be able to see how its presence and form could emerge in conjunction with the evolution of bodily forms as a consequence of the survival advantages that it confers upon organisms that possess it. Insofar as classical mechanics is taken to be the basic mechanics, the existence of human consciousness could never be explained in this sense because the classical principles do not specify how consciousness enters: one can vary at will one's idea of how consciousness is connected to the physical properties of some organism, and even hold it to be absent altogether from that organism's life, without contradicting the principles of classical mechanics. On the other hand, consciousness does enter efficaciously into the Bohr/Heisenberg/von Neumann/Wigner formulation of quantum mechanics, and so this conception of the basic dynamical theory does provide at least a toehold for a possible naturalistic explanation of how consciousness evolved. For in this theory consciousness is tied tightly to the causally efficacious collapse process. But invoking quantum mechanics does not automatically provide a natural explanation for the evolution of consciousness. The mind/brain dynamics depends critically upon the details of how the collapse process operates in the brain. In the simplest scenario, the dynamics would be indistinguishable from what would be predicted by Bohm's model, which involves no collapses and no consciousness. If the naturalistic program is to succeed, then the collapse process in human brains must be more complex than that which the simplest possible quantum scenario would yield.

One approach, that of Penrose and Hameroff, depends on difficult-to-achieve long-range quantum-coherence effects that extend over a large part of the brain. Moreover, Penrose ties this model to Platonic ideals, not intrinsically connected to physical structure, but rather more free-floating, and prior to their physical embodiments. Naturalistic science, on the other hand, would have each thought tied intrinsically to some physical substrate, such as a brain.

Some technical foundations for a naturalistic approach to these questions appear in two earlier versions (Stapp 1996a,b) of this chapter that did not meet the space limitations imposed on contributions to these proceedings. The point in those papers is that if the "good-measurement" condition is lifted, and the collapses are taken to be collapses to patterns of neurological activity of the kind identified in Stapp (1993) as the brain images of thoughts, but without demanding that these patterns be disjoint from similar but slightly different patterns (specified by slightly earlier or later, or stronger or weaker, pulses on some neurons), then a significant speedup can occur— compared to classically described or Bohm-described processes—of brain processes that are searching for abductive solutions to typical problems that organisms must face in their struggle for survival. This speedup can confer survival advantage. A reason for top-level brainwide events being favored over lower-level events is given in Stapp (1994).

ACKNOWLEDGMENTS

This work was supported by the Director, Office of Energy Research, Office of High Energy and Nuclear Physics, Division of High Energy Physics of the U.S. Department of Energy under Contract DE-AC03-76SF00098.

REFERENCES

Bohm, D. 1952. A suggested interpretation of quantum theory in terms of "hidden" variables, I and II. *Physical Review* 85:166–193.

Bohm, D., and B. Hiley. 1993. *The Undivided Universe: An Ontological Interpretation of Quantum Theory*. London: Rutledge.

Everett, H. III 1957. Relative state interpretation of quantum mechanics. *Reviews of Modern Physics* 29:463–462.

Stapp, H. P. 1993. *Mind, Matter, and Quantum Mechanics*. New York: Springer-Verlag, Ch. 6.

Stapp, H. P. 1996a. Chance, choice, and consciousness: A causal quantum theory of the mind/brain. http://www-physics.lbl.gov/~stapp/stappfiles.html.

Stapp, H. P. 1996b. Science of consciousness and the hard problem. *Journal of Mind and Brain* forthcoming. http://www-physics.lbl.gov/~stapp/stappfiles.html.

Stapp, H. P. 1994. Quantum mechanical coherence, resonance, and mind. In: Proceedings of the Norbert Weiner Centenary Congress 1994, Proceedings of Symposia in Applied Mathematics 52. http://www.physics.lbl.gov/~stapp/stappfiles.html.

Squires, E. 1990. *The Conscious Mind in the Physical World*. Bristol: Adam Hilger.

von Neumann, J. 1932. *Mathematical Foundations of Quantum Mechanics* (English translation 1955). Princeton: Princeton University Press, Ch. 6.

Wigner, E. 1967. *Remarks on the Mind-Body Problem: Symmetries and Reflections*. Bloomington: Indiana University Press.

52 Why Are Quantum Theorists Interested in Consciousness?

Euan J. Squires*

A possible answer to the question in the title of this chapter would be that we can explain consciousness. That would be false; we have no more idea how to explain consciousness than anyone else; that is, we have *no* idea! In fact, the whole idea of trying to *explain* consciousness is probably a mistake; consciousness just is (see last section).

The proper answer to the question is that we cannot understand quantum theory without invoking consciousness.[1]

Quantum theory is a wonderful, elegant theory that, at least in principle, allows us to calculate the properties of all physical (and chemical) systems. It gives correct results for the probabilities in particular results from an enormous range of experiments. It is accurate and universal, and no violations of its predictions are known, even where those predictions are highly counterintuitive.

If quantum theory really applies to all systems however, except in very special circumstances, there can never be any observations—that is, no events for which the aforementioned statistical predictions could apply.

This statement is so important, though straightforward, that it deserves an example. We imagine that a system to be "measured" is in a state that I describe as $|+\rangle$. (No need to worry what this symbolism means or why I use this funny notation.)

This system is measured with an apparatus A, and let us suppose that after the measurement the combined system can be described by $|+, A^+\rangle$. This expression means that the $+$ reading on the apparatus corresponds to the system being described in the state of $+$. Generally the apparatus is not isolated but interacts with an environment (air, microwave background, black holes, strings, etc.). If we call all this E, then the full state is $|+, A^+, E^+\rangle$. Of course this statement will in general change with time, but I do not need to indicate this condition explicitly.

Next, let us suppose that Melinda looks at the apparatus. This act puts her brain, denoted Me, into a specific state. Hence the state of the relevant

*Sadly, Euan Squires died in the Summer of 1996. He was a lively man of great depth who contributed significantly to quantum theory and consciousness studies. We hope his one-mind idea is correct.

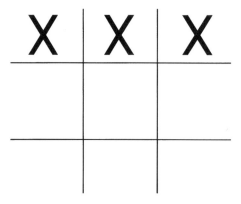

Figure 52.1 A hypothetical neural pattern that Melinda interprets as the result +.

system is now

$$|+, A+, E^+, Me^+\rangle \tag{52.1}$$

Everything up to here is perfectly straightforward. Assuming that I knew the physical structure of the apparatus (not too difficult to imagine), of the environment (a bit harder), and of Melinda's brain (harder still), then the evolution of this final state could be calculated from the Schrödinger equation.

Notice that the precise nature of the physical brain is totally irrelevant here; we need make no assumptions whatever about that subject, except that the brain is a physical thing and is therefore described by the laws of quantum theory.

Now we need to introduce the concept that none of us knows anything about. Presumably the Me^+ state of Melinda's brain corresponds to some sort of "pattern" that her consciousness, knowing something about apparatus A, interprets as meaning that the system was in the state +. To be concrete, suppose the pattern is as given in Figure 52.1.

We can then repeat the discussion thus far with some other state of the system. Let us call this state $|-\rangle$. In an obvious generalization of the notation used above, the state after the measurement will now be

$$|-, A^-, E^-, Me^-\rangle. \tag{52.2}$$

Again, there will be some pattern in Melinda's brain that her consciousness recognizes as meaning that the system was in the state −. Suppose that this time the pattern is as in Figure 52.2.

At this stage we have nothing that differs from classical physics. The calculation yields a result that that is interpreted by consciousness. These, however, are the "special circumstances" referred to above, where we have no measurement problem.

The problem arises because it is possible, and indeed sometimes very easy, to prepare a state that is not + or −, but a "bit of each." We write this state $a|+\rangle + b|-\rangle$, where the relative magnitudes of a and b tell us something about how much of + compared to − the state contains. In practice, most

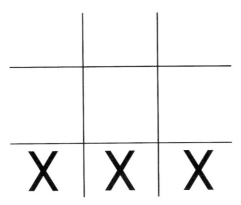

Figure 52.2 A hypothetical neural pattern that Melinda interprets as the result −.

states that are observed will have this form. (To prevent any possible mis-understanding here we emphasize that this new state is not just a way of saying that the state might be + or it might be −, and that we do not know which. Quantum theory allows us to discuss this situation—the state is then called a *mixed state*—but it is not what we have here.)

What happens when we measure this new state using the same apparatus as before? Here is another piece of quantum magic. From the results of the previous calculations, it is a trivial matter to calculate what happens. In fact, the final state becomes

$$a|+, A^+, E^+, Me^+\rangle + b|-, A^-, E^-, Me^-\rangle. \tag{52.3}$$

We do not get one pattern or the other, but something that is a bit of one and a bit of the other. Nothing is obviously remarkable about that; we started with the system in a state that we wrote as a "sum" of system states, and we finish with a similar type of sum of observed states.

Now come the surprises.

1. It is a simple matter of fact that Melinda will experience either the + state or the − state. According to her experience, the state shown in Figure 52.3 will be exactly the same as if it were either Figure 52.1 or 52.2.

Being careful, I specify that this statement is what Melinda will tell us. To be sure (see below), we can check by doing the observation ourselves. Then I will be aware of the pattern in either Figure 52.1 or Figure 52.2—certainly not the "sum" of the two patterns, as in Figure 52.3.

Notice that this one result of which I am aware exists in consciousness, but not in "physics,"—that is, no one result is present in the state of the physical world as it is calculated according to quantum theory. If this is "dualism," then I am happy to be called a dualist.

2. The reasoning in item 1 follows from orthodox quantum theory, in the sense that I will clarify immediately. Because I sometimes read statements that seem to deny this orthodoxy, because we must be precise about what we mean, and because, if we think about it, this reasoning is amazing, I shall derive it mathematically.

Euan J. Squires: Why Are Quantum Theorists Interested in Consciousness?

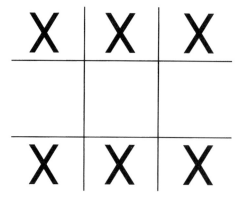

Figure 52.3 A possible "sum" of neural patterns corresponding to the superposed states. But Melinda's experience corresponds either to the pattern in Figure 52.1 or in Figure 52.2.

Suppose Melinda had agreed to write a 0 on a piece of paper as soon as she knew whether the system was in the state + or the state −. Notice that she does not write down *what* it is, only that she *knows* what it is. Clearly, both where the system was in the + or − state, as soon as she had looked at the apparatus, she would have written the 0. It follows trivially from standard quantum theory that where the state was the sum of the two, she would again write down the 0. Thus she would tell the world that she had become aware of the pattern in either Figure 52.1 or Figure 52.2. Every physical action she took would convey this message. I think she would therefore have become aware of one result, as indeed we know happens in practice. Otherwise she would consistently be telling the world, and herself, a lie. In other words, I know from orthodox quantum theory that Melinda's brain state does not correspond to a definite result; I also know from orthodox quantum theory that she will consistently tell me she is aware of one result.

This thinking seems to imply that orthodox quantum theory has told us something about how consciousness actually works. Of course, this interpretation relies on the assumption of consistency that we have used. All Melinda's physical actions, as long as they are governed by quantum theory, will imply that she knows a unique result. The assumption is that she really does know such a result. One could imagine (just about) that, on the contrary, she was not aware of any result, but that nevertheless she put the 0 on the paper, and in all other ways behaved as though she did.

We cannot run this argument with a computer (try it). It works because Melinda is conscious and it therefore makes sense to talk about "knowing." Computers, on the other hand, do not *know* anything, and we would have no way of giving the essential instruction to write a 0 as soon as the result is known.

3. Here is something that does not follow from the simple evolution equation of quantum theory—that is, the Schrödinger equation—which is all we have used so far. In a large set of identical runs of the experiment above the number of times Melinda would see + and − would be in the ratio of

$|a|^2/|b|^2$. This relation is a "rule" that is added to quantum theory. It is called the Born rule (after Max Born, who first proposed it), and it has been confirmed repeatedly in myriad experiments.

Where then is the problem, and what has all this reasoning to do with consciousness?

The complete description of the "physics" in orthodox quantum theory is the state displayed above, which includes both terms, that is, both "results." The unique result of which I am aware does not exist in physics—but only in consciousness. The Born rule has nothing to say about physics—it says something about consciousness.

I must qualify this statement by emphasizing that I am speaking of orthodox quantum theory. I could add something to physics (e.g., the Bohm hidden-variable model) or I could change it (e.g., the explicit collapse models of GRW/Pearle, etc.), so that the result would be in the physics. Even then the properties of consciousness would appear, but all that is another story that we shall not follow here.

NAÏVE MANY-MINDS INTERPRETATION

To continue, we notice that the simplest possibility for what is happening would be that after the measurement we have two "Melindas," one of whom has one experience, and one has the other. We need not worry that this description does not appear to Melinda to be what is happening, because it is guaranteed by quantum theory that each "Melinda" will be unaware of the other's existence, and will indeed have no possibility of knowing about the other (this condition is true for all practical purposes, though if she were sufficiently clever she could perhaps devise means for checking whether the other Melinda really existed.) We have here the "naïve" many-worlds interpretation of quantum theory; it is better called the "many-views" or "many-minds" interpretation (Zeh 1981, Squires 1987, Albert and Loewer 1988, Lockwood 1989) because the physical world, described by the quantum state, for example, as displayed above in our simple example (equation 52.3) is always *one* thing.

Notice two points. First, the experienced world is precisely that—*the world as experienced*. It is not identical to the physical world. When we "measure" something, we experience a particular result, but, in general, that result does not refer to anything that was there before our experience of it, or even after the experience; it exists only in consciousness. Second, all this knowledge has been achieved with nothing beyond orthodox quantum theory.

Although it is superficially very attractive, however, this naïve interpretation *does not work*. The reason is simple—it includes no probabilities, that is, no Born rule. It has no "degrees of existence"; everything will exist regardless of how small its probability should be according to the Born rule. In other words, probabilities are meant for something to "happen," and here nothing has actually happened. Now I am aware that the foundations of the whole theory of probability are very uncertain, even in the classical domain, but this insecurity should not prevent us from recognizing that at this stage we do not have a satisfactory theory of the quantum world.

ONE-MIND INTERPRETATION

To make progress, we can propose instead that, although the description of the physics is as given by the state above, with both terms, consciousness actually *selects* one term (Squires 1990, 1991, 1993) Normally this selection will happen at random with the weights given by $|a|^2$ and $|b|^2$, so that the Born rule is guaranteed. (In general, saying that something happens at random requires that we give a weight, and we really have no other possibilities, and so the Born rule is very natural.)

We now have, I believe, an acceptable solution to the measurement problem in quantum theory. It has several merits.

1. In principle the solution allows for consciousness to be "efficacious"—that is, it can change the experienced world. In other words, it can help explain what consciousness is for. The point here is that we may find circumstances in which a quantum superposition in the brain is not correlated to things outside the brain (like the displayed state above). Then the selection, which perhaps need not be random, could determine the action that a person takes. This condition would correspond to our experience of free will, and it would affect the experienced world, although it would not alter the total wave function. In other words, it would not violate the requirement (for some people) that physics be "closed."

Of course, at this stage in our discussion (but not before), we must make some assumptions about physical brains. To make it possible for the condition we are describing here to happen, we have to accept that brains are genuinely *quantum* systems that cannot be described by classical physics. I do not find accepting this statement difficult. Although surgeons may see brains as warm, wet matter, which from their point of view can be described perfectly well by classical physics, it remains true that there is no such thing as classical matter. To say that quantum effects, such as those we describe here, cannot occur in brains, would be like telling a nineteenth-century physicist who had just happened to invent quantum theory that, even if it were true, it would never be possible to detect the theory's effects in the real world.

Let me be more precise here: the requirement is that particular superpositions of microscopic systems should occur in the brain in such a way that selecting one "term" in the superposition (or "region," because the superposition need not include only discrete elements), becomes magnified to correspond to one specific macroscopic action. In other words, the brain is able to make quantum measurements. Because quite simple mechanical devices can make such measurements, this requirement does not seem to be expecting too much of a brain.

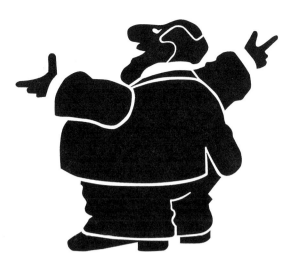

Figure 52.4 A template that produces a pink man from a sheet of pink paper. Is the man already present without the template?

2. Associating consciousness with "selection" seems to be something that others, using very different arguments, want to make. A recent example is Cotterill (1995), who writes, "consciousness is *for* … evaluation and choice."

3. We would have a unique "real"—that is, experienced—world. The non-selected parts of the wave function would not really exist. For an analogy, imagine a sheet of white paper. By putting a suitable mask on this sheet we could have a picture of, say, a person—see Figure 52.4. Now different masks would produce different pictures (worlds)—indeed, all possible pictures. It would be misusing language, however, to say that the sheet of white paper *contained* all the pictures—only the one selected by the mask would exist.

4. As with most versions of the "many-worlds" interpretations, this one allows us to use anthropic arguments to explain the apparent coincidences necessary for our existence, but here it is with a unique world, rather than a scenario in which conceivably all things actually exist. The argument would be that in some sort of universal wave function, consciousness selects a part in which consciousness can exist.

ALTERNATIVE MANY-VIEWS MODELS

Several attempts have been made to give meaning to probability when all experiences occur. For example, Albert and Loewer (1988) and Albert (1992) suggest that associated with every person are many minds, and that each selects at random, as in the single-experience proposal above. Again this system seems to work, but clearly the number has to be very large, otherwise we will face the possibility of meeting "zombies." In fact, Albert and Loewer suggest an infinite number, an idea that I find hard to accept because I am not sure I really know what it means to have an infinite number of "objects" associated with a given person. Even worse, they want a continuous infinity. This condition runs into the problem that no natural measure occurs on a continuous infinity: it just means nothing to say, for example, that "more" minds see one result than another. The same problem is met by Lockwood (1989, 1996), who proposes instead to have all "minds" labeled by a continuous parameter, such as $0 < \lambda < 1$, so that a fraction of the line goes to one result, and another fraction to another, and so on, to give the Born rule. Again, this line suffers, it seems to me, from the insuperable problem that no natural measure occurs on such a line.

On aesthetic grounds, I am more comfortable with the idea that we have one world, rather than having to accept that all things that *can be* actually *are*, however improbable the Born rule would make them. It just seems too much to have to believe that people really are holding conferences on physics, consciousness, and so on, who have never experienced interference, or read about it, or met anyone who had. They will have an awful shock next time they see a thin film of oil on water (or at least "a large part," whatever that may mean in this context, of them will).

NONLOCALITY

Finally, we must discuss nonlocality. It is sometimes stated that one advantage in the "many-worlds" style of solutions to the measurement problem is that they do not suffer from the nonlocality that is all too evident in the Bohm model or in collapse models. To some extent this statement is accurate: the nonlocality is removed from the physics because it arises only from the results of measurements, and so does not occur if no such results are achieved. It is still around, however; it has simply been removed to "consciousness."

We can see this condition if we consider how consciousness can take note of the quantum probability. We need to think more about how we locate the "patterns" that correspond to an experience. Suppose the quantum state is given by $|\Psi(x, y, t)\rangle$, where x stands for the variables of particles in the brain and y for particles in the system, the apparatus, and the environment. The displayed state equation (52.3) is just one example of such a state. To see a pattern we must project this condition onto a state of some presumed "consciousness basis" in the brain. If we denote this condition by states $|C_n(x)\rangle$, where the n labels possible experiences, then the probability of the nth experience is, according to quantum theory, $|C(x)|\Psi(x, y, t)\rangle|^2$. This expression, however, is not a number but a function of the positions of all the other particles (some of which may well be thousands of miles away). To get a number we must integrate over all these positions. This procedure of course is horrendously nonlocal in realistic measurements. In other words, consciousness, if it is to "know about" probabilities, as it must if we are to obtain the Born rule, cannot be a local thing.

This requirement is very important because it means the selection model will have only one selection, not one for every person, ensuring the essential property that all observers will make the same selection. In other words, consciousness must be thought of as *one* thing. Schrödinger firmly believed in this stricture, and it may be a contribution that quantum physics can make to the study of consciousness, thereby guaranteeing that quantum physics will continue to have a place at consciousness meetings and in books about consciousness.

RELATED IDEAS

The idea that consciousness has to be introduced if we are to understand quantum theory has been around since the 1920s. Apart from the work mentioned above, recent contributions are due to Hodgson (1989), Mavromatos and Nanopoulos (1995), Penrose (1989), Page (1995), and Stapp (1993). These models have many features in common, and in common with the model I advocate here (specifically, the selection model shares many features Stapp discusses in his recent articles and this volume, Chapter 51). The principal difference is that in varying ways these authors have models in which the operation of consciousness is associated with some sort of explicit wave-function collapse, so that the physics is not given exactly by the Schrödinger equation. It seems to follow that differences will be observable between predictions by these models and those by standard quantum theory (cf., for example, Pearle and Squires 1994). This variation is not necessarily a bad thing, but the models need to be made more precise so that these differences can be calculated.

A more serious objection may be that properly describing the collapse requires a replacement for the Schrödinger equation. Such equations are already available, of course (see Ghirardi et al. 1990 and references therein), but at least in this context they suffer because the collapse effect has nothing to do with consciousness.[2] Rather, the collapse is a universal phenomenon, and the rate is very small—that is, negligible—for microscopic systems, but is proportional to something like the number of particles, so that it is large in the macroscopic world. If we follow this line too closely, we are in danger of saying that consciousness arises, like rapid collapse, simply from having large systems. I believe Stapp, at least, would reject this suggestion—rightly, in my opinion. Maybe things look different if the stochasticity of the collapse arises from something that is noncomputable. This condition might provide a link with possible nonalgorithimc aspects of conscious thought.

SUMMARY

Orthodox quantum theory requires "something else." It is a plausible hypothesis to say that this something is a primitive ingredient of the world—that is, not reducible to other things in physics—and to identify it with consciousness. It includes or perhaps we should say *is*, the quale of experience. The model naturally shows us why this consciousness is causally effective.

To identify the mechanisms in the brain where the required quantum "measurements" that magnify quantum selections into macroscopic effects take place, is a problem for the future.

NOTES

1. The interpretation problem of quantum theory and the hard problem of consciousness also share the property of attracting articles that claim to provide a solution but in fact do not address the problem.

2. Some people would regard this quirk as a virtue of these models, but they would be unlikely to read this book.

REFERENCES

Albert, D. 1992. *Quantum Mechanics and Experience*. Cambridge: Harvard University Press.

Albert, D., and B. Loewer. 1988. Interpreting the many-worlds interpretation. *Synthèse* 77:195–213.

Cotterill, R. M. J. 1995. On the unity of conscious experience. *Journal of Consciousness Studies* 2:290–311.

Ghirardi, G. C., P. Pearle, and A. Rimini. 1990. Markov processes in Hilbert space and continuous spontaneous localisation. *Physical Review A* 42:78–89.

Hodgson, D. 1989. *The Mind Matters*. Oxford: Oxford University Press.

Lockwood, M. 1996. Many-minds interpretations of quantum mechanics. Oxford preprint; *Journal for the Philosophy of Science*, forthcoming.

Lockwood, M. 1989. *Mind, Brain and the Quantum*. Oxford: Blackwell.

Mavromatos, N., and D. V. Nanopolous. 1995. Noncritical string theory formulation of micro-tubule dynamics and quantum aspects of brain function. CERN preprint TH/95–127.

Page, D. 1995. Sensible quantum mechanics: Are only perceptions probabilistic? University of Alberta preprint.

Pearle, P., and E. J. Squires. 1994. Bound state excitation, nucleon decay experiments, and models of wave function collapse. *Physical Review Letters* 73:1–5.

Penrose, R. 1989. *The Emperor's New Mind*. Oxford: Oxford University Press.

Squires, E. J. 1990. *Conscious Mind in the Physical World*. IOP: Bristol.

Squires, E. J. 1987. Many views of one world—An interpretation of quantum theory. *European Journal of Physics*. 8:171–174.

Squires, E. J. 1991. One mind or many? *Synthèse* 89:283–286.

Squires, E. J. 1993. Quantum theory and the relation between conscious mind and the physical world. *Synthèse* 97:109–123.

Stapp, H. P. 1996. The hard problem: A quantum approach. Berkeley preprint, LBL-37163MOD; *Journal of Consciousness Studies*, forthcoming.

Stapp, H. P. 1993. *Mind, Matter and Quantum Mechanics*. Berlin: Springer-Verlag.

Zeh, H. D. 1981. The problem of conscious observation in quantum mechanical description. *Epistemological Letters* 73.

53 Synaptic Transmission, Quantum-State Selection, and Consciousness

Friedrich Beck

Nerve impulses are stochastic processes that are always present in the living brain (Freeman 1995). Recent investigations suggest that the neural net stays close to instability, and in this way can be switched between different states by minute action. To control such a system, a stable regulator has to be present that generates a coherent pattern in the active cortical unit. We argue here that the decisive unit in this regulator is a quantum trigger that determines the onset of synaptic exocytosis upon an incoming nerve impulse.

A nerve impulse propagating into a synapse causes exocytosis, that is the release of transmitter substance across the synaptic membrane, resulting in a brief excitatory postsynaptic depolarization (EPSP). Many of these milli-EPSPs are required to generate a discharge of an impulse by a pyramidal cell. Exocytosis is an all-or-nothing process, occurring with a probability of much less than one per incoming nerve impulse. Synaptic transmission therefore qualifies as a basic regulator of brain activities. This function has been demonstrated in biochemical studies on how drugs and anesthesia influence the ion-channel properties of the synaptic membrane (Flohr 1995, Louria and Hameroff 1996).

To be robust against thermal fluctuations, a quantum trigger has to function on an atomic level, as we show (page 621). Quantum processes that regulate charge transport through biological membranes have been observed in photosynthesis with bacteria (Vos et al. 1993). The observations can be explained by electron-transfer processes between states of the membrane proteins, as described by Marcus theory (Marcus 1956, Marcus and Sutin 1985). Quantum effects in biological membranes, however, are a much more general phenomenon, and we conclude on page 624 that assuming such a mechanism is also consistent with the known data for synaptic exocytosis. The quantum amplitudes of the corresponding tunneling process determine the small exocytosis probabilities, and in this way form a regulating pattern for the coupled cortical unit. Our hypothesis calls for experimental testing by ultrahigh-frequency spectroscopy.

Quantum processes are important in the relation between brain activity and conscious action. Several authors emphasize that the noncomputable performance of a conscious brain can be understood only by evoking a quantum-mechanical state collapse, or state-selection mechanism (Stapp 1993, Eccles

1994, Penrose 1994). We argue that state selection is possible only if a well-defined quantum state is present that collapses into one of its components upon filtering. This condition is fulfilled for the tunneling amplitudes in electron transfer but is hard to establish for macroscopic quantum states at room temperature, which may, however, produce large-scale coherence (Fröhlich 1968) but no state collapse. Apart from the physiological question, then, if a quantum trigger is responsible for the all-or-nothing character and the low probabilities for synaptic exocytosis, such an element in controlling the neural network could also bring us closer to a science of consciousness.

WHY IS QUANTUM MECHANICS INTERESTING?

The remarkable progress in brain research over the past decades has revived vivid discussion of the old problem of mind–brain relationships. The first rational formulation was given by Descartes (1644), and since then has been called *Cartesian dualism*. In this formulation of the mind–brain relationship the immaterial mind controls the material brain by acting upon the latter according to conscious will. With the triumphant progress of classical physics and its strict determinism, dualism came into ever-heavier waters, and was finally abandoned by many scientists.[1] The notion that the mind acts on the material brain would require either exertion of a force (Popper, Lindahl, and Århem 1993), implying that the mind is not really immaterial, or it would force one to give up at least one of the global physical-conservation laws based on strict space-time symmetries. Neither is acceptable from a purely scientific standpoint. We emphasize, however, that the seemingly contradictory notions of *dualism* and *identity theory* ("the mind is the brain") is itself deeply rooted in the logic of a world view based on classical physics. We are so used to our daily experience of macroscopic events surrounding us that are well described by classical physics, that we can hardly appreciate a world in which determinism is not the rule of the game. "If–then" lies deeply in our conscious experience. And yet the quantum world, governing microphysical events, has a different logic.

The basic difference between *classical* and *quantum* dynamics can be made clear in a simple diagram, without entering into the theory's subtleties. Generating a physical process consists of preparing an *input* (the initial conditions) followed by a more or less complicated *process*, and a possible *output* (the result) that can be observed. For simplicity, we restrict the distinguishable outcomes to two states (Figure 53.1). In classical dynamics the output is *unique* (strict determinism), which means we have *either* state I *or* state II: *excluding* states (Figure 53.1A). The *essence* of a quantum process is, contrary to this condition, that the output is *not unique* (no strict determinism); we have *neither* state I *nor* state II but a coherent superposition of both states: *interfering* states.

In both cases the system's time development is given by partial differential equations of first order in the time variable (Newton's or Maxwell's equations in the classical case, the Schrödinger equation in the quantum case),

(A) Classical Dynamics

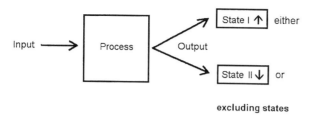

(B) Quantum Dynamics

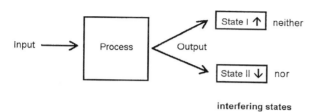

Figure 53.1 Schematic diagram of classical and quantum evolution. Equal preparation leads to different outputs: (A) excluding states, (B) interfering states.

which describe the dynamics in a strictly *causal* way: the initial conditions *uniquely* determine the output. The *noncausal* element in the quantum case enters through the famous *von Neumann state collapse*, which occurs if one tries to realize the output state, either by a measurement or by letting the output state undergo a successive process. Then the coherent superposition

$$\alpha \cdot |state\ I> + \beta \cdot |state\ II>$$

collapses into

either	$\|state\ I>$	with probability $|\alpha|^2$,
or	$\|state\ II>$	with probability $|\beta|^2$,
and	$|\alpha|^2 + |\beta|^2 = 1$	

For the *single event* (and we emphasize that quantum mechanics is a theory for the single event and not, as sometimes claimed, an ensemble theory) the outcome is *completely unpredictable*, provided not all but one of the probabilities are zero, which would imply that the one left is one. This result constitutes the *noncomputable* character in quantum events (Penrose 1994). It is evident that the deterministic logic underlying Cartesian dualism, which runs so heavily into conflict with the material world of classical physics, no longer applies if elementary quantum processes are decisive in brain dynamics.

QUANTUM OR CLASSICAL BRAIN DYNAMICS?

As pointed out in the preceding section, a science of consciousness has to be built on a different logic than the usual classical one if quantum events and

Friedrich Beck: Synaptic Transmission, Quantum-State Selection, and Consciousness state collapse are decisive in regulating brain processes. To qualify as science, the quest for quantum events cannot, however, come from philosophical reasoning, or from the wishful demand for the existence of a "free will," but rather has to rely on physiological studies of the brain structure, and ultimately on experimental evidence. We therefore ask next where in the brain quantum selection could possibly take place.

Figure 53.2 is a three-dimensional sketch of the cortical structure—the brain's neural switchboard—from Szentagothai (1978). Figure 53.2A shows the six laminae with two large pyramidal cells in lamina V and their apical dendrites, finishing in tuftlike branching in lamina I. There is agreement (Schmolke and Fleischhauer 1984; Peters and Kara 1987) that apical bundles of dendrites form the basic anatomical units in the neocortex. The synaptic connectivity of the apical bundles is established mainly by spine synapses, covering in large amounts (on the order of a few thousands) the apical dendrites. Figure 53.2B shows the structure of a spine synapse in close contact with the dendritic shaft. The basic unit in a spine synapse is the presynaptic membrane, which is able to release transmitter molecules, stored in vesicles, into the spine apparatus. This release results in a brief excitatory post-synaptic depolarization (EPSP), which generates an electrotonic signal in the microtubules. Coherent summation of such signals leads to impulse discharge of the pyramidal cell into its axon, connecting the neural net. This is the conventional macro-operation of a pyramidal cell, and it can be satisfactorily described by classical electrochemistry and network theory (Mountcastle 1978, Edelman 1989). The all-important regulatory function of the spine synapse results from exocytosis, the release of transmitter molecules across the presynaptic membrane, occurring only with a probability much less than one upon each incoming nerve impulse (Redman 1990). We therefore regard exocytosis as a candidate for quantum processes to enter the network, and thus regulate its performance (Beck and Eccles 1992).[2]

In the brain exists an interplay between micro- and macrostructures. The latter consist of dendrites, pyramidal cells, electrochemical transitions, while, on the other hand, microstructures involve membranes and microtubules. Both are clearly separated by time scales or, correspondingly, energy scales. The macrostructure is typically characterized by the brain's living in *hot and wet* surroundings of $T \approx 300°$K. This environment immediately raises the question of quantum coherence versus thermal fluctuations. It is well known that, as soon as thermal energies surpass quantal energies, classical thermal statistics prevails.

To answer this question, we can define two characteristic energies:

1. the thermal energy per degree of freedom

$$E_{th} = \frac{1}{2} k_b T \qquad \text{with } k_b : \text{Boltzmann's constant.}$$

2. the quantal energy, defined as zero-point energy of a quasi-particle of mass M

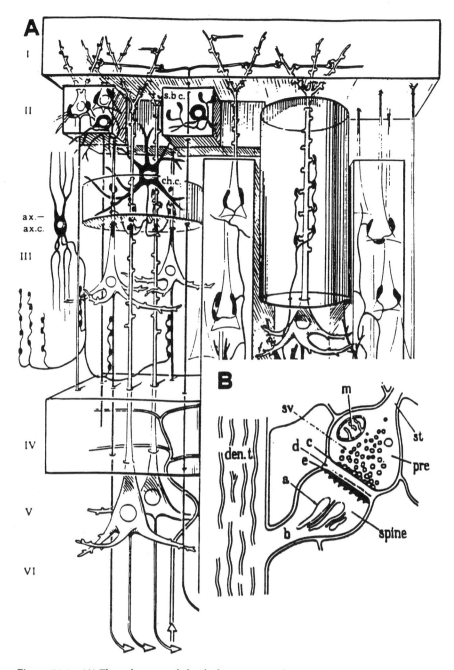

Figure 53.2 (A) Three-dimensional sketch showing cortical neurons of various types (Szenta-gothai 1978). (B) Detailed structure of a spine synapse (Gray 1982).

which is localized over a distance Δq. From Heisenberg's uncertainty relation $\Delta p \cdot \Delta q \geq 2\pi\hbar$ it follows (using the equals sign)

$$E_{qu} = \frac{(\Delta p)^2}{2M} \cong \left(\frac{2\pi\hbar}{\Delta q}\right)^2 \frac{1}{2M} \quad \text{with } \hbar : \text{Planck's constant.}$$

These relations define *two energy regimes*

$E_{qu} \gg E_{th}$:   *the quantal regime*

$E_{th} \gg E_{qu}$:   *the thermal regime*

An estimate with typical numbers: $T = 300\,\text{K}$, localization distance $\Delta q \sim 1\text{Å}$, and $E_{qu} = E_{th} = E_c \approx 1.3 \cdot 10^{-2}\,\text{eV}$, results in a *critical quasi-particle mass*

$M_c \approx 6M_H$ with M_H : mass of a hydrogen atom.

This estimate indicates that the dynamical mass of a quantum trasition, if robust against thermal fluctuations, has to be on the order of the hydrogen atomic mass, or less. Biomolecules whose mass is in the range of kD do not qualify *as a whole.*

We can also derive a *critical frequency*, $\hbar\omega_c = E_c$, and a *signal time*, $\tau = 2\pi/\omega_c$,

$\omega_c \approx 2 \cdot 10^{13}\text{s}^{-1}$; $\tau \approx 30\,\text{ps}$

These results show unambiguously that quantum processes at room temperature involve frequencies smaller than the picosecond scale. This condition, in turn, means they correspond to electronic transitions, like electron transfer or changes in molecular bonds (e.g., breaking of a hydrogen bridge).

Our analysis leads to the consequence that in brain dynamics two well-separated regions with different time scales exist:

1. The *macroscopic*, or cellular dynamics with time scales in the millisecond range, and down to nanosecond range.

2. The *microscopic*, or quantal, dynamics, with time scales in the picosecond to femtosecond range.

The large difference in time scales makes it possible to deal with quantum processes in the individual microsites, and decoupled from the neural net. On the other hand, it explains why the usual biochemical and biophysical studies do not show the need for introducing quantum considerations. To uncover them one has to employ ultrashort time spectroscopy (Vos et al. 1993).

SYNAPTIC EMISSION: THE QUANTUM TRIGGER

We regard signal transmission at spine synapses as an important regulating process in the cortical activity (cf., however, note 2). It is achieved by *exocytosis* of transmitter substance upon incoming nerve impulses. This regulation has two characteristic features:

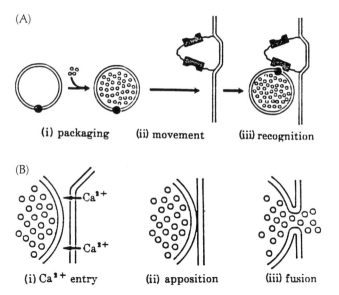

(i) packaging   (ii) movement   (iii) recognition

(B)

(i) Ca²⁺ entry   (ii) apposition   (iii) fusion

Figure 53.3   Different stages of synaptic vesicle development: (A) filling, movement towards the presynaptic membrane, docking. (B) Stages of exocytosis. Note the essential role of Ca^{2+} after depolarization by a nerve impulse (Kelly et al. 1979).

1. It is an *all-or-nothing* (quantal) process of vesicular release—that is, at most one of the vesicles docked at the presynaptic vesicular grid opens upon a nerve impulse (see Figure 53.3).

2. Exocytosis occurs with probabilities $\ll 1$ after stimulation.

The low exocytosis probability has been established by fluctuation analysis on motoneurons of isolated Ia nerve fibers (Jack, Redman, and Wong 1981), and more recently in CA1 neurons of the hippocampus (Sayer, Friedlander, and Redman 1990).

Based on these observations we propose this model:[3] Because our estimates (cf. the preceding section) allow for the quantal regime only processes on the electronic level, though exocytosis as a whole involves macromolecular dynamics (cf. Figure 53.3), we assume a *quantum-trigger mechanism*: An incoming nerve impulse excites some electronic configuration to a metastable level that is separated energetically by a potential barrier $V(q)$ from the state that leads unidirectionally to exocytosis. Here, q is a *collective coordinate* representing the path along the coupled electronic and molecular motions between two states. The motion along the path is described by a *quasi-particle* of mass M that is able to tunnel through the barrier quantum mechanically. These simplifications allow the complicated molecular transition to be treated as an effective one-body problem whose solution follows from the time-dependent Schrödinger equation

$$i\hbar \frac{\partial}{\partial t} \Psi(q;t) = -\frac{\hbar^2 \partial^2}{2M \partial q^2} \Psi(q;t) + V(q) \cdot \Psi(q;t)$$

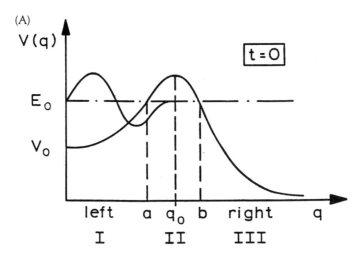

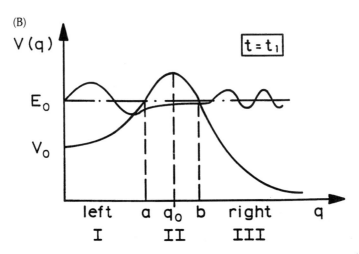

Figure 53.4 (A) the initial state $(t = 0)$ of the quasiparticle in the potential well $V(q)$. The wave function is located to the left of the barrier. E_0 is the energy of the activated state which starts to tunnel through the barrier. (B) After time t_1 the wave function has components on both sides of the barrier. a, b: classical turning points of the motion inside and outside the barrier (Beck and Eccles 1992).

Figure 53.4 shows schematically the initial state at $t = 0$ (after activation by the incoming impulse), and at the end of the activation period, $t = t_1$. Here it is assumed that the activated state of the presynaptic cell lasts a finite time t_1 only before it recombines. t_1, however, is of the macroscopic time scale (microsecond to nanosecond), as discussed in section three. At $t = t_1$ the state has evolved into a part still sitting to the left of the barrier in region I, and the part in region III has tunneled through the barrier.

We can now separate the total wave function at time t_1 into two components, representing the left and the right parts:

$$\Psi(q; t_1) = \Psi_{\text{left}}(q; t_1) + \Psi_{\text{right}}(q; t_1),$$

and this expression constitutes the two *interfering amplitudes* for the *alternative results of the same process*, as discussed in section two: exocytosis has happened (Ψ_{right}), *or* exocytosis has not happened (Ψ_{left}) (inhibition).

State collapse transforms this expression into

exocytosis: probability $p_{\text{ex}}(t_1) = \int |\Psi_{\text{right}}|^2 \, dq$

inhibition: probability $p_{\text{in}}(t_1) = \int |\Psi_{\text{left}}|^2 \, dq$

Using the WKB approximation (Messiah 1961) to solve the tunneling problem, we can once more evaluate the process with characteristic numbers:

input	mass of quasi-particle:[4]	$M \approx 500 \times$ electron mass
	spatial extension:	$\Delta q \approx 1\,\text{Å}$
	effective barrier height:	$V - E \approx 0.5\,\text{eV}$
	effective barrier width:	$b - a \approx 1\,\text{Å}$
	activation time:	$t_1 \approx 10\,\text{ns}$
result	energy of tunneling state:	$E_0 = 0.3\,\text{eV}$
	barrier-penetration coefficient:	$T \approx 10^{-7}$
	exocytosis probability:	$p_{ex}(t_1) \approx 0.5$

The numerical estimate with realistic numerical input leads to meaningful results for the quantum trigger regulating exocytosis!

As a result, we can describe brain dynamics by two scales:

microscopic scale (femtosecond):	*quantum synaptic dynamics*
macroscopic scale (nanosecond):	*(coherent) cell dynamics*
coupling:	*microtublar structure*

As a *possible realization* we can consider *electron transfer* (ET) between biomolecules. In biological reaction centers such processes lead to *charge transfer* across *biological membranes*. The quasi-particle describes the electron coupled to nuclear motion according to the Franck-Condon principle. The theory has been worked out by Marcus (1956), and was later put into a quantum-mechanical version by Jortner (1976). The initializing step of ET is excitation of a *donor D*, usually a dye molecule with subsequent transport of an electron to *acceptor A*, producing the polar system D^+A^-. This system is accompanied by rearrangement of the molecular coordinates leading to unidirectional charge separation, and over several further electronic transitions with increasing time constants to the creation of an action potential across the membrane. The energetics is shown in Figure 53.5. Figure 53.5A shows the potential energy curves separately for electrons and nuclear conformations, Figure 53.5B gives the combined potential in the quasi-particle picture (Marcus and Sutin 1985). The latter form closely resembles the effective potential assumed in the quantum-trigger model.

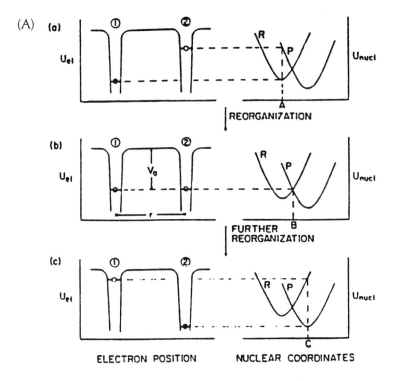

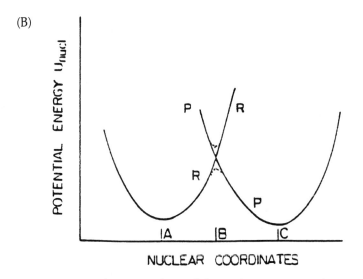

Figure 53.5 (A) Electron transfer coupled to nuclear motion. *Left*: electronic potential energy curves, *right*: corresponding nuclear potential curves. (a), (b), (c): electronic energies in the two wells for the nuclear positions A, B, C. The transition proceeds from (a) over the barrier (b) to the final state (c). (B) The same situation in the quasiparticle picture. The potential energy surfaces of donor (R) and acceptor (P) are shown. The positions correspond to A, B, C in (A). The dotted lines indicate splitting due to electronic interactions between donor and acceptor (Marcus and Sutin 1985).

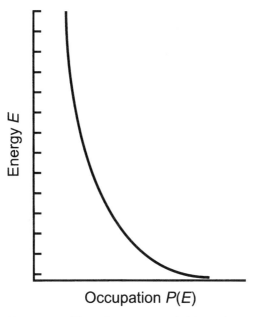

Figure 53.6   Thermal occupation probabilities of excited states.

COHERENCE AND STATE SELECTION

In the *thermal regime* (page 624), thermal fluctuations activate a canonical spectrum according to the Boltzmann distribution (Figure 53.6)

$$P(E) = \mathrm{Exp}\left(-\frac{E}{k_b T}\right).$$

Thermal fluctuations destroy phase coherence by couplings to the heat bath.

Long-range coherence in biological systems at room temperature can be established either by classical nonlinear dynamics (e.g., self-organized criticality, Bak, Tang, and Wiesenfeld 1988), or by macroscopic quantum states (Fröhlich coherence, Fröhlich 1968). The ingredients necessary for macroscopic quantum states at room temperature are *dissipation* and *energy supply* ("pumping"). Pumping *stabilizes* against thermal fluctuations, and phase synchronization is achieved by *self-organization*. The latter is mediated by *classical fields* (electromagnetic, phonons, molecular), which implies that the quantum spectrum becomes *quais-continuous*. Quantum-state selection and state collapse, however, need few discrete states, and consequently are not possible with long-range coherent states.

Synaptic selection, of course, has to be combined with cooperative processes in cortical units, consisting of bundles of pyramidal cells bound together to produce *spatiotemporal patterns*. They couple the synaptic switches by long-range coherence in microtubular cell connections. It establishes the *nonalgorithmic* units of consciousness ("awareness"). Figure 53.7

Friedrich Beck: Synaptic Transmission, Quantum-State Selection, and Consciousness

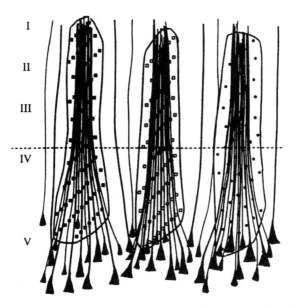

Figure 53.7 Coherent couplings of bundles of pyramidal cells (dendrons) to form a spatial pattern (Eccles 1994).

gives a schematic sketch of three bundles of pyramidal cells ("dendrons"), surrounded by the spatial pattern that is produced temporarily by coherent couplings of the individual pyramidal cells (Eccles 1994). (He calls the patterns "psychons" and relates them to a dualist concept.) The physiological mechanism for pattern production is not yet fully understood. It relates to perceptions and intentions, as well as to learning and memory. It could be produced by Fröhilich coherence, as suggested by Hameroff and Penrose (1996) or by self-organization in classical nonlinear dynamics. The important function of quantum events in brain dynamics does not, however, depend on these large-scale processes, but rather is due to microscopic molecular transitions. Even with classical coherence, quantum events could and will influence organization of the spatiotemporal patterns.

CONCLUSIONS

Quantum-state collapse is the decisive process that distinguishes quantum mechanics from classical physics. In a *single event* it is *nonpredictable*. By this condition it qualifies for the nonpredictable and noncomputable aspect of brain functioning. We emphasize that this description introduces a new logical concept, different from the classical determinism underlying the struggle among dualism, identity theory, and the call for "free will." Interpreting of quantum mechanics as a succession of *single events* produces in a natural way the fundamental difference between past and future, insofar as the past is *known* (by events having manifestly occurred), and the future is *not known* (by the unpredictability of state reduction).

These important concepts for understanding consciousness on a scientific basis lead us to investigate in this work if present knowledge about the cortical structure allows for implementing quantum events into brain dynamics. The basic results and assumptions are:

• Spine synapses are important regulators in brain activity, filtering the everpresent firings of nerve impulses.

• Exocytosis, the release of transmitter substance across the presynaptic membrane, is an *all-or-nothing* event, occurring with probability $\ll 1$.

• A model, based on electron transfer, relates exocytosis with a two-state quantum trigger, leading to superposition of the two states, subject to collapse.

• The coherent coupling of synapses via microtubular connections (the "binding problem") is still an open problem. Quantum coherence is not needed to couple the microsites that bear the quantum transitions with definite phase relations to produce a spatio-temporal pattern. The quantum trigger can, however, switch between coherent modes (limit cycles?).

• The quantum trigger opens a doorway for better understanding the relationship between brain dynamics and consciousness.

ACKNOWLEDGMENTS

This work was stimulated by intensive discussions with John C. Eccles, whose great knowledge of the brain and its physiology made it possible for a theoretical physicist to enter that field of research. Stimulating discussions with Dr. H. P. Stapp and Dr. K. Pribram, as well as with many colleagues at a recent Fetzer Institute Round Table, are also acknowledged.

NOTES

1. For the present status of the discussion on dualist-interactionism, identity theory, and materialism, see Eccles (1994).

2. An alternative regulative process by tubulin molecules comprising the cylindrical walls of microtubules has been proposed by Hameroff and Penrose (1996). We emphasize that the basic quantal event postulated by these authors, a two-state conformational transition in the tubulin, is rather similar to the synaptic quantum-trigger model presented here, and its realization by electron transfer.

3. A quantum model of synaptic firing was presented by Walker (1970). His mechanism for electron transfer across the presynaptic membrane is, however, quite different from the one proposed here, and would violate the conditions given in section two above.

4. The estimate for the quasi-particle mass respects that coupling the electron transition to the molecular motion increases the mass considerably.

REFERENCES

Bak, P., C. Tang, and K. Wiesenfeld, 1988. Self-organized criticality. *Physical Review A* 38:364–374.

Beck, F., and J. C. Eccles. 1992. Quantum aspects of brain activity and the role of consciousness. Proceedings of the National Academy of Science of the U.S.A. 89:11,357–11,361.

Descartes, R. 1644. *Principia philosophiae*. Amsterdam.

Eccles, J. C. 1994. *How the Self Controls Its Brain*. New York: Springer-Verlag.

Edelman, G. M. 1989. *The Remembered Present: A Biological Theory of Consciousness*. New York: Basic Books.

Flohr, H. 1995. An information processing theory of anesthesia. *Neuropsychologia* 33:1169–1180.

Freeman, W. 1996. Random activity at the microscopic neural level in cortex ("noise") sustains and is regulated by low-dimensional dynamics of macroscopic cortical activity ("chaos"). Proceedings of the International Workshop, "The role and control of random events in biological systems, Sigtuna, Sweden, September 1995; *International Journal of Neural Systems* 7:473–480.

Fröhlich, H. 1968. Long-range coherence and energy storage in biological systems. *International Journal of Quantum Chemistry* 2:641–649.

Gray, E. G. 1982. Rehabilitating the dendritic spine. *Trends in Neuroscience* 5:5–6.

Hameroff, S., and R. Penrose, 1997. Orchestrated reduction of quantum coherence in brain microtubules: a model for consciousness. In *Toward a Science of Cousciousness II—The 1996 Tucson Discussions and Debates*, Eds. S. Hameroff, A. Kaszniak, A. Scott. Cambridge: MIT Press.

Jack, J. J. B., S. J. Redman, and K. Wong, 1981. The components of synaptic potentials evoked in cat spinal motoneurons by impulses in single group Ia afferents. *Journal of Physiology* 321:65–96.

Jortner, J. 1976. Temperature dependent activation energy for electron transfer between biological molecules. *Journal of Chemical Physics* 64:4860–4867.

Kelly, R. B., J. W. Deutsch, S. S. Carlson, and J. A. Wagner. 1979. Biochemistry of neurotransmitter release. *Annual Review of Neuroscience* 2:399–446.

Louria, D. and Hameroff, S. 1997. Computer simulation of anesthetic action. In *Toward a Science of Consciousness II—The 1996 Tucson Discussions and Debates*, Eds. S. Hameroff, A. Kaszniak, A. Scott. Cambridge: MIT Press.

Marcus, R. A. 1956. On the theory of oxidation-reduction reactions involving electron transfer. I. *Journal of Chemical Physics* 24:966–978.

Marcus, R. A., N. Sutin, 1985. Electron transfer in chemistry and biology. *Biochimica et Biophysica Acta* 811:265–322.

Messiah, A. 1961. *Quantum Mechanics*, vol. I, Amsterdam: North Holland, pp. 231–242.

Mountcastle, V. B. 1978. An organization principle for cerebral function: The unit module and the distributed system. In *The Mindful Brain*. Cambridge: MIT Press.

Penrose, R. 1994. *Shadows of the Mind*. London: Oxford University Press.

Peters, A., and D. A. Kara. 1987. The neuronal composition of area 17 of the rat visual cortex. IV. The organization of pyramidal cells. *Journal of Comparative Neurology* 260:573–590.

Popper, K. R., B. I. B. Lindahl, P. Århem. 1993. A discussion of the mind-brain problem. *Theoretical Medicine* 14:167–180.

Redman, S. J. 1990. Quantal analysis of synaptic potentials in neurons of the central nervous system. *Physiological Review* 70:165–198.

Sayer, R. J., M. J. Friedlander, and S. J. Redman. 1990. The time-course and amplitude of EPSPs evoked at synapses between pairs of CA3/CA1 neurons in the hippocampal slice. *Journal of Neuroscience* 10:626–636.

Schmolke, C., and K. Fleischhauer. 1984. Morphological characteristics of neocortical laminae when studied in tangential semi-thin sections through the visual cortex in the rabbit. *Anatomy and Embryology*. 169:125–132.

Stapp, H. P. 1993. *Mind, Matter, and Quantum Mechanics*. New York: Spring-Verlag.

Szentagothai, J. 1978. The neuron network of the cerebral cortex: A functional interpretation. *Proceedings of the Royal Society of London* B 201:219–248.

Vos, M. H., F. Rappaport, J. C. Lambry, J. Breton, and J.-L. Martin. 1993. Visualization of coherent nuclear motion in a membrane protein by femtosecond spectroscopy. *Nature* 363:320–325.

Walker, E. H. 1970. The nature of consciousness. *Mathematical Biosciences* 7:131–178.

54 A Sonoran Afternoon

Stuart R. Hameroff and Alwyn C. Scott

EDITOR'S NOTE: Late one summer afternoon in Arizona's Sonoran Desert, Stuart Hameroff and Alwyn Scott awoke from their siestas to take margaritas in the shade of a ramada. On a nearby table, a tape recorder had accidentally been left on, and this is a lightly edited transcript of their conversation.

Stuart: Tell me, Al, why are you so negative about quantum theories of the mind?

Al: Before trying to answer that, let's remember where we are in agreement. We both feel uncomfortable with the notion that the mind is nothing more than the switchings off and on of the brain's neurons, and we are both looking for something more. But we're looking in different places. Furthermore, I don't have anything against quantum theory. From the perspective of applied mathematics, it's really interesting to consider how Schrödinger's linear-wave dynamics manages to mimic the experimentally observed properties of, say, molecular vibrations. But I don't see any need for quantum theory to explain the strongly nonlinear dynamics that are observed in the brain.

Stuart: What needs to be explained are the tough questions of consciousness—particularly qualia, or conscious experience: Chalmers's hard problem—as well as binding and other enigmatic features. I agree that nonlinear dynamics is necessary, but why not quantum theory *also* if it can answer these tough questions?

Al: Sure, we need to understand the riddle of subjective experience. I completely agree with you there. But quantum theory doesn't help much because the binding of stable and globally coherent states is a phenomenon that arises more naturally in classical *nonlinear* systems than in the *linear* theory of quantum mechanics. You simply don't need quantum theory to explain global coherence.

Stuart: I agree that consciousness is a globally coherent state, but globally coherent *classical* states are merely couplings and correlations of separate individual activities. Classical states don't necessarily solve the binding problem. On the other hand, macroscopic quantum states such as super-conductors, Bose-Einstein condensates, superfluids, and the proposed preconscious "Orch OR" microtubule states Roger Penrose and I have been suggesting (Penrose and Hameroff 1995; Hameroff and Penrose 1996a, 1996b) are qualitatively different. These are globally coherent in the sense of "being one entity."

Al: There's lots more to classical nonlinear dynamics than neurons firing synchronously. A generic feature in classical nonlinear dynamics is the emergence of stable dynamic entities at each level of description to provide a basis for the nonlinear interactions at the next higher level of description. You don't need to assume that quantum theory is required for such behavior, examples of which abound. Benzene molecules emerge from the nonlinear forces between hydrogen and carbon atoms, just as proteins emerge from the nonlinear attractions among amino acids. Tornadoes emerge from the nonlinear dynamics of air and sunshine, just as cities and cultural configurations emerge from the *very* nonlinear interactions among human beings. Each of these is indeed "one entity." You can't have half a benzene molecule.

Stuart: But benzene, tornadoes, and individual proteins are not conscious— and I would argue that quantum effects *are* necessary for certain activities of benzene rings, and proteins.

Al: Benzene, proteins, tornadoes, and cities emerge as globally coherent entities from classical nonlinearities. That's what I'm saying. You are right that quantum theory is needed to compute the attractions between atoms, but once calculated, these can be treated as classical forces.

Stuart: Classical nonlinearity *is* needed in biology and consciousness; I just think quantum effects too are required. And though it's true that a quantum state evolves linearly according to the Schrödinger equation, highly nonlinear events occur in Penrose's "objective reduction" (OR). In OR, a quantum-coherent superposition state (if isolated from environmental decoherence) will continue linearly only until a specific threshold is reached. (The threshold is related to quantum gravity, and is expressed by $E = \hbar/T$). At that instant, "self"-collapse of the wave function occurs, and specific classical states are chosen noncomputably. Thus the Orch OR model is nonlinear. In fact, Orch OR describes consciousness as a sequence of discrete events rather than a continuum. Penrose's noncomputable OR (Penrose 1989, 1994, 1996) seems to me the ultimate manifestation of nonlinearity.

Al: I can't argue with Roger's theory because I don't understand it. And it would really be neat if the Orch OR model turns out to be a useful description of reality, but—to repeat—I don't see the *need* for it to explain the many nonlinearities that are observed at the various levels in biological dynamics.

Stuart: Perhaps not. But what about consciousness?

Al: The special thing about consciousness—it seems to me—is that it emerges from all the levels in the brain's dynamics; not just one (the neurons, for example) but *all* of them.

Stuart: Including quantum coherence at the level of intraneural microtubules?

Al: I don't have any philosophical problem with quantum coherence playing a role in conscious phenomena, but there is no theoretical need for it. Look, the fundamental dynamics of the brain are dissipative. We can't even construct Schrödinger's equation for a nerve impulse that is traveling along an axon. A nerve impulse is a *completely classical phenomenon.*

Stuart: Yes, and we both agree that nerve impulses per se can't explain consciousness. About dissipation, a quantum state in the brain must be cleverly (and transiently) isolated. In the Orch OR model, quantum coherence in microtubules emerges during preconscious, nondissipative phases, which are isolated by actin gelation. At instantaneous collapse, gel is dissolved to "sol" (solution), information is communicated, and energy dissipates.

Al: To the extent that I can understand what you are saying, I'm not convinced. Are quantum effects to be anticipated in the dynamics of your microtubule solitons?

Stuart: Not necessarily. Classical signaling along microtubules is stipulated in Orch OR theory, and classical microtubule solitons may be involved in the "sol" open phases. The idea is that quantum (gel) isolation phases alternate with classical signaling (sol) open phases at frequencies such as 40 Hz, for example.

Al: Because the mass of an individual tubulin molecule runs easily into the tens of thousands of atomic mass units, the minimum length of the waves from which Schrödinger's wave packets are constructed is a very small fraction of an atomic diameter (Scott 1996). Much too small for biochemists too worry about.

Stuart: A quantum superposition—an actual separation of mass distribution—of a very small fraction of an atomic diameter is more than enough. In Hameroff and Penrose (1996a), we consider the displacement distance for superposed tubulin protein molecules "separated from themselves" in three ways: as separated protein spheres, as separations of component atomic nuclei, and as separations of component nucleons (protons or neutrons). We determined that the earliest collapse (hence the predominant effect) comes with separation at the level of atomic nuclei. The entire protein is superposed, but at the level of each of its 10^5 atomic nuclei being separated from themselves by their 10^{-6} nanometer diameter. This diameter is much smaller than the wave packet. The implications of quantum-coherent superposition for consciousness are irrespective of the distance of separation. The significance comes from the quantum-coherent binding, from the self-collapse events that are processes in fundamental space-time geometry (akin to Whitehead's "occasions of experience"), and from noncomputable selection of postcollapse states.

Al: Well, I'm not talking about anything as complicated as all that. The key point is that for tubulin at biological temperatures, the size of a quantum-wave packet is much less than the size of a protein molecule. For the same reason, one would not use quantum mechanics to calculate the trajectory of a howitzer round.

Stuart: Then this question pertains to the classical soliton case, but not the quantum phase, during which the relevant mass movement is superposition.

Al: Let's consider how quantum theory *does* enter the picture. I agree that it is definitely necessary to describe the motions of the electrons that hold a molecule together, because the mass of an electron is more than four orders of magnitude less than that of a typical atom, which is small enough that its quantum-wave packet can extend over several atoms. To separate the electronic motions from those of the atomic nuclei, quantum chemists use the Born-Oppenheimer approximation (Born and Oppenheimer 1927), taking advantage of the electrons' moving about much more quickly than the atomic nuclei because they are so much lighter. Thus one assumes in the first approximation that the atomic nuclei are stationary. Then the forces between nuclei are calculated from the structures of electronic-wave functions, which can be regarded as a nonlinear "rubber cement" that holds a molecule together. An important feature in Born's formulation is that one can estimate the errors involved so that it becomes clear when quantum effects can be ignored. At the biochemistry level, these effects are very small.

Stuart: Michael Conrad points out that the Born–Oppenheimer approximation assumes that an electron and its nucleus behave like a football and the earth. The gravitational field (mass) of the football is negligible compared to that of the earth, and so the ball follows the earth very rapidly. But the electromagnetic field of an electron and a proton are the same, independent of the mass. Delocalized electrons accelerate relative to their nuclei, and may affect nuclear motion and conformation. In superconductors, motions of the electrons clearly affect the nuclear lattice.

Al: Yes, that's right, and in ways that can be calculated.

Stuart: As Conrad describes it, proteins and nucleic acids are extremely complicated nonlinear systems, each with tens of thousands of electrons, protons, and neutrons (Conrad 1996). Some intraprotein electrons are very delocalized and are now known to tunnel long distances through hydrogen-bond pathways. Electron delocalization also occurs in surface electrons (which cannot closely follow any specific nuclei) and in aromatic (electron-resonance) ring structures in the amino acids tyrosine, phenylalanine, tryptophan, and histidine. These may comprise water-free "hydrophobic pockets" within protein interiors, precisely where general anesthetics act (apparently by limiting electron delocalizability). Conrad observes that significantly delocalized electrons that accelerate relative to their nuclei must then absorb and emit photons whose frequencies cannot be precisely accounted for by the rotational and vibrational transitions of the nuclei. Conrad's model of quantum protein computing argues that superposition of electron states contributes to interference effects that "jiggle the nuclei," particularly the hydrogen bonds, and thereby open up new pathways of conformational self-organization. Parallelism of the electronic-wave function is thereby converted to a speedup of protein-conformational dynamical function.

Al: Sure, proteins are very complicated objects; that's why they can do so many neat things.

Stuart: And they may use quantum superposition to do them.

Al: Well, that may be so, but it's not obvious. Quantum descriptions of protein dynamics are often convenient, but that doesn't mean they are necessary. [Pause.] Taking another tack, let me try to express my position in this way. Brains are composed of neurons, synapses, and glial cells in the same sense as living organisms are composed of chemical atoms, and the functional organization is equally intricate. Just as one would not attempt to describe an organism's life in terms of the motions of its constituent atoms, one cannot describe the mind in terms of switchings by its constituent neurons. But the intricacy in this picture doesn't require quantum effects. Life and mind emerge from the immensely complicated nonlinear and hierarchical structures of body and brain. *That's* where the mystery lies.

Stuart: How would you explain the intelligent, adaptive behavior of a single-cell organism like a paramecium, which leads a rich existence without a neural network or synapses?

Al: That's a good point. Sherrington suggested that these little guys could be using their cytoskeletons to compute.

Stuart: We don't necessarily know all the brain's hierarchical levels, or how they interact—we don't understand life. Nor do we know precisely *how* brains are composed of neurons. Factors like electrotonic synapses, dendritic microprocessing, the function of glia and cytoskeletal processes are generally ignored.

Al: I completely agree. And just as one would not try to describe a bacterium in terms of the Born–Oppenheimer force field between its constituent atoms....

Stuart: One might need something like quantum theory to describe a fundamental life process in the bacterium. How do we know? What *is* life?

Al: ... one cannot think of the brain merely in terms of individual neurons. Neurons organize themselves into assemblies of neurons, each of which exhibits global coherence, binding, and threshold phenomena, as does an individual neuron. Thus assemblies of neurons can organize themselves into assemblies of assemblies, which in turn organize themselves into assemblies of assemblies of assemblies—and so on—up to the functional dynamic entities that provide the basis for the immensely complicated behaviors that underlie human consciousness (Scott 1995).

Stuart: Granted. But what is it that these behaviors are underlying? What *is* consciousness?

Al: Stuart, if I knew, I would certainly share it with you, but these statements about the functional organization of the brain—which are supported by many experimental studies—are far removed from the considerations of quantum mechanics. No need to cast about for sources of mystery here; fully organized thoughts are immensely (in a precise technical sense) complicated entities, and the experiments of present-day electrophysiology tell us little about how they might interact.

Stuart: And they tell us nothing about the nature of conscious experience—the "hard problem." We do need to cast about for something.

Al: Yes, and I'm suggesting that the immensely intricate nonlinear structure of the brain's dynamics is a much richer source of mystery than quantum theory will ever be. In my opinion, physicists who turn to quantum theory for explanations of such intricate phenomena are looking in the wrong direction. Quantum theory tells us how atoms interact, but little about protein dynamics and nothing about the electrophysiology of the brain.

Stuart: I disagree. Regulation of protein conformational dynamics is not understood, and some evidence supports quantum effects: For example, quantum coherence apparently does occur in certain proteins (e.g., BPTI, ferritin—Roitberg et al. 1995, Tejada et al. 1996), and quantum-spin correlations are preserved in cytoplasm (Walleczek 1995). Michael Conrad has extensively considered quantum effects in proteins.

Al: Well, yes, protein dynamics are very complicated. That's also *my* point. But—I repeat—it's not clear that you really need quantum theory to describe this intricacy. I spent about ten years studying quantum theories of polaronic effects in protein and at the end of the decade it was difficult to point to anything of experimental significance that could not be just as well described classically (Scott 1992).

Stuart: That's not to say that quantum effects in proteins may not be experimentally shown subsequently, as the Roitberg and Tejada papers suggest. It's an extremely tricky business—quantum effects are, in general, unobservable.

Al: If physicists are truly interested in contributing to our understanding of phenomena related to consciousness, they should acquaint themselves with the relevant neurological facts, which are far more intricate than can be expressed in a quantum formulation.

Stuart: I think a theory of consciousness must integrate philosophy, physics, and neurobiology, and so I basically agree. The "relevant neurological facts" may, however, turn out to include quantum effects.

Al: It's my view that physics and mathematics will have minor parts in this integration. [Pause.] And I have the impression that some physicists cling to the quantum approach because they are subconsciously aware that their knowledge is of limited value for understanding really interesting questions—like the nature of life and mind. Physics is a science of the past.

Stuart: Not being a physicist, I don't take this claim personally, but I do think it's unfair and incorrect. Face it—neither the hard problem of experience nor the nature of the universe is understood. Physics may offer solutions for both, particularly if experience is a fundamental property of the universe, as Chalmers concludes.

Al: On this point, I'm much more conservative than David. I don't feel comfortable with blithely assuming the existence of some new force field (or whatever) without experimental evidence for it.

Stuart: Experimental evidence points to the fact that reality exists. There *is* some fundamental makeup of the universe; we just don't know precisely what it is. The Casimir force of quantum fluctuations—the quantum "foam"— has just been measured (Lamoreaux 1997). Penrose's quantum-spin networks (Rovelli and Smolin 1995) are one approach to describing reality at its most basic (Planck-scale) level. This is where ("funda-mental") experience may reside.

Al: And though I would have no problem with a quantum theory of neural behavior if there were some experimental evidence to support it, there is none that I know of. Thus I prefer to concentrate my very limited powers of analysis on the vast and unexplored realms of hierarchical dynamics.

Stuart: Your work on hierarchical emergence is extremely important. And it is true that there is currently no hard evidence for quantum coherence and OR in microtubules. Orch OR is a model. I might add, however, that there is currently no experimental evidence for consciousness. It is unobservable (except in ourselves). Also, the isolated quantum states predicted in Orch OR will require clever, directed experiments. It's not at all surprising—assuming they do indeed exist—that they haven't been verified. In a recent paper (Hameroff 1997), nineteen specific testable predictions of the Orch OR model are suggested.

Al: Isn't the fact that we are having this conversation clear experimental evidence for consciousness?

Stuart: Not necessarily. I could be a zombie. In fact after another margarita or two, I may *be* a zombie.

Al: Ah …! Don't get started on zombies; the whole idea is kooky! Why worry about something that doesn't exist?

Stuart: Chill out, Al. Zombies are a useful philosophical concept. For example, if one were able to pinpoint a threshold for consciousness in the course of evolution, nonconscious organisms below that threshold—still capable of intelligent, adaptive behavior—would be zombies. Wouldn't they?

Al: H'm, that's an interesting idea.

Stuart: Actually, now that I think of it, having another glass or two would put me in a state quite opposite that of a zombie. I would be having a rather pleasant experience, but be relatively incapable of intelligent, adaptive behavior. Quite the opposite of the "zombie" state in which I'm driving my car but thinking of something entirely different.

Al: In his *Varieties of Religious Experience*, William James lists bibulosity as the first level of transcendental experience. But get back to evolution. When and how do you think consciousness emerged?

Stuart: I'd bet on small worms and spiny urchins in the early Cambrian sea floor 540 million years ago. The reasoning is explained in my chapter for the Tucson II book.

Al: Look, we agree that consciousness exists as an aspect of reality; the question is: how do we characterize it? Ten to a hundred billion nerve cells, each of which is locally described by the Hodgkin-Huxley equations, provide the basis for a very intricate nonlinear field theory. Immensely intricate. Such a system is not a product of theoretical imagination; it is supported by many thousands of carefully reviewed experimental research papers in electrophysiology. And a really intricate nonlinear lattice theory—with functional significance at many levels of dynamic reality—is our best bet for ultimately comprehending consciousness.

Stuart: How do we know that neural-membrane firing activities describable by Hodgkin-Huxley equate to consciousness?

Al: I'm not claiming that, and I don't think they do. As I've said, the real nonlinear picture is much more intricate. One has many levels of activity—from active patches of nerve membrane to action potentials on nerve fibers to behaviors of whole neurons to assemblies of neurons to assemblies to assemblies to ... the mind boggles ... to the complex behaviors that characterize a fully developed brain. But it doesn't stop even there. Each brain is a component—an atom, if you will—in a particular human culture. As a classical nonlinear field theory, this picture can easily explain global coherence, binding, threshold phenomena, free will, and so on. As I've said, it's *much* richer and more intricate than linear quantum theory will ever be.

Stuart: But why not also look *down* the hierarchical organization to the quantum level? Why arbitrarily pick membrane patches as the fine grain?

Al: At the end of the day, I suppose, it comes down to intuition. My whole professional life—thirty-five years—has been devoted to the study of classical nonlinear dynamics. [Pause.] My little finger tells me that quantum effects aren't important. [Pause.] Of course, that's not an argument, is it?

Stuart: Perhaps not, but I have great respect for intuition. It's a noncomputable process. It's just that *my* intuition—and Roger's—is that quantum effects in microtubules are necessary to explain difficult issues.

Let's look at five enigmatic features of consciousness: [Counting on his fingers.] (1) the nature of experience, (2) binding, (3) free will, (4) noncomputability, (5) transition from preconscious processes to consciousness. You are claiming that classical nonlinear effects, or "emergence," can explain 2 through 5, but without 1—the hard problem of experience—2 through 5 are empty. For example, in the transition from preconscious processes to consciousness, you are saying that nonlinear threshold phenomena can explain the transition. But transition into what? If the hard problem of experience isn't explained, then nonlinear threshold transitions are not necessarily explanatory. The same is true of binding and global coherence. Synchronization of neural firing activities doesn't solve anything unless a mechanism for conscious experience is attached. It's just a correlate of consciousness. A macroscopic quantum-coherent state, however, does truly "bind" its components into a unified entity.

Al: Classical nonlinear dynamics also truly binds components into unified entities. Think of a tornado or Jupiter's Great Red Spot.

Stuart: As I said before, tornadoes and the Great Red Spot are not conscious. But why not? Tornadoes and the Great Red Spot are self-organizing processes in a medium (atmospheric gases) that happens *not* to bear an intrinsic property or component of experience. The emergent property is wind, not mind.

Al: The emergent property of much of our neurophilosophy is also wind.

Stuart: Yes [chuckle], but philosophy *can* be useful in attempting to understand consciousness. For example, a line of panpsychist and panexperiential philosophers have suggested that experience is a fundamental feature of reality—Spinoza, Leibniz, Whitehead, Wheeler, and now Chalmers. Leibniz's "monads" are fundamental geometric regions of reality that bear experiential qualities. Whitehead's "occasions of experience" are events that occur in a wider field of raw experience.

The Orch OR model links these purely philosophical positions with the physics of reality at its most basic level. The Planck scale (10^{-33} cm) is where space-time geometry is no longer smooth. The best description of space-time at this level may be Penrose's quantum-spin networks (Rovelli and Smolin 1995) and this could be where "protoconscious" raw experience resides. We label this "funda-mental" geometry. Orch OR events are self-organizing quantum events at the Plank scale that select and reconfigure funda-mental geometry. This is an inescapable—if seemingly bizarre—conclusion.

Al: I still don't see how your quantum state gets to be conscious.

Stuart: It's not the state, it's a sequence of self-collapse events in a postulated protoconscious medium. Funda-mental experience is accessed and selected with each Orch OR event. Consciousness is stepwise rather than continuous. Don't you agree?

Al: I know only what goes on in my head, and that seems continuous.

Stuart: Movies seem continuous, but they are actually sequences of frames.

Al: And you can't claim that your conclusion is inescapable because so many see it differently. [Pause.] Shall we mix another pitcher?

Stuart: Well, it's inescapable to me. Yes, *más margaritas*! Let's find that bibulous "antizombie" state of pure experience.

REFERENCES

Born, M., and J. R. Oppenheimer. 1927. Zur Quantentheorie der Molekeln. *Annalen der Physik* 84:457–484.

Conrad, M. 1996. Percolation and collapse of quantum parallelism: A model of qualia and choice. In S. R. Hameroff, A. Kaszniak, and A. C. Scott, eds., *Toward a Science of Consciousness—The First Tucson Discussions and Debates*. Cambridge: MIT Press, pp. 469–492.

Hameroff, S. R. 1997. Funda-mental geometry: The Penrose-Hameroff Orch OR model of consciousness. In N. Woodhouse, ed., *Geometric Issues in the Foundations of Science: Proceedings of a Conference Honoring Roger Penrose*. Oxford: Oxford University Press. In press.

Hameroff, S. R., and R. Penrose 1996a. Orchestrated reduction of quantum coherence in brain microtubules: A model for consciousness. In S. R. Hameroff, A. Kasziak, and A. C. Scott, eds., *Toward a Science of Consciousness—The First Tucson Discussions and Debates*. Cambridge: MIT Press, pp. 508–540. Also published in *Mathematics and Computers in Simulation* 40:453–480. http://www.u.arizona.edu/~hameroff/penrose1

Hameroff, S. R., and R. Penrose. 1996b. Conscious events as orchestrated spacetime selections. *Journal of Consciousness Studies* 3(1):36–53. http://www.u.arizona.edu/~hameroff/penrose2

Lamoreaux, S. K. 1997. Demonstration of the Casimir force in the 0.6 to 6 micron range. *Physical Review Letters* 78:5–8.

Roitberg, A., R. B. Gerber, R. Elber, and M. A. Ratner. 1995. Anharmonic wave functions of proteins: Quantum self-consistent field calculations of BPTI. *Science* 268:1319–1322.

Rovelli, C., and L. Smolin. 1995a. Spin networks in quantum gravity. *Physical Review D* 52:5743–5759.

Rovelli, C., and L. Smolin. 1995b. Discreteness of area and volume in quantum gravity. *Nuclear Physics B* 442:593–619.

Scott, A. 1992. Davydov's soliton. *Physics Reports* 217:1–67.

Scott, A. 1995. *Stairway to the Mind*. New York: Springer-Verlag (Copernicus).

Scott, A. 1996. On quantum theories of the mind. *Journal of Consciousness Studies* 3: 484–491.

Tejada, J., A. Garg, S. Gider, D. D. Awschalom, D. P. DiVincenzo, and D. Loss. 1996. Does macroscopic quantum coherence occur in ferritin? *Science* 272:424–426.

Walleczek, J. 1995. Magnetokinetic effects on radical pairs: A possible paradigm for understanding sub-KT magnetic field interactions with biological systems. In M. Blank, ed., *Electromagnetic Fields: Biological Interactions and Mechanisms. Advances in Chemistry*, No. 250. Washington, DC: American Chemical Society Books.

XII Time and Consciousness

OVERVIEW

Whatever else the realities of mental life may be, we can probably agree that they are *dynamic*, our thoughts and feelings changing from moment to moment. To understand consciousness, therefore, it seems necessary to appreciate the nature of time.

What then is time?

Does time have direction? Some physicists tell us that time is one of the independent variables appearing in the fundamental equations describing the universe: Maxwell's electromagnetic equations, Einstein's equations for special and general relativity, Schrödinger's equation for an evolving quantum-wave function, and so on. Interestingly, in all these formulations, time has no direction; it runs as well in either direction.

The second law of thermodynamics, which was formulated in the nineteenth century to explain limits in designing and operating steam engines, suggests to other physicists that randomness and disorder (entropy) must inexorably increase until everything in the universe arrives at a uniform temperature. Because this "heat-death" scenario ignores gravity and black holes (Coveney and Highfield 1990), still other physicists suppose, the expanding universe will begin to shrink some day and eventually collapse; thus the Big Bang may eventually be followed by a Big Crunch. During the contraction phase, some physicists go so far as to speculate, time may flow backward, rivers will flow uphill and light will be emitted by our eyes to be absorbed by distant stars. Roger Penrose (1989) maintains, however, that even during the Big Crunch, entropy would be increasing, the Second Law would still hold, and the direction of time would be preserved. (For an alternative view, see Price 1996.)

Just as some physicists refuse to describe time as something that "flows" (in the theory of relativity, time is merely one coordinate in 4-dimensional space-time), some philosophers characterize as "mythical" our sense of time's flow. "If time flows past us, or if we advance through time, this would be a motion with respect to a hypertime ... which would lead us to postulate a hyper-hypertime and so on ad infinitum" (Edwards 1967). Despite all the evidence from our subjective sense, such sages assert, time does not really flow.

Although biologists and psychologists have appropriate respect for physicists' and philosophers' vast theoretical insights, they are rightly disturbed by characterizations of time as reversible, static, or relativistic. In the realms of life and mind, time does appear to have both direction and flow, whether one considers development in an individual organism, a metabolic process, or the course of evolution. Life runs inexorably away from the past and toward the future, and consciousness involves a sense of time's direction and flow: a "specious present," William James observed, a momentary "now" through which the future moves to become the past.

How might we describe mental time? We have, of course, a mechanical clock on the wall, skillfully designed by engineers to keep account of the hours in the day, but is that machine up to the task of measuring mental time? Take ten minutes of clock time and imagine two rather different situations. In the first, you are sitting in a quiet bar, chatting with a dear old friend after a separation of some years. In the second, you are crouched in your dentist's office having a root canal excavated. On the wall, the engineer's clocks record exactly ten minutes in both scenes. Are these two time intervals *really* the same? Be honest.

Dealing as they do with dynamic problems at many levels of description, applied mathematicians are inclined to view time from a more flexible perspective than that of physicists. Given a problem in which the telltale symbol t appears, one must consider how it is to be characterized. Does it go in one direction only (implying a dissipative or diffusive process), or does it go in both directions (indicating that energy is conserved under the dynamics)? Or does it expand and contract, or jump about in some manner that is more difficult to describe?

To whom does one turn for an answer to such questions? Surely one asks the experimentalists who have gathered and organized the data from which the description of a particular dynamics has arisen. This flexible attitude is carefully discussed in an important book entitled *The Genesis and Evolution of Time*, by J. T. Fraser (1982), which deserves a careful reading by every serious student of consciousness. The author convincingly argues that the nature of time—the meanings that we assign to it and the ways in which we describe it—depends strongly on the hierarchical level of description at which the concept is being employed. Why? Because we conceive of time in the context of some dynamic process, and such processes are not the same at different levels of description.

The sort of time that is useful for describing the dynamics of the universe in the first 15 femtoseconds after the Big Bang, for example, is far different from that governing the dynamics of one's thoughts and feelings while seated in Doctor Fell's chair. And the great basketball player Michael Jordan, when asked to explain his inspired maneuvering through a host of menacing defenders, explained that "time slows down" for him. Patients awakening from general anesthesia have no conception of how long they were unconscious; for them, time did not pass. From such examples we see a characteristic variability in the subjective passage of time. Perhaps consciousness comprises a sequence of distinct events, of which Jordan has more per move than his opponents (Hameroff and Penrose 1996).

It is clear, in any case, that life and consciousness operate on a vast range of time scales, and the authors in this part describe attempts to characterize time in two rather different contexts. The first is that of a bat, flying through the night air, guided by auditory responses to its singing toward a crisp and tasty insect. In the second example, time is seen from the perspective of a Trappist monk, immersed in a discipline that most of us would find impossible to abide, as he searches for the Presence of God.

Neurobiologists Prestor Saillant and James Simmons have studied the big brown bat *Eptesicus fuscus*, paying attention to the creature's startling ability to measure time delays on the engineer's clock to an accuracy of about 20 *nanoseconds* (Simmons 1996). Why "startling"? Because the transition time for switching a patch of neural membrane is about one millisecond, which is inadequate for the bat's temporal precision by several orders of magnitude. To explain this experimental finding, the authors propose a neural means for signal processing that may provide the brown bat with the ability to expand and contract the scale of its temporal perceptions.

In Chapter 56, anthropologists Van Reidhead and John Wolford present an experimental study on temporal perceptions in a Trappist monastery that suggests two qualitatively different concepts of time in human experience. The first is that of clock and calendar times, which are commonly used to organize affairs in Western cultures, and this time is characterized by the monks as "profane, linear, abstract," and not particularly useful. The second sort of time perception seems related to an altered state of consciousness, arising over a period of years under the practiced discipline and leading to sharpened awareness of Divine Presence.

Although this section is exploratory, the editors find such studies on the nature of time extremely significant, pointing in a direction that is most important for future research in the science of consciousness.

REFERENCES

Coveney, P., and R. Highfield. 1990. *The Arrow of Time*. New York: Fawcett Columbine.

Edwards, P. 1967. *The Encyclopedia of Philosophy*, vol. 8. New York: Collier-Macmillan, p. 126.

Fraser, J. T. 1982. *The Genesis and Evolution of Time*. Sussex: Harvester Press.

Hameroff, S. R., and R. Penrose. 1966. Conscious events as orchestrated space-time selections. *Journal of Consciousness Studies* 3(1):36–53.

Penrose, R. 1989. *The Emperor's New Mind*. Oxford: Oxford University Press.

Price, H. 1996. *Time's Arrow and Archimedes' Point: New Directions for the Physics of Time*. New York: Oxford University Press.

Simmons, J. A. 1996. Formation of perceptual objects from the timing of neural responses: Target-range images in bat sonar. In R. Llinás and P. S. Churchland, eds., *The Mind-Brain Continuum*. Cambridge: MIT Press, pp. 219–250.

55 Time Expansion and the Perception of Acoustic Images in the Big Brown Bat, *Eptesicus fuscus*

Prestor A. Saillant and James A. Simmons

Most of the time, the neural correlates of perception are measured in time scales ranging roughly from 1 to 100 msec. In the mammalian auditory system, however, information processing occurs on a completely different time scale, extending down to 1 to 10 μsec. For example, human subjects can discriminate differences in the time of arrival of 1-kHz tones at their two ears of 11 μsec (Klump and Eady 1956) and the big brown bat can detect changes in the arrival time of echoes in the sub-μsec range (Simmons et. al. 1990). How is it possible to integrate information on such vastly different time scales into a unified, behaviorally relevant perception? Consider the uniform perception of 3-D space that comes from both auditory and visual processing. In each sensory modality the brain is challenged to generate a perception of 3-D space from lower-dimension inputs. Sensory fusion then requires the two representations to be linked. It has been shown that synchronized timing of neural activity in the msec range may have important implications for perception of visual objects (Gray et. al. 1989). Thus, neurons with nonoverlapping receptive fields demonstrate higher synchronization when simultaneously stimulated by one object then when simultaneously stimulated by two separate objects. These findings reveal why it is important to think of the brain as a time machine rather than simply as a series of topological or functional neuronal maps.

Relatively new findings on bat sonar at Brown University suggest that μsec-scale information present in auditory stimuli can affect the timing of local evoked potentials on a μsec scale (Simmons et. al. 1996). Several fascinating possibilities are associated with this discovery. First, the idea that the brain can extract information present at μsec and sub-μsec time scales and expand the temporal representation of this information requires mechanisms of neural information processing that are not as yet identified. This time-expansion effect may function as a temporal "zoom lens" that provides signal-processing advantages to the mammalian auditory system. Time-expanded representations with ratios of 1:10 to 1:100 have been found in the auditory system of the big brown bat, and the ratios increase as we traverse from lower brain centers, such as the inferior colliculus, to higher brain areas, such as the auditory cortex. This variable time expansion may provide a substrate for wavelet-like processing strategies in the bat auditory system, conferring

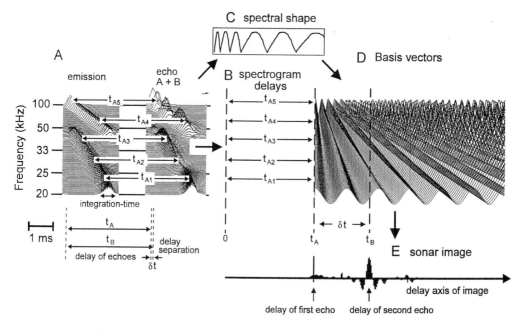

Figure 55.1 Formation of SCAT images. (A) Cochlear block. (B) Temporal block. (C–D) Spectral block. (E) Final sonar image of two surfaces.

upon them additional scale and rotation invariance, as well as sparse 3-D matrix compression, and the integration of μsec-scale processes with other msec-scale processes in the brain.

SCAT AND TIME EXPANSION

The time-expansion phenomenon was first predicted by the model of bat echolocation known as the SCAT model (Saillant et al. 1993). This prediction is described in Figure 55.1. The SCAT model consists of three blocks, which model at differing degrees of abstraction the neural information processing believed to occur in the bat's auditory system. For simplicity, the bat's broadcast is modeled as a pair of downward-sweeping harmonics from 100 kHz to 40 kHz, and 50 kHz to 20 kHz. The cochlear-block outputs (Figure 55.1A) represent outputs from hair cells along the basilar membrane in the inner ear. The vertical axis represents 81 hair cells organized tonotopically from 100 kHz to 20 kHz. The horizontal axis represents time. The left side of Figure 55.1A labeled "emission" shows frequency-modulated (FM) echolocating bat's emitted sound as it would appear in the inner ear. The second half of this figure (labeled "echo $A + B$") represents an echo from a target including two surfaces separated by 60 μsec. The presence of the second surface is encoded into the spectrum of the echo and appears as a pattern of peaks and notches in the spectrum. It is clear from psychophysical experiments, however, that the bats perceive the position of the two surfaces in space, rather than only one surface plus spectral coloration or timbre. The two subsequent blocks in the SCAT model explain the bats' perception of two separate surfaces in terms of plausible neural mechanisms. The second block (spectrogram correlation block) consists of neuronal delay lines that carry impulses generated by simulated auditory afferent fibers. These delay lines extract the delay between the emitted sound and the returning echoes by measuring coincidences of neural impulses across frequencies and within each frequency (Figure 55.1B). The spectrogram correlation block is sufficient for registering the returning echo's overall delay (t_a), but it cannot provide information about the position of the secondary surface 60 μsec away. The third block in the SCAT model (transformation block) converts the spectral information in the echo back into position information (Figure 55.1E). This process can be modeled as the multiplication of the spectral shape vector (Figure 55.1C) by an oscillatory matrix (Figure 55.1D). The oscillatory matrix can be thought of as real-time oscillations in the brain that are linked to detection of the first surface in the returning echo. A precise relationship must connect these oscillations and the center frequency of the corresponding afferent hair cells, as shown in Figure 55.1D. The actual oscillatory frequencies, however, need not be in the bat's ultrasonic range of 100 kHz to 20 kHz. For example, these oscillatory frequencies could conceivably be scaled down to between 4 kHz and 800 Hz, a 25:1 reduction. Frequency reduction leads to time expansion, however, so that a secondary surface 60 μsec away would be reconstructed as a surface 1.5 msec away.

Have we any evidence for this type of time expansion in the brain? In the big brown bat, the neural representations of binaural time differences on the order of 10 to 50 μsec have been shown to result in shifts in the timing of local evoked potentials in the range of several msec (Simmons et al. 1996). In these experiments, sounds were presented to each ear by a separate miniature speaker. Only the delay difference between the sounds was altered. Figures 55.2A and B show the time-expansion effect found for interaural time differences when recording local evoked potentials from the auditory cortex. It is clear that time expansion has occurred, with a ratio of about 16:1. The SCAT model as shown, however, is a monaural model. In the binaural experiment, no interference pattern is imposed on the actual sounds arriving at the two ears as it would in an echo from a target with two closely spaced surfaces, and so the interference must occur between the neural responses for the two ears. Another experiment (data not shown) yields results that are more like predictions by the SCAT model. In this experiment, the distance between two overlapping echoes presented as auditory stimuli results in a time-expanded linear change in the temporal location of local evoked potentials in the auditory cortex. Here, spectral information related to target structure is present in each echo, and the expansion ratio obtained is about 13:1 (Simmons et al. 1996). Although the actual mechanism of time expansion needs to be further explored, the phenomenon exists, and may have important implications for understanding neural information processing, mechanisms of attention, and perception in the auditory system.

Prestor A. Saillant and James A. Simmons: Time Expansion and Acoustic Images in the Bat

(A)

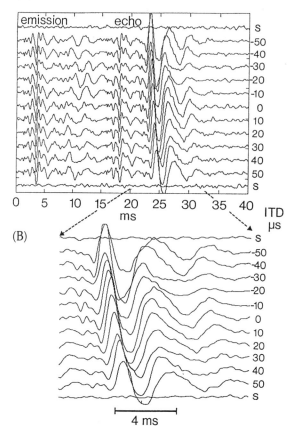

(B)

4 ms

Figure 55.2 Time-expanded representations in the cortex. Local evoked potentials are shown for various interaural time delays (ITDs). Changes in ITD of 100 μsec overall results in a local evoked-potential shift of about 1.6 msec. (B) is zoomed-up version of (A).

INVARIANT PROCESSING AND 3-D DATA COMPRESSION WITH TIME EXPANSION

If the dimensions of 3-D objects are converted from spatial units into temporal units, then it is easier to see how time expansion may allow invariant representations of scaled or rotated objects. Figure 55.3 shows a SCAT image of three wires as they are rotated in space. The upper and lower plots show the same SCAT image, but in the upper plot lines have been drawn to help clarify the results. The spacing between the wires is shown in the inset on the right side. The graph's vertical axis represents the distance in time between the wire pairs for different orientations along the horizontal axis from 0° to 30° (time and distance are interchangeable when dealing with sonar echoes). At 0° all three wires are at nearly the same distance from the artificial bat's ear that was used for acquiring the sonar data. Clearly, as we rotate the wires the effect is similar to what would happen if we were to take

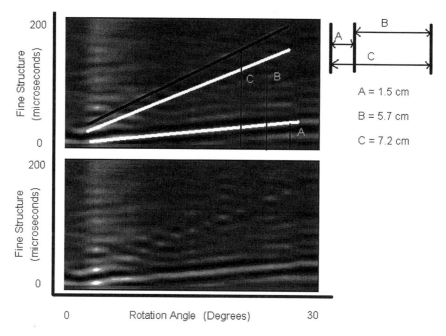

A = 1.5 cm

B = 5.7 cm

C = 7.2 cm

Figure 55.3 SCAT image of 3 wires rotated through 30 degrees, showing how the target's features expand. Distance and time are equivalent to each other in sonar processing. The upper plot is a replica of the lower plot, with lines drawn through it.

the vertical axis and stretch it. Stretching the vertical axis would be the equivalent of time expansion. Thus a rotation-invariant representation of the three wires could be achieved by variable time expansion of the input representation. One could simply choose the largest rotation as the target's invariant representation, and then expand the data obtained at other orientations until a match was found. Of course, this is not a new idea: time expansion and contraction is the basis for wavelet processing. Figure 55.4 shows another example of invariance that can be obtained from time expansion. Again the plots have been duplicated so that lines could be added to the upper plot. Here SCAT images of two hex nuts of different sizes were generated. Again, it is clear that the images could be thought of as stretching or compressing the vertical time axis.

Time-expansion processing lends itself naturally to data compression in two ways. First, data compression can be achieved by reducing the number of templates that are stored in memory. Thus, one time-series template may be enough to represent a range of an object's orientations. The dynamic time expansion occurring on sensory data can then be used to match the signal to the stored template. A second form of data compression also results from expanded representations. For example, in the visual system only the retinal fovea has an expanded representation in the visual cortex. As a result, high spatial resolution is possible in a central region, without overwhelming the visual system with high-resolution information from the much larger retinal periphery. This is a form of data compression, allowing a greater expanse of

Prestor A. Saillant and James A. Simmons: Time Expansion and Acoustic Images in the Bat

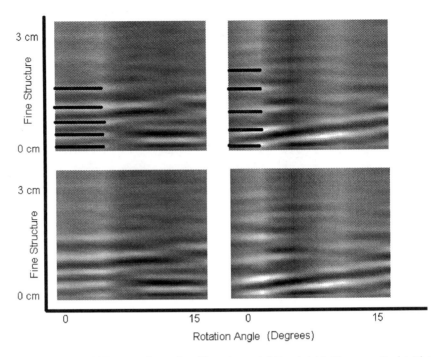

Figure 55.4 SCAT image of a small and large hex nut (left and right sides, respectively). Plots show that size of objects can be represented by time expansion. The upper plot is a replica of the lower plot with lines drawn through it.

space to be represented then would be possible at very high resolution. Time expansion may also lend itself to this type of data compression. Consider how a clock ticking in the night can suddenly seem very loud and disturbing when previously it had remained unheard. The need to process sensory data at close to real time prevents continuous time expansion of all sensory data. Thus only selected input streams can have time-expansion processing. It seems plausible, then, that the time-expansion phenomenon could provide the auditory system with an acoustic fovea-like phenomenon, allowing it to zoom in on important stimuli while minimizing representation of stimuli arriving from uninteresting portions of space. Like the topographical expanded representations in the visual system, this mechanism could provide expanded representations in the time domain.

REFERENCES

Gray, C. M., P. Konig, A. K. Engel, and W. Singer. 1989. Oscillatory responses in cat visual cortex exhibit intercolumnar synchronization, which reflects global stimulus properties. *Nature* 338:334–337.

Klumpp, R. G., and H. R. Eady. 1956. Some measurements of interaural time difference thresholds. *Journal of the Acoustical Society of America* 28:859–860.

Saillant, P. A., J. A. Simmons, S. P. Dear, and T. A. McMullen. 1993. A computational model of echo processing and acoustic imaging in FM echolocating bats: The spectrogram correlation and transformation receiver. *Journal of the Acoustical Society of America* 94:2691–2712.

Simmons, J. A., P. A. Saillant, M. J. Ferragamo, T. Haresign, S. P. Dear, J. Fritz, and T. A. McMullen. 1996. Auditory computations for biosonar target imaging in bats. In H. L. Hawkins, T. A. McMullen, A. N. Popper, and R. R. Fay, eds., *Auditory Computation*. New York: Springer-Verlag, pp. 401–468.

Simmons, J. A., M. Ferragamo, C. F. Moss, S. B. Stevenson, and R. A. Altes. 1990. Discrimination of jittered sonar echoes by the echolocating bat, *Eptesicus fuscus*: The shape of target images in echolocation. *Journal of Comparative Physiology A* 167:589–616.

Context, Conditioning, and Meaning of Time-Consciousness in a Trappist Monastery

Van A. Reidhead and John B. Wolford

In this chapter, we set out to understand the development of shared perception and experience of time—time-consciousness. Our case is a Trappist monastery in the United States. Key questions are: Can a community intentionally reenculturate adults to a specialized kind of time-consciousness? How are alternative experiences of time conditioned? Do alternate forms of time-consciousness have measurable effects?

LITERATURE

The literature makes clear that the philosophy, organization, and experience of time varies among cultures, documenting alternative kinds of time-consciousness. Eliade (Beane and Doty 1976) identified alternate kinds of time: "profane" and "sacred." Profane time is linear, and sacred time is neither homogeneous nor continuous. For Eliade, each form of time-consciousness is experienced in its corresponding space, sacred time in sanctified and profane time in routine spaces. Sacred time is inexhaustible, always present, never changing, always equal to itself, and is purely ontological, but profane time is bounded by birth and death. "Religious man" lives both kinds of time simultaneously. Such a person, nonetheless, experiences time boundlessly, unbothered by its existential implications. Ontologized time becomes a sacred value, the domain in which God, ultimate reality, is encountered and reconciled (Beane and Doty 1976).

Turner (1969) developed a symbolic anthropology that is focused on "ritual process" as a methodology for transporting people to alternate perceptions of time–space relationships, whence they gain renewed perspective on sociohistorical reality. Ritually invoked consciousness bridges experience of the ineffable with normal social conditions, informing the latter with creative insight, thus renewing historical time. Historical time is redeemed, cyclically, by infusions of creative energy from ritually evoked antistructural time-consciousness (Turner 1974).

Hall (1983) delineates nine types of time-experience, including categories for profane and sacred, with definitions similar to those of Eliade, and seven other types—biological, personal, physical, micro- (culture-specific), sync- (harmonizing personal and cultural), meta- (intellectual abstractions), and metaphysical. Hall's approach is a helpful though undeveloped theoretical enterprise.

These three approaches parallel the postmodernist cultural critique. Using deconstruction, discourse analysis, reflexivity, antirepresentationalism, and chaos theory, postmodernism has undertaken a critique of standard Western notions of time and space. Linear time is no longer an objective reality. Time is anarchic and disconnected, although (following the affirmative postmodernists) inhering in relational significance (Baudrillard 1987, Derrida 1976, 1981, Foucault 1973, 1980, Megill 1989, Rosenau 1992).

For Hall and Eliade, time-consciousness is more than an adaptive expression in the sum of cross-cultural, evolved traits. It defines consciousness and distinguishes it from other categories in perception. The cyclically structured, ritualized life of Trappist monks describes a method for conditioning a specific kind of time-consciousness and corresponding experience.

TIME IN A TRAPPIST MONASTERY

Time, in a Trappist monastery, is spent with little variation. Any change repeats itself on a 24-hour, biweekly (the time required to recite the Psalms), seasonal (liturgical seasons), and annual (complete liturgical cycle) schedule. Although monks make long-range plans and commitments, time is predominantly lived cyclically, and the same sensory experiences repeat themselves daily, biweekly, seasonally, and, at most, annually. One monk describes the Trappist routine as purposely "monotonous" (Reidhead 1996a).

Monks rise at 3:15 A.M. daily, begin the day together in choir (community prayer), to which they return seven times, the last ending at 7:30 P.M., followed by silence and sleep.[1] The seven choir times, collectively referred to as the Divine Office or the Order of the Hours, are broken by set times for meals, ordinary labor, private prayer, and personal needs. The life is one of prayer and labor—*ora et labora* is the governing dictum (Fry et al. 1980).

In a Trappist monastery, all time is sacred. Nonetheless, it is nested in profane, historical, linear time, in which monks maintain competence.

PRESENT CASE

In 1993, Reidhead launched an ethnographic study at the monastery that continues today. Prior to October 1995, when ten monks were interviewed for this study, Reidhead had spent ninety days of in-residence participant observation in the monastery. The decision to investigate time grew out of Reidhead's personal experience of chronological blurring following prolonged periods at the monastery and Wolford's (1992) interest in time-space experience among nineteenth-century Shakers.

The October 1995 interviews were designed to ascertain beliefs, interpretations, and experiences of time. Reidhead's interviews were overlapped, during a five-day period, by informal interviews by Wolford. The findings from the *Time Interviews* corroborate in-depth knowledge of individual monks and the community, acquired since 1993. Reidhead returned to the monastery in July 1996, to conduct interviews on health and aging (Hanna 1996) and power (Loesel 1996). He added further time questions to clarify issues relevant to preparation of this chapter.

The intent in the interviews was twofold: (1) Determine a monk's unconscious levels of awareness of time. Does ritual participation cause a qualitative difference in time perception? Do general or specific (or both) differences appear in time conceptualization? What are the qualitative differences between work time and time dedicated to religious practice? (2) Understand how time-consciousness is conditioned.

RESULTS

Six questions were designed for statistical assessment using consensus analysis (CA), a technique that factors correlation coefficients to measure agreement in very small populations (Romney, Weller, and Batchelder 1986, Hurwicz 1995). The six primary questions, designed to collect nominal data for factor loading in CA, were supported by open-ended discussion, a necessary method in ethnographic anthropology (Geertz 1973, pp. 6–16). Consensus was documented at the 90 percent confidence level.[2] Numerical values for the six factored variables and data from discussions follow.

QUESTIONS AND DISCUSSION

1. *Are you normally aware of the date? If yes or no, explain.* Five monks professed general unawareness and five reported awareness. Three who reported date awareness have administrative duties; one reported not having been date conscious until assuming editorship of a journal; the fifth attributed date awareness to his attentiveness to the liturgy, which operates on a dated cycle. It seems significant that half of those questioned reported being generally unaware of, and furthermore, unconcerned about the date. One monk who was immediately aware of the date explained:

Many [monks] won't even know the day of the week. It's all kind of one. But there are dates of significance ... like one's profession date ... that give you something to focus on.... It is probably meant to be that way, because it helps us live in mindfulness of God, here and now. Everything is here in the present (Reidhead 1995).

Another, also aware of the date, reported:

The only way that I am aware of past and future is in terms of my work. In terms of my prayer, past and future are ... unnecessary distractions. The whole point of a person's prayer life—his religious, spiritual life—is to focus on the present, because that is the only thing that exists ... (Reidhead 1995).

No convergence appears between the kind of spirituality a monk practices and awareness or unawareness of the date. One especially contemplative monk supplied the date, day of week, month, and year without hesitation.

Van A. Reidhead and John B. Wolford: Time-Consciousness in a Trappist Monastery

He explained this seeming contradiction by reference to his emphasis on the liturgical cycle's structure and content; it is nested in standard time. Contemplative consciousness is conversant with normal, linear time (Geertz 1973, pp. 389–391). Another monk, of mystical reputation, confirmed this connection, saying, "Time and space is everything, because that is the gift of God. Man is a limited being."

2. *Do you focus most on the past, present, or future? How often do you have thoughts in these three domains? Explain.* One of ten monks reported persistent preoccupation with the past, a disturbing phenomenon causing cognitive dissonance. A second monk reported thinking often, though not usually, about the past, explaining that he has regrets about how he used his time.

Explaining the importance of present focus, the newly commissioned editor said:

Since becoming editor I have felt the pressure of time as never before. If that were to continue for an indefinite period it could be very stressful, with repercussions for health and other things (Reidhead 1995).

3. *Where does a person encounter God, in the past, present, or future? Explain.* All ten monks agreed that God is encountered only in the present, for the present is the only time that is real. A monk known for contemplative practice but formerly an abbot explained:

"Mindfulness of God" means living here and now, and that applies to everything. A monk will say, "Well, I don't want to be washing dishes, I want to be in choir, praying." But that is wrong. It is all the same (Reidhead 1996b).

4. *Does your participation in choir affect your experience of time? If yes, how? If no, what is your experience of the choir, temporally?* Agreement was unanimous that participation in choir focuses on the present. This statement should not, however, be taken to indicate that a monk's mind never wanders. Five monks said their thoughts regularly stray to things other than choir. Because CA is designed to analyze belief, attitude, and perception, and not behavior, the finding that monks' minds stray from choir was not factored.

One monk explained the relationship between choir and the rest of the monastic enterprise simply:

Over a period of time you have work and you have private prayer, and these [revolve] around the Divine Office (Reidhead 1995).

5. *Does your experience of choir affect your experience of work? Explain.* Agreement on this question too was unanimous. One monk explained the conditioning effect of choir time on time outside choir:

The life is structured to facilitate continual mindfulness of God.... The various times when we go to church [choir] can be seen as highlighting that mindfulness of God. There are ways to bring it to sharp consciousness and awareness, and then, in the times outside of that, the mindfulness continues (Reidhead 1995).

He further explained:

... [I]t is helpful to me to have [choir times] spaced periodically throughout the day and the night, rather than having them all together in one clump. It's not that time spent outside the choir is not sacred, because it is ... but it is a different quality of sacred time (Reidhead 1995).

A monk, most of whose life has been spent on the monastery farm, explained:

Human nature is related to animals, in the way of structure, physically. If you have ever worked with animals, you know that they respond to routine.... It is the same with us.... The offices [choir] should be at the same time every day, not scattered around, [so that] you have the expectation that Terce, Sext, or None is coming up (Reidhead 1995).

6. Does your personal time focus—past, present, future—affect your productivity in work? Explain. Nine of ten monks reported that their focus on the present yields tangible results in improved efficiency and productivity at work. Analyzing data from the same monastery, Hanna (1996) documents lower morbidity, later mortality—regionally normed—and greater productivity in work throughout old age, until death, than in the general population, findings that tangentially support the monks' claims of heightened productivity.

Explaining how their present focus improves performance in work, one monk said:

Regularity is an essential component in the mindfulness of God. A person needs a sense of regularity, predictability, and stability. You can do a tremendous amount, even though you are only working in chopped-up intervals, because you are assured of having those intervals (Reidhead 1995).

Referring to the Rule of St. Benedict, and thus to the monks' obligation to obedience, another monk said:

There shouldn't be any conflict between the two. Like St. Benedict says, *ora et labora*. There is a time for prayer and a time for work.... You are continually reminded that work is another form of prayer, that you are working for God. You are doing it not just as something else to do, but to serve the community, and in serving the community you are serving God (Reidhead 1995).

Far from treating the method as a purely physical structure, every monk emphasized the role of God. Primary emphasis on mindfulness of God, the understanding that God is encountered exclusively in the present, and the conviction that a monk must put the "work of God" first, permeates the system. Monks place belief in God squarely at the center of their method. One monk explained what keeps the brothers coming back to choir:

The Rule of Benedict says nothing is to be preferred to the Work of God, which is the Divine Office [choir], community, choir prayer. A key criterion in discerning [if a person has a] vocation [to be a monk] is, does the individual love the Divine Office (Reidhead 1995)?

To love something so utterly repetitious, the monk must first believe in it, without which act he can never hope to relinquish his own will to the obedience required for the monastic method to work.

About space, the monks reported that no space is more sacred than any other. Space is sanctified by consciousness of God's presence, a time-dependent phenomenon, for God can be experienced only in the present. Time, not space, is the key physical variable in the monastic system.

This statistical convergence, like that found with CA, does not detract from the broader finding that the individual monks' behavior, attitudes, and interpretive systems vary widely. General agreement prevails on important issues, such as how a monk orders his life, but little effort is made to structure his individual belief system, preferences, and expressions of personality. The twenty-five monks enjoy many individualized interpretations about experience and meaning in their lives, but, as the interview responses confirm, all have a shared core of ideas, practices, and mental experiences of time.

St. Augustine, writing a century before St. Benedict, understood time, experientially defined, as a mental phenomenon (Sherover 1975). Saints Augustine, Pachomius, Jerome, Basil, John Cassian, and others, in the centuries preceding St. Benedict, worked to develop theologies and programs to condition men and women to a "more authentic," present-centered consciousness (Fry et al. 1980). St. Benedict benefited from this diverse enterprise.

MODEL

The major finding is that a specific kind of time-consciousness—measured by mental perception and experience—is conditioned by a person's self-subjection to a strict, cyclically structured social order. The key conditioning agent for Trappists is the cyclically structured, repetitive use of time. A hermit from another Trappist community explained, "The Trappist ideal is for an unvarying, monotonous routine" (Reidhead 1996a). A repetitive routine blocks mental diversions, leaving the mind free to focus on the immediate context, resulting in a shift from "normal" linear (past–present–future) time-consciousness to one that is rooted in the present.

Without disciplined observance of the monastic structure, the order could achieve no measurable result. St. Benedict's call to "The labor of obedience ... " (Fry et al. 1980) is not only an eschatological admonition but a conditioning directive, without which the intended effect cannot be experienced in time-space reality. Neophytes who do not submit to the conditioning do not persevere long enough to become monks. One monk, known for methodical rigor, estimated that an average of three years is required for successful—internalized, enculturated, unselfconscious—conditioning of "Trappist time-consciousness" (Reidhead 1995).

Belief, however, precedes obedience in the conditioning system, making it possible for the novice monk to bend his will to that of his "superiors" (Fry et al. 1980) in living the intense, physically structured life of a Trappist.

We suggest, then, that the conditioning "formula" or model required to alter time-consciousness among Trappists proceeds:

Belief > Time structure > Discipline > Altered consciousness

It appears, though stronger confirmation is required, that Trappist time-consciousness yields a byproduct in high-quality, high-yield "work" productivity. Hanna's (n.d.) work corroborates this impression, as do Reidhead's firsthand observations for nearly five years, and observations from historical evidence (Lekai 1977). Hanna's research further indicates that monks live longer, healthier lives than their age mates in the same geographic region. If validated, these observations yield an expanded model:

Belief > Time structure > Discipline > Altered consciousness > Beneficial byproducts.

Nonetheless, research designed to assess this assumption is needed.

CONCLUSIONS

This analysis, and the resulting model, inevitably oversimplify a complex consciousness-conditioning system. The monks' individual mental systems, abilities, and interests are, we suggest, as variable as those in the population at large.

Moreover, people understand time by the standards of the culture to which they are enculturated. Western cultures demand an abstract, linear relationship to time (Hall 1983). This dominance imposes itself on any alternative or subordinate temporal reality. Thus, Trappist monks, though they contextualize time by Western norms for linearity—profane, linear, and abstract—consciously structure their internal cultural time in nested cycles that repeat themselves endlessly. Manipulating time-consciousness thus, Trappists use the Western standard as a gateway for enculturating their own antistructural temporal orientation (see Reidhead 1993).

Human beings accommodate many temporal orientations. To achieve individual normalization and broader cultural adaptability, monks accept the profane, linear pattern, but restructure it to gradually enculturate a different, indigenous, dominant form of time-consciousness. Nonetheless, nothing in our research confirms the postmodernist dismissal of the objectifiable reality of historical time, linearly structured. Despite the monks' choosing to enculturate to sacred time, they remain, like Geertz's Balinese (Geertz 1973), conversant in and dependent for survival upon linear time.

Finally, the mutually supporting methodologies we have used in this research, integrating quantitative and qualitative approaches, serve as a trope for the complex, holistic experience of time, place, individuality, community, and divinity that monks experience. Using standard research methods, we want to understand what it is that the monks already know, consciously and unconsciously. Nearly fifteen centuries ago, St. Benedict understood that individuals in search of the divine must integrate standard cultural and social understanding with religious life. Through their individual diversity, the monks reveal the complexity of this interplay. At the very least, the belief that they are consecrated, by choice and calling, to God, is a crucial part of the method that sustains discipline until they achieve the conditioning effect of present time-consciousness. Methodologically speaking, belief is a domain in ethnographic analysis, and phenomenologically (Husserl 1964), God exists inside it. Profound belief in God structures the way in which monks interpret experience, consciously by obedience to the Rule and, eventually, if they persevere, unself-consciously as enculturated members of Trappist society.

ACKNOWLEDGMENTS

We thank the monks of Holy Trinity Abbey and of other abbeys who have contributed to this research. Dr. Margo Lea Hurwicz, Erin Doucette, Lynn Davis, and Timothy Hogan, all of the University of Missouri–St. Louis Anthropology Department, deserve special thanks.

NOTES

1. The Office follows a general pattern common to all Trappist monasteries. The Order of the Hours at Holy Trinity is:

3:30 AM	Vigils
6:00 AM	Lauds
6:20 AM	Community Mass
7:45 AM	Terce
12:15 PM	Sext
2:15 PM	None
5:30 PM	Vespers (On Sundays and holy Holidays, Benediction follows Vespers.)
7:30 PM	Compline

2. The first part of each question was coded to produce nominal data, for factoring, yielding the consensus analysis results.

REFERENCES

Baudrillard, J. 1987. Modernity. *Canadian Journal of Political and Social Theory* 11:63–72.

Beane, W. C., and W. G. Doty, eds. 1976. *Myths, Rites, Symbols: A Mircea Eliade Reader*, 2 vols. New York: Harper Colophon.

Derrida, J. 1976. *Of Grammatology*, trans. G. Spivak. Baltimore: Johns Hopkins University Press.

Derrida, J. 1981. *Positions*. Chicago: University of Chicago Press.

Foucault, M. 1973. *The Birth of the Clinic*. London: Tavistock.

Foucault, M. 1980. *Power/Knowledge*. C. Gordon, ed., C. Gordon, L. Marshall, J. Mepham, and K. Soper, trans. Pantheon.

Fry, T., I. Baker, T. Horner, A. Raabe, and M. Sheridan. 1980. *The Rule of St. Benedict in Latin and English, with notes*. Liturgical Press.

Geertz, C. 1973. *The Interpretation of Cultures*. New York: Basic Books.

Hall, E. T. 1983. *The Dance of Life: The Other Dimension of Time*. New York: Anchor Press/Doubleday.

Hanna, J. 1996. "Lifestyle and vitality in a Trappist monastry: The plasticity of aging." Unpublished manuscript.

Hurwicz, M. L. 1995. Physicians' norms and health care decisions of elderly medicare recipients. *Medical Anthropology Quarterly* 9:211–235.

Husserl, E. 1964. The phenomenology of internal time-consciousness, J. S. Churchill, Trans. Bloomington: Indiana University Press.

Loesel, J. 1996. "Investigating the relationship between position and influence in a Trappist monastery." Unpublished manuscript.

Lekai, L. J. 1977. *The Cistercians: Ideals and Reality*. Kent, OH: Kent State University Press.

Megill, A. 1989. Recounting the past: "Description," explanation, and narrative in historiography. *American Historical Review* 94:627–653.

Reidhead, V. A. 1993. Structure and anti-structure in monasticism and anthropology: Epistemological parallels and models. *Anthropology of Consciousness* 4:11–20.

Reidhead, V. A. 1995. Unpublished field notes, October.

Reidhead, V. A. 1996a. Unpublished field notes, April.

Reidhead, V. A. 1996b. Unpublished field notes, July.

Romney, A. K., S. Weller, and W. H. Batchelder. 1986. Culture as consensus: A theory of culture and informant accuracy. *American Anthropologist* 88:313–338.

Rosenau, P. M. 1992. *Post-Modernism and the Social Sciences: Insights, Inroads, and Intrusions*. Princeton: Princeton University Press.

Sherover, C. M. 1975. *The Human Experience of Time: The Development of Its Philosophic Meaning*. New York: New York University Press.

Turner, V. 1969. *The Ritual Process*. Ithaca: Cornell University Press.

Turner, V. 1974. *Dramas, Fields, and Metaphors*. Ithaca: Cornell University Press.

Wolford, J. B. 1992. The South Union, Kentucky, Shakers and tradition: A study of business, work, and commerce. Ph.D. diss., Indiana University.

XIII Transpersonal Psychology

OVERVIEW

Transpersonal experiences have been defined as nonordinary states of consciousness in which the sense of self extends beyond the individual "to encompass wider aspects of humankind, life, psyche, and cosmos" (Walsh and Vaughan 1996, p. 17). Founded in the 1960s, transpersonal psychology is the study of such experiences and their causes and correlates, as well as disciplines that they inspire (e.g., meditation and other forms of systematic spiritual practice). Of course, any theory of consciousness meant to be comprehensive must in some way account for transpersonal experiences. Further, as some theorists (e.g., Wilber 1997) have argued, transpersonal perspectives may be capable of providing a unique and coherent integration of many diverse fields of human knowledge. The two chapters in this section describe major methodologies and observations by which transpersonal psychologists have sought a comprehensive science of consciousness.

Charles Tart opens by describing a spontaneous transpersonal experience that a colleague reported, thereby setting the stage for a discussion of methodology needed to understand such experiences. Tart challenges the reader to consider an enlarged scientific methodology that is not limited by a "scientistic commitment to reductionism." He closes by reiterating Tart's (1972) earlier plea for state-specific sciences to study altered states of consciousness.

Roger Walsh sets out to give a conceptual history and to assess the study of altered states and stages in consciousness. He contrasts Asian and Western views of consciousness, emphasizing our modern Western world's resisting both validity and significance of multiple conscious states. Illustrating a phenomenological mapping of transpersonal states, he demonstrates how common features can be identified and types of states coherently clustered.

These authors show why a science of consciousness must account for transpersonal experiences, and deeply question whether the metaphysical assumptions of a "Newtonian–Cartesian paradigm and ... the materialistic philosophy that has dominated Western science for the last three hundred years" (Grof 1996, p. 45) are up to the task.

REFERENCES

Grof, S. 1996. Theoretical and empirical foundations of transpersonal psychology. In S. Boorstein, ed., *Transpersonal Psychotherapy*, 2nd ed. Albany: State University of New York Press, pp. 43–65.

Tart, C. 1972. States of consciousness and state-specific sciences. *Science* 176:1203–1210.

Walsh, R., and F. E. Vaughan. 1996. Comparative models of the person and psychotherapy. In S. Boorstein, ed., *Transpersonal Psychotherapy*, 2nd ed. Albany: State University of New York Press, pp. 15–30.

Wilber, K. 1997. *The Eye of Spirit: An Integral Vision for a World Gone Slightly Mad.* Boston: Shambhala.

57 Transpersonal Psychology and Methodologies for a Comprehensive Science of Consciousness

Charles T. Tart

Transpersonal psychology is the study of experiences that seem to take us beyond, *trans*, our ordinary personal boundaries. As we have recently defined it in the catalog of the Institute of Transpersonal Psychology,

Transpersonal psychology is a fundamental area of research, scholarship, and application based on people's experiences of temporarily transcending our usual identification with our limited biological, historical, cultural, and personal self and, at the deepest and most profound levels of experience possible, recognizing/being "something" of vast intelligence and compassion that encompasses/is the entire universe. From this perspective our ordinary, "normal" biological, historical, cultural, and personal self is seen as an important, but quite partial (and often pathologically distorted) manifestation or expression of this much greater "something" that is our deeper origin and destination ...

A COSMIC-CONSCIOUSNESS EXPERIENCE

Although the "mystical-experience" label is so widely and vaguely applied that it is almost useless for scientific work, we are slowly learning how to describe some such events more specifically. One such experience is *cosmic consciousness* (CC) (Bucke 1961, p. 2). This experience of the ground of being goes well beyond mere intellectual insight: "The prime characteristic of CC is, as the name implies, a consciousness of the cosmos, that is, of the life and order of the universe."

A scholar at the Tucson II meeting, Dr. Allan Smith, had a spontaneous experience of CC that we are about to publish (Smith and Tart in press). The care and precision in his description, which I quote only in part, clarifies that which we mean by transpersonal experience. Smith, thirty-eight at the time of his experience, was an academic researcher in anesthesiology, scientist, and materialist. Here is what happened:

My CC event began with some mild tingling in the perineal area, the region between the genitals and anus. The feeling was unusual, but was neither particularly pleasant nor unpleasant.... I then noticed that the level of light in the room as well as that of the sky outside seemed to be increasing slowly. The light seemed to be coming from everywhere ... it gave the air a bright, thickened quality that slightly obscured perception rather than sharpened it. It soon became extremely bright, but the light was not in the least unpleasant.

Along with the light came an alteration in mood. I began to feel very good, then still better, then elated. While this was happening, the passage of time seemed to become slower and slower.... It is difficult to estimate the time period over which these changes occurred, since the sense of time was itself affected.... Eventually, the sense of time passing stopped entirely.... Only the present moment existed. My elation proceeded to an ecstatic state, the intensity of which I had never even imagined could be possible. The white light around me merged with the reddish light of the sunset to become one all-enveloping, intense, undifferentiated light field. Perception of other things faded....

At this point, I merged with the light and everything, including myself, became one unified whole. There was no separation between myself and the rest of the universe. In fact, to say that there was a universe, a self, or any "thing" would be misleading—it would be an equally correct description to say that there was "nothing" as to say that there was "everything." All words or discursive thinking had stopped and there was no sense of an "observer" to comment or to categorize what was "happening." In fact, there were no discrete events to "happen"—just a timeless, unitary state of being.

Perhaps the most significant element of CC was the absolute knowingness that it involves. This knowingness is a deep understanding that occurs without words. I was certain that the universe was one whole and that it was benign and loving at its ground....

Eventually, the CC faded. The time changed, light, and mood elevation passed off. When I was able to think again, the sun had set and I estimate that the event must have lasted about twenty minutes. Immediately following return to usual consciousness, I cried uncontrollably for about a half hour. I cried both for joy and for sadness, because I knew that my life would never be the same....

Cosmic consciousness had a major impact on the course of my life. I had received a national prize for my research and had a grant funded for five years, but any interest I had in becoming a famous academician evaporated. My research seemed more like an interesting puzzle than work of immense importance to the world. I left my secure and successful university faculty position and supported myself as a part time free lance clinician. I needed time to explore spirituality and to integrate the CC experience into my life.

Dr. Smith's experience is an especially dramatic and powerful transpersonal event completely illustrating the earlier definition. Those of us who are academics recognize the power of any experience that would make a person give up certain tenure. Most transpersonal experiences are less striking, such as those bringing quiet, meditative spaciousness, but many people's lives change dramatically after one such experience, a primary reason for studying them, for they are often more life-changing than most of life's other phenomena. Understanding these experiences also requires us to be very clear about the methodology of study.

SOME METHODOLOGICAL CONSIDERATIONS FOR A SCIENCE OF CONSCIOUSNESS

To establish transpersonal psychology as a science, we must first review basic scientific method, both to make methodological points and to distinguish genuine science from something too often mistaken for it—scientism. These ideas are covered in more detail in Tart (1972).

In my understanding of science, a primary goal and absolute rule is *factuality*: we must accurately and honestly describe the data to the best of our ability, regardless of our preferences or biases. Then we can go on to create theories to explain and make sense of our data and derive more and more comprehensive and elegant theories—*as long as they continue to be true to data.*

In basic scientific method, we start with some subject that interests us. Whether that subject touches on aspects of the external world or internal experience matters not. We observe the phenomenon as well and fully as we can, humbly aware that we may not be the most accurate or objective of observers, constantly seeking to improve our observational ability. Relentless observation gives us the initial data on which to build a science.

We are seldom satisfied, though, with raw data, and so we construct theories to make sense of the data and relate them to other areas of knowledge. Here we try to be "logical" in our thinking, but philosophically we recognize that the world has many "logics," many systems of thinking according to rules based on assumptions (and our state of consciousness—see later discussion). No one logic has ultimate validity, but we specify the system of logic we are using (such as arithmetic or a version of non-Euclidean geometry) and try to think in accordance with the rules and assumptions—with this technique we are being "logical." A good theory accounts for all the data we have collected.

The third stage distinguishes science from much ordinary thinking. It starts with our recognizing that *all* logics are semiarbitrary and that something that makes perfect sense to us may fail to fit subsequent data: we must continue to work the inherent logic of our theory and make predictions about new situations, then test those predictions against new observations. If the predictions are confirmed, good: continue developing the theory. But if they are not confirmed, it does not matter how "logical," "elegant," or otherwise wonderful our theory is: it must be modified or rejected. Data are *always* primary.

The fourth step in science, pivotal to and interacting with all others, is open and honest communication with colleagues. Any scientist can be a flawed and biased observer, theorizer, and predictor. It is less likely that all one's colleagues will be flawed and biased in exactly the same way, so that as others check one's observations, theoretical logics, and predictions, they can both expand data and theory and check for errors. Thus science becomes a collective activity with mutual enrichment that evolves, a cycling of information in the steps discussed above. We start with rough data and crude ideas, these are constantly checked and refined, and, *in the long run*, more and more data are conceptualized more and more accurately.

SCIENTIFIC METHOD VERSUS SCIENTISM

A primary function of consciousness is to create simulations of reality (Tart 1975) and it is too easy to mistake our simulations of reality for reality itself.

Sociologists long ago (Wellmuth 1944) recognized *scientism*, a widespread and institutionalized form of behavior in which current scientific findings, married to a philosophical commitment to materialism, start to be psychologically treated as if they were final and absolute truth, like a dogmatic religion.

Interacting with contemporary cultural prejudices, scientism renders some subjects of inquiry acceptable and others forbidden. An example relevant as we study consciousness is parapsychology. In spite of methodological standards routinely much higher than those applied in most accepted areas of science (see, e.g., this volume, Chapters 59 and 61), it is almost impossible to get research funding or to·publish results in mainstream journals. Thus as science slides over into scientism, some kinds of observations are readily accepted because they fit the consensus on that which is likely, but others are a priori rejected. Theories that result from biased observations are themselves biased. Indeed, only specific kinds of logic are allowed and others, such as those from meditative disciplines, are rejected a priori rather than examined for potential usefulness. Methodologies that apparently test the consequences of various theories are also subject to scientistic bias, meaning that we have approved and disapproved ways of proceeding.

In reviewing basic scientific method above, one strong point is communication, peer review, and collaboration, with the result mentioned earlier that *"in the long run,* more and more data are conceptualized more and more accurately." When scientism distorts the basic scientific method, however, the communication aspect becomes a tool for social approval and control. Let us continue with our parapsychology example, considering the late Charles Honorton (personal communication 1975). For a decade he followed the fate of manuscripts on parapsychology that were submitted to *Science*. Among other problems with ignorant and biased refereeing, he found that *empirical* papers reporting ESP data were rejected, the referees saying that no *theoretical* foundation allowed ESP to occur. Authors of *theoretical* papers who attempted to establish such foundations were rejected on the grounds that the referees had seen no *empirical* data creating the need for any theories. Similarly, in consciousness research, some theorists ignore transpersonal experiences, as if "rational" problem solving were the only function of consciousness.

If you will reflect on your reactions to my mentioning parapsychology in these paragraphs, consider if we have an immediate example of a tendency to scientism—that is, unthinking rejection of data without comprehensive knowledge about empirical data on the subject. A colleague did advise me not to mention parapsychology in this chapter (even though I have devoted part of my career to empirical research on the subject and can claim expert status). He felt that we have enough prejudices among scholars to overcome in asking them to take an open-minded look at transpersonal psychology without waving the "red flag" of parapsychology. We request your honest observation about your attitude.

I firmly believe that, in the long run, the process of science is self-correcting, but in the short run, the span of our lifetimes, we must be very sensitive to bias and scientism in our attempts to construct a science of consciousness.

FURTHER METHODOLOGICAL CONSIDERATIONS: HISTORY

Hoping to create a scientific understanding of consciousness that is more than a scientistic commitment to reductionism, we must face the fact that most consciousness data are introspective. And yet many feel that such data are inherently inferior and will get us nowhere. After all, did not early psychology at the turn of the century attempt to be a "science of the mind," using introspection, but fail so miserably that behaviorism replaced it? Reviewing why introspective psychology failed in the past will be helpful in avoiding mistakes in our own efforts.

Training Observers

First, following the absolute dictum that science must true to the data, it progresses with accurate observation, but introspective psychology had observers with grossly inadequate training. "Trained observer" often meant an assistant who had spent perhaps a dozen hours being trained to report in a few categories. From all we now know about training in meditation, however, the normal mind is extremely restless and agitated. Judging from conversations I have had with Buddhist meditation teachers, becoming a good observer of one's own mental processes probably requires something like 5000 hours of meditation training, not a dozen. I can report that it took me years of concentrative and practice in insight meditation before I could start to see more accurately what I was experiencing moment by moment, as opposed to my *ideas* about what I was experiencing.

Simulation and Pseudo-Validation

Second, my own thinking (see, e.g., Tart 1975, 1993) and that of others now makes it clear that the mind automatically and continuously creates an internal *simulation* of the world that is usually experienced as if it were a direct perception of external reality. Although minimal fidelity to external physical reality is usually required simply for survival, we have much latitude in how many other aspects of existence are simulated (such as, who is "attractive"). Thus the simulation that usually we automatically take for reality, our continuing experience of world, self, and others, is often highly biased and distorted. Introspective psychology was little aware of this distortion, instead naively believing that these (untrained) observers were getting directly at fundamental data about Mind. The more likely truth is that beliefs were being pseudo-validated by pseudo-data.

Biased Experimenters

Third, no one saw that *bias among experimenters* (see, e.g., Silverman 1977) was a major factor, a factor I believe is well established in psychological research, but still too often ignored by psychologists (Rosenthal 1994).

Experimenters can subtly convey to subjects the results they expect, and subjects, usually eager to please and to make the scientific research succeed, semiconsciously or unconsciously alter their mind's world simulation to experience things and behave in the "scientifically correct" way. I believe this factor was especially prominent in early introspective psychology, when research assistants' jobs depended on being "good observers" as determined by the Herr Doktor Professor in charge of the laboratory. The literature on experimenter bias is extensive.

Individual Differences

Finally, a belief was prevalent that psychology could quickly discover the fundamental Laws of the Mind, just as chemists and physicists were discovering fundamental laws of the material world. Just give a research assistant a preparation of "standard mind," a few hours of training, and observe the fundamental data. In retrospect, we now know the ordinary state of consciousness in "normal" people can differ enormously in one culture, and even more between cultures. The lack of agreement among observers seeming to imply that as a method introspection had no scientific value reflected a lot of unrecognized but real differences among individuals, not necessarily the method's failure.

A primary task for a comprehensive science of consciousness will be adequately describing the phenomena of experience. Lest we stumble in the same way as the early introspectionists did, we must be sensitive to (1) the need for really extensive training, and we must find out what that training should be like; (2) the difference between that which happens "naturally" (if such events ever happen) in experience and the events that we mainly create; (3) biased experimenters; and (4) individual differences, to be recognized and studied rather than suppressed.

ALTERED STATES AND STATE-SPECIFIC SCIENCES

As both transpersonal psychology and the study of altered states of consciousness (ASCs) make clear, consciousness can function in radically different ways and it is incorrect to dismiss variations as neural malfunctions. We need to experientially investigate for ourselves Allan Smith's transpersonal knowledge that "the universe was one whole and that it was benign and loving at its ground ... " and then ask how we can further test the truth in this experience rather than just dismiss it.

Space does not permit me to develop this idea, but I argue elsewhere (Tart 1972) that basic scientific method, discussed above, can be applied in various ASCs, with the altered perceptions, logics, predictions, and interpersonal cross-checks and validations used as tools for a wider spectrum of knowledge, leading to *state-specific sciences*—that is, sciences in which the investigator is capable of functioning well in an ASC as part of his or her working methodology. This proposal was premature in 1972, although it has been applied in some lucid-dreaming studies, but it will grow more and more important as we ask basic questions about consciousness.

CONCLUSIONS

Consciousness includes many varieties of experience that require methodologies specifically appropriate to consciousness. These include such transpersonal experiences as CC, which may more deeply influence a person's life in five minutes than will a lifetime of ordinary experiences. In Chapter 58, Walsh discusses in more detail the developing field of transpersonal psychology. We must study this whole spectrum, being sensitive to issues like adequate training for observers, bias in experimenters and individual differences to develop our field.

REFERENCES

Bucke, M. 1961. *Cosmic Consciousness: A Study of the Evolutions of the Human Mind*. New Hyde Park, NY: University Books.

Rosenthal, R. 1994. On being one's own case study: Experimenter effects in behavioral research—30 years later. In W. Shadish and S. Fuller, eds.), *The Social Psychology of Science*. New York: Guilford Press pp. 214–229.

Silverman, I. 1977. *The Human Subject in the Psychological Laboratory*. New York: Pergamon Press.

Smith, A., and C. Tart. In press. A spontaneous cosmic consciousness experience. *Journal of Consciousness Studies*.

Tart, C. 1972. States of consciousness and state-specific sciences. *Science* 176:1203–1210.

Tart, C. 1975. *States of Consciousness*. New York: Doubleday.

Tart, C. 1993. Mind embodied: Computer-generated virtual reality as a new, dualistic-interactive model for transpersonal psychology. In K. Rao, ed., *Cultivating Consciousness: Enhancing Human Potential, Wellness and Healing*. Westport, CT: Praeger, pp. 123–137.

Wellmuth, J. 1944. *The Nature and Origin of Scientism*. Milwaukee: Marquette University Press.

58 States and Stages of Consciousness: Current Research and Understandings

Roger Walsh

If the two Tucson conferences on consciousness have made one thing clear it is that we have no clear agreement on a definition for consciousness.

Even though people may not know what consciousness is, they have gone to enormous efforts throughout recorded history to try to change it. Physiological methods such as fasting, sleep deprivation, exposure to heat or cold; environmental approaches such as solitude and retreats in nature; sensory stimulation by music and dance; pharmacological means such as psychedelics; disciplines such as yoga, meditation, or contemplation; all have been used for thousands of years to alter consciousness.

The prevalence and importance of altered states of consciousness (ASCs) may be gathered from Bourguignon's (1973, p. 11) finding that 90 percent of cultures have institutionalized forms of them. She concludes that this is "a striking finding and suggests that we are, indeed, dealing with a matter of major importance, not merely a bit of anthropological esoterica."

And yet in the West, systematic study of ASCs began just recently, undertaken primarily by transpersonal psychologists. Our understanding of ASCs therefore has developed mostly in parallel with the transpersonal movement.

This movement began in the late 1960s when a small group of people met in the San Francisco Bay area seeking to expand the scope of Western psychology and culture, which seemed to be overlooking some of the most meaningful and important aspects in human existence. Born in the laboratory and clinic, Western psychology and psychiatry had been dominated by behaviorism and psychoanalysis. These disciplines had contributed a great deal, but by focusing on simple, measurable behavior and on pathology they had also overlooked a great deal, including psychological health and exceptional well being. Worse still, they had reduced or pathologized crucial parts of human experience such as alternative states of consciousness to neurotic processes or neuropathology.

Abraham Maslow was a leader in giving birth to the transpersonal movement. Maslow (1968) was increasingly interested in psychological health as opposed to pathology and concluded that, "to oversimplify the matter, it is as if Freud supplied to us the sick half of psychology and we must now fill it out with the healthy half".

One characteristic in Maslow's exceptionally healthy subjects—"self-actualizers," he called them—was to prove crucial for the transpersonal movement's birth. These subjects tended to have peak experiences: spontaneous, ecstatic, unitive states of consciousness akin to the mystical experiences widely reported and highly valued in many centuries and cultures. Here was an indication that psychological health and potential might include possibilities undreamed of by mainstream psychology. Transpersonal psychology arose to explore these possibilities. The name *transpersonal* was chosen to reflect a characteristic common to many of these possibilities: the sense of self or identity could extend beyond (trans-) the personality or individual person, beyond the entity Alan Watts called the skin-encapsulated ego, to encompass larger aspects of humankind, life, and cosmos.

Initially it was thought that peak experiences were inevitably spontaneous, brief, and almost overwhelming. Subjects regarded these experiences as the high points of their lives but also doubted if they could stand them for more than brief periods (Maslow 1971).

It was therefore a shock when the pioneers turned eastward. For they found that Asian psychologies, philosophies, religions, and contemplative disciplines have been systematically studying consciousness and its states for centuries and have detailed accounts, not just about peak experiences, but whole families of peak experiences. Moreover, they seemed to have disciplines—such as yoga and meditation—capable not only of inducing peak experiences but of sustaining them. In other words, they claimed that peak experiences could be transformed into plateau experiences and altered states of consciousness could be stabilized as altered traits of consciousness. Knowing the long history and remarkable richness of the Asian traditions' study of consciousness, it seems essential that future conferences on consciousness ensure that those perspectives be represented.

THE MANY STATES OF CONSCIOUSNESS

Multiple States

As research continued, more and more alternate states of consciousness were recognized and many appeared beneficial. This abundance contrasted starkly with the conventional Western view, which had long considered altered states to be relatively few and primarily pathological, such as delirium and intoxication. Indeed, our culture has long resisted even recognizing the existence, let alone the value, of alternate states.

A most dramatic example of this resistance was the reaction to hypnosis and the British physician James Esdaile. While stationed in India more than a century ago, Esdaile discovered the remarkable capacity of hypnosis to reduce pain and mortality in surgical patients. So startling were Esdaile's findings that medical journals refused to publish his reports. On his return to Britain, Esdaile therefore, arranged a demonstration before the British

College of Physicians and Surgeons, where he amputated a gangrenous leg while the hypnotized patient lay smiling calmly. His colleagues' conclusion? Esdaile had paid a hardened rogue to pretend he felt no pain. Charles Tart (1986, p. 80) comments, "They must have had very hard rogues in those days."

The cause and result of this resistance is that our modern Western world view is the culture that anthropologists call *monophasic*, as opposed to *polyphasic* (Laughlin, McManus, and Aquile 1992, Laughlin, McManus, and Shearer 1993). That is, we value and derive our world view almost exclusively from one state: the usual waking state. By contrast, polyphasic cultures value and derive their world views from multiple states such as waking, dreaming, and various contemplative states. One goal for the transpersonal movement therefore has been to try to open psychology and other disciplines to polyphasic perspectives.

Let us summarize the story thus far. Some of the transpersonal pioneers' earliest discoveries centered on the value and variety of alternate states of consciousness. Specifically they discovered whole families of potential transpersonal states, that these states have been recognized and valued for centuries by many cultures, but by contrast that all have generally been denied or pathologized in the West (Walsh 1993).

THE TASK OF DIFFERENTIATING STATES

Once this richness and plasticity of consciousness were recognized, the obvious question was: How can these alternate states, and the disciplines that produce them, be categorized and compared? One response was to put them all together and say of diverse states and disciplines that they are just equivalent roads up the same mountain. General systems thereby would call this an argument for equifinality, the claim that diverse states and paths will invariably culminate in the same state.

This interpretation was very neat but unfortunately very naive. Indeed it became ever more apparent that the truth is far more complex. Significant differences distinguish the states produced by different disciplines, but also we have ways of categorizing and clustering these states. Phenomenological mapping and deep structural analyses would provide the necessary methods.

In the past, most who made comparisons attempted only to say whether specific states were identical or different. Phenomenological mapping, though, is a method for mapping and comparing states of consciousness on multiple experiential dimensions and it therefore allows more precise and multidimensional comparisons. For example, it has been claimed that shamanic, yogic, and Buddhist practices result in identical states of consciousness: "shamans, yogis and Buddhists, alike are accessing the same state of consciousness" (Doore 1988, p. 223) and that the shaman "experiences existential unity— the samadhi of the Hindus or what Western mystics and spiritualists call enlightenment and illumination, *unio mystica*" (Kalweit 1988, p. 236).

Table 58.1 Transpersonal States: Distinctions and Similarities (from Walsh 1993)

Dimension	Shamanism	Buddhist (Vipassana) Insight Meditation	Patanjaji's yoga
Control	↑ Partial	↑ Partial	↑↑ Extreme control in some samadhis
Awareness of environment	↑ Decreased	↑ Increased	↓↓ Greatly reduced
Concentration	↑ Increased, fluid	↑ Increased, fluid	↑↑ Increased, fixed
Arousal	↑ Increased	↓ Usually decreased	↓↓ Greatly decreased
Affect	+ or −	+ or − (positive tends to increase)	Ineffable bliss
Identity	Separate self-sense, may be a nonphysical "soul"	Self-sense is deconstructed into a changing flux: "no self"	Unchanging transcendent self, or *purusha*
Out-of-body experience	Yes, controlled ecstasy ("ecstasis")	No	No, loss of body awareness ("enstasis")
Experience	Organized, coherent imagery determined by shamanic cosmology and purpose of journey	Deconstruction of complex experiences into constituent stimuli and flux	Single-object ("samadhi with support") or pure consciousness ("samadhi without support")

In fact, however, we find major differences when we map states from these disciplines on multiple experiential dimensions. When we compare such vital aspects as control, awareness of the environment, concentration, arousal, emotion, self-sense, and content of experience, many differences among shamanic, yogic, and Buddhist states become apparent (see Table 58.1).

The point in phenomenological mapping is that it allows us to map, compare, and differentiate states of consciousness on not one, but many experiential dimensions, with greater precision than has heretofore been possible. The result is that we can better appreciate the richness and variety of transpersonal states and also clearly differentiate them from pathological states such as schizophrenia, with which they have sometimes been confused (Walsh 1990, 1993; Walsh and Vaughan 1993a).

COMMON DEEP STRUCTURES

Once we discover these many states, several questions come up. Can we make sense of this multiplicity of states? Can we identify commonalities and cluster states in some coherent manner? Are they related in some developmental sequence? And can we find a framework to provide coherent understanding of their roles and relationships? In recent years the answer to all these questions has been yes, thanks mainly to Ken Wilber, who has used the principles of developmental structuralism to identify similarities among states and to cluster them accordingly (Walsh 1993, 1996; Walsh and Vaughan 1994; Wilber 1995, 1996, 1997; Wilber, Engler, and Brown 1986).

A major concept in Wilber's work is the "deep structure," which was introduced first in linguistics but is perhaps easiest to clarify by analogy with the human face. Underlying the billions of unique human faces are a few deep structures, such as ears, eyes, nose, mouth, and hair. These few structures allow for vast numbers of different faces (surface structures) and allow us to distinguish one from another.

Wilber's contribution is in applying this kind of deep structural analysis to states of consciousness. He suggests that underlying the vast array of states of consciousness are relatively few deep structures. For example, the shaman seeing power animals, the Buddhist contemplative envisioning Buddha images, and the Hindu practitioner merging with her Ishta deva clearly are all having different experiences. And yet at a deep structural level they are all seeing archetypal religious figures: figures that symbolize and "embody" specific desired qualities such as wisdom, compassion, or power.

Likewise, the Buddhist in nirvana and the Vedantist in nirvikalpa samadha are both experiencing states in which no objects or images arise into awareness. The deep structure of their experiences is therefore similar or identical. It is also clearly distinct, though, from the deep structure of an archetypal religious figure and from nondual experiences.

This kind of deep structural analysis makes clear that it may be possible to cluster contemplative experiences and states and identify a finite number of underlying deep structures. This analysis in turn may allow a map of contemplative experiences and states, which Wilber in fact provides.

Although applying deep structural analyses to transpersonal experiences is a remarkable innovation, Wilber goes further, combining it with developmental analyses, thus yielding a powerful developmental structuralism. Wilber (1995, 1996) suggests that transpersonal deep structures and their corresponding states of consciousness may take form in a specific developmental sequence in several major stages. Among these stages are (1) recognizing increasingly subtle realms of mind, (2) going beyond all objects and appearances to pure consciousness, and (3) recognizing all objects and phenomena as creations or projections of consciousness. Wilber calls these stages subtle, causal, and nondual.

Subtle

When contemplative practices work their effects, when the usual raucous mental activity is stilled, when the mind quiets and becomes more sensitive, then, say various traditions, an inner world of subtle mental phenomena comes to awareness. These mental phenomena may be formless, as in the light and sound of shabd and nad yoga or the emotions of love and joy in the Buddhist *brahma viharas*. On the other hand, the mental phenomena in these subtle stages may take specific forms such as the archetypal images described above or also random forms.

Causal

After subtle states have deepened and stabilized, causal states devoid of objects, images, or phenomena may arise. This is the unmanifest realm called, for example, pure consciousness, Mind, spirit, or geist. This causal condition is described as the abyss of Gnosticism, the Atman of Vedanta, the nirvana of Buddhism, and the Tao of Taoism.

The Nondual

In the nondual condition, objects and images reappear but are immediately and spontaneously perceived as projections, or modifications of consciousness (Wilber 1995, 1996). Now it seems that consciousness manifests itself as the universe. This state is described as Zen's One Mind, Aurobindo's Supermind, Hinduism's Brahman-Atman or *sat-chit-ananda* (being-consciousness-bliss).

Contemplatives who reach this stage experience consciousness in a radically new way. For them, consciousness seems to have awakened and seems to see itself in all things; to recognize itself in and as all worlds, realms, and beings of the universe; unbound by space, time, and limits of any kind because it creates space, time, and limits. This, so it is said, is the final realization or awakening variously known as enlightenment, liberation, wu, moksha, or fana, which these traditions regard as one of the highest goals in human existence (Walsh 1993; Wilber 1995, 1997)

Here I describe phenomenological accounts and I do not try to argue for one ontology. I do, however, argue for open-mindedness about ontologies.

For example, the nondual experience obviously suggests a radical philosophical idealism: a world view that sees consciousness as primary and matter as derivative. Most participants in the Tucson conferences have been wedded to philosophical materialism, the belief that matter is primary. Remember that this world view has never been proved by science or philosophy; rather it is a presupposition. Indeed, neither science nor philosophy has ever been able to prove the existence of an outside world, a problem that Immanuel Kant referred to as "the scandal of philosophy."

From the contemplative's viewpoint, philosophical materialism is the world view that follows naturally in the absence of ASCs. Contemplatives suggest that the deeper one's meditation, the richer the array of ASCs experienced; the further one has explored the mind contemplatively, the more likely one is to recognize the remarkable creative capacity of consciousness and to move toward a philosophical idealism.

For those who object that consciousness could not possibly create an apparently external, objective, material, independent world, not to mention bodies, please remember that we do it every night. We call it dreaming.

LABORATORY SUPPORT

Enlightenment sounds like a nice idea, but do we have supporting evidenced for it, or is it merely a pleasant fantasy? In recent years both supportive analogies and laboratory findings have become available.

From laboratory studies of meditators comes evidence of heightened awareness in both waking and sleeping states. Tachistoscopic studies of advanced meditators who had reached at least the first in the four classic Buddhist stages of enlightenment revealed enhanced perceptual processing speed and sensitivity (Brown, Forte, and Dysart 1984a, b).

Rorschach tests showed a particularly interesting pattern. They suggested that these enlightened subjects were not necessarily free of normal psychological conflicts about dependency, sexuality, and aggression. Strikingly, however, they showed little defensiveness and reactivity to these issues (Brown and Engler 1986; Murphy and Donovan 1997).

Enhanced awareness may also occur during sleep. In the transcendental-meditation tradition the first stage in enlightenment is named cosmic consciousness and is defined by unbroken continuity of awareness—which Ken Wilber calls subject permanence—during waking and sleeping states. Recent EEG studies of advanced TM practitioners who claimed to have reached this state were supportive (Mason et al. 1997).

The awareness that one is dreaming during dreams, known as lucid dreaming, may offer an excellent analogy or metaphor for enlightenment. Lucid dreaming has been advocated for hundreds of years by yogic, sufi, and Tibetan Buddhist traditions. Western psychologists dismissed the state as impossible, however, until the 1970s, when it was demonstrated in the laboratory (LaBerge 1985, Gackenbach and Bosveld 1989, Walsh and Vaughan 1992, 1993a).

During lucidity, subjects "awaken" in their dream. At that moment they are startled to recognize that the world that formerly seemed unquestionably external, objective, material, and independent is in fact an internal, subjective, immaterial, and dependent mental creation and that they are the creators, not the victims of the dream. They can then, if they choose, begin various meditative practices within the dream (LaBerge 1997; Surya Das 1997).

Just how far this discipline can be taken is indicated by advanced practitioners such as Aurobindo (1993) and Tibetan dream yogis. In Tibetan dream yoga, practitioners are first taught to become lucid in their dreams and then to use dreams as part of their meditative practice. Lucidity is then cultivated in nondream sleep so that the yogis seek to remain continuously aware 24 hours a day. Meanwhile, during daylight hours, they cultivate the awareness that their waking experience is also a dream (Dalai Lama 1983, LaBerge 1985, 1993). The ideal result is unbroken awareness around the clock and the sense that all experience is a creation of mind (La Berge 1997)

OUR USUAL STATE OF CONSCIOUSNESS

Clearly, then, the human condition offers possibilities far beyond those usually recognized. It follows that the condition we have called "normality" is not the peak of human development but rather may represent an arbitrary, culturally determined form of developmental arrest. Maslow (1968, p. 16) summarized the situation well by saying "Certainly it seems more and more clear that what we call 'normal' in psychology is really a psychopathology of the average, so undramatic and so widely spread that we don't even notice it ordinarily."

Indeed, the world's contemplative traditions widely agree that our usual state of consciousness is not only suboptimal but significantly distorted and dreamlike. In the East the dreamlike characteristics of our usual state have been called maya or illusion, and in the West they have been called a consensus trance (Charles Tart), a verbal trance (Fritz Perls), hypnosis (Willis Harman), or a collective psychosis (Roger Walsh).

Usually the dream goes unrecognized for several reasons. We all share in it, we have been hypnotized since infancy, and we live in the biggest cult of all: cult-ure.

Let us summarize the contemplative traditions' primary claim. A state of consciousness is available to us that is related to our ordinary waking state as lucid dreaming is to ordinary dreaming.

We can therefore very easily summarize the great contemplative traditions' message. It is "Wake up!" Wake up from your suboptimal entranced state of consciousness; wake up to your postconventional developmental possibilities; wake up to your transpersonal nature.

SUMMARY

What then has been achieved in our understanding of states and stage of consciousness?

We started by recognizing that there is more to human beings and the human possibility than had been recognized, and that this more includes multiple states of consciousness.

From thinking that there was only one type of peak experience we have come to recognize whole families of such experiences and have devised ways of mapping and comparing them.

We have recognized that ours is a monophasic culture, which may constrict and distort our world view.

We have identified common structures underlying experiences that apparently differ widely and thereby have been able to cluster transpersonal experiences and states into classes.

We have mapped development beyond the limit that was formerly thought the ceiling of human possibility and have found preliminary evidence of common transpersonal, transconventional developmental sequences in many traditions.

We have discovered common elements and processes in many of the world's authentic contemplative disciplines and recognized that these disciplines form an art and technology for catalyzing postconventional development. Moreover, we have gathered laboratory evidence that these disciplines are efficacious and now have several hundred studies just on meditation.

We have also begun to understand the achievement that for centuries has been considered the summum bonum—enlightenment or liberation—and have found laboratory support for some classical claims.

Most of these discoveries have been made during the last thirty years. Who can guess what the next thirty will bring? But they may bring most if we combine the best of Eastern and Western perspectives and combine the best of science with the best of contemplative inquiry.

ACKNOWLEDGMENTS

The author thanks the Tucson conference committee, Bonnie L'Allier for secretarial assistance, and the *Journal of Transpersonal Psychology* for permission to use portions of a previous article as a basis for this chapter.

REFERENCES

Aurobindo. 1993. Continuous consciousness. In R. Walsh and F. Vaughan, eds. *Paths Beyond Ego: The Transpersonal Vision*. Los Angeles: J. Tarcher, pp. 83–84.

Bourguignon, E., ed. 1973. *Religion, Altered States of Consciousness, and Social Change*. Columbus: Ohio State University.

Brown, D., and J. Engler. 1986. The stages of mindfulness meditation: A validation study. In K. Wilber, J. Engler and D. Brown, eds. *Transformation of Consciousness: Conventional and Contemplative Perspectives on Development*. Boston: New Science Library/Shambhala, pp. 191–218.

Brown, D., M. Forte, and M. Dysart. 1984a. Differences in visual sensitivity among mindfulness meditators and non-meditators. *Perceptual and Motor Skills* 58:727–733.

Brown, D., M. Forte, and M. Dysart. 1984b. Visual sensitivity and mindfulness meditation. *Perceptual and Motor Skills* 58:775–784.

Dalai Lama. 1983. Talk given at the International Transpersonal Association. Davos, Switzerland.

Doore, G. ed. 1988. *Shaman's Path*. Boston: Shambhala.

Gackenbach, J., and J. Bosveld. 1989. *Control Your Dreams*. New York: Harper Collins.

Gackenbach, J., and J. Bosveld. 1993. Beyond lucidity: Moving towards pure consciousness. In R. Walsh and F. Vaughan, eds., *Paths Beyond Ego: The Transpersonal Vision*. Los Angeles: J. Tarcher, pp. 81–83.

Kalweit, H. 1988. *Dreamtime and Inner Space*. Boston: Shambhala.

LaBerge, S. 1985. *Lucid Dreaming*. Los Angeles: J. Tarcher.

LaBerge, S. 1993. From lucidity to enlightenment: Tibetan dream yoga. In R. Walsh and F. Vaughan, eds., *Paths Beyond Ego: The Transpersonal Vision*. Los Angeles: J. Tarcher.

LaBerge, S. 1997. *Report to the Fetzer Institute on Dream Yoga*.

Laughlin, C., J. McManus, and E. D'Aquile. 1992. *Brain, Symbol and Experience*. New York: Columbia University Press.

Laughlin, C., J. McManus, and J. Shearer. 1993. Transpersonal anthropology. In R. Walsh and F. Vaughan, eds., *Paths Beyond Ego: The Transpersonal Vision*. Los Angeles: J. Tarcher.

Maslow, A. H. 1968. *Toward a Psychology of Being*, 2nd ed. Princeton: Van Nostrand.

Maslow, A. 1971. *The Farther Reaches of Human Nature*. New York: Viking.

Mason, L., C. Alexander, F. Travis, G. Marsh, D. Arme-Johnson, G. Sackenbach, D. Mason, M. Rainforth and K. Walton. 1997. Electrophysiological correlates of higher states of consciousness during sleep in long term practitioners of the Transcendental Meditation program. *Sleep* 20:102–110. Murphy, M., and S. Donovan. 1997. *The Physical and Psychological Effects of Meditation*, 2nd ed. Sansalito, IONS.

Surya Das. 1997. *Awakening the Buddha Within*. New York: Riverhead.

Tart, C. 1986. *Waking up: Overcoming the Obstacles to Human Potential*. Boston: New Science Library/Shambhala.

Walsh, R. 1990. *The Spirit of Shamanism*. Los Angeles: J. Tarcher.

Walsh, R. 1993. The transpersonal movement. *Journal of Transpersonal Psychology* 25:123–140.

Walsh, R. 1996. Developmental and evolutionary synthesis in the recent writings of Ken Wilber. *ReVision* 18(4): 9–18.

Walsh, R., and F. Vaughan. 1992. Lucid dreaming. *Journal of Transpersonal Psychology* 24:193–200.

Walsh, R., and F. Vaughan. 1993a. *Paths Beyond Ego: The Transpersonal Vision*. Los Angeles: J. Tarcher.

Walsh, R., and F. Vaughan. 1993b. The art of transcendence. *Journal of Transpersonal Psychology* 25:1–9.

Walsh, R., and F. Vaughan. 1994. The worldview of Ken Wilber. *Journal of Humanistic Psychology* 34(2):6–21.

Wilber, K. 1993. The spectrum of transpersonal development. In R. Walsh and F. Vaughan, eds., *Paths Beyond Ego: The Transpersonal Vision*. Los Angeles: J. Tarcher, pp. 116–117.

Wilber, K. 1995. *Sex, Ecology, Spirituality*. Boston: Shambhala.

Wilber, K. 1996. *A Brief History of Everything*. Boston: Shambhala.

Wilber, K. 1977. *In the Eye of Spirit*. Boston: Shambhala.

Wilber, K., J. Engler, and D. Brown, eds. 1986. *Transformations of Consciousness: Conventional and Contemplative Perspectives on Development*. Boston: New Science Library/Shambhala.

XIV Parapsychology

OVERVIEW

The shadow side in consciousness studies has to do with claims of "anomalous" effects that do not seem to fit into a mechanistic, classical picture of reality. These effects include claims and descriptions of such unexpected phenomena as extrasensory perception, mental telepathy, precognition, remote viewing, and psychokinesis, which are collectively labeled "parapsychology" or simply "psi."

Although most scientists ignore these phenomena or deride them as little more than primitive belief in magic, many reasonable people find parapsychology's claims credible, a point that was emphasized from the floor in the closing critique at the Tucson I Conference in April 1994. For this reason, the Organizing Committee for the Tucson II Conference decided to invite a panel of plenary speakers who were charged to present and debate both sides of this contentious issue.

In the collective mind of conventional science, parapsychology's claims are often lumped with observations recording altered mental states in exotic cultures—shamanic journeys, ecstatic visions, healing by incantation, and so on—but we must make an important distinction. The evidence for such mystical experiences is clear and bold, if subjective, and the question for a science of consciousness is how to explain them in a context that fits a theory of the mind. For parapsychology proponents, on the other hand, the first problem is to present a credible demonstration that the data are not artifactual but real. Considering that the effects observed are often the same order of magnitude as experimental noise, this proof is not a trivial matter.

In Chapter 59, Marilyn Schlitz and Edwin May present the argument for parapsychology. According to public-opinion polls, half or more than half of Americans believe in extrasensory perception (ESP) or claim to have experienced it. Parapsychology has been held to a much higher standard of proof than other scientific subjects, they say, which is reasonable because "exceptional claims require exceptional proof." Third, they relate the discovery of psi effects to that of meteorites: for centuries, scientific academies laughed away the peasants' claims reporting rocks that fell from the sky.

Schlitz and May survey the types of parapsychological studies (ESP; forced-choice ESP; ganzfeld; remote viewing; psychokinesis; mechanical, electrical, and biological targets; and so on), considering the pitfalls that await interpreters and discussing some notable results. One example is the CIA-sponsored review of 20 years of ganzfeld and remote-viewing experiments, which claimed 95 percent confidence in positive results. Schlitz and May also describe statistical meta-analyses of parapsychological studies similar in significance and conclude that psi effects are established. They believe parapsychological data bear important implications for the science of consciousness.

Susan Blackmore, a well-known skeptic about and critic of parapsychology, presents her views in Chapter 60, asking two questions:

1. Are the data supporting paranormal phenomena credible?

2. Assuming that paranormal phenomena are not experimental artifacts, would they help us to understand consciousness?

To address the first question, Blackmore recounts her own efforts as a parapsychologist: she found only negative results. Visiting a successful lab, she claims to have observed both fraud and incompetence, and asserts that data from the accused laboratory comprise a significant portion of those in the meta-analyses reported by Schlitz and May. Although Blackmore concedes that recent results in ganzfeld and remote viewing appear substantial, her answer to the first question is, Probably not. To the second question, she contends that psi effects act at subconscious levels, and so the answer is no.

Recognizing parapsychology's dualist origins, physicist Dick Bierman suggests that accepting its claims may depend on tolerance for paradox, and mentions John Beloff's observation that "if mind can influence intentionally the behavior of an object ... It seems futile to doubt that a mind can interact with its own brain...."

Bierman describes "retropsychokinesis" studies. In ordinary psychokinesis (PK) experiments, subjects attempt to alter a random-number generator's output from some distance away. In *retro*-PK, a *previously recorded* generator's output is the target. Bierman claims positive results with probability of random chance 1 in 10,000, and discusses the implications of these observations for consciousness studies. How could effect precede cause? Whither time reversal and nonlocality? He concludes that classical mechanisms fail, and that psi effects are acausal connections like the Einstein-Podolsky-Rosen (EPR) nonlocal correlations in quantum physics. From this perspective, Bierman looks forward to a unifying framework for both quantum physics and consciousness.

How is the interested and intelligent layperson to untangle this web of claims and counterclaims?

Proponents of parapsychology must first recognize that their data remain less than totally convincing to unbiased practitioners of experimental science. If a person reports (say) a mystical experience, leading to a change in spiritual perspective, a psychic event of some sort undoubtedly has occurred, and the challenge is to explain it. Conventional scientists do seem justified in questioning many claims simply because the data rise so little above experimental noise. Whenever this doubt arises, experimenters in many scientific disciplines—from specious observations of biological resonances (Scott 1992) to a carefully reported failure to confirm Albert Einstein's theory of special relativity (Miller 1925)—have learned that in the laboratory shadows lurk an unholy host of ways in which quite honest people can be led astray.

Assuming on the other hand that some of the psi data are not artifactual, much more effort should be expended in explaining them. Why? Because experiments could·be done, turning on and off some element in the proposed explanation, thereby improving the statistical validity of the observations by many orders of magnitude.

Bierman has moved the discussion in this direction by suggesting an explanation for psi phenomena arising from quantum-theory, but the human being's subtle ways—which are widely observed at the cultural-anthropology level—should not be ignored. Biologist Lewis Thomas (1974) said a generation ago:

It is in our collective behavior that we are most mysterious. We won't be able to construct machines like ourselves until we've understood this, and we're not even close.

REFERENCES

Miller, D. C. 1925 *Proceedings of the National Academy of Sciences. U.S.A.* 11:306–314.

Scott, A. C. 1992. Davydov's soliton. *Physics Reports* 217:1–67.

Thomas, L. 1974. *The Lives of a Cell.* New York: Viking Press.

59 Parapsychology: Fact or Fiction? Replicable Evidence for Unusual Consciousness Effects

Marilyn Schlitz and Edwin May

Parapsychology is the scientific study of psi phenomena, unusual exchanges of information or energy, such as extrasensory perception, or psychokinesis (mind over matter), which are currently not explainable by known biological or physical rules. Psi is just a descriptive label—it does not suggest that such anomalous phenomena are "psychic," or that they can be explained by a specific underlying mechanism (Bem and Honorton 1994).

Are parapsychological topics fact or fiction? According to recent surveys, many Americans believe they are fact. In a recent Gallup poll (Gallup and Newport 1991), nearly half (49%) of the 1236 respondents reported that they believe in extrasensory perception. In a survey of college professors, more than half the 1100 in the sample reported that they believed ESP was either an established fact or a likely possibility (Wagner and Monnet 1979). Likewise, a 1987 survey published by the University of Chicago's National Opinion Research Center canvassed 1473 adults, of whom 67 percent claimed they had experienced ESP (Greeley 1987).

Public beliefs and attitudes are poor arbiters of "objective" science, however, and anecdotes do not carry the same reliability as the scientific method. For more than a century, a few researchers have been applying scientific standards in studying psi phenomena. But how do we evaluate the evidence from laboratory experiments? Do they produce a replicable effect? And what implications does parapsychology have for nascent consciousness studies? These are the questions we aim to address.

ISSUES FOR EVALUATION

Before we can evaluate the evidence for extrasensory perception or psychokinesis, it is prudent to remind ourselves about the criteria that must be satisfied to indicate that the phenomenon we question is or is not real. Belief versus evidence is not a straightforward choice. We have all heard that "exceptional claims require exceptional proof." Of course, claims are exceptional only when they do not fit within a specified frame of reference. We need not look far into our past, however, to see how scientific beliefs about reality have shifted from one view to another. How science discovered meteorites comes to mind. For centuries, peasants reported stones falling from the sky. At the time the French Academy of Science dismissed their reports as incredible, and yet today's science has no difficulty in accommodating meteorites. Contemporary evidence that calls into question the divide between mind and matter raises provocative empirical challenges, just as meteorites once did—or radioactivity, atomic fission and fusion—and the anomalous motion by Mercury's perihelion, which the General Theory of Relativity finally explained.

Parapsychology has always been controversial. Strong views frequently resist change even in the face of data; indeed, many people, scientists included, make up their minds about whether psi is fact or fiction without examining any data at all (Collins and Pinch 1994, Hess 1993). One critic wrote a review: "The level of the debate during the past 130 years has been an embarrassment for anyone who would like to believe that scholars and scientists adhere to standards of rationality and fair play" (Hyman 1985, p. 89). Much of the skeptic versus proponent debate has been useful, leading to stronger research designs and more sophisticated analyses, but at other times it has limited the chances for clear and unbiased evaluation. Cosmologist Carl Sagan (1991) articulated the problem: "It is the responsibility of scientists never to suppress knowledge, no matter how awkward that knowledge is, no matter how it may bother those in power; we are not smart enough to decide which pieces of knowledge are permissible and which are not...."

EVALUATING REPLICATION WITHIN THE PSI DATABASE

Fortunately, we do not have to rely on arbitrary criteria to credibly evaluate the evidence for ESP or PK. Throughout its history, parapsychologists have devised techniques for assessing probabilities so that chance expectation can be determined and criteria can be established for rejecting the null hypothsis. Recently, parapsychologists have been using meta-analysis as a tool for assessing large bodies of data. A meta-analysis is a critical and technical review of a body of published literature (Rosenthal 1991). Going beyond the format generally considered a "review" article, in a meta-analysis we apply statistical inference techniques to the reported data and attempt to draw general conclusions. Here, we emphasize determining the degree of replication among parapsychological experiments of a specific type (Rosenthal 1986).

A good description of the issues pertinent to evaluating statistical replication can be found in Utts (1991), but they include these ideas:

• File-drawer. Often in social and psychological sciences the measure of success is a p-value equal to or less than 0.05. That is, if the null hypothesis is true, we have a 5 percent chance of observing a deviation as large in an independent test. Although the trend is changing, many researchers and technical journals have treated this value as a sharp threshold; a study quoting a *p*-value of 0.55 is not published and another quoting a value of 0.45 is published. The file-drawer represents studies that were conducted but failed to meet the 0.05 threshold and were not published. Obviously, if researchers were publishing only one in twenty studies in the literature, a nonexistent effect would look "real" according to these standards. Any review of evidence must estimate the number of studies in the file-drawer.

• *Statistical power.* *p*-values strongly depend on the number of trials in a study. An experiment may "fail to replicate" not because the phenomenon in question is not real, but because the study had too few trials. Rosenthal (1991) and others have addressed this question by proposing a trial-independent measure of success called *effect size*. Reviewers must be cognizant of such "threshold" problems.

• *A replication issue.* The evidence for a phenomenon's existence cannot rest on one investigator or one laboratory. How other laboratories attempt to replicate an earlier experiment is a general problem for the social sciences. For example, an exact replication is one in which independent investigators duplicate the original protocol as closely as possible. These studies contribute to the overall evidence, but are complicated by the risk that some undetected artifact may be subtly embedded in the protocol that could cause the result to be misinterpreted. A conceptual replication, in which experimenters address the broad goal but include significantly different methodological details, protects against such misinterpretations, lessens the chances for fraud, and guards against inappropriate techniques. In reviewing evidence in the social sciences, conceptual or "heterogeneous" replications carry much more weight than homogeneous, or "exact" replications.

This context established, let us examine the evidence for ESP and PK.

EXTRASENSORY PERCEPTION (ESP)

"Passively" acquiring information without help from the known senses is an operational definition of ESP. Experiments are of two broad types, depending on whether the participant is constrained to respond within known possibilities or is completely free to respond with his or her impressions. Classically, these are called the forced-choice and free-response methodologies.

For each trial, the protocol or plan for gathering data in each methodology is similar.

• A target is chosen randomly from defined possibilities.

• An individual blind to the target chosen is asked to register his or her impressions of the target.

• In a series of trials, a statistically valid technique is applied to determine if the result exceeds chance.

The theme is open to much variation, and the experimenter usually takes significant care to ensure that no information "leaks" from target to participant via recognized senses. A complete protocol covers such details as procedures for randomizing, keeping target and data secure, and number of trials and participants.

Forced-Choice ESP Testing

Although current parapsychologists seldom use the technique, most data collected in the forced-choice methodology use Zener cards as targets. The cards carry five symbols: circle, square, star, wavy lines, and cross. A deck consists of 25 cards, five for each symbol. Experimenters using Zener cards published two reviews describing their results. Data are analyzed by statistically clean methods. Most often, the probability of observing x hits (i.e., correct answers) in n trials when the chance hit probability is 0.2 is done by exact binomial calculation.

Before meta-analytical techniques were available, Honorton (1975) critically reviewed Zener card-guessing experiments that had been conducted between 1934 and 1939. In almost 800,000 individual card trials in which targets had been specified, the effect size was 0.013 ± 0.001, corresponding to an overall combined effect of 12.7 sigma. Honorton, discussing criticisms aimed at this body of evidence, concluded that they had been adequately addressed. He did not, however, include today's formal meta-analytical criteria.

Using modern meta-analytical tools, Honorton and Ferrari (1989) reviewed the precognition card-guessing database (in which the target was randomly generated after the trial data were gathered). They examined 309 studies reported by 62 investigators. Nearly 2 million individual trials were contributed by more than 50,000 subjects, The combined effect size was 0.020 ± 0.002, corresponding to an overall effect of 11.4 sigma, a high level of confidence with which to reject the null hypothesis.

The analysis produced two important results. First, many critics say that the best results are from studies with fewest methodological controls. To check this hypothesis, Honorton and Ferrari devised an eight-point measure of quality. The categories included whether or not researchers employed automated recording of data or proper randomizing techniques. Researchers scored each study with these measures and found no significant correlation between study quality and study score. Thus, lack of quality and controls cannot account for the effect. Second, if researchers gradually improved their experiments, one would expect significant correlation between quality of study and data on which the result was published. They found a correlation of 0.246 with 307 degrees of freedom ($p = 2 \times 10^{-7}$). Finally, applying the criteria described above, Honorton and Ferrari concluded that a statistical anomaly in this database cannot be explained by poor study quality, file-drawer, or fraud. Although the effect sizes in these studies are quite small, the results are statistically robust and stable.

Free-Response ESP Testing

Most free-response experiments are of the ganzfeld and remote-viewing types. They differ from the forced-choice methodology in that their target material can be almost anything: video clips from movies, photographs from national magazines, and geographic locations.

The ganzfeld technique (the German word means "whole field") was designed at the turn of the century by introspective psychologists who sought to induce imagery experiences in experimental volunteers. Their idea was that once somatosensory information is reduced, one's ability to detect the psi-mediated information is enhanced (Bem and Honorton 1994). When behaviorism took hold, introspective psychology was marginalized and the ganzfeld technique fell into disuse. But the psi researchers, attempting to test the model that internal somatic and external sensory information normally mask one's perception of weak psi-mediated signals, rediscovered the technique.

In a typical ganzfeld trial subject, sequestered in a soundproof room, is placed in a mild state of sensory isolation. The condition is induced by providing a uniform visual field by taping translucent Ping-Pong-ball halves over each eye and illuminating them with a soft red light. They create an audio equivalent with white noise. Subjects report that after a few minutes the red glow and static noise appear to vanish from conscious awareness. Honorton implemented the idea to test the hypothesis that incorrect ESP perception arises because of somatosensory noise. The experiment followed naturally from successful dream studies at Maimonides Medical Center in New York (Child 1985).

A complete description of the ganzfeld protocol appears in Honorton et al. (1990). At the time of the evaluation the subject is blind to the correct target picture. After the impressions are complete, the subject is presented a defined target pack including the intended target and three decoys. The four targets are as different from one another as possible. Under the null hypothesis (no ESP), the probability of guessing the correct answer is 0.25. The observed hit rate for nearly 500 trials is from 0.32 to 0.41, with 95 percent confidence, again allowing researchers to reject the null hypothesis.

The remote-viewing protocol differs from the ganzfeld procedure in two ways. First, the viewer (subject) is not placed in an overt altered state but sits, business like, frequently across a table from a monitor, who is also blind to the target choice. The monitor is to facilitate drawing as much information from the viewer as possible. The second change from the ganzfeld protocol is in the analysis. Instead of having the viewer decide which target best matches the impressions, an independent analyst, also blind to the correct target, performs that function.

As part of an invited talk at the 20th Congress of Skeptics, which was organized by the Committee to Scientifically Investigate the Claims of the Paranormal, Professor Utts (1996), a statistician from the University of California at Davis, described the current state of the free-response experiments.

She analyzed both the published ganzfeld studies and, as part of a CIA-sponsored investigation, the government-supported remote-viewing studies. Besides the historical ganzfeld database, she found five additional ganzfeld replications from worldwide laboratories. For remote viewing, she included in her analysis only the data generated at SRI International and at Science Applications International. She estimated the size of the hitting fraction and computed the 95 percent confidence interval for the individual studies as well as for the combined remote-viewing and ganzfeld databases. Of the eight individual analyses, five of the confidence intervals do not overlap the chance hitting rate of 0.25 for the intended target embedded among three decoys. The combined (ganzfeld and remote-viewing) hit rate for 2878 trials was in the range 0.33 ± 0.02 with 95 percent confidence.

PSYCHOKINESIS (PK)

Interacting with the physical world by mental means alone operationally defines psychokinesis. One unintended consequence of such a definition is the difficulty of ensuring that nothing normal happened. It is relatively straightforward to ensure for ESP that no sensory leakage by traditional methods has occurred. With physical effects, however, it is difficult and expensive to gain equal assurance, for results are more problematic as the apparatus grows more sensitive.

Generally, PK phenomena are categorized in four groups. Were the target systems electromechanical or biological, and how large was the effect? Micro-PK effects cannot be seen without sophisticated statistical analysis, as in the roll of a die that is slightly biased, putatively by PK. Macro-PK is detectable by visual inspection, as of an iron rod bent by that means. Because macro-PK on either target system is problematic, we focus on the substantial micro-PK database.

Mechanical or Electrical Targets

Most published studies on micro-PK involve true devices for generating random numbers. In a typical study, a carefully designed binary-bit generator that devises its randomness either from electronic noise or by detecting radioactive particles, produces a binary data stream. Interspersing active with control periods, the subject attempts to modify the output stream solely by mental means.

Radin and Nelson (1989) carefully meta-analyzed the historical database. They assigned a 16-point quality rating to more than 800 studies conducted by 68 investigators from 1959 to 1987. They computed an overall weighted-effect size of approximately $(3.0 \pm 0.5) \times 10^{-4}$. As in the ESP analysis, they found no correlation between quality of study and outcome from study. In their meta-analysis, Radin and Nelson were able to show that the results from highly heterogeneous studies could not be accounted for by poor protocols, inappropriate statistical analyses, the file-drawer effect, or fraud.

Biological Targets

The case for PK on biological targets, or Direct Mental Interactions with Living Systems (DMILS), is developing. These studies have been fewer than those using mechanical targets, but the evidence is compelling and worthy of future research. The best replications arise from a class of experiments using electrodermal potential as the target system. Results in 25 experiments indicate that the average amount of electrodermal activity differs statistically when a remote individual intends to calm or activate the distant person's physiology compared with randomly selected and counterbalanced control periods (Braud and Schlitz 1991, 1989). This work is seen as a possible trigger for a distant-healing response and so is seen as having potential for direct application (Schlitz 1996). A formal meta-analysis of this database is currently under way (Schlitz and Jonas n.d.).

CONCLUSIONS ON THE PSI DATABASES

Now that we have reviewed the evidence for psi phenomena, it is clear from meta-analyses of ESP and PK databases that the statistical results are far beyond those expected by mean chance. Finding high-level scientific consistency from different laboratories and heterogeneous protocols among studies, the results are not likely to result from systematic flaws in methodology. Parapsychologists are therefore able to confidently reject the null hypothesis. The effect sizes are small, but they are comparable to those reported in recent medical studies heralded as breakthroughs (Honorton and Ferrari 1989, Utts 1991). In short, if we take the standards applied to any other scientific discipline, psychic functioning has been thoroughly established (Bem and Honorton 1994, Utts 1995). As in any progressive research program, one must move beyond proof-oriented science. The next question is the work's implications for the science of consciousness?

TOWARD AN EXPANDED SCIENCE OF CONSCIOUSNESS

One of the great questions facing the scientific community as we enter the twenty-first century is whether or not nature can be nonlocal and nontemporal at the macro level, not merely at the quantum level. The data from parapsychology apply to this fundamental question, suggesting a faculty for perceiving and interacting with the physical world that lies beyond the reach of ordinary senses. The data further suggest links between the objective world and the inner world of human experience that currently do not fit accepted views of science.

The scientific world has much faith that explanations for the results claimed by parapsychology will be forthcoming once our current scientific models are modified (Stapp 1994, Stokes 1987). It is equally possible that the data will help us to reflect upon and potentially revise the epistemological and ontological assumptions that guide modern science. In this way, psi research may lead us to a new way of knowing about the world and our place in it.

Following the relativistic views of science recently explicated by works in the history, sociology, and philosophy of science, we recall that science deals with models and metaphors representing aspects of experienced reality (Harman and Schlitz n.d.). Any model or metaphor may be permissible if it helps order knowledge, even if it seems to conflict with another model that is also useful. (The classic example is the history of wave and particle models in physics.) A peculiarity in modern science is that it allows some kinds of metaphors and disallows others. It is perfectly acceptable, for example, to use metaphors directly derived from our experience of the physical world (such as "fundamental particles," or "acoustic waves"), as well as metaphors representing that which can be measured only by its effects (such as gravitational, electromagnetic, or quantum fields). It has further become acceptable in science to use holistic and nonquantifiable metaphors such as *organism, personality, ecological community*, and *universe*. But nonsensory "metaphors of mind"—metaphors that call up images and experiences familiar from our own inner awareness,—are taboo. We are not allowed to say (scientifically) that some aspects of our experience of reality are reminiscent of our experience of our own minds—to observe, for example, that psi phenomena make it appear that there may be some supraindividual nonphysical mind.

Social philosopher Willis Harman (1994) speaks of the need for a new epistemology that employs broader metaphors and recognizes that all scientific concepts of causality are partial. (For example, the "upward causation" of physiomotor action resulting from a brain state does not necessarily invalidate the "downward causation" implied in the subjective feeling of volition.) In other words, a new epistemology would implicitly question the assumption that a nomothetic science characterized by inviolable "scientific laws" can in the end adequately deal with causality. Varvoglis (1996, p. 594), writes "In our search for a scientific basis for consciousness,' the primary, most fundamental issue is whether or not consciousness is, in some nontrivial sense, "real." Can it be "causal"? Parapsychological data suggest that consciousness may be causal, or that ultimately there may be no causality but only a whole system evolving (Wilber 1996). Then psi might be not an anomaly but part of another order of reality.

CONCLUSIONS

We began by asking if parapsychology were fact or fiction. Having reviewed various meta-analyses, we conclude that the data from parapsychology are robust and therefore warrant that we reject the null hypothesis. It may be that psi data will eventually be accommodated by our current scientific models of reality, or that those data will force us to reevaluate the assumptions on which we have built contemporary science. Apollo 14 astronaut Edgar Mitchell said, "There are no unnatural or supernatural phenomena, only very large gaps in our knowledge of what is natural.... We should strive to fill those gaps of ignorance" (1986). This is the challenge, and the opportunity.

ACKNOWLEDGMENT

We thank Professor Utts for allowing us to use some of her presented material.

REFERENCES

Bem, D. J., and C. Honorton. 1994. Does psi exist? Replicable evidence for an anomalous process of information transfer. *Psychological Bulletin* 115(1):4–18.

Braud, W. G., and M. J. Schlitz. 1983. Psychokinetic influence on electrodermal activity. *Journal of Parapsychology* 47:95–119.

Braud, W. G., and M. J. Schlitz. 1989. Possible role of intuitive data sorting in electrodermal biological psychokineses (bio-PK). *Journal of Scientific Exploration* 3(1):43–63.

Braud, W. G., and M. J. Schlitz. 1991. Consciousness interactions with remote biological systems: Anomalous intentionality effects. *Subtle Energies* 2(1):1–46.

Child, I. 1985. Psychology and anomalous observations: The question of ESP in dreams. *American Psychologist* 40(11):1219–1230.

Collins, H. M., and T. Pinch. 1994. *The Golem: What Everyone Should Know about Science*. Cambridge: Cambridge University Press.

Gallup, G. H., and F. Newport. 1991. Belief in paranormal phenomena in adult Americans. *Skeptical Inquirer* 15:137–146.

Greeley, A. 1987. Mysticism goes mainstream. *American Health* 7:47–49.

Harman, W. 1994. A re-examination of the metaphysical foundations of modern science: Why is it necessary? In W. Harman and J. Clark, eds., *New Metaphysical Foundations of Modern Science*. Sausalito: Institute of Noetic Sciences, pp. 1–15.

Hess, D. J. 1993. *Science in the New Age: The Paranormal, Its Defenders, and Debunkers, and American Culture*. University of Wisconsin Press.

Honorton, C. 1975. Error some place. *Journal of Communication* 103–116.

Honorton, C., R. E. Berger, M. P. Varvoglis, M. Quant, P. Derr, E. L. Schechter, and D. C. Ferrari. 1990. Psi communication in the ganzfeld: Experiments with an automated testing system and a comparison with a meta-analysis of earlier studies. *Journal of Parapsychology* 54:99–139.

Honorton, C., and D. C. Ferrari. 1989. Future telling: A meta-analysis of forced-choice precognition experiments, 1935–1987. *Journal of Parapsychology* 53:281–308.

Hyman, R. 1985. A critical overview of parapsychology. In P. Kurtz, ed., *A Skeptic's Handbook of Parapsychology*. Buffalo, NY: Prometheus Books, pp. 1–96.

Mitchell, E. 1986. *Noetic Sciences Review*. Winter.

Radin, D. I., and R. Nelson. 1989. Evidence for consciousness-related anomalies in random physical systems. *Foundations of Physics* 19(12):1499–1514.

Rosenthal, R. 1986. Meta-analytic procedures and the nature of replication: The ganzfeld debate. *Journal of Parapsychology* 50:315–336.

Rosenthal, R. 1991. *Meta-Analytic Procedures for Social Research*. London: Sage Publications.

Sagan, C. 1991. UCLA Commencement Speech. June 14.

Schlitz, M. 1996. Intentionality and intuition and their clinical implications: A challenge for science and medicine. *Advances* 12(2):58–66.

Schlitz, M., and W. Harman. 1998. The implications of alternative and complementary medicine for science and the scientific process. In W. Jonas and J. Levin, eds., *Complementary and Alternative Medicine*. Baltimore: Williams Wilkins.

Schlitz, M., and W. Jonas. n.d., A systematic review of the database on direct mental and spiritual interactions between living systems. Work in progress.

Stapp, H. P. 1994. Theoretical model of a purported empirical violation of the predictions of quantum theory. *American Physical Society* 50(1):18–22.

Stokes. D. M. 1987. Theoretical parapsychology. In S. Krippner, ed. *Advances in Parapsychology Research* 5. Jefferson, NC: McFarland Press, pp. 77–189.

Utts, J. 1991. Replication and meta-analysis in parapsychology. *Statistical Science* 6(4):363–403.

Utts, J. 1995. An evaluation of remote viewing: Research and applications. In M. D. Mumford, A. M. Rose, and D. A. Goslin, eds., *The American Institutes for Research Report*. September 29.

Utts, J. 1996. Statistical evidence for psychic functioning. 20th Congress of Skeptics.

Varvoglis, M. 1996. Nonlocality on a human scale: Psi and consciousness research. In S. R. Hameroff, A. Kaszniak, and A. Scoff, eds., *Toward a Science of Consciousness: The First Tucson Discussions and Debates*. Cambridge: MIT Press, pp. 589–596.

Wagner, M. W., and M. Monnet. 1979. Attitudes of college professors toward extrasensory perception. *Zetetic Scholar* 5:7–17.

Wilber, K. 1996. *A Brief History of Everything*. Boston: Shambhala.

60 Why Psi Tells Us Nothing About Consciousness

Susan Blackmore

I wish to ask two questions about the relationship between consciousness and psi.

1. Are there any paranormal phenomena?
2. If there are, do they help us to understand consciousness?

For the first I would like to be able to provide a fair and unbiased assessment of the evidence for psi, however briefly. This is simply impossible. Many people have tried and failed. In some of the best debates in parapsychology proponents and critics have ended up simply agreeing to differ, for the evidence can be read either way (e.g., Hyman and Honorton 1986). The only truly scientific position seems to be to remain on the fence, and yet to do science in practice demands you have to decide which avenues are worth pursuing. I do not think psi is.

My reasons are not an objective evaluation of the evidence but more than twenty years of working in and observing the field of parapsychology. During that time various experimental paradigms have been claimed as providing a repeatable demonstration of psi, and several have been shown to be false. For example, it took more than thirty years to show that Soal had cheated in his famous experiments with the special subject Basil Shackleton (Markwick 1978). The promising animal precognition experiments were blighted by the discovery of fraud (Rhine 1974) and the early remote-viewing experiments were found to be susceptible to subtle cues that could have produced the positive results (Marks and Kammann 1980).

The most successful paradigm during that time, and the one I shall concentrate on, has undoubtedly been the ganzfeld. Subjects in a ganzfeld experiment lie comfortably, listening to white noise or seashore sounds through headphones, and wear half ping-pong balls over their eyes, seeing nothing but a uniform white or pink field (the ganzfeld). Meanwhile a sender in a distant room views a picture or video clip. After half an hour or so the subject is shown four such pictures or videos and is asked to choose which was the target. It is claimed that they can do this far better than would be expected by chance.

The first ganzfeld experiment was published in 1974 (Honorton and Harper 1974). Other researchers tried to replicate the findings and there followed many years of argument and of improving techniques followed, including the "Great Ganzfeld Debate" between Honorton (1985), one of the originators of the method, and Hyman (1985), a well-known critic. By this time several other researchers claimed positive results, often with quite large effect sizes. Both Hyman and Honorton carried out meta-analyses combining the results of all the available experiments, but they came to opposite conclusions. While Hyman argued that the results could all be ascribed to methodological errors and multiple analyses, Honorton claimed that the effect size did not depend on the number of flaws in the experiments and that the results were consistent, did not depend on any one experimenter, and revealed certain regular features of extrasensory perception (ESP).

The ganzfeld reached scientific respectability in 1994 when Bem and Honorton published a report in the prestigious *Psychological Bulletin*. They reviewed Honorton's earlier meta-analysis, and reported impressive new results with a fully automated ganzfeld procedure claiming finally to have demonstrated a repeatable experiment. So had they?

My own conclusion is biased by my personal experience. I tried my first ganzfeld experiment in 1978, when the procedure was new. Failing to get results myself, I went to visit the laboratory in Cambridge where some of the best results were being obtained. When I found there on my confidence in the whole field and in published claims of success.

These experiments, which looked so beautifully designed in print, were in fact open to fraud or error in several ways, and indeed I detected several errors and failures to follow the protocol while I was there. I concluded that the published papers gave an unfair impression of the experiments and that the results could not be relied upon as evidence for psi.

Eventually the experimenters and I all published our different views of the affair (Blackmore 1987, Harley and Matthews 1987, Sargent 1987), and the main experimenter left the field altogether. I turned to other experiments.

I would not be bringing up this depressing incident again but for one fact. The Cambridge data are all there in the Bem and Honorton single laboratory, review. Indeed, out of 28 studies included, nine came from the Cambridge lab, more than any other single laboratory, and they had the second highest effect size after Honorton's own studies. Bem and Honorton point out that one of the laboratories contributed nine of the studies, but they do not say which one. Not a word of doubt is expressed, no references are given, and no casual reader could guess there was such controversy over a third of the studies in the database.

Of course the new autoganzfeld results appear even better. Perhaps errors from the past do not matter if there really is a repeatable experiment. The problem is that my personal experience conflicts with the successes I read about in the literature, and I cannot ignore either side. I cannot ignore other people's work because science is a collective enterprise and publication is the main way of sharing our findings. On the other hand I cannot ignore my own findings—there would be no point in doing science at all if I did. The only honest reaction is to say, "I don't know."

Since then the CIA has released details of more than twenty years of research into remote viewing (Hyman 1995, Utts 1995), and the spotlight has left the ganzfeld. Perhaps the ganzfeld will go down in history as evidence for psi, but I am left with my personal doubts about this, here as about other paranormal claims. I have had many experiences of hearing about a new finding, spending a lot of time and effort investigating it, and ending up disappointed—whether it be an experiment, a haunting, an incredible coincidence, or a new psychic claimant. Of course that is no proof that psi is not there. I might really be a "psi-inhibitory experimenter" and so be unable to observe the psi that is there. Or I might just have been looking in the wrong places.

This is why I cannot give a definitive and unbiased answer to my question, "Are there any paranormal phenomena?" I can give only a personal and biased answer—that is, probably not.

But what if I am wrong and psi really does exist? What would this tell us about consciousness?

The popular view seems to be something like this—if ESP exists, it proves that mental phenomena are nonlocal, or independent of space and time, and that information can get "directly into consciousness" without all that nasty messing about with sensory transduction and perceptual processing. If PK (psychokinesis) exists, it proves that mind can reach beyond the brain to affect things at a distance—that consciousness has a power of its own.

I suspect that it is a desire for this "power of consciousness" that fuels much enthusiasm for the paranormal. Parapsychologists have often been accused of wanting to prove the existence of the soul, and yet convincingly denied it (Alcock 1987). I will instead accuse them of wanting to prove the power of consciousness. In Dennett's terms you might say they are looking for skyhooks rather than cranes. They want to find that consciousness can do things all by itself, without depending on that complicated and highly evolved brain.

I have two reasons, for doubting that they will succeed. First, parapsychologists have yet to demonstrate that psi has anything to do with consciousness, and second, there are theoretical reasons why I believe the attempt is doomed. But note that by consciousness I am referring to the really interesting aspects of consciousness—that is, subjectivity, or "what it is like?" to be something.

First, to make their case that psi effects actually involve consciousness, experiments rather different from those commonly done will be needed. Let us consider the ganzfeld. Do the results show that consciousness, in the sense of subjectivity or subjective experience, is involved in any way?

I would say no. There are several ways in which consciousness might, arguably, be involved in the ganzfeld, but there appears to be no direct evidence that it is. For example, even in a very successful experiment the hits are mixed with many misses and the subjects themselves cannot say which is which (if they could, the successful trials could be separated out even better results obtained.). In other words, the subject is unaware of the ESP even when it is occurring.

The ganzfeld does involve a kind of mild altered state of consciousness. Indeed, Honorton first used the technique as a way of deliberately inducing a "psi-conducive state." However, it has never been shown that this is a necessary concomitant of ESP in the ganzfeld. Experiments to do this might, for example, compare the scores of subjects who reported entering a deep altered state with those who did not. Or they might vary the ganzfeld conditions to be more or less effective at inducing altered states and compare the results. These kinds of experiments have not been done. Without appropriate control conditions we have no idea what it is about the ganzfeld that is the source of its success. It might be consciousness, it might be the time spent in the session, the experimenter's personality, the color of the light shining on the subject's eyes, or any of a huge number of untested variables. There is simply no evidence that consciousness is involved in any way.

Another example is recent experiments on remote staring (Braud and Schlitz 1989). It has long been claimed that people can tell when someone else is looking at them, even from behind their head. Ingenious experiments now test this claim with video cameras and isolated subjects. Results suggest that the staring and nonstaring periods can be distinguished by physiological responses in the person being stared at. In other words, they are able to detect the staring—but not consciously. These experiments may be evidence that something paranormal is going on, but whatever it is it appears to be unconscious rather than conscious.

In psychokinesis (PK) experiments, the claim that consciousness is involved is made explicitly. For example, a well-known paper is entitled, "The effects of consciousness on physical systems" (Radin and Nelson 1989). And yet as far as I can see, there is no justification for this title.

In these experiments a subject typically sits in front of a computer screen and tries to influence the output of some kind of random-number generator (RNG), whose output is reflected in the display. Alternatively, they might listen to randomly generated tones, with the intention of making more of the tones high, or low, as requested, or they might try to affect the fall of randomly scattered balls or other systems. The direction of aim is usually randomized and appropriate control trials are often run. It is claimed that, in extremely large numbers of trials, subjects are able to influence the output of the RNG. Is this influence an effect of consciousness on a physical system?

I don't see why. The experiments demonstrate a correlation between the output of the RNG and the direction of aim specified to the subject by the experimenter. This is certainly mysterious, but the leap from this correlation to a causal explanation involving "the effect of consciousness" is so far unjustified. The controls done show that the subject is necessary, but in no way do they identify what it is about the subject's presence that creates the effect. It might be their unconscious intentions or expectations; it might be some change in behavior elicited by the instructions, it might be some hitherto unknown energy given off when subjects are asked to aim high or aim low. It might be some mysterious resonance between the RNG and the subject's pineal gland. It might be almost anything.

As far as I know, no appropriate tests have been made to find out just what it is. For example, does the subject need to be conscious of the direction of aim at the time? Comments in the published papers suggest that some subjects actually do better when not thinking about the task, or when reading a magazine or being distracted in some other way, suggesting that conscious intent might even be counterproductive.

Perhaps this is not what is meant by consciousness here, but if not, then what is intended? Perhaps it is enough for the person to be conscious at all, or perhaps they have to be in an appropriate state of consciousness. In any case, to identify the effect is actually due to consciousness, relevant experiments will have to be done. They might compare conditions in which subjects did or did not consciously know the target direction. In some trials subjects might be asked to think consciously about the target and in others they might be distracted, or they might be put into different states of consciousness (or even unconsciousness) to see whether this affected the outcome. Such experiments might begin to substantiate the claim that consciousness is involved. Until then, the findings remain an unexplained anomaly.

Some parapsychologists have suggested to me that when they talk about consciousness affecting something they mean to include unconscious mental processes as well. Their claim would then be equivalent to saying that something (anything) about the person's mind or brain affects it. However, if the term "consciousness" is broadened so far beyond the subjective, then we leave behind the really interesting questions it raises and, indeed, the whole reason so many psychologists and philosophers are interested in consciousness at all. If we stick to subjectivity, then I see no reason at all why paranormal claims, whether true or false, necessarily help us understand consciousness.

The second reason I doubt that the paranormal power of consciousness will ever be proven is more theoretical. As our understanding of conscious experience progresses, the desire to find the "power of consciousness" sets parapsychology ever more against the rest of science (which may, of course, be part of its appeal). The more we look into the workings of the brain, the less it looks like a machine run by a conscious self and the more it seems capable of getting on without one. There is no place inside the brain where consciousness resides, where mental images are "viewed," or where instructions are "issued" (Dennett 1991). There is just massive parallel throughput and no center.

Then there are Libet's experiments, suggesting that conscious experience takes some time to build up and is much too slow to be responsible for making things happen. In sensory experiments he showed that about half a second of continuous activity in sensory cortex was required for conscious sensation, and in experiments on deliberate spontaneous action he showed that about the same delay occurred between onset of the readiness potential in motor cortex and timed decision to act (Libet 1985)—a long time in neuronal terms. Though these experiments are controversial (see the commentaries on Libet 1985 and Dennett 1991) they add to the growing impression that actions and decisions are made rapidly and only later does the brain weave a story about a self who is in charge and is conscious. In other words, consciousness comes after the action; it does not cause it.

This is just what some meditators and spiritual practitioners have been saying for millennia: our ordinary view of ourselves as conscious, active agents experiencing a real world, is wrong—an illusion. Now science seems to be coming to the same conclusion.

Parapsychology, meanwhile, is going quite the other wat. It is trying to prove that consciousness really does have power; that our minds really can reach out and "do" things, not only within our own bodies but beyond them as well. Odd, then, that so many people think of parapsychology as more "spiritual" than conventional science. I think it could be quite the other way around.

With the welcome upsurge of interest in consciousness, and the many scientists and philosophers now interested in the field, I look forward to great progress being made out of our present confusion. I hope it will be possible to bring together the spiritual insights and the scientific ones, so that research can reveal the kind of illusion we live in, how it comes about, and perhaps even help us to see our way out of it. As far as this hope is concerned parapsychology seems to be going backward, hanging on to the idea of consciousness as an agent. This is the second reason why I doubt that evidence for psi, even if it is valid, will help us understand consciousness.

I will therefore answer my two original questions with "probably not," and definitely "no."

REFERENCES

Alcock, J. E. 1987. Parapsychology: Science of the anomalous or search for the soul? *Behavioral and Brain Sciences* 10:553–643 (plus commentaries by other authors).

Bem, D. J., and C. Honorton, 1994. Does psi exist? Replicable evidence for an anomalous process of information transfer. *Psychological Bulletin* 115:4–18.

Blackmore, S. J. 1987. A report of a visit to Carl Sargent's laboratory. *Journal of the Society for Psychical Research* 54:186–19.

Braud, W., and M. Schlitz. 1989. A methodology for the objective study of transpersonal imagery. *Journal of Scientific Exploration* 3:43–63.

Dennett, D. 1991. *Consciousness Explained*. Boston: Little, Brown.

Harley, T., and G. Matthews, 1987. Cheating, psi, and the appliance of science: A reply to Blackmore. *Journal of the Society for Psychical Research* 54:199–207.

Honorton, C. 1985. Meta-analysis of psi ganzfeld research: A response to Hyman. *Journal of Parapsychology* 49:51–86.

Honorton, C., and S. Harper. 1974. Psi-mediated imagery and ideation in an experimental procedure for regulating perceptual input. *Journal of the American Society for Psychical Research* 68:156–168.

Hyman, R. 1985. The ganzfeld psi experiment: A critical appraisal. *Journal of Parapsychology* 49:3–49.

Hyman, R. 1995. Evaluation of the program on anomalous mental phenomena. *Journal of Parapsychology* 59:321–351.

Hyman, R., and C. Honorton, 1986. A joint communiqué: The psi ganzfeld controversy. *Journal of Parapsychology* 50:351–364.

Libet, B. 1985. Unconscious cerebral initiative and the role of conscious will in voluntary action. *Behavioral and Brain Sciences* 8:529–539; Commentaries 8:539–566 and 10:318–321.

Marks, D., and R. Kamman. 1980. *The Psychology of the Psychic*. New York: Prometheus Books.

Markwick, B. 1978. The Soal-Goldney experiments with Basil Shackleton: New evidence of data manipulation. *Proceedings of the Society for Psychical Research* 56:250–277.

Radin, D. I., and R. D. Nelson, 1989. Evidence for consciousness related anomalies in random physical systems. *Foundations of Physics* 19:1499–1514.

Rhine, J. B. 1974. Comments: A new case of experimenter unreliability. *Journal of Parapsychology* 38:215–225.

Sargent, C. 1987. Sceptical fairytales from Bristol. *Journal of the Society for Psychical Research* 54:208–218.

Utts, J. 1995. An assessment of the evidence for psychic functioning. *Journal of Parapsychology* 59:289–320.

61 Do Psi Phenomena Suggest Radical Dualism?

Dick Bierman

Near the end of the nineteenth century, the founding fathers of psychical research were driven by the idea that reality transcends the material world and were convinced that the successful Western scientific method could be used to prove this belief (Beloff 1977). Furthermore, the founder of empirical parapsychology, Dr. J. B. Rhine, who started to explore psychic phenomena in the laboratory in the 1930s, was a dualist and considered that these apparent phenomena supported his world view.

More recently, the physicist Wigner suggested that to solve the measurement problem in quantum physics, one had to give a special status to the measuring entity (Wigner 1967). This interpretation would imply that consciousness should be different from matter. This essentially dualistic notion was taken as a starting point for a whole family of theories dealing with psi phenomena that are labeled observational theories. And finally, the psychologist and philosopher John Beloff wrote in the very first issue of the *Journal of Consciousness Studies* (Beloff 1994) a defense for his radical dualist position, and I quote from that article:

... Results [of meta-analyses on parapsychological experiments] show ... the over-all significance of [psi] phenomena is astronomical.... The relevance of parapsychology to the problem at issue [i.e., dualism vs. epiphenomenalism] should now become apparent ... if it is the case that mind can influence intentionally the behavior of an object other than its own brain it would be futile to doubt that a mind can interact with its own brain....

It becomes clear that throughout the history of research on psi phenomena the status of human consciousness has been crucial. Although many present-day researchers are attracted to this field out of curiosity rather than some dualistic world view, many from the outside and some from the inside still consider parapsychology a quest to prove the transcendence of mind over the material world.

Assuming that the phenomena reported are not due to deception or to some hitherto undetected methodological flaw—in other words that these phenomena are "real" anomalies—the question that we have to ask ourselves is: Does that really support the idea that consciousness is in part or completely different from matter and can never be reduced to it? And

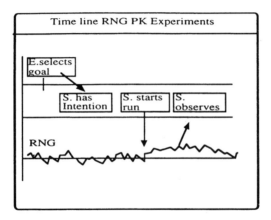

Figure 61.1 Time-line RNG (random-number generator) PK (psychokinesis) experiments.

implicitly: Can those (immaterial) mental states be a cause of change in material systems?

EMPIRICAL DATA

At first sight the meta-analytical findings to which Beloff refers, such as those reported by Radin and Nelson (1989), seem to confirm this idea: Intentional states of the subject in the experiments are manipulated by the experimenter according to some random decision, and subsequently, more often than can be expected by chance, a material state will be observed that corresponds to the subject's mental intention (see Figure 61.1).

It seems straightforward to claim that the induced mental state (possibly through its corresponding physical brain state) "caused" a bias in the observed material states corresponding to the subject's intention. In principle the results still allow for an explanation where in the brain states "influence" the random physical system through some physical field. It is generally assumed (though not well tested), however, that the distance between the subject and the "affected" material system does not matter and that therefore physical fields may be ruled out as an explanatory vehicle for the effects observed. Hence the idea that consciousness has properties that transcend space and time.

Even if one is willing to accept that these parapsychological data reflect some underlying reality, however, the interpretation as given by Beloff is premature because of his selective use of parapsychological data.

In the early 1970s, E. H. Walker proposed the first observational theory (Walker 1975), which essentially extended the original idea put forward by Wigner that consciousness was involved in the "collapse" of the state vector. Assuming that consciousness was instrumental in bringing about the singular state that we observe, then, according to Walker, it would follow that consciousness should be considered the "hidden variable" that other theoretical physicists had postulated to get rid of this measurement problem. It had

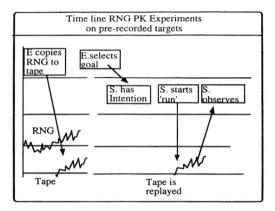

Figure 61.2 Time line RNG PK experiments on prerecorded targets.

been shown, however, that such a "hidden" variable should have nonlocal properties. Walker argued that the Lorentz-invariance constraint demanded nonlocality in time, too. Combining Walker's argument with the evidence that a conscious observation could "result" in biasing a random physical system, one could postulate that it should not matter if such observations were to be postponed. This very idea was tested by an arrangement that differs from the original psychokinesis test arrangements in that the random physical systems' behavior is stored *before* an intention corresponding to a wished-for outcome is formulated. At a later time the hitherto unobserved data are fed back to the subject (Figure 61. 2).

These types of experiments have been done and indeed resulted in significant correlations between behavior of the RNG and an observers' intention *at a later time!*

These results, if real, should also be taken into account if one wants to discuss how relevant parapsychological data are for a dualistic perspective.

To assess the reality of the results, a review of all published experiments with prerecorded targets was performed. In all, 26 experiments were located in the literature (Table 61-1).

We counted nine main experimenters from seven institutions. They used several target systems with different a priori probabilities, precluding statistical analysis at the level of individual trials or samples. At the level of the experiments, however, it turned out that 18 of the 26 experiments gave results that corresponded to the intentions of the participants. The combined z-score (Stouffer-z) was 5. 3. The probability therefore that these data are due to chance is smaller than 1 in 10,000. Given the limited number of studies, these odds are certainly as impressive as those reported by Radin and Nelson (1989).

If psychokinesis on prerecorded targets is a real phenomenon, then the empirical evidence's apparent support for psychokinesis for an interactionist dualist's position becomes rather confusing. To maintain the position that mental states have causal effects on matter, one would have to accept that

Table 61.1 Review of all published PK experiments with prerecorded targets.

Authors	Year	Journal	Z-score
Bierman et al.	1975	EJP, 1–1	0.89
Schmidt	1976	JA5PR, 70	3.14
Schmidt	1976	JA5PR, 70	4.22
Schmidt	1976	JA5PR, 70	2.90
Millar et al.	1976	RIP 1976	0.00
Houtkooper	1977	EJP, 1–4	1.15
Houtkooper	1977	EJP, 1–4	−0.28
Broughton et al.	1977	RIP 1977	0.00
Terry et al.	1977	RIP 1977	−3.07
Terry et al.	1977	RIP 1977	−1.60
Braud et al.	1979	JSPR	−0.10
Gruber	1980	EJP, 3–2	1.90
Gruber	1980	EJP, 3–2	3.08
Houtkooper	1980	EJP, 3–3	3.23
Houtkooper	1980	EJP, 3–3	0.37
Houtkooper	1980	EJP, 3–3	−2.45
Schmidt	1985	JOP, 49	1.82
Schmidt	1985	JOP, 49	1.96
Bierman	1985	EJP, 5	−1.90
Bierman	1985	EJP, 5	1.54
Schmidt et al.	1986	JOP, 50	2.71
Schmidt et al.	1988	RIP 1988	1.66
Schmidt et al.	1990	RIP 1991	0.62
Schmidt et al.	1992	JOP, 57	1.88
Michels	1993	Skepsis, 6	1.64
Schmidt and Stapp	1993	JOP, 57	1.23
		Total	5.31

effects may precede causes. The most cautious way to describe the data in all psychokinesis studies is by avoiding causal reasoning and merely stating that, within some system constraints, anomalous correlations are found between mental states and the behavior of random physical systems.

CONCLUSION

If psi phenomena as referred to by Beloff are real (Bem and Honorton 1994, Radin and Nelson 1989), then we may need to reconsider whether they support his dualistic perspective on the relation between mind and matter because of the new data presented in this chapter because the latter data most prominently reflect the metacausal character of psi phenomena. This connection complicates considerably the naive picture of mental states driving material states, as proposed in the dualist perspective. Of course these new data do not fit in any mechanistic framework whatsoever. In fact, both the dualistic and the materialistic perspectives are based on traditional cause-and-effect sequences, which do not apply to the phenomenon of psychokinesis on prerecorded targets.

The centrality of "time reversal" or "time independency" in all theoretical approaches to psi phenomena (e. g., Stokes 1987) seems not coincidental but rather supports the idea that parapsychological data do require understanding that transcends traditional materialistic and some dualistic perspectives, both of which assume that effects follow from causes and are mediated by some classical signal or force.

It may be preferable to interpret the parapsychological data as correlations without a cause, much like the (EPR) nonlocal correlations in physics. The latter correlations allow for no explanation such as signals traveling from one part of the system to another.

Von Lucadou (1994) explicitly proposes that: *psi correlations are an emergent property of macroscopic complex self-referential systems which are phenomenologically equivalent to non-local correlations in Quantum Physics.* Such a view, in which quantum physics and a theory of mind may arise from an underlying unified theoretical framework, would support nonreductionistic identity theories rather than dualistic theories on the relation between mind and matter.

REFERENCES

Beloff, J. 1994. Minds and machines: A radical dualist perspective. *Journal of Consciousness Studies* 1:32–37.

Beloff, J. 1977. Historical overview. In Benjamin B. Wolman, ed., *Handbook of Parapsychology*. New York: Van Nostrand Reinhold, pp. 3–25.

Bem, D. J., and C. Honorton. 1994. Does psi exist? Replicable evidence for an anomalous process of information transfer. *Psychological Bulletin* 115:4–19.

Radin, D. I., and R. D. Nelson. 1989. Evidence for consciousness related anomalies in random physical systems. *Foundations of Physics* 19:1499–1514.

Stokes, D. M. 1987. Theoretical parapsychology. In S. Krippner, ed., *Advances in Parapsychological Research* vol. 5. Jefferson, NC: McFarland, pp. 77–189.

von Lucadou, W. 1994. The endo-exo-perspective: Heaven and hell of parapsychology. In D. J. Bierman, ed., *Proceedings of the 37th Parapsychology Convention*, University of Amsterdam, August. (Similar ideas can be found in next entry.)

von Lucadou, W. 1994. Wigner's friend revitalised? In H. Atmanspacher and G. Dalenoort, eds., *Inside versus Outside*. New York: Springer-Verlag, pp. 369–388.

Walker, E. H. 1975. Foundations of paraphysical and parapsychological phenomena. In L. Oteri, ed., *Quantum Physics and Parapsychology*. New York: Parapsychology Foundation, pp. 1–53.

Wigner, E. 1967. *Symmetries and Reflections*. London: Indiana University Press, pp. 172–179.

XV Aesthetics and Creative Experience

OVERVIEW

Perhaps the most characteristic and effective expression of human consciousness is the creative act, in which something formerly unimagined comes to be realized. If consciousness is shrouded in mystery, then the poet—who seems to make something arise from nothing—shows us the fleeting magic toward which this mystery can lead.

In the first chapter in this final section, Lis Nielsen presents a model to guide creative problem solving that unites Bernard Baars's global-workspace theory with an appraisal theory of emotion, providing a framework for interplays among cognition, emotion, and motivation. From this perspective, a creative act is motivated by the need to resolve an emotionally significant mismatch (or discord) between internal assumptions and externally available information. Aaron King and Alwyn Scott augment Nielsen's model in the penultimate chapter with an arithmetic discussion of creative dynamics, demonstrating that the mathematical dimension of the conceptual space from which William Shakespeare carved his plays is: (1) much greater than the dynamic dimension of his brain's synapses, and (2) larger than will ever be explored.

The book's final chapter, by Paul Johnston, illustrates the myriad discordances in human existence by examining one Shakespearean play—Troilus and Cressida—in which the principal characters are sorely beset by incompatible aspects of their respective realities. Poetry's biological function, Johnston suggests, is to deal with life not by turning a blind eye to its inevitable discord but by exercising the transcendent powers of a song.

62 Modeling Creativity: Taking the Evidence Seriously

Lis Nielsen

In reflecting on the creative process, the Danish poet Søren Ulrik Thomsen writes: "Although there is a part in every artist that desires nothing more than to be free to create all the time, what one encounters in practice is something quite different. Just as truly as the completion of a work of art requires—in fact, *demands*—the death of those experiences that brought it into being, so too does artistic practice demand everything from the creator. Perhaps this can explain that violent resistance against the mysterious un-pleasantness of writing, which every writer knows is just as tightly bound up in the artistic process as is the ecstasy of successful creation. The process swings unceasingly between work and procrastination, playing itself out as an eternal struggle between a desire to create and a terror of the process" (Thomsen 1994, author's trans.).

Subjective reports such as Thomsen's account of the motivational and emotional demands made by the creative enterprise tell us much about the intricate interplay between subjective feelings and creative cognition. Poet and scientist alike attest to feeling deep insecurity, uncertainty, and anxiety, combined with a sense of having relinquished or lost control when faced with a creative problem as a task. They also attest to intuitive and sometimes elusive feelings of knowing or warmth—of being pulled or guided in clear directions on the path to the solution; and to feeling joy, ecstasy, and right-ness when at last a solution is achieved (May 1980, Thomsen 1994, 1995, Csikszentmihalyi 1990). Such evidence is supported by careful studies on problem solving and the intimate connections between the systems support-ing cognitive and emotional activity in the brain (Holyoak 1995, Scardamalia and Bereiter 1991, Holzkamp-Osterkamp 1991, Damasio 1994, LeDoux 1993).

In this chapter I propose a general information-processing model of cre-ative problem solving that incorporates emotional aspects, as a preliminary effort to fill a gap left by purely cognitive theories. The model unites Baars's global-workspace theory of conscious experience (Baars 1988), employing both its terminology and symbolism, with an appraisal theory of emotion, a theoretical coupling that makes explicit the intimate connections among cognition, emotion, and motivation in creative problem-solving. My primary claim is that these connections apply in the creative process because they are intrinsic to all conscious processing. This interpretation can thus be seen as extending Baars's arguments explaining how and why information gains access to consciousness.

The model rests on two presuppositions. First, consciousness evolved to help solve problems in surviving and adapting in changing environments. I understand problem solving broadly as including everything from simple decisions about where to look next, to complex tasks that require creative reasoning (see, e.g., Baars 1988, Ch. 6, Damasio 1994, Ch. 8, Cotterill 1995). The second is that creative problem solving can usefully be modeled as the search within and restructuring of a conceptual space (Holyoak 1995, Boden 1990). These points are not argued here.

We can consider creative activity as the cognitive and emotional dialectic between an individual and a conceptual space. This dialectic arises when the individual who is motivationally engaged with that space or aspects of it searches for adaptive and valuable solutions to more or less well-defined problems that arise within the space. Following Boden's suggested criteria, we find that creative solutions are those which transform the structure of the space, expand its boundaries, reveal previously uncharted areas, or change the heuristics, thereby enabling novel solutions to be generated that could not previously have been conceived (Boden 1990).

Here I adopt these (admittedly controversial) working definitions:

Cognition: The construction, comparison, or alteration of mental representations.

Emotion: A psychological process consisting of a phenomenological experience and associated tendency toward action aroused by cognitive appraisal of some information's personal significance.

Motivation: The more or less stable psychological contexts that structure individual behavior and conscious experience according to their personal significance.

THEORETICAL COUPLING

Baars's global-workspace theory and an appraisal theory of emotion lend themselves to a natural coupling. That which the former says in the language of cognition, the latter states in emotional language.

Following Baars's theory, consciousness is modeled as a global workspace, a blackboard on which globally broadcast messages can be displayed *if and only if* they fulfill the remaining criteria for conscious experience. Among others, these criteria require that they be *informative* and *accessible by a self-system*. Conscious content is constrained by a nonrigid hierarchy of *contexts* comprising the individual's complete psychological makeup. These contexts are the innate and acquired information-processing schemata that have been found useful for dealing automatically with various tasks. Contexts in turn are composed of *automatic unconscious processors*. Deeper levels of context represent more stable aspects of the self (Baars 1988). I call this nest of contexts a *motivational hierarchy* because it represents the individual's goals, knowledge, and behavioral potential, from which all experience and activity derive their meaning.

To our adaptive advantage, many complex behaviors can be carried out automatically and unconsciously. But violations of expectations in an active context will be *informative*, interrupt automatic processing, and gain access to consciousness, where planning and decision making can take place (Baars 1988).

The criterion that only informative contents can gain access to conscious awareness implies that conscious content must be both *relevant* to activated contexts in the motivational hierarchy, and *significant* in that it indicates challenges to context stability. Consciousness, at any given time, will include the piece of information that currently is most personally significant, that which poses the greatest *challenge to the stable self-system* (Baars 1988).

From here the link to emotion theory is straightforward. Appraisal theories of emotion consider how a piece of information's personal significance is cognitively appraised, (its valuation as positive or negative for personal goals) to be a necessary condition for emotional arousal (Lazarus 1991, Frijda 1993). Moreover, evidence is strong that unless the relevant context is active, the event's significance will not be appraised, and no emotion will be aroused (Frijda 1993). When they do occur, however, appraisals need not be conscious. Very simple, unconscious appraisals based on innate or overlearned emotional schemata may be enough to direct our attention to a piece of information (Frijda 1993, Damasio 1994). But once aroused, the emotion itself involves feelings and tendencies toward action, as well as continuing appraisals that play themselves out in time.

Using Baars' terminology we can describe the cognitive process of appraisal as the *subjective evaluation* of the recognized mismatch between an individual's motivational contexts and some piece of information. The stronger claim is that because it is informative and accessible to the self-system, *every content of consciousness will be an appraisal of personal significance, a potential elicitor of emotion.* According to the model, the aspects of the creative process that are conscious will necessarily be those which involve appraisals. Though some appraisals may be unconscious, it is nonetheless appraisals of goal-relevance, characteristic of emotions, that give information access to consciousness. Without this emotional component, searches may break down or be aborted. Emotional feedback may provide a crucial motivational element driving the search (Damasio 1994, Holzkamp-Osterkamp 1991).

Thus consciousness is seen as having both a cognitive and an emotional aspect. The cognitive processes are modeled as the construction, comparison, and alteration of conscious representations, resulting from activation, decomposition, and restructuring of contexts at various levels in an individual's motivational hierarchy. The emotional aspect of consciousness will involve subjective feelings and continuing appraisals that are aroused when an activated context decomposes and restructures to accommodate incompatible information. Formerly stable ways of dealing with the environment are challenged by the demands presented by new information. The more significant the information (the deeper the context(s) it challenges and restructures are nested in the motivational hierarchy, the stronger one might expect the emotion to be.

Consciousness can be operationally defined as *the cognitive and emotional awareness of problems relevant to one's motivational contexts*, in which problems are broadly defined as informative challenges to stable context. By their mutual connection to the motivational hierarchy, the cognitive and emotional aspects of conscious experience are intrinsically linked.

THE MODEL

Figure 62.1 depicts my model of creative problem solving. With the model I attempt to accommodate the phenomenological evidence about emotion's function in the creative process. If creative solutions require restructuring of conceptual spaces, and if our ways of conceptualizing these spaces are constrained by the contexts now in our stable self-system, then restructuring of spaces will challenge that system's very stability. Informative content of consciousness poses just such challenges. How we deal with it may turn out to make the difference between routine and creative problem solving.

Figure 62.1A illustrates a problem being recognized. Consciousness of a problem within a conceptual space occurs when the individual's motivation and expectation to (1) move smoothly and freely through the space, (2) have desirable experiences within the space, (3) have a consistent or complete model of the space, or (4) challenge the boundaries of the space, encounter an obstacle.

The problem is recognized as mismatch between the individual's contextually constrained representation of the conceptual space and some internal or external state of affairs. These can be data that do not fit a theory, an incomplete phrase in a composition, or presentation of a task (the creative imperative). Challenges to personal contexts are informative and appraised as personally significant. Emotional appraisals may be unconscious, not yielding full-blown emotional episodes. Instead they may give rise to subtle feelings or "somatic markers" (Damasio 1994). These feelings direct attention, focus consciousness, and enlist processing and search mechanisms, some of which are conscious and others unconscious.

Figure 62.1B depicts the initial processes in searching for a solution. Consciously, the search involves exploring the conceptual space revealing further aspects of the mismatch between context and content that cannot be readily accommodated in the space as conceived, and creating a demand for restructuring. Unconsciously, activated contexts decompose and additional contexts relevant to the problem are activated and gain access to consciousness. As contexts decompose and are activated, they guide cognitive processing, giving rise to appraisals of personal significance that lend an emotional quality to consciousness.

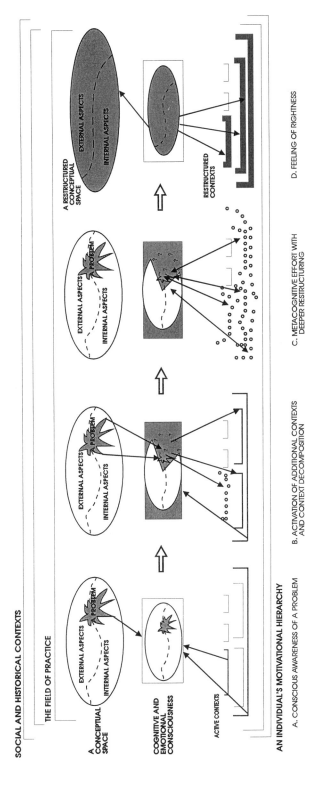

Figure 62.1 A model of creative problem solving within a conceptual space. Consciousness of a problem arising within a conceptual space is jointly constrained by the social and historical contexts in which that space is embedded—including the context for the field of practice in which the problem arises—and by the individual problem solver's psychological contexts. Active contexts in the individual's motivational hierarchy are in bold. Unconscious automatic processors into which activated contexts decompose are shown by circles. Consciousness is modeled as a blackboard on which global cognitive and emotional messages are broadcast because of their relevance to the motivational hierarchy. The conceptual space is modeled as encompassing both internal representations and thinking styles and external phenomena, objects, and contexts in the creative environment. The creative process is modeled as a dialectic between the individual and the space, rather than as a mere restructuring of representations in the individual's mind.

Figure 62.1C illustrates the conscious effort that is often required if adaptive or novel solutions are to be found, and the resulting decomposition of contexts, with accompanying negative feelings such as uncertainty and anxiety. Metacognitive processes may be employed in response to these feelings to direct or focus attention, to enlist effort, or to select strategies, leading to further and deeper restructuring. Restructuring of contexts may yield positive emotional feedback in the form of feelings of knowing or warmth that suggest one is on the right track.

A typical report by writers and artists is that they experience both attraction to and avoidance of the creative task. The avoidance may derive from recognizing the need to access deeper layers of context to address the problem or awareness that stable aspects of the self must be destroyed if creative solutions are to be found. Because the self consists of a stable contextual hierarchy, violations of deeper contexts, whether imposed from outside or purposefully sought in creative efforts, can cause anxiety. It has been argued that expert writers tolerate more anxiety and purposely frame problems in challenging, difficult ways to arrive at more creative solutions (Scardamalia and Bereiter 1991).

Unconsciously, contexts may be decomposing and restructuring in response to both awareness of the initial problem and persisting conscious effort. Unconscious processing leads to changes in the contextual framework, allowing solutions that could not arise prior to the restructuring to arise later. The phenomenon referred to as "incubation" in the creativity literature is often similarly described.

In general, emotions can be aroused by cognition of both the problem and the solution. They can be aroused by the conscious effort of restructuring the conceptual space, as well as by the unconscious restructuring of contexts. Activating and decomposing contexts at deeper layers in the motivational hierarchy, which involve challenging some more comprehensive and stable aspects of the self, might arouse stronger emotions.

Figure 62.1D represents the way in which discovering a solution leads to a change in the conscious state. Cognitively, it will involve changing the representation of the conceptual space, now encompassing a solution to the problem, and will correspond to restructuring contexts, without which the change in representation is impossible. The emotional character of this state may depend on whether the restructuring is experienced as a sudden achievement (insight) or a gradually worked-out solution. Creative individuals report feeling ecstasy and a product's rightness or goodness-of-fit with the goal aimed at.

Changes in conceptual spaces bring about changes in an individual's motivational and contextual hierarchy, as necessitated by restructurings to accommodate the solution. Restructured contexts then constrain future conscious contents. When contexts restructure, changes are lasting and former ways of representing the space are altered or destroyed. It is speculated that deeper restructurings of context will correspond to more radical reframing of conceptual spaces, yielding more novel solutions. Accordingly, we might expect that more creative solutions will have stronger emotional correlates.

If the solution arrived at by the individual is deemed both novel and useful or valuable within the field of practice or by society at large, it may be incorporated into the field, leading to changes in the external field structure. Transfers at this stage occur at levels of explanation beyond our scope here.

CONCLUSIONS

From the phenomenological evidence, it is clear that emotions and motivations are essential in creative problem solving. They initiate the process and drive it, step by step, to completion—sometimes leading the way, sometimes indicating that the right way has been found. The model provides a framework within which we can make sense of phenomenological reports on this intimate interplay between cognition and emotion in the creative process. The model also illustrates how consciousness binds cognition, emotion, and motivation. It suggests that all conscious experience will have cognitive and emotional aspects, intimately related by their relation to motivational contexts. It makes clear too why the emotional stakes in creativity are so high. Without sufficient motivation and tolerance for change, creative activity may pose challenges to the self-system that are experienced as simply too formidable.

The creative process is fraught with tension between pleasure and pain, fear and absorption, will and aversion. For that very reason, it involves the whole person, not just the cognitive mind. For many, this is one of creative activity's strongest attractions. Thomsen writes, "Only those who are prepared to risk miserable defeat will be given the chance to reach extraordinary heights and produce true works of art" (Thomsen 1994, author's trans.). Without emotional courage and motivational commitment, creative cognitions have little chance of getting off the ground.

REFERENCES

Baars, Bernard J. 1988. *A Cognitive Theory of Consciousness*. Cambridge: Cambridge University Press.

Boden, Margaret A. 1990. *The Creative Mind: Myths and Mechanisms*. London: Weidenfeld and Nicolson.

Cotterill, Rodney. 1995. On the unity of conscious experience. *Journal of Consciousness Studies* 2:290–312.

Csikszentmihalyi, Mihaly. 1990. *Flow: The Psychology of Optimal Experience*. New York: Harper Perennial.

Damasio, Antonio R. 1994. *Descartes' Error*. New York: G. Putnam's Sons.

Frijda, Nico H. 1993. The place of appraisal in emotion. *Cognition and Emotion* 7:357–387.

Holyoak, Keith J. 1995. Problem solving. In E. E. Smith and D. N. Osherson, eds., *Thinking: An Invitation to Cognitive Science*, vol. 3. Cambridge: MIT Press.

Holzkamp-Osterkamp, Ute. 1991. Emotion, cognition, and action potence. In C. W. Tolman and W. Maiers, eds., *Critical Psychology*. New York: Cambridge University Press.

Lazarus, Richard S. 1991. *Emotion and Adaptation*. New York: Oxford University Press.

Le Doux, J. E. 1993. In search of an emotional system in the brain: Leaping from fear to emotion to consciousness. In Gazzaniga, Ed., *The Cognitive Neurosciences*. Cambridge: MIT Press.

May, Rollo. 1980. *The Courage to Create*. New York: Bantam Books.

Scardamalia, M., and C. Bereiter. 1991. Literate expertise. In K. A. Ericsson and J. Smith, eds., *Toward a General Theory of Expertise*. Cambridge: Cambridge University Press.

Thomsen, Søren Ulrik. 1994, 1995. A dance on words: Reflections on the artistic creative process, parts 1 and 2. *Kritik* 110:31–51 and 116:1–21.

63 Dimensions of Creativity

Aaron King and Alwyn C. Scott

In his recent book *The Astonishing Hypothesis*, Francis Crick (1994) boldly asserts the philosophical position called functionalism with the words

"You," your joys and your sorrows, your memories and your ambitions, your sense of identity and free will, are in fact no more than the behavior of a vast assembly of nerve cells and their associated molecules.

Our aim is to show—using a simple counting argument—that this view is unable to describe essential features in creative brain activity. Although the argument we present is mathematical, it does not require abstract notation for precise presentation. Thus the results can be understood—if not accepted—by the general reader.

To follow the discussion, however, three basic concepts must be appreciated. The first is the *phase space*, as the theater for describing a system that changes with time, and the dimension of that space. Second is the *hierarchical organization* of information that is stored in the brain. Finally, one must grasp the notion of a finite number of items that is in fact too large to be listed. Finite numbers of this magnitude have been labeled *immense* by the physicist Walter Elsasser (1969).

Here is the gist of the argument. The number of dimensions of a phase space that is large enough to embrace or realize the dynamics of creative brain activity is immense. From this immensity we draw two conclusions. First, the dynamics of creative brain activity cannot be represented in the phase space of neuronal activity because the phase-space dimension of creative brain activity is much larger than that of the neurons. Second, because the dimension of the phase space of creative brain activity is immense, this activity is inherently unpredictable.

Such a criticism of functionalism is not new. More than a century ago William James (1890) archly described the "automaton-theory" in his *Principles of Psychology*:

If we knew thoroughly the nervous system of Shakespeare, and as thoroughly all his environing conditions, we should be able to show why at a certain period of his life his hand came to trace on certain sheets of paper those crabbed little black marks which we for shortness' sake call the manuscript of *Hamlet*. We should understand the rationale of every erasure and alteration therein, and we should understand all this without in the slightest degree acknowledging the existence of the thoughts in Shakespeare's mind. The words and sentences would be taken, not as signs of anything beyond themselves, but as little outward facts, pure and simple.

Thus James anticipates our quantitative argument, with which we aim to show that any theory modeling only the neurons in Shakespeare's brain—ignoring the thoughts in his mind—is unable to describe the writing of *Hamlet*.

Think of a billiard table with one ball on it. How much information does one need to specify the state of this simple system as the ball moves? Certainly it is necessary to specify the position of the ball upon the table, which requires two quantities, one for the position along the long axis of the table, another for that along the short axis—and one must also record the ball's speed in each of these directions. Thus four quantities are required.

This is an example of the system mathematicians call *dynamical*; its state is specified by four quantities (the positions and velocities) that depend on time. The mathematician sees these quantities as coordinates in a *phase space* of four dimensions. The key concept is that each point in the phase space can be identified with a possible state of the system. The system is "dynamical" because the phase point moves as time goes on.

Suppose now that we put nine more balls on the table. For each ball we need four quantities, making 40 in all. Thus, this new system has a phase space of 40 dimensions. If the balls are put in motion, the way the system changes in time can be described by the motion of a phase point in a 40-dimensional space.

Assuming that the balls do not interact with one another, it is possible to calculate exactly what the behavior of the system will be. Each ball's position and velocity at the next moment will depend only on its position and velocity at the current moment. Thus we can think of the system as 10 independent 4-dimensional subsystems, and the whole is equal to the sum of its parts. Such a system is called *linear*.

But of course the balls do interact with each other whenever they collide. To make the example more interesting, suppose each ball carries a positive or negative electrical charge, so that they attract or repel each other as do the atoms in a molecule. Then it is clear that the position and velocity of a ball in the next instant will depend in a complicated way upon the present positions and velocities of all the balls. Thus we have no way of decomposing the system into independent subsystems; its dynamics are inherently *nonlinear*. Furthermore, it is clear that the nonlinear motion in the full 40-dimensional space of the ten balls cannot be described in the 4-dimensional space of one ball. What would the behavior of such a system be like? It is not difficult to see that complicated behavior would be the rule rather than the exception.

As an example not too far from our ten charged billiard balls, consider one protein molecule, say of myoglobin, as a dynamical system. It is composed of 2318 charged atoms, much like the billiard balls above. Because the motion of these atoms is not restricted to the planar surface of a billiard table, we need six dimensions for each atom, or 13,908 dimensions of the phase space that specifies the possible states of the myoglobin molecule.

Now consider the brain's neurons as a dynamical system. What might be an appropriate phase space for this system? To specify the state of the neurons in the brain, we could indicate the activity level at each synapse (neural interconnection) at each moment in time. If the brain has 10 billion neurons, each making 10,000 synaptic connections with other neurons, this assumption implies rougly 100 trillion variables that specify the state of the brain. Thus the phase space of the dynamics of the brain's neurons has a dimension of about 100 trillion.

In the realm of biology, hierarchical organization is the rule. At the lowest level of life, functional proteins undergo intricate nonlinear vibrations to carry out their roles as enzymes, facilitating biochemical transformations. On the next level, bewilderingly varied biochemical cycles are busily transforming both energy and molecular structures into more useful forms. Higher levels involve intricate combinations of DNA, RNA, and proteins that are able to replicate themselves. At a yet higher level, all these activities combine to form a living organism, which can forage for food, reproduce itself, and evolve into ever more interesting forms.

Turning to the human brain's organization the Canadian psychologist Donald Hebb (1949) made an important contribution, introducing this concept—a *cell assembly* of the brain's neurons—in his classic *Organization of Behavior*:

Any frequently repeated, particular stimulation will lead to the slow development of a "cell-assembly," a diffuse structure comprising cells ... capable of acting briefly as a closed system, delivering facilitation to other such systems and usually having a specific motor facilitation. A series of such events constitutes a "phase sequence"—the thought process. Each assembly may be aroused by a preceding assembly, by a sensory event, or—normally—by both. The central facilitation from one of these activities on the next is the prototype of "attention."

To understand Hebb's cell assembly, consider that it can be portrayed by a social metaphor. We can compare the brain to a city and the individual neurons to its citizens. A citizen might be a member of several assemblies such as a political association, a church, a bowling league, a parent-teacher's group, a hiking club, the Junior League, and so on. Each social assembly's members are interconnected by the lists of addresses and telephone numbers that allow an organization to activate its own members—or even those in a like-minded assembly—should an appropriate occasion arise. Members of the hiking club could become active to encourage the 4-H club to resist development of a theme park near their farms. Or the Junior League might enlist teachers' support to close a pornographic bookstore. Just as an individual could be a member of both the hiking club and the League, a nerve cell participates in many assemblies in the brain.

Aaron King and Alwyn C. Scott: Dimensions of Creativity

Hebb describes how the interconnections in a cell assembly form a sort of "three-dimensional fishnet," which "ignites" when a sufficient (threshold) number of its constituent neurons become active. Because an assembly of neurons shares the individual neuron's essential properties—threshold behavior and all-or-nothing response—one can imagine an assembly of assemblies, which Hebb called a "second order assembly," or an assembly of assemblies of assemblies, called a "third order assembly," and so on up through the brain's organization.

At the highest level in this hierarchy, the activity of each higher-order assembly is associated with its own dimension in an appropriate phase space. The phase point's motion in this space represents the flow of thought, which we experience as our brains go from one concept to the next and then on to the next. How shall we describe the dynamics of this many-layered system?

At the neuron level, we have no theoretical difficulty, although many practical problems lie in dealing with a phase space of 100 trillion dimensions. But what of the higher levels? Clearly, the higher-order assemblies that have actually developed (representing ideas that have been thought) can be considered real objects. But what of assemblies that have not yet developed? These cannot be ignored in any comprehensive study of the brain because any of them might come forth in the next moment. Thus the dimensions of the phase spaces in which are staged the dynamics of the higher-order assemblies must be large enough to include these yet unrealized possibilities. How large are these spaces?

Astronomers tell us that we live in a finite universe. From this premise, the physicist Walter Elsasser shows that the number of actual events is bounded. He writes,

One can estimate an "upper bound of events" in a crude fashion by multiplying the estimated number of, say, protons in the universe [one followed by 80 zeros] by the estimated number of sufficiently short time intervals [say, one followed by 30 zeros of picoseconds] that make up the lifetime of the universe (Elsasser 1969).

In this way he estimates the maximum number of real events that can occur in the universe as one followed by 110 zeros; larger numbers are called *immense*. Consider the basis for this number. The first factor (one followed by 80 zeros) is the atomic weight of the universe. At the level of ordinary chemistry, no finer subdivision of the mass of the universe is possible. The second factor (one followed by 30 zeros) is the age of the universe measured in picoseconds (1 picosecond equals 1 trillionth of a second). Why picoseconds? Because this is the time scale of a molecular vibration. At the level of ordinary chemistry, there is no finer subdivision in the age of the universe. Because biological and computing systems operate at or above the level of ordinary chemistry, the product of these two numbers (one followed by 110 zeros) provides a generous upper bound on both the number of things that can be constructed and the number of events that can transpire.

Remember that immense numbers are finite; we are not dealing with infinities here. Intuitively, we can think of the difference between ordinary, nonimmense numbers and immense numbers as the difference, for example, between the number of tick-tack-toe games and the number of chess games. Anyone can play out the few possible games of tick-tack-toe in just a few minutes. Chess is altogether another story because the number of possible chess games is immense. Thus, only a tiny fraction of the possible chess games have ever been played or ever will be, and there will always be interesting chess games that have never been played.

Although no real process can involve an immense number of events, immense numbers of possible events are easy to come by. Take proteins. A protein molecule is a polymer chain of amino acids. Each amino acid can be one of 20 types. Thus, we have 20 possibilities for the first amino acid in the chain. For each of these choices, we again have 20 possibilities for the second amino acid. Thus, we have 20 times 20 equals 400 possible arrangements for the first two amino acids. For the first three, we have 20 times 20 times 20 equals 8000 possibilities. Because a typical protein has about 200 amino acids in its chain, the number of possible proteins of this size is equal to 20 multiplied by itself 200 times. Because this result is larger than 10 multiplied by itself 110 times, there are an immense number of such protein molecules. All the proteins that have ever been made, or ever will be, are but a minute fraction of these possibilities. In other words, there will be always be interesting and useful proteins that have not been invented. Moreover— like a bright idea or a novel chess game—a new one might appear at any moment.

Let us now consider the dynamics in William Shakespeare's brain as he works on the play *Hamlet*. From the hierarchical perspective sketched above, the neurons in his neocortex are organized into first-order cell assemblies representing (say) letters of the alphabet. These might be organized into second-order assemblies representing words, which in turn are organized into third-order assemblies representing lines in the play, and so on up through the structures of scenes in the complete play. In somewhat greater detail, the counting might go like this:

Neural variables: Assuming, as above, 10 billion neurons in Shakespeare's neocortex with an average of 10,000 synaptic inputs to each, the phase space at this level has a dimension of 100 trillion, which is one followed by 14 zeros.

Letters: Of the many stable assemblies in the neocortex, 26 correspond to letters in the English alphabet. Thus the phase space at this level must have a dimension of at least 26.

Words: Assuming 5 letters for a word, there are more than 10 million letter combinations, of which (say) 100,000 are words in Shakespeare's vocabulary. Each of these words corresponds to an assembly that is already formed in his brain. Thus the dimension of the phase space at this level is 100,000.

Lines: With 10 words to a line, we have a number of lines equal to about one followed by 50 zeros, many being nonsensical. At this level, his brain

Aaron King and Alwyn C. Scott: Dimensions of Creativity

will be considering some of this large—but not yet immense—number of possible lines to find those appropriate for a scene in the play. Each line that is considered is represented by an assembly that involves a specific combination of word assemblies. Let us conservatively suppose that Shakespeare finds only 100 usable candidates for each line in each scene.

Scenes: To keep the arithmetic simple, assume that each scene has 100 lines and—as estimated above—100 candidate assemblies for each line in Shakespeare's brain. This estimate implies a number of possible ways to construct a scene that is equal to 100 multiplied by itself 100 times, or one followed by 200 zeros. By Elsasser's definition, this is an immense number of possibilities.

Thus Shakespeare cannot think of them all, and yet, as mentioned above, none can be excluded from consideration. A poetic jewel may lie just below the surface of the conscious mind. The dimension of the dynamics at this level is therefore immense.

Because the number of possible scenes is larger than the number of synapses in the brain by a factor of about 10 followed by 180 zeros, it is not possible to represent Shakespeare's creative activity by counting the neurological switchings that occur at the neuron level. Just as the 40-dimensional motion of 10 billiard balls cannot be represented in the 4-dimensional phase space of one ball, the immense dimensional phase space that Shakespeare explores as he constructs a scene for *Hamlet* cannot be reproduced in the merely large phase space of the cortical synapses. Remember that the phase-space dimension of the cortical neurons cannot be immense because neurons are real, physical objects. Most of the possible cell assemblies at the level of creative thought, on the other hand, will never be realized; there is not "world enough and time." One must therefore conclude that functionalism must fail to represent Shakespeare's creative activity as "the behavior of a vast assembly of nerve cells and their associated molecules."

Let us be clear about what this argument shows. We have demonstrated that the number of higher-order assemblies that could form is immense. This result follows from the hierarchical structure of the brain's organization into cell assemblies and the combinatory relationship between number of possible assemblies at the highest level and that of the actual assemblies at the next lower level. Of course, only a few of the possible assemblies actually do form at the highest level, and only one is selected for the final version of the play, but any theory that attempts to completely describe the dynamics of this selection must be couched in terms of the highest-order variables and not solely in terms of the neural variables.

Having reached these conclusions, let us consider that which has not been proven. The foregoing argument does not imply that it is impossible for engineers to construct a system (out of silicon transistors, say) that could engage in creative activity. If the construction of such a creative computing system were to be attempted, however, it should be designed to take advantage of hierarchical structure as does the human brain. Furthermore, we have no assurance that its unpredictable activities would please us.

REFERENCES

Crick, Francis. 1994. *The Astonishing Hypothesis.* New York: Simon and Schuster.

Elsasser, Walter. 1969. Acausal phenomena in physics and biology, *American Scientist* 57:502–516.

Hebb, Donald. 1949. *Organization of Behavior.* New York: Wiley.

James, William. 1890. *Principles of Psychology.* New York: Holt.

64 Poetry, Mental Models, and Discordant Consciousness

Paul K. Johnston

In his contribution to consciousness studies, *Stairway to the Mind*, Alwyn Scott (1995) admonishes that "Physical scientists considering consciousness should not start out by discussing the brain of William Shakespeare." Because I am not a physical scientist, but an English professor, I hope I can be forgiven for ignoring this advice, for in this chapter I present the brain of William Shakespeare as indeed the place to begin thinking about human consciousness. More specifically, I consider William Shakespeare's brain as it presents to us another brain, or at least another mind—that of an imaginary youth named Troilus, son of Priam, king of Troy during its assault by the Greeks, and brother of Paris, lover of Helen, and of Hector, the hero of Troy who is finally defeated in battle by the Greek hero Achilles.

I pause a moment, though, to fully acknowledge the limitation on my thoughts, suggested in passing by my use of the phrase "human consciousness," rather than the less restricted "consciousness" found in Professor Scott's admonition. In considering the peculiar nature of human consciousness, I must leave alone the hard problem of how biological creatures can be conscious of the world at all, for this level of phenomenal awareness human beings no doubt share in some fashion with other species. The more specific problem I address—the peculiarities in human consciousness distinct from that of other creatures—I became interested in while I was a farmhand on a small dairy farm in western New York. This was a time in my life when the thought of my lifeless body hanging from a rafter in the barn was a source of peculiar satisfaction, and my mind continually mulled over making this thought reality. It occurred to me that, though the means of self-destruction were available to the cows as well as to me, I had never heard of a cow committing suicide, and I wondered why that was. My own mind at that time was troubled by disappointments in romantic love, disappointments that I knew from Freud were fundamentally sexual, however they might seem to me. And yet the cows too were sexual beings. Despite Freud's emphasis on the sexual origins of love and neurosis, I concluded that my troubled mind could not simply be a product of my being a sexual creature, for if it were then I should have found a similarly troubled cow someday hurling herself off the barn's second floor to her destruction.

The true difference between myself and the cows, I soon realized, was my capacity for language, a capacity not shared by the cows, but one that I did share with all other members of my species. I became interested in how this seeming evolutionary advantage should bring with it the misery and the impulse to self-destruction I was then experiencing. A great deal of subsequent reading has confirmed what I came to suspect there in the barn, that human language serves first as a tool for thinking, and just secondarily as a tool for communication. Language gives us increased power to think about ourselves and the world, to organize our sensory input in complex ways, or, as Kenneth Craik (1943) wrote, to create a more complex internal model of ourselves and the world.

The evolutionary advantages from this increased modeling capacity do not need enumeration. Among other things, it has allowed us to domesticate the cow, rather than vice versa. We understand the cow better than the cow understands us. This powerful tool comes at a cost, however—the mental disturbances resulting from models so powerful as to include mutually incompatible information. The brain experiences this incompatibility as incapacitating emotion, and searches for ways to resolve it. Our neural nets, themselves temporarily discordant, cannot long abide disarray.

Poets and other creative writers have often been aware of the sometimes unbearable neural discordancies that beset the human mind as a result of its capacity for language. In the twentieth century, T. S. Eliot's Prufrock (Eliot 1917) expresses the language-empowered mind's paradoxical desire to escape language when he exclaims, "I should have been a pair of ragged claws/ Scuttling across the floors of silent seas," echoing the anguish felt nearly a century earlier by Frederick Douglass (1845) when, still a slave, he learned to read and thus found for the first time a language powerful enough for him to reflect on his condition: "In moments of agony, I envied my fellow slaves for their stupidity. I have often wished myself a beast. I preferred the condition of the meanest reptile to my own. Anything, no matter what, to get rid of thinking!" Reflecting more analytically on the problem, the novelist F. Scott Fitzgerald (1945) observed that "the test of a first-rate intelligence is the ability to hold two opposed ideas in the mind at the same time and still retain the ability to function." That Fitzgerald's observation comes in a story called "The Crack-Up" suggests that this test is not always passed.

The brain's consciousness—its internal representation of its "self" and the world outside itself—cannot be just anything, of course: for it to be biologically useful it must correspond to some degree with the world. For human beings this conformity becomes more complicated, for part of their external world is the world of culture created by the increased modeling capacity of human brains enabled by human language. This added layer of complexity greatly increases the problem of opposition and discordancy, placing an even greater burden on human consciousness, as does (perhaps even more so) the added complexity of the human individual's ability, again enabled by language, to create a sense of self in relationship to the world of culture as well as the world of nature, a sense of self with hopes and anxieties, capable of pride and capable of embarrassment.

Shakespeare's play *Troilus and Cressida* (1601–1602)[1] expresses most fully how complex is the consciousness made possible by human language. If *Troilus and Cressida* is less familiar than other Shakespeare plays, it is nonetheless fruitful in what it comprehends. Its setting is the Trojan War in classical legend, the war in which the Greeks retrieve from Troy the beautiful but adulterous Helen, who has fled there with Paris, one of the Trojan king Priam's many sons. This legendary war is itself emblematic of the struggle by human consciousness to establish ordering norms within which it can flourish, norms not only for sexual behavior but for civic behavior and for personal behavior. And language is essential to this struggle. Debate runs through the play: the Trojans debate whether Helen, a beautiful but also unfaithful woman, is worth the staggering sacrifice of life required to keep her. The Greeks debate how to bring the great but sulking Achilles out of his tent to fight the Trojans. In this setting unfolds the story of Troilus and Cressida, secret lovers who become separated by the fortunes of war, Cressida forced to go over to the Greeks on the very morning after her first night with Troilus, one half of an exchange demanded by her father, who has gone over to the Greeks voluntarily.

Shakespeare is both swift and brutal in presenting the sea of oppositions this double story unleashes in the thoughtful brain. In the play's opening scene, Troilus reflects on the battlefield discordancies outside Troy: "Peace, you ungracious clamors!" he exclaims. "Peace, rude sounds!/Fools on both sides! Helen must needs be fair,/When with your blood you daily paint her thus." Troilus' verb "paint" reminds us that Helen's beauty is at least in part created by paint—that is, makeup—rather than being wholly nature's endowment; yet worse, her visage in Troilus' image is painted not with makeup but with the blood of those young men on both sides daily dying in the battle whose only justification is the beauty of her face. And at the play's end, when the two great heroes finally meet, Hector is slain by Achilles not because Achilles is even momentarily the greater fighter in this battle for honor, but because Hector, having killed a weaker opponent because he liked his armor, has removed his own to try it on, and because Achilles, coming then suddenly upon him, has his band of Myrmidons about him, who hold Hector helpless while Achilles delivers the fatal blow. Such is the honor won on the battlefield.

It is to the plot of the lovers Troilus and Cressida I want to turn, however, to approach nearer to the peculiar nature of human consciousness. In an elaborate bit of staging in the play's fifth act, Troilus, accompanied by the Greek general Ulysses, spies upon Cressida as she betrays the pledge she had made to him, giving to the Greek Diomedes the token Troilus had given her just before her exchange. A third party, Thersites, a cynical Greek slave, also hidden, watches both, and we, the audience, watch Thersites watching Ulysses watch Troilus watching Cressida.

Visibly distraught with the opposed realities that his visual system now presents to his conscious awareness—the face of Cressida is both the face that fills him with pleasure and the face that fills him with pain—Troilus resists Ulysses' urging to turn away, saying, "Fear me not, my lord;/I will not be myself, nor have cognition/Of what I feel." But such detachment proves impossible, and when Diomedes and Cressida retire, Troilus exclaims,

This she? No, this is Diomed's Cressida.
If beauty have a soul, this is not she;
If souls guide vows, if vows be sanctimonies,
If sanctimony be the gods' delight,
If there be rule in unity itself,
This was not she. O madness of discourse,
That sets up with and against itself:
Bifold authority, where reason can revolt
Without perdition, and loss assume all reason
Without revolt. This is, and is not,
    Cressid.
Within my soul there doth conduce a fight
Of this strange nature that a thing
    inseparate
Divides more wider than the sky and earth;
And yet the spacious breadth of this division
Admits no orifex for a point as subtle
As Ariachne's broken woof to enter.
Instance, O instance, strong as Pluto's
    gates;
Cressid is mine, tied with the bonds of
    heaven.
Instance, O instance, strong as heaven
    itself;
The bonds of heaven are slipped, dissolved
    and loosed,
And with another knot, five-finger tied,
The fractions of her faith, orts of her love,
The fragments, scraps, the bits and greasy
    relics
Of her o'ereaten faith, are given to Diomed.

O madness of discourse, which sets up both with and against itself! Here we have presented to us the discord that both disables and reveals the mechanism of human consciousness. When the rule of unity that our internal models of ourselves and the world demands, that one thing be not both itself and its opposite, confronts opposing ideas that are both nevertheless true, human consciousness falters. Such opposed realities become more common, paradoxically, with greater powers of modeling, greater powers of comprehension such as those made possible by language, as Donald Hebb (1980) observed. One response by the brain is hinted at by the end of Troilus' speech, where he begins with language to devalue Cressida, to let go of one of the two opposing ideas, although letting go of it entails letting go of the love that gives his soul elevation. The cynicism of Thersites—throughout the play he has characterized the combatants on both sides as "those who war for a placket," thus reducing all to Helen's genital gratification—the cynicism of Thersites is but a fully developed example of this response, protecting the cynic from having to deal with any opposed thoughts. The sulking of Achilles, the sensuousness of Paris, the scheming single-mindedness of Ulysses, the faith of Hector in the honor of others—all these are strategies of consciousness to be less conscious, to become more like the obtuseness of Ajax and less like the madness of all-knowing Cassandra. Like drink or like drugs, they so diminish the capacity of human consciousness that it can be maintained without the anguish Troilus suffers.[2] When these do not avail, we have the option of battle itself, where in one will either kill or be killed, shutting down, if the latter, the consciousness that has become disordered.

The brain's reaction to such neural discord as Troilus here suffers is either to eliminate the discord or to shut itself down. Elimination often involves discounting in some way or dismissing information about the world—that is, it involves becoming less conscious. Shutting down, however, whether by means of alcohol or other drugs or by suicide, diminishes even more our modeling capacity, and thus our humanity, than even willful stupidity. Such responses move us away from our special human consciousness. Thersites observes that he would rather be a dog, a mule, a cat, a toad, a lizard, a herring, than be Menelaus, Helen's cuckolded husband, burdened with the consciousness of himself and the world that that cuckoldry entails. He would, he says, conspire against destiny. He would, in other words, retreat to a consciousness free from the burden of words. But this escape does conspire against our human destiny. A biologically more effective response to the brain's discordancies is poetry, which at its best fully retains the discordant elements that create discordancy while nevertheless resolving their incompatibility by containing those disordered elements within the formal structures of art.[3]

Troilus and Cressida is one such response, produced by Shakespeare's brain defying the discordancies in human existence. In it the opposed realities that test our human consciousness are present, fully and undiminished. Cressida is a being whose essence is at once physical and nonphysical, an embodied mind who also embodies the soul's beauty and the soul's betrayal. Troilus is both given to beauty and obsessed with sex. War is both pointless and necessary. Death is both avoidable and inevitable. And yet our minds survive their encounter with these discordancies because they reside within the greater order of art. It is poetry's task not to lie about the world and make it more ordered than it is, nor to give in and simply repeat its disorder, but to fully contain the world's disorder within the order imposed by art, to transform chaos into beauty, to more effectively arrange our neural nets' bloom and buzz. In doing so our minds are strengthened. Our language capacity is strengthened. Our consciousness is strengthened, better able to contain the contradictions our consciousness inevitably creates. Such is poetry's biological function, enabling discordant human consciousness to continue its special development in all its self-awareness and all its vulnerability.

NOTES

1. This date is scholarship's best conjecture about when *Troilus and Cressida* was composed. Its subsequent publication history is complex, as for Shakespeare's plays in general. For our general purpose here, any modern edition will serve as a reference source.

2. Changeux (1985), similarly discussing how drugs reduce the neural discordances in human culture, comments on Western society's increasing use of benzodiazepines, drugs that enhance the effects of gamma-aminobutyric acid, an inhibitory neurotransmitter.

3. Thersites' observation suggests that Nagel (1974), in putting forth the bat's mental world to contrast human consciousness, underestimates language's function in human consciousness. The phenomenal world of mammals whose visual systems are closer to our own must nevertheless be extraordinarily alien to human consciousness. To have had present in the mind for a lifetime a phenomenal world forever and utterly unmediated by language is by definition unimaginable, as what we imagine is the absence of words, which begins with a notion of their presence. The testimony that comes closest to presenting such a world is perhaps that of Helen Keller (1902), who is able to recall her mental existence during the years following her childhood illness when she was completely devoid of language, and to contrast this existence with her mental life after she restarted acquiring language, "when I was restored to my human heritage."

REFERENCES

Changeux, J.-P. 1985. *Neuronal Man: The Biology of Mind*. New York: Pantheon.

Craik, K. J. W. 1943. *Consciousness Explained*. Cambridge: Cambridge University Press.

Douglass, Frederick. 1845. *Narrative of the Life of Frederick Douglass, An American Slave, Written by Himself*. Freq. reprinted.

Eliot, T. S. 1917. *The Love Song of J. Alfred Prufrock*. Freq. reprinted.

Fitzgerald, F. Scott. 1945. *The Crack-Up*. New York: New Directions.

Hebb, D. O. 1980. *Essay on Mind*. Hillsdale, NJ: Lawrence Erlbaum.

Keller, Helen. 1902. *The Story of My Life*. Freq. reprinted.

Nagel, T. 1974. "What is it like to be a bat?" *Philosophical Review* 83(4)435–450.

Scott. A. 1995. *Stairway to the Mind: The Controversial New Science of Consciousness*. New York: Springer-Verlag.

Shakespeare, William. 1601–1602. *Troilus and Cressida*.

Appendix

These are the categories in which consciousness studies were arranged at the Tucson II conference, along with their number of presentations.

Philosophy (95)

1.1 Content of consciousness (11)
1.2 Ontology of consciousness (12)
1.3 Knowing what it is like and the knowledge argument (2)
1.4 Qualia (6)
1.5 Machine consciousness (5)
1.6 The function of consciousness (4)
1.7 The "hard problem" and the explanatory gap (20)
1.8 Higher-order thought (1)
1.9 Epistemology and philosophy of science (14)
1.10 Personal identity and the self (7)
1.11 Free will and agency (6)
1.12 Intentionality and representation (5)
1.13 Miscellaneous (2)

Neuroscience (85)

2.1 Neural correlates of consciousness (5)
2.2 Vision (8)
2.3 Other sensory modalities (7)
2.4 Motor control (1)
2.5 Memory and learning (1)
2.6 Neuropsychology (10)
2.7 Anesthesiology (7)
2.8 Cellular and subneural processes (5)
2.9 Quantum neurodynamics (10)
2.10 Pharmacology (3)
2.11 The binding problem (8)
2.12 Language (see 3.6)

2.13 Emotion (1)
2.14 Time (3)
2.15 Specific brain areas (7)
2.16 Miscellaneous (9)

Cognitive Science and Psychology (87)

3.1 Attention (6)
3.2 Vision (5)
3.3 Other sensory modalities (3)
3.4 Memory and learning (3)
3.5 Emotion (5)
3.6 Language (4)
3.7 Mental imagery (2)
3.8 Implicit and explicit processes (1)
3.9 Unconscious and conscious processes (5)
3.10 Sleep and dreaming (5)
3.11 Cognitive development (5)
3.12 Artificial intelligence and robotics (3)
3.13 Neural networks and connectionism (14)
3.14 Cognitive architectures (9)
3.15 Ethology (7)
3.16 Task performance and decision making (1)
3.17 Theory of mind
3.18 Intelligence and creativity (3)
3.19 Miscellaneous (6)

Physics and Mathematics (66)

4.1 Quantum theory (22)
4.2 Space-time relativity (4)
4.3 Integrative models (20)
4.4 Emergent and hierarchical systems (3)
4.5 Nonlinear dynamics (3)
4.6 Logic and computational theory (6)
4.7 Holography (1)
4.8 Bioelectromagnetics and resonance effects (4)
4.9 Thermodynamics
4.10 Miscellaneous (3)

Biology (9)

5.1 Evolution of consciousness (5)
5.2 Biophysics and living processes (4)

Experiential Approaches (72)

6.1 Phenomenology (15)
6.2 Meditation, contemplation, and mysticism (10)
6.3 Hypnosis (2)
6.4 Biofeedback (2)
6.5 Other altered states of consciousness (1)
6.6 Transpersonal and humanistic psychology (23)
6.7 Psychoanalysis and psychotherapy (17)
6.8 Lucid dreaming (2)

Anomalies of Consciousness (29)

7.1 Parapsychology (20)
7.2 Medicine, healing, and placebo studies (5)
7.3 Spiritual healing
7.4 Psychoneuroimmunology
7.5 Out-of-body experiences (2)
7.6 Miscellaneous (2)

Humanities (29)

8.1 Literature, hermeneutics, and linguistics (10)
8.2 Art (5)
8.3 Music (2)
8.4 Religion (6)
8.5 History
8.6 Aesthetics (4)
8.7 Mythology (2)

Culture and Society (35)

9.1 Sociology and political science (11)
9.2 Anthropology (8)
9.3 Information technology (2)
9.4 Ethics and legal studies (1)
9.5 Education (4)
9.6 Business and organizational studies (4)
9.7 Miscellaneous (5)

Index

Canadian Charter of Rights and Freedom, 162
Capacitor model for learning, 384
Cariani, P., 587
Cartesian dualism, 620
Cartesian Materialism, 101, 138–139
Cartesian Theater, 102–103
Casimir, Hendrick, 199–200
Cat-in-a-box experiment, 428, 594
Categorization in visual perception, 345
Cats, REM sleep in, 477, 479
Causal accounts in study of consciousness, 19–20
Causal laws in criminal law, 160
Causal states of consciousness, 682
Causation argument in reductionism, 48–49
Cell assemblies of neurons, 727–728
Cellular automata, emergence in, 586–592
Central state materialism, 87
Centrencephalon concept, 242
Centrioles, 424–425
Centripetal force, representational, 508–509
Chalmers, David J.
  analysis of Hard Problem of, 109–116
  compared to Searle, 116–117
  on experience and consciousness, 199
  on life, 75
  at Tucson conference, 2–3, 8, 106
  on zombies, 172, 176
Changeux, J.-P., 516
Chaotic attractors, 488–489, 588
Charge transfer in microtubules, 408–410
Chemicals in conscious state paradigm, 479–480
Chemotaxis in bacteria, 399–400
Children, word learning by, 568
Chimpanzees, language learning by, 390–391, 524–527, 536–539
Chinese box, 183–184
Choices. See also Decisions; Free will
  consciousness for, 426–427
  in criminal law, 160, 164–165
  in dream experiences, 500
  in evolution, 75
  in human rights, 161
Churchland, Patricia
  theory reduction by, 50
  at Tucson conference, 7
Churchland, Paul, 8
Cilia
  in Euglena gracilis, 410–417
  microtubules for, 424–425
Clark, Thomas, 58
Clarke, Cris, 64
Classical fields in quantum states, 629

Classical mechanics
  for brain dynamics, 621–624
  inadequacy of, 597–598
  physical processes in, 620–621
Classification in active seeing, 300
Clever Hans (horse), 526, 529
Clifford, William, 88
Codetermination in neurophenomenology, 40
Cognition
  in animals, 523–529
  in conscious state paradigm, 481
  in creativity models, 718–723
Cognitive development, representational redescription in, 248
Coherence
  quantum, 429
  and state selection, 629–630
Coherent oscillations in bacteria, 403
Collapse
  in evolution of consciousness, 604–607
  in quantum triggers, 627
Collective coordinates in quantum triggers, 625
Collective psychosis, 684
Collective states in unity of consciousness, 91
Color
  and achromatopsia, 303
  in blindsight, 373
  in synesthesia, 286–289
Comatose patients, vision reflexive responses in, 298
Commentary-key paradigm, 373–375
Commonality among states of consciousness, 680–682
Communication. See also Language
  by animals, 523–529
  by bacteria, 402–403
  by dolphins, 551–559
Comparative neurophysiology, 552
Comparative psychology, 383
Comparator hypothesis, 284–286
Complex attractors, 588
Complexes, 491
Complication part in dreams, 498
Compositional effect of language, 564, 567
Comprehension in language, 539–541, 543–544
Computational ETM (CETM), 586
Computer functionalism, 76
Computers
  consciousness in, 181–182
  quantum, 92
  sentience in, 83–84
Concept formation, language in, 567

Conceptual question of consciousness, 79
Concreteness, 131
Congenital factors in criminal law, 160
Conrad, Michael, 638–639
Conscience in fetal development, 160
Conscious I, 271
Conscious state paradigm, 473
  historical background of, 476
  input-output gating in, 477–479
  models for, 480–483
  modulation in, 479–480
  REM sleep discovery in, 476–477
  reticular activation concept in, 476
  state-dependent features in, 474–476
Conscious vision, 299–301
Consciousness modules, 225–226
Consensus trances, 684
Consent in criminal law, 158
Contemplation, 53
Content of consciousness, 93
  relational features in, 271–274
  vs. subjectivity, 237–238
Context
  in creativity models, 722
  in dolphin whistles, 555–556
  for time, 646
Contextual systems in global-workspace
    framework, 269–270
Contrast enhancement in perceptual-retouch,
    351–353
Convenience description levels, 577–578
Copenhagen interpretation, 428, 594
Correlation argument in reductionism, 48–49
Corssen, G., 459
Cortex in NCC, 220
Cortical blindness, 299, 301
Cosmic-consciousness experiences, 669–675
Cosmic-level consciousness, 401
Cotterill, R. M. J., 615
Cowey, A., 376
Craik, Kenneth, 125, 734
Creative discontent, 518
Creativity, 715
  dimensions of, 725–730
  models of, 717–723
Credit ratings, machine calculations for, 188
Crick, Francis
  on a- and p-consciousness, 330–331, 333–
    337
  Astonishing Hypothesis of, 255
  on blindsight, 275
  on functionalism, 725
  on NCC, 219, 224, 226

on thought experiments, 110–111
  at Tucson conference, 8
Criminal law, 157–168
Criterion problem in threshold experiment,
    361–362
Cross-linguistic comparisons, 564
Crystals in quantum mechanics, 192–196
Cultures
  monophasic vs. polyphasic, 679
  time in, 657
Cyclic attractors, 588
Cytoskeleton, 197–199, 639
  in differentiation, 424–426
  information processing by, 423
  origin of, 421

D. B. (blindsight subject), 373
Damasio, A., 516
Dantzig solvers, 517–518
Darlington, R. B., 389
Darwin, Charles
  on animals, 533
  and animism, 379–380
  on language, 561–562
  on thought, 562
Data compression with time expansion, 652–
  654
Day-residue in dreams, 498
de Quincey, C., 66
de Vries, R., 462
Debate in *Troilus and Cressida*, 735–738
Decisions. *See also* Choices; Free will
  heuristics in, 514–515
  neural systems in, 515–516
  styles in, 517–518
Deep structure analysis of states of conscious-
    ness, 680–682
Defenses in criminal law, 158
Definitions in study of consciousness, 17–18
Dehaene, S., 516
Deikman, A., 59
Delbruck, Max, 73
Dement, William, 477
Democritus, 86
Dennett, Daniel C.
  on birth of agency, 423
  on blindsight, 373–374
  on functionalism, 136, 138–139
  on habits, 127
  on language, 561
  on neurophenomenology, 32–33
  on reaction to animal learning, 525
  at Tucson conference, 3–5

Goodale, M. A., 331
Grain problem, 88–89
Grammar, 534–538
Gravity, representational, 506
Gray, Jeffrey
  on conscious content, 271–272
  on reactions, 98, 103
  at Tucson conference, 3, 93
Great Chain of Being, 533
Green, J. P., 205
Greenberg, J. P., 300
Greenfield, Susan, 3–4
Griffin, David Ray, 130
Griffin, Donald, 129–130
  on animal thought, 523–524
  at Tucson conference, 5
Groenewegen, J. J., 241
Grossman, R. G., 237
Group-level properties, 580–581
Group minds, economies as, 154
Grouping
  in active seeing, 300
  qualia in, 302
Guilt in criminal law, 157
Gurwitsch, Aaron, 33

Habitual thought and behavior, 566
Hall, E. T., 657–658
Hall, George, 200
Hallucinations from occipital-lobe destruction, 304
Hallucinogenic drugs, 205
Hameroff, Stuart
  analysis of approach by, 119–121
  and collapse conditions, 606–607
  on psychedelic drugs, 205
  Sonoran Desert discussion with Scott, 635–644
  at Tucson conference, 7
Hanna, J., 661
Hard Problem
  analysis of, 109–116
  divisions in, 110–113
  experience as answer for, 143–148
  ignorance as premise in, 113–116
  NCC in, 279–289
  Tucson conference discussions on, 3, 7
Harlow, Harry, 385–387
Harlow, M. K., 385
Harman, Willis, 698
Harvy, J. H., 490
Hawking, Stephen, 71
Healing, 7
Heat-death scenario, 645

Heat experiments by Florentine Experimenters, 336
Hebb, Donald O.
  on cell assemblies, 727–728
  on mental representations, 463–464
Heisenberg, Werner
  and quantum vacuum, 199
  Wave-Function-Collapse ontology, 600, 602–606
Helen (monkey), blindsight in, 301–303
Hemispheres, subjectivity in, 239
Herman, Louis, 525
Heterophenomenological approach, 87
Hierarchical organization in creativity, 725, 727
Hierarchical systems, 573–575
Hilbert space, 90
Hillis, Danny, 4
Hinkley, R. E., 204
Hippocampus
  in conscious content, 271
  in memory processes, 264, 515–516
Hobbes, Thomas, 6
Hobner, M., 367
Hobson, J. Allan
  activation-synthesis hypothesis by, 490–491
  on dreamlike consciousness, 235
  on meaning in dreams, 491–492
  at Tucson conference, 3
Hodgson, David, 4
Honorton, Charles
  ganzfeld test methods by, 695
  in Great Ganzfeld Debate, 701–702
  psi manuscript study by, 672
  Zener card analysis by, 694
Honzik, C. H., 384
Hopi language, 564
Hubbard, T. L.
  displacement studies by, 506–508
  on representational momentum, 505
Hubel, David, 309–310
Human rights in criminal law, 157–158, 161–163
Humanists, 72
Hume, David, 88
Husserl, H. 33
Hut, Piet, 3
Hutchinson, J. E., 566
Hydrophobic regions
  anesthesia effects on, 203
  quantum effects in, 204–206
Hyman, R.
  in Great Ganzfeld Debate, 701–702
  on science and parapsychology, 692

Hypnosis
  and culture, 684
  resistance to, 678–679

Ideas, existence of, 120, 199
Identity theory, 86
Ignorance in Hard Problem, 113–116
Illusions in conscious experience, 282
Imagery
  in dream consciousness, 490
  memory and conscious awareness in, 321–327
Immediacy in neurophenomenology, 35
Immense numbers in creativity, 725, 728–730
Impaired perceptual awareness, digit
  identification under, 339–343
Incompatible information, 734–738
Inductive reasoning, language in, 567
Inequalities in criminal law, 167
Infants
  conscious states in, 475
  consciousness in, 231–232
  mental life of, 568
  spatial recall in, 568–569
Infinite lattices, cellular automata with, 587
Information-bearing account. *See* Functionalism
Information dissemination, 238
Information processing
  in bacteria, 399–400
  in scientific study of consciousness, 27–28
Inkplot tests, dreams as, 499
Inner speech, 46
Inner stillness, 54
Input
  in dream consciousness, 490, 497
  in ganzfeld tests, 695
  in waking consciousness, 490
Input-output gating in REM sleep, 477–479
Insanity in criminal law, 158
Instrumental conditioning
  in animal signing, 538
  in capacitor model, 384
Intelligence
  artificial. *See* Artificial intelligence
  differentiation in, 424–426
Intelligent Agents, 189
Intensity in mystical states, 54–55
Intention
  in behavior, 534
  in consciousness, 50
  in criminal law, 158, 160
  determining, 551–552
  in dolphin play, 557–558

in meaningfulness, 86
and prehension, 133
in zombies, 176–177
Interfering states
  in quantum mechanics, 620
  in quantum triggers, 627
Interoceptive stimulation in waking
  consciousness, 490
Interpretation
  of consciousness, 220–221
  of dreams, 499
Intimacy in neurophenomenology, 35
Intralaminar nuclei, thalamic, 237–243
Intraoperative awareness, 440
Intrinsic meaning, 91
Introspectionism vs. neurophenomenology,
  36–37
Intuition in neurophenomenology, 35, 37
Invariant processing with time expansion,
  652–654
Invariants in neurophenomenology, 35
Ion channels in anesthesia, 447–451
Irreducibility
  of brain, 117
  in neurophenomenology, 32–33
Isoflurane, 261, 439

Jackendoff, R., 280
Jackson, Frank, 122
James, William, 1
  on abstraction, 567
  automaton-theory by, 725–726
  on awareness, 64
  on bibulosity, 642
  on experience, 35
  on hemianopic disturbance, 303
  on "now", 646
  on thought, 487
  Tucson conference discussions on, 6
Jasper, H. H.
  and centrencephalon concept, 242
  on subjectivity, 239
Jerison, H. J., 389
Jessel, D., 166
John of the Cross, St., 63
Johnson, J. Q., 510
Johnson, M., 514
Johnston, Paul, 10
Jokes in dreams, 146–147
Jones, K. T., 509
Jouvet, Michel, 477
Judgment-making machines, 188–189
Jung, Carl
  and complexes, 491
  on dreams, 499

Perihelion precession of Mercury, 115
Perky effect, 321, 324–325
Personal responsibility, machines for avoiding, 188–189
Personality disorders in criminal law, 157
Pettit, P., 167
Phase space in creativity, 725–727
Phencyclidine, 459
Phenomenal consciousness. *See* Access (a-) and phenomenal (p-) consciousness
Phenomenal individuals and boundaries, 149–155
Phenomenological approach. *See* Neurophenomenology
Phenomenological mapping of states of consciousness, 679–680
Phenomenological reduction (PhR), 34–36
Philosophy
  in consciousness analysis, 125
  and machine consciousness, 183
  relation to science, 16–17
Phonons
  pumped, 92
  in quantum mechanics, 192–193
Photons, virtual, 199–200
Photoreceptors
  in Cambrian period, 430
  of *Euglena gracilis*, 407–419
Physical principles, nonconscious knowledge of, 505–511
Physical systems, 89–90
Physical variables in classical mechanics, 597–598
Physicalism
  in causality, 50
  and zombies, 171
Physiology in criminal law, 166
Pilot-Wave Ontology, 600, 602, 605–606
Pinker, S., 562
Piore, M. J., 514
Place, Ullin, 49–50
Planck, Max, 199
Planck constant and classical levels, 195
Planck scale and reality, 199–201, 643
Plato
  on ideas, 120, 199
  on reality, 89
Play by dolphins, 557–558
Plotinus, 65
Plots in dreams, 498–499
Poets, 734
Pollen, D., 330
Polyphasic cultures, 679
Pontine system in transition to sleep, 473

Pontogeniculo-occipital (PGO) waves in REM sleep, 477–479, 490–491
Poppel, E., 367
Positive reinforcement in instrumental conditioning, 384
Positron emission tomography (PET)
  for anterior cingulate cortex blood flow, 248–250
  for brain imaging, 256–263
  in synesthesia study, 287
Potency, anesthetic, 444
Power of consciousness, 703
Pragmatic description levels, 577–580
Pragmatics of neurophenomenology, 38–39
Precession of perihelion of Mercury, 115
Preexperimental bridging principles, 220–221
Prefrontal cortex in decisions, 516
Prehension, 131–133
Premack, David, 525, 539
Pribram, K. H., 515
Prigogine, Ilya, 379
Principles of Psychology (James), 1
Proactive enhancement of contrast in perceptual-retouch, 351–353
Probability in quantum ontologies, 601
Probability learning, maximizing in, 386
Process philosophies, 151
Process thinking, 487
Profane time, 657
Prokaryotic cells, 398–399
Propofol, 257–261
Prosopagnosia, 301
Protein molecules
  anesthesia effects on, 203
  immense number of, 729
  as nonlinear systems, 726–727
Protoconscious experience, 199, 643
Pseudo-validation in scientific studies, 673
Psychedelic drugs, 205
Psychokinesis (PK)
  criticism of, 704
  evidence for, 696–697
  Tucson conference discussions on, 9
Psychology in consciousness analysis, 125
Psychometric functions, 362–364
Psychons, 630
Psychophysics, 361
Pumped phonon systems, 92
Pumping in quantum states, 629
Punishment
  in criminal law, 161, 167
  in instrumental conditioning, 384
Pure awareness, 59